DENTOFACIAL ORTHOPEDICS
WITH FUNCTIONAL APPLIANCES

DENTOFACIAL ORTHOPEDICS WITH FUNCTIONAL APPLIANCES

THOMAS M. GRABER, D.D.S., M.S.D., Ph.D.

Former Professor and Chairman, Section of Orthodontics, Pritzker School of Medicine,
University of Chicago; Director, Kenilworth Dental Research Foundation
and G.V. Black Institute for Continuing Education, Kenilworth, Illinois;
Research Scientist, American Dental Association Research Institute,
Chicago; Visiting Professor, University of Michigan, Ann Arbor;
Editor, American Journal of Orthodontics; Recipient,
Albert Ketcham Award

THOMAS RAKOSI, M.D., D.D.S., Ph.D.

Professor and Head, Department of Orthodontics and Jaw Orthopedics,
University of Freiburg, Freiburg, Germany

ALEXANDRE G. PETROVIC, M.D., D.Sc.

Director of Research, National Institute of Health and Medical Research, France;
Director, Laboratory for Craniofacial Cartilage and Bone Growth Regulations
(INSERM-U.213), Louis-Pasteur University Medical School, Strasbourg, France;
Visiting Professor, Department of Orthodontics, Louisiana State University
Medical Center, New Orleans

with 1180 *illustrations*

The C. V. Mosby Company

ST. LOUIS • TORONTO • PRINCETON   1985

A TRADITION OF PUBLISHING EXCELLENCE

Editor: Darlene Warfel
Assistant editor: Melba Steube
Manuscript editor: George B. Stericker, Jr.
Book design: Jeanne Genz
Cover design: Tilford Smith
Production: Kathy Teal, Barbara Merritt, Mary Stueck

The C.V. Mosby Company
11830 Westline Industrial Drive, St. Louis, Missouri 63146

Library of Congress Cataloging in Publication Data

Graber, T.M. (Thomas M.), 1917-
    Dentofacial orthopedics with functional appliances.

    Bibliography: p.
    Includes index.
    1. Orthodontics.   2. Orthodontic appliances.
3. Malocclusion—Treatment.   I. Rakosi, Thomas.
II. Petrovic, Alexandre G.   III. Title.   [DNLM:
1. Malocclusion—therapy.   2. Orthodontic Appliances.
3. Orthodontics, Corrective.   WU 400 G728d]
RK521.G688   1985   617.6′43   84-19061
ISBN 0-8016-1937-8

C/MV/MV   9 8 7 6 5 4 3 2 1   03/B/362

To
Doris, Edith, and Suzanne
and to woman power

PREFACE

The welter of clinical reports in the dental literature and the profusion of short courses being given on so-called functional appliances have engendered great interest in this approach to orthodontic-orthopedic therapy. The popularity and large number of sales of the book *Removable Orthodontic Appliances* by one of the authors are testimony to the enhanced desire to learn more about these appliances on the American side of the Atlantic. Functional jaw orthopedics has been used (and misused) for many years in Europe. As in America, cultism, dogma, and arbitrary follow-the-leader approaches have too often dominated the scene. The results have been spotty. There is an old saying, "It is not the tool but how you use it that counts." Well, this can be rephrased to cover one facet of the topic at hand: Although functional appliances may provide dramatic examples of stable and balanced corrections of severe malocclusions, on the one hand, they also may, on the other, show cases in which only partial correction was achieved or excessive lower incisor tipping was the result.

It is unfortunate that the glowing functional appliance "successes" have been emphasized and oversold by some American proponents, also that weekend "motel courses" have been given too often by poorly trained orthodontists, pedodontists, or would-be orthodontists who were interested more in the financial returns from these courses, or the ego inflation that goes with standing behind a podium with a captive audience. Thus, what has become a "hot number" for orthodontics has effectively burned more than a few orthodontists and, to our discredit, many patients who have been promised too much.

Despite the admonitions in *Removable Orthodontic Appliances,* and from superbly qualified course leaders such as McNamara, Fränkel, Eirew, Rakosi, Schmuth, Shaye, Bimler, Ahlgren, and others, hundreds of clinicians have grabbed an appliance and used it indiscriminately on their patients. The inexorable unfavorable patient response from excessive use by inadequately trained orthodontists, and totally unqualified pedodontists and general practitioners, has produced a wave of frustration and antagonism to functional appliances in many quarters. Yet, if the clinician has realized that diagnosis is as demanding for functional jaw orthopedics as it is for fixed appliances, that case selection is critical, that construction bite details can make or break a treatment regimen (no matter how perfectly the appliance is constructed), that it takes time to learn how to manipulate these appliances, that mistakes will be made, that growth direction and growth amount as well as growth timing are major factors in the ultimate success or failure of a treatment regimen, and that patient cooperation and motivation demand constant reinforcement after careful initial patient selection—if all these have been absorbed into the clinician's *modus cogitandi,* then they cannot help engendering a warm glow of success and pride in the beautiful results attained on many patients, results not possible from fixed appliances alone.

It is the purpose of this book to present those essential details of diagnosis for functional appliances, to give detailed instructions on how to obtain a correct construction bite, to describe fabrication and use of various types of functional appliances, and to particularize the specific treatment regimens for different malocclusion categories. We hope we will be able to offset the unfavorable backlash against functional appliances engendered by the mixed experiences of the past 5 or 6 years.

It might appear a bit unseemly that the qualifications of the authors to tackle this challenge should be extolled. However, this aspect is vitally important if the objectives elaborated in the previous paragraph are to be achieved.

Professor Rakosi is head of one of the finest orthodontic departments in the world. The University of Freiburg has an eminent reputation and its orthodontic specialty training program has turned out some of the top clinicians in Europe, a number of whom head other departments as well. Professor Rakosi has had a rich clinical and research experience, teaching and practicing orthodontics in Czechoslovakia and Switzerland, before assuming the professorship at the University of

Freiburg. His recent book, *Cephalometric Radiography,* is widely used by clinicians around the world and is considered the best and most current diagnostic volume in this subject area. Freiburg is also a center for highly successful continuing education courses in fixed and removable appliance mechanotherapy for practitioners from Europe, America, and Asia.

Professor Petrovic heads what many observers consider the top craniofacial growth and development research center in the world. The prolific, innovative, and meticulous clinically oriented basic research emanating from Louis Pasteur Medical School in Strasbourg has profoundly affected all phases of orthodontics. The team of Petrovic, Stutzmann, Oudet, Gasson, Lavergne, Meyer, and others has produced a multitude of chapters in various books and articles in the professional literature of Europe and the United States on histochemical response to various appliances and to the ramification of force values, treatment timing, and effect on the various tissues of the maxilla, mandible, etc. This book brings together the unique, exciting, and provocative research of the past 15 years and allows the clinician to understand the raison d'être for all orthodontic and orthopedic therapy.

Professor Graber has spent a lifetime practicing and writing about many aspects of orthodontics. He has published more books and articles than any author in orthodontic history. He continues to teach, practice, write, direct research, and guide continuing education programs, as well as serve as an editor or editorial advisor for a number of journals and as an orthodontic education advisor for institutions around the world. His busy private practice is a blend of fixed and removable appliance techniques that provides biologically oriented optimal service to his patients.

A generation of orthodontists has been surfeited with cephalometrics. The majority of orthodontic graduate student research projects have been related to cephalometrics in one form or another. Although mensuration is commendable if it means more objectivity, making diagnostic decisions solely on the basis of linear and angular measurements gleaned from a two-dimensional profile radiograph has resulted in overly simplistic solutions to complex biologic problems. It is fair to say that the craniofacial complex, despite the thousands of graduate theses gathering dust on library shelves, is an imperfectly observed variable.

Diagnosis requires manifold approaches to a multisystem involvement. A broader approach to both research and diagnosis is imperative, if we are to advance beyond the "numbers racket" of traditional cephalometrics.

Chapter 1, by Professor Petrovic, is a fresh insight into the potential of a cybernetically oriented approach to progress in orthodontics. Via this approach, that mythical "black box" is bound to become smaller. This chapter needs to be read and reread so it will input into the reader's own biologic computer the systematic analysis of oral physiology, growth and development, and the effects and counterreactions engendered by orthodontic treatment.

Chapter 2, also by Professor Petrovic, summarizes the most important research that has been done in his laboratory, specifically with regard to the modus operandi of functional appliances. This chapter alone justifies the existence of the book and is unique. Clinical implications and applications abound.

Chapter 3, by Professor Rakosi, provides a thorough analysis of the principles of functional appliances so necessary for a full understanding of which appliances to use and when and how. Not all functional appliances employ the same "functional orthopedic" approach, yet there are common denominators for most appliances. Many a clinician would not have had the sad experiences of partial or iatrogenic failure if Chapter 3 had been available and read before placing a functional appliance that was recommended in a weekend course.

Cephalometrics, properly used, is a valuable diagnostic and treatment adjunct. Based on his recent widely used book on cephalometric analysis, Professor Rakosi has synthesized the best combination of cephalometric criteria for functional appliance use specifically in Chapter 4. The functional appliance is not the proverbial Procrustean bed, into which all Class II malocclusions are crammed whether or not they fit. Certain cephalometric measurements, taken together, provide insight into both current morphology and future pattern expression, as well as the likely treatment response. Using the tool properly is the name of the game, and Chapter 4 takes the clinician a long way toward that goal.

In Chapter 5 Professor Rakosi continues the diagnostic and analytical steps necessary before embarking on the functional appliance approach. A functional analysis makes eminently good sense for the use of a functional appliance; and yet, far too many clinicians have neglected this aspect of patient assessment before treatment. The various steps in this assessment are described in a manner permitting immediate clinical application.

Chapter 6, on the activator, is the first of a number of chapters on functional appliances per se. In it Professor Rakosi describes the philosophy, the physiologic justification, and the development of the basic appliance, which is the progenitor of all functional appliances. The minutiae of the all-important construction bite, along with the rationale and variances of vertical and horizontal jaw positioning, are detailed for specific cases. Treatment planning and the use of and problems encountered with the instrument are all-important aspects to be found in this chapter, which serves as a prerequisite for subsequent activator appliance variations.

In Chapter 7, on fabrication and management of the

activator, Dr. Rakosi illustrates "how to do it." The information contained herein will be invaluable to both the neophyte and the experienced clinician as specific details based on years of experience are elucidated.

Continuing the management aspects of activator use, Dr. Rakosi discusses in Chapter 8 the trimming of the acrylic portions of the activator to better guide the teeth into their proper positions after jaw posturing is achieved by the construction bite.

Chapter 9 describes the Bionator, which is a widely used modification of the activator, and gives the rationale for the changes that have been made in it. The justification of full-time wear and the appliance modifications recommended are important aspects of functional appliance use. Here again, Dr. Rakosi's great experience and knowledge come to the fore.

Chapter 10, by Dr. Graber, is a detailed and lengthy discussion of the Fränkel appliance. Because of the tremendous exposure and usage of this device in the past 10 years, as well as the relatively more demanding aspects of its fabrication and management, specific step-by-step details are described and illustrated so the clinician can avoid the pitfalls commonly encountered by the uninitiated, and even the experienced, clinician. Great care has been taken to weed out the propaganda and to present the approach most likely to be successful for the various categories of malocclusion. This is the most complete presentation in English on the Fränkel appliance. Professor Fränkel's assistance in the chapter is specially recognized.

Chapter 11, also by Dr. Graber, offers a viable combination of fixed and functional appliances that will likely point the way in the treatment of most basal sagittal malrelationships for Class II and Class III malocclusions. It is a practice-tested approach that melds the best of American and European technologies, permitting the attainment of the achievable optimum with a minimum of mechanotherapy and potential iatrogenic interference. Selected case reports by outstanding clinicians demonstrate the possibilities of combination therapy.

Chapters 12 to 15, by Dr. Rakosi, deal with malocclusion treatment. In Chapter 12 the all-important and detailed aspects of actual treatment of Class II malocclusions are described. This is the type of case in which the functional appliance has its greatest application and success. In the final analysis, the functional appliance serves best as a deficiency appliance. This and the subsequent chapters by Dr. Rakosi are unequaled in the literature and show the effects of long years of clinical experience and patient management. Of great importance is the variation of appliance construction and use for different types of growth patterns.

Chapters 13, 14, and 15 present the same careful and detailed treatment rationales for deep overbite cases, Class III malocclusions, and open bite problems as is done in Chapter 12 for Class II malocclusions. Treatment specifics most likely to assure achievement of the best possible result are presented in detail. Although these four chapters are not "cookbook," they do give the applied biologist the details for successfully employing functional appliances in a great number of cases.

Chapter 16 is a philosophical epilogue of sorts. What is the future of functional appliances? Clearly, despite their misuse because of poor indoctrination, oversell, inadequate clinician attention to treatment details, and unwillingness to combine fixed and functional appliances for the highest degree of correction, the future is bright—provided clinicians are willing to apply themselves assiduously to the principles and techniques expounded in this text. No book can be all things to all people. The sheer enormity of available information makes it impossible for a single or even a multiple volume text. Yet, the research justification and validation of functional appliance procedures presented in this book and the techniques described will go a long way toward assuring the type of success we have come to demand of ourselves in America; and the results can be achieved with less pain and less effort, more routinely, and with less likelihood of root resorption, bone loss, decalcification, soft tissue damage, and TMJ problems.

All good books these days are the result of a team effort. Contributions from the research staff of Professor Petrovic are significant. The many line drawings and photographs in this profusely illustrated atlas of treatment procedures required the artistic efforts of authors as well as technicians. The production demands of this type of book are prodigious. Nevertheless, The C.V. Mosby Company and its superbly trained staff rose to the occasion. Darlene Warfel helped conceptualize the book and direct its progress. Melba Steube did a meticulous job of organizing, made more difficult by a multinational and multiauthored use of the English language. George Stericker gave his usual perfectionist attention to the editing of manuscript, galleys, and page proofs, to the illustrations, tables, and all those details that go unnoticed unless there is a mistake or an omission. And countless others have contributed along the way by example, precept, suggestions, actual work, or sacrifice of personal time to the cause. To all of them we are most grateful. Editorial excellence goes hand-in-hand with clinical excellence. For those who read the book, the dedication of all who had a hand in its production and the successful blending of efforts will be obvious.

Thomas M. Graber
Thomas Rakosi
Alexandre G. Petrovic

CONTENTS

INTRODUCTION

There can be no doubt about the fervent, almost messianic, zeal of Edward Angle when he told his students: "All you can do with an appliance is push, pull, or turn a tooth. I have given you the best possible appliance. Now use it!" In the halcyon days of orthodontics, when cultism was at its peak, the disciples knew they were on the righteous road to orthodontic salvation. When Charles Tweed intoned, "There is only one way to treat malocclusions properly, and I am giving it to you," the followers saw the light. Course participants nodded in acquiescence when Harold Kesling gave one of his many courses at La Porte, Indiana, on the Begg technique and admonished, "This is the precise way to go. Don't vary the technique one bit, because you will fail if you do. Anyway, I have tried other variations and they failed!" And on the other side of the Atlantic, devotion to dogma held adherents of Andresen, Häupl, Korkhaus, Schwarz, and Petrik together with rapt attention to removable appliance systems that supposedly cured all orthodontic ills.

One common denominator in all these orthodontic "religions" was the worship of the appliance. Mechanistically oriented techniques and cookbook approaches to treatment appealed to the majority of orthodontists, who preferred to have others do their thinking for them. Too often the leaders paid only lip service to the biologic and physiologic aspects of treatment, and the disciples could not disguise their contempt for other orthodontic philosophies and for those who had the temerity to deviate from the dictums of "der Führer." American orthodontists, with a higher level of specialization and more intensive university graduate training, looked upon removable appliances as a "cop-out" or ineffectual compromise approach to treatment by those who were not able to move teeth with fixed appliances. Biologically oriented European orthodontists saw potential tissue damage and inordinate attention to the minutiae of tooth movement by fixed appliance adherents, who largely ignored the basal sagittal relations and neuromuscular aspects of malocclusion.

This dichotomy was deep and seemingly irreconcilable, and it has remained thus until the last decade or so. Then orthodontists on both sides of the Atlantic began to see the fatal flaws of this "either-or" approach and to seek answers to their technique-oriented problems in the camp of the "enemy." A considerable number of young European dentists received graduate orthodontic training in the United States and demonstrated their prowess with European confrères, or they took courses and read books on removable appliances and found answers to some of the problems inherent in multibanded mechanotherapy. The change in orthodontic approaches has been profound on both sides of the Atlantic, and the patient has been the ultimate beneficiary of this melding of ideas and techniques; but with change have also come additional or different problems. Although short courses stimulate interest and willingness to try other approaches, they do not begin to tell the whole story. Weak links exist in "hands-on" indoctrination, wherein actual experience under proper supervision over an appreciable time is the only way to do justice to a new technique. Diagnosis is the no. 1 priority; yet it is a subjective cogitative assessment of diagnostic records that is seldom presented adequately or really understood at the level demanded by the new orthodontic philosophy. Lectures simply cannot do justice to such important pretreatment considerations or to the continuing needs for therapeutic diagnosis during appliance manipulation. The proliferation and use of removable appliances, and the "oversell" of certain name-oriented appliances in 1- and 2-day short courses in the United States, have made the situation even more critical now. Because of inadequate diagnostic and therapeutic indoctrination, coupled with improper clinical and laboratory techniques, there has been a significant backlash against functional appliances.

The real need now is for a comprehensive, objective, problem-oriented textbook that will give adequate attention to the philosophic, biologic, diagnostic, therapeutic, and stabilizing aspects of orthodontic treatment. It cannot be a substitute for expert-oriented and supervised clinical experience, but it can go a long way toward making the reader understand the raison d'être of a specific approach and it can serve the neophyte well in facing the problems of a new technique. This book is our answer to the long-overdue need. We have tried to combine the best of all orthodontic worlds. Diagnostic and tissue reaction aspects are common denominators in both fixed and removable appliance techniques. Both demand an equal amount of diagnostic acumen, and both fixed and removable appliances can and should be used in the correction of most orthodontic problems today.

Careful consideration was given to the makeup of the team of authors and the material to be covered in the book. Drs. Rakosi and Graber are both professional teachers and clinicians of long experience who have written extensively on fixed and removable appliances, with prior textbooks as well as articles in the periodical literature. Neither "sells" any appliance or technique. Their contributions to this book are based on their successes and failures. The net result is a problem-oriented text that can save the reader many heartaches and hours of clinical time. Professor Petrovic is one of the world's greatest scientists in craniofacial growth and development. He and his research team have exhaustively tested various appliances under controlled laboratory conditions and have produced the most comprehensive and objective research data on these appliances in the world. Indeed, all three of the authors have been engaged in experimental research on fixed and removable appliances, so they are well qualified to write this textbook on orthodontics for a global professional use.

In our initial discussions about the feasibility of a book of this type, another point was made that served as a stimulus for a successful end product—the way some graduate orthodontic students are being indoctrinated today. Too often, graduate programs are primarily clinically oriented, learned from examples (or case reports) represented as more or less authentic procedures that have been selected on a trial-and-error basis from treatment regimens applied to various malocclusions. Whereas many instructors express their support of the scientific method and research, and may even guide a graduate student through a cephalometric study of some aspect of orthodontics, very few have been genuinely impregnated with the scientific know-how and philosophy based on a broad foundation and system of knowledge. In all fairness, this is true not only of orthodontics but also of most clinical aspects of medicine, wherein arbitrary surgical, pediatric, or medical ministrations are the result of treatment-oriented procedures based on specific patient complaints; and some of our so-called researchers, who espouse the "scientific method" but concentrate on a minor facet of the problem while ignoring the overall picture, are not advancing the science and art of dentofacial orthopedics, either.

Holistic dentofacial orthopedics is more than recognition that the mouth is part of the face, which is part of the head, which is part of the body, etc. If we are to prevent the overwhelming clinical preoccupation with "straightening teeth," the graduate student must be inculcated with a scientific approach that will permit a critical look at all clinical procedures and their explanations, an approach that will not only allow improved "treatment philosophies" but also stimulate a search for other answers in the biologic continuum. Otherwise, like most inadequately prepared professionals facing competent colleagues, the semiqualified orthodontist will search for "cookbook" answers, joining peer groups of malcontents looking for some kind of vocational monolithism. This approach will ultimately lead to vocational deterioration and decadence.

More than learning how to run a computer is involved. As Chapter 1 points out, a cybernetic manner of thinking is essential, based on scientifically established and confirmed facts. Equally important, the information must be organized in a manner that favors communication with colleagues both in and out of the specialty of orthodontics—with all members of the health sciences. Sadly, even today, there are clinicians who ignore the work of their contemporaries. The first chapter, on the scientific method, bolstered by Popperian as well as cybernetic analysis, will prepare the graduate student to take his place in the orthodontics of tomorrow with an inquiring mind and the ability to analyze, synthesize, and speculate about the clinical realities, developing new insights to answer old problems.

Chapter 1 discusses the need for a broad-based research methodology and a recognition of the multiplicity of factors if we are to understand and use functional appliances properly. The chapter is unique in orthodontic literature and will require more than one reading for the full impact of cybernetic theory and its application to both fixed and removable appliance orthodontic therapy to be absorbed. Written by a world-renowned physician, researcher, and conceptualizer, it not only embodies the best approaches for the present but also gives guidelines for future research that are most likely to be productive in our studies of multifaceted mechanisms of tissue response, growth guidance, and appliance choice and manipulation.

In Chapter 2 Professor Petrovic discusses the theoretical and research justification of functional orthopedics at the cellular level. When is the treatment biologic? How can we influence and guide the natural forces such as tooth eruption, growth increments, growth direction, and function to favor the correction of various malocclusions? Why is biologic treatment necessary? Since each orthodontic tooth movement means a stressing of the tissues, with a potential acceleration of the aging process, how can we provide the optimal forces? Based on basic and clinical research, just what *are* the possibilities of influencing the tissues by stimulating, inhibiting, or guiding the natural processes? To answer these questions, there is a full accounting of the intensive ongoing research from the Petrovic Laboratory at the Louis Pasteur University Medical School in Strasbourg. The continuing research of Petrovic, Stutzmann, Oudet, Meyer, Gasson, and Lavergne serves as the basis for this integration of important aspects of functional appliance use and tissue response. Bone physiology, the temporomandibular joint, tooth eruption, the various growth processes, and form and function are discussed in the proper context. Treatment timing, force magnitude, force direction, force duration, and appliance design are critical considerations for the clinician. Yet, as noted already, most current techniques are founded on arbitrary principles based on anecdotal clinical use by a small group of clinicians who have developed their precepts on a trial-and-error basis. Have many orthodontic and orthopedic techniques been carefully and exhaustively tested on animal models, varying specific modalities and their mode of application? The rhetorical negative answer makes this chapter even more important, helping the would-be user of functional appliances understand the biologic justification as well as the limitations. As with Chapter 1, Chapter 2 will require more than one reading. It will continue to serve as a valuable and specific source of information on the most important aspects of appliance utilization and tissue response; but if the orthodontist truly wants to be considered an applied biologist and not a glorified mechanic, a full appreciation of this chapter is essential. In so many instances, when listening to a lecture or reading a new book, the clinician will comment, "Let's get the preliminaries over and get on with the main bout. How do we *use* the appliances?" It is this very response that has led to poor case selection, to misuse and overuse of functional appliances, and to the inevitable disenchantment encountered. In this book it is imperative that the reader thoroughly understand Chapters 1 and 2 if the balance of the book is to offer the most that it can, for much of it is based on the first two chapters. Surely a fuller appreciation of the significant research that has been done can only enhance the reader's enthusiasm for further exploratory "feedback."

Chapter 3 is a melding of the research of many investigators and the practical patient treatment experiences of countless clinicians to develop the principles of functional appliances. A major section deals with force application and biomechanics. An important part delineates the differences between so-called mechanical treatment and functional treatment. In the discussion of force application are the various types of force as well as the principles of force application to and tissue reaction in the periodontal ligament, alveolar bone, condyle, and sutures. General principles of orthodontic treatment

are touched upon, not only the basic principles but also the elimination and application of force. Functional forces, muscle forces, and mechanical forces are described with particular reference to removable appliances. The elements of causal and compensatory therapy play an important role and are given. Absent from this chapter are the all too frequent arbitrary pronouncements, based on cultist dogma and historical precedence. The chapter, instead, presents the current understanding of just what functional appliances can and cannot do for a variety of malocclusions.

Chapter 3 also deals with the methods of force elimination. Conventional fixed orthodontic mechanotherapy relies on the *delivery* of force, and the concept of doing away with force seems untenable. Yet the fundamental physiologic principles discussed in Chapter 2 make it apparent that force removal systems can be as important as force delivery systems. The Fränkel buccal shields and lip pads and the Bionator buccal wire configurations are good examples of the mechanisms used with great success. This portion of the chapter deals with the objectives of inhibitory treatment, the indications of the deciduous and mixed dentition use of this approach, the possible side effects, the theory and action of the Fränkel and Bionator appliances, and the actual design of such appliances.

The next part of the book, dealing with vital process stimulation, delineates the objectives of stimulating-type therapy, the indications for and contraindications against this therapy, and the practical application and construction of various appliances.

Chapters 4 and 5, on diagnostic presuppositions, first elucidate the functional significance and then describe in extenso the diagnostic criteria themselves. The specifics on postural resting position, the temporomandibular joint, and neuromuscular function are described, with special emphasis on clinical examination. The section on cephalometrics is based on the recent book by Professor Rakosi and is most complete, elaborating on needed aspects of growth forecasting specifically for functional appliances and on the soft tissue evaluations that are so important for functional appliance use. With all the countless theses, articles and book chapters on cephalometrics that have been written in the past 40 years, it is exciting to read two chapters that specifically apply to a chosen technique. Again, these chapters are unique in orthodontic literature. They will help the clinician pick the proper cases, assure a reasonable degree of success, and provide a pragmatic means of ongoing treatment assessment.

The bulk of the book deals with combination inhibition-stimulation therapy. The activator exemplifies this approach.

Chapters 6, 7, and 8 are a complete and pragmatic discourse on the objectives of activator treatment, its mode of action, its skeletal effectiveness, its construction, variations, and uses, and the indications for and contraindications against its use in different types of problems. The dentoalveolar aspects of management are discussed, with instructions for trimming to get the best possible guided and differential eruption to correct the malrelationships. Step-by-step instructions are given for actual therapy for different conditions. Side effects are also discussed to alert the operator to potential pitfalls.

Chapters 9 and 10 are equally comprehensive discussions of the most important modifications of the original activator appliance—the Bionator (the skeleton activator) and the Fränkel Function Regulator, again going over indications and contraindications, construction, and step-by-step use. When and how to change appliances in midcourse, based on treatment response, is also discussed.

A comprehensive chapter (Chapter 11) on combination functional appliance–extraoral force treatment is included, because of the importance of using extraoral force inhibitory-type treatment in specific types of malocclusion or when functional appliance treatment alone has achieved only part of the treatment goals. It is a "marriage" of fixed and functional appliance philosophies and techniques—combining the best possible correction of sagittal and vertical dysplasias with (as in other appliance sections) the indications, contraindications, modifications, and step-by-step management of these types of problems. It is a classic example of the "inhibition-stimulation" approach, allowing the application of optimal control on the particular part of the face and dentition where it is needed. The use of multibanded therapy with supportive functional appliances at one phase of treatment is also described. For the fixed appliance orthodontist, this chapter may well be a good starting point in combining conventional therapy with muscle control mechanisms for the manipulation of mandibular malrelationships.

The next four chapters (Chapters 12 to 15) deal with specific types of malocclusion and their treatment with functional appliances. Class II, Division 1, Class II, Division 2, deep overbite problems, and Class III and open bite cases are discussed in detail, and specific treatment recommendations and details are elucidated. Illustrations and examples are given for various treatment rationales. The scope of treatment with removable and combination appliances is again discussed in the light of differential diagnoses using patients to illustrate the various points.

Chapter 16 is an epilogue, fittingly done by the author of the first two chapters. In the eyes of the medical researcher, what does the future hold for functional appliances? Where will we turn for appliance enhancement of ongoing research in this dynamic and changing field? How will we further combine fixed and removable appliance techniques to produce the best possible result for the greatest number of patients?

An enormous amount of time was spent by the three authors exploring all possible facets and ramifications of functional appliance therapy. So many "cookbooks" exist in orthodontics, bordering on dogma and cultism, that it was our sincere desire to avoid leading the clinician by the nose. Rather we felt that if one understands the background and physiologic implications it is possible to follow the procedures outlined and let the biologic computer, the brain, process the information and make the necessary alterations demanded by the laws of biologic variability and the infinite shades of live tissue response. The book is the culmination of three lifetimes of experience, in which the authors have evolved an efficient and successful clinical approach that takes minimum time, with achievable optimal results. It is not the final word, not is it possible to provide all the answers within the confines of one book. However, we are confident that it will serve the clinician as a usable chairside guide for a significant portion of his practice and make his professional life more interesting, rewarding, and successful.

CHAPTER 1

RESEARCH METHODOLOGY IN CRANIOFACIAL GROWTH

The last two decades have witnessed the extraordinary evolvement of the science and art of orthodontics, resulting mainly from the awareness and propensity of researchers to ask a new set of questions concerning the relationship between the craniofacial growth mechanisms and the modus operandi of orthodontic and dentofacial orthopedic appliances. The use of modern conceptual and instrumental tools in such investigations made the quest for answers to the new questions conceivable and feasible.

The real progress, however, lies less in the technology than in the questions investigators were and are asking. Most of all, the investigator is no longer restricted by the arbitrary limits of the specialty. The present-day orthodontist is confronted with a challenging and interdisciplinary situation, ranging from anatomy and physiology to molecular biology. Orthodontists are involved in more and different realms of knowledge than are any other dentists or stomatologists. The wide spectrum of research direction is now bringing them closer to understanding both the pathogenetic and the therapeutic aspects of this field.

Recent progress in orthodontics has resulted more from critical and exacting research than from the anecdotal and armchair speculations of the first 50 years of the specialty.

The *first event* was related to the finding concerning the biologic peculiarities of the mammalian condylar cartilage. In 1967-1969, Petrovic and co-workers (Charlier and Petrovic, 1967b; Charlier et al., 1968, 1969ab) published the first rigorous demonstration that the condylar cartilage growth rate and amount could be modified by using appropriate functional and orthopedic appliances. Since then, many researchers and experimenters have been involved in inquiries pertaining to the possibility of modulating the condylar cartilage growth rate. Clinicians also directed their investigative energies to the problem.

In the 1960s also it was shown that the lateral pterygoid muscle plays a regulating role in the control of the condylar cartilage growth rate (Petrovic and Stutzmann,

1972; Stutzmann and Petrovic, 1974ab, 1975c). This finding was further investigated and confirmed by McNamara et al. (1975) in the early 1970s. At about the same time Stutzmann et al. (1976) discovered that the retrodiscal pad plays a mediator role in the efforts of the lateral pterygoid muscle to control condylar growth. Now there is little doubt that, regardless of the findings and opinions, no experimental or clinical investigation relative to the effect of functional appliances is ignoring the condylar cartilage. In an attempt to provide as broad and precise a representation as possible for the many interdisciplinary findings that have become accepted as part of modern orthodontics and dentofacial orthopedics, Petrovic employed the phraseology of cybernetics and control theory to account for the craniofacial growth mechanisms and the modus operandi of the functional and orthopedic appliances. The cybernetic viewpoint supplies sophistication to orthodontic concepts by displaying qualitative and quantitative relationships between observationally and experimentally collected findings. This is a momentous step toward providing a conceptual tool for a broader understanding of the clinical orthodontic problems, particularly since the rigorous language of cybernetics is the most appropriate way to lead to the current use of the computer. More recently the molecular biology approach to the modus operandi of functional appliances has shed a new light on the clinical meaning of experimental investigations.

The *second major event* pertained to the emergence of orthodontics as a major field of biomedical sciences. In the mid-1970s, using the cellular, tissue culture, and organ culture methods of studying human alveolar bone taken from the distal and mesial sides of the premolars and molars both before and during treatment with orthodontic or functional appliances, Jeanne Stutzmann and various co-workers (1979, 1980) introduced precise quantitative evaluations of different parameters of the bone turnover rate. Speculations about when, how, and how much various appliances modulate the human alveolar bone on the distal and mesial surfaces of premolars and molars gave way to rigorous observations

5

and findings. However, sophisticated procedures and technical difficulties confined this research approach to the highly specialized laboratories connected with clinical departments. Of course, some previous research efforts had already disclosed certain basic findings and others had analyzed the qualitative tissue reactions, in periodontium and alveolar bone, linked to physiologic migration or to orthodontically induced tooth movements; but no systematic inquiry on the quantitative aspects had been performed before the investigations of Stutzmann's groups.

The *third major event* in recent years was represented by the chronobiologic aspects of cartilage and bone growth and the effectiveness of functional and orthodontic appliances. Claudine Oudet and co-workers demonstrated that the effect of these appliances on condylar cartilage growth and on alveolar bone turnover, in both the rat and the human, produces significant variations during the day-night cycle and the seasonal sequence (Oudet and Petrovic, 1978a, 1982; Petrovic et al., 1981ce, 1984). These researchers also discovered that the reduced rate of growth in the rat lateral pterygoid muscle, as produced during treatment with functional appliances, is significantly higher in the resting phase than in the activity phase of the individual. This diminished rate of increase (along with analogous variations in other masticatory muscles) plays an important role in the mechanism of action of some functional appliances by maintaining the mandible in a more forward position, even during the daily period when the appliance is not worn (Petrovic et al., 1982ab).

It is obvious that these interesting chronobiologic aspects of orthodontic treatment not only will have a striking impact on future research but also should be routinely considered by orthodontists in their everyday practice (Petrovic et al., 1982a; Oudet et al., 1984).

With the rapid increase in research efforts, a new vision of the mechanism of action of functional appliances has developed. Above all, the constant interplay and cross fertilization between clinical and biologic research have changed orthodontic knowledge and thinking. The flood of assumptions is receding. In the place of small islets, continents of solid well-grounded knowledge are emerging. Yet much about the etiology and pathology of major dentofacial malrelations is still unknown, and the answers are not likely to come solely from observations of the patient but from biomedical research. Undoubtedly the biologic analysis of craniofacial growth mechanisms and the modus operandi of orthodontic appliances is assuming a more important role in treatment decision making. The benefits of this newer knowledge and thinking will depend on its assimilation and application by orthodontists and dentists who are taking care of the individual patient. Whole populations may bene-

fit. Such utilization of these newer masses of information should have a positive "feedback" effect, psychologically and socially, on biomedical investigation.

This chapter is based primarily on the experimental research investigations pursued in the Laboratory for Craniofacial Growth Mechanisms, together with cognitive assistance of several leading clinically oriented researchers and research-oriented clinicians from around the world. Their names will be frequently mentioned in the following pages. The purpose of the chapter is not only to provide the reader with newer information but also to help him master the structure and the meaning of the knowledge. Indeed, words like *science, theory, hypothesis, explanation, meaning, cause, effect,* and *mechanism of action* are often used in a way that may be equivocal, irrelevant, and misleading, the result being confusion and misunderstanding.

COGNITIVE STATUS OF BIOMEDICAL AND MEDICAL CONCEPTS, PROPOSITIONS AND THEORIES

What is the goal of research? It is the increase of knowledge; but, then, what is the knowledge and how does the knowledge grow?

Epistemologic features

The branch of philosophy that deals with the possibility, nature, origin, structure, and validity of knowledge is called *epistemology.* In biomedical sciences, epistemology concerns mainly the relations between the "subject" and the "object," between the thinking and the normal or pathologic reality.

The biomedical researcher makes the following distinctions: *Logic* is a formal discipline of inquiry relative to the principles guiding legitimate reasoning. *Epistemology* is a philosophical branch inquiring into the nature and validity of knowledge. *Psychology* investigates the conscious aspects of the cognitive process exclusively as a part of the mental life, epistemology dealing rather with the reference of cognitive processes to reality.

Epistemology may be divided into several basic areas: the possibility and limits of knowledge, the origin of knowledge (empiricism versus rationalism), the methodologic* problems of acquiring knowledge, the varieties of knowledge (non-inferential apprehension of data by perception and inferential knowledge, including scientific knowledge insofar as it involves inference from ob-

---

*Methodology should not be mistaken for technology or techniques. Methodology refers to the analysis of conceptual, observational, and experimental principles and processes that are guiding a scientific, biomedical, or clinical inquiry. In addition to general problems of such an inquiry, each branch of science, medicine, or dentistry has specific methodologic problems that should be investigated.

servational data), the structure of knowledge, and the problem of truth (the correspondence theory, in which the criterion of truth concerns the relation between the statement and its object, versus the coherence theory, in which the criterion of truth concerns the logical consistency of an individual statement with a wider and well-organized system of statements). The orthodontist and any other dentist or physician may be tempted to consider epistemologic problems as something that has no actual connection to his specialty and his activity. In fact, at every step of biomedical and clinical research and activity, one is confronted with problems of epistemologic and methodologic essence. Nothing is worse than when the researcher and the clinician are not even aware that they are dealing with an epistemologic or methodologic obstacle or difficulty.

The first step for the orthodontist is thus to analyze the proper object of his specialty (both the knowledge and the activity), the manner in which orthodontics develops, the characteristics of statements, the generalizations, theories, and paradigms that orthodontics involves, and the nature of its methodologic and conceptual foundations or assumptions as well as its relations to other scientific, technologic and biomedical branches.

There is little doubt that the epistemologic situation of biomedical sciences corresponds, for the most part, to the philosophical vision of Karl Popper (Petrovic, 1977, 1982, 1983). Indeed, according to Popper, science is not a static acceptance of truth but rather the permanent search for truth. No theory, no statement, may be really verified; but when efforts to refute a working hypothesis fail, a proposition is then corroborated. However, "corroborated" means that a theory or a concept is strengthened and not that it is definitely, unmistakably, true. In other words, the criterion of validity is the resistance to refutation. For the orthodontist this means that not only should support for a working hypothesis be looked for but also one should be especially alert to biomedical concepts and clinical cases which *could* refute the concept.

In *Conjectures and Refutations, the Growth of Scientific Knowledge* (1963), Popper states:

> Clinical observations, like all other observations, are interpretations in the light of theories; and for this reason alone they are apt to seem to support those theories in the light of which they are interpreted. But real support can be obtained only from observations undertaken as tests (by attempted refutations); and for this purpose, criteria of refutation have to be laid down beforehand: it must be agreed which observable situations, if actually observed, mean that the theory is refuted.

This statement may be considered as a "guiding rule" in any medical (or orthodontic) research. It also implies that any theory, any concept, in orthodontics is neces-

sarily *conjectural* and—to use Kuhn's language (1962)—based on a paradigm (i.e., on a model that is used as a thinking pattern). A paradigm-free fact just does not exist.

In compliance with Popper's thinking, Petrovic (1982) affirms that any "refutation-corroboration" process in medicine and orthodontics is not a cognitive act but a decision-making procedure; even the distinction between what is normal and what is pathologic results rather from an operational definition than from an appreciation of the biomedical reality.

According to Popper, the degree of refutability is the measure of the heuristic fruitfulness of a working hypothesis. As a corollary, the irrefutability of a theory or concept is the mere expression of its informational emptiness or at least its meagerness. Unquestionably, the decisional analysis in medicine and orthodontics implies, in both diagnosis and therapeutics, the progressive refutation of what appears to be erroneous.

Therefore, in line with Petrovic's conception (1977, 1982, 1983), the Popperian epistemology is a powerful intellectual tool in ordering and structuring the experimental and clinical research data (Popper, 1963).

Methodologic features

Some preliminary statements are necessary:

1. Biomedical theories and concepts shed light on only part of the clinical reality. Hence, the "decision-making" procedures in orthodontics are based on both scientific biomedical knowledge and empirical clinical evidence. Therefore Petrovic and Stutzmann (1980a) make the epistemologic distinction between
   a. Biomedical knowledge—established according to the rigorous rules of scientific inquiry; in this case the reasoning validates the basis of the orthodontic decision making
   b. Clinical know-how—a collection of clinical procedures and guidelines established and evaluated according to the criterion of effectiveness; in this case the reasoning is only an intellectual attempt to account for the clinical effectiveness (it cannot either validate or invalidate the orthodontic decision making)
2. The causal explanation of dentofacial malrelations and the modus operandi of functional appliances is to be searched for much more in the morphophysiologic peculiarities of different growth sites than in the agents or events playing a triggering role (Petrovic, 1972).
3. The distinction between the *normal* and the *pathologic* is an operation of decision rather than a cognitive act. Indeed, for an isolated morphologic or physiologic parameter, the *limit* between

the normal and the pathologic is apprehensible or ascertainable only very occasionally. However, a discontinuity may be detectable on the level of a system (e.g., during the transition phase from the optimal stable occlusal relationship to a suboptimal one). Needless to say, such a discontinuity is not necessarily the threshold of the pathologic!

4. In orthodontics, founded mainly on empirical procedures, the *explanation* has the form of doctrine. In biomedical orthodontics the *explanation* has the form encountered in biologic sciences, with four main categories:
   a. Deductive type
   b. Deductivoprobabilistic type
   c. Functional type
   d. Phylogenetic type

5. Formally the biomedical explanation is the process of fitting a factual statement into the framework of systematically organized knowledge. As for the so-called clinical explanation, it consists mostly of accounting for a singular phenomenon by reference to corresponding general statements (theories, concepts) together with the specific conditions under which the involved biomedical statements operate. Indeed, the orthodontist is necessarily interested in forecasting (i.e., attributing an explanatory scheme for future occurrences), theorizing that if the conjecture and the appropriate set of initial requirements are fulfilled the anticipated event will actually happen.

6. The research investigator (experimenter or clinician) faces individual variability of the sample, uncontrolled or even unknown disturbing factors, unexpected secondary effects, etc.; hence, the necessity of a carefully prepared research design including, whenever possible, the quantitative variation of input variables (e.g., a functional appliance) and the quantitative evaluation of output parameters (e.g., growth rate, amount, and direction and the lengths and angles of specific cephalometric criteria). Methodologically the causal research is, in fact, a factor search with identification and analysis.

7. The word *theory* has two meanings:
   a. It may refer to systematically organized knowledge (e.g., the cybernetic theory of craniofacial growth).
   b. It may refer to a set of assumptions, logically formulated but yet to be tested (e.g. the "functional matrix" theory).
   In epistemology the distinction is made between *laws* (valid, corroborated, empirical generalizations) and *principles* (axioms, postulates [i.e., sets of unproved or undemonstrable propositions], theories).

Now, which types of biomedical and clinical explanation are we encountering in scientifically based orthodontics? It is superfluous to emphasize the inappropriateness of bare, unsupported, verbal statements, even if they still survive in the literature. It is sometimes amusing to observe how often ambiguous words or inarticulate sentences may be successful. Perhaps it is because everyone can introduce his own orthodontic fantasies into such vague words and sentences.

From a formal viewpoint, four basic types of explanation are current in the literature dealing with craniofacial growth and orthodontic questions (Petrovic, 1982, 1984ab):

1. *Deductive type*
   In this case the explicandum appears as a necessary consequence of certain premises. Such an explanation may be used for description and classification of observations as well as for the forecast of future events, including the degree of probability. The deductive explanation requires a logically organized framework of knowledge (e.g., a cybernetic diagram containing precise quantitative data).

2. *Deductivoprobabilistic type*
   In this type of explanation at least one of the premises consists of probabilistic statements (theories or concepts) relative to specific categories of individual occurrences. The deductivoprobabilistic type concerns not the degree of validity of the premise(s) but the relationship between the premises and the explicandum.
   This type of explanation is the most common in medicine, including orthodontics. It is at the basis of rules in differential diagnosis and prognosis. The computer-based orthodontic decision is an illustration of such reasoning.

3. *Functional type*
   In this case the explanation takes the form of specifying the function that an element performs in maintaining, against random variations and intrinsic or extrinsic disturbances, some major characters of the system *as a whole* to which it belongs.
   This type of explanation corresponds to the so-called goal-seeking description of the technologic systems. Various components of the system controlling craniofacial growth and development stand with each other in precise causal interdependence and responsiveness, involving interactions and feedbacks. Thus the functional explanation presupposes a cybernetically organized knowledge.
   One point should be emphasized: Since morphophysiologic systems are almost always nonlinear, quantitative descriptions may only exceptionally be restricted to differential equations; "discontinuities" must be taken into account. Practically, the so-called mathematical theory of catastrophe is an excellent to-

pologic tool to account for discontinuities (i.e., the bifurcation type of situations during growth and development, p. 59).

4. *Evolutionary type*

A morphophysiologic entity, like the temporomandibular joint, that characterizes mammalians may be accounted for by describing how it has evolved from some earlier phylogenetic forms.

In the evolutionary type of explanation, the first step is to set out the sequence of major events through which an earlier system has been transformed into a later one. The second step is to discover events that are causally pertinent to the transformation of the system. The third step is to give reason for the transformation by detecting the morphophysiologic appropriateness of the newly evolved system. The fourth step is to elucidate the evolutionary successfulness of one versus some other transformation. An evolutionary explanation is, at best, presumptive; because an evolutionary transformation is generally a nonrecurring event, its hypothetical explanation is hard to test.

Yet the evolutionary explanation for the peculiarities of the condylar cartilage (Petrovic et al., 1975b) is intellectually tempting.

In reptiles the joint between the skull and the lower jaw is formed by two bones originating from the primary-type cartilages, the quadratus and the articular. In mammals this joint is formed by two dermal bones, the squamosal and the dentary (i.e., mandible), the latter developing from three posterior secondary-type cartilages (coronoid, condylar, angular—the last one differentiating only in small mammals).

According to Symons (1951), in the mammalian embryo the condylar cartilage also develops independently of the chondrocranium. Thus phylogenetic data throw light on ontogenetic data. At the same time, phylogenetically and ontogenetically, the prechondroblastic zone of the condylar cartilage (and of *any* secondary cartilage) appears to be closer to craniofacial sutures and to the subperiosteal zone than to epiphyseal cartilage.

Obviously the responsiveness of the condylar cartilage growth to *local* factors may explain the extraordinary success of the, phylogenetically new, mammalian joint between the skull and the lower jaw (Petrovic, 1970, 1972; Petrovic, et al., 1975). The condylar cartilage growth is integrated into an organized *functional* whole, having the form of a servosystem and able to modulate the lengthening of the condyle in such a way that the lower jaw adapts to the upper jaw during growth. Indeed, the operation of confrontation between the positions of the upper and lower dental arches is the "comparator" of the servosystem. The comparator is at the origin of the correction signals intended to modulate the postural activity of the lateral pterygoid muscle

so as to place the mandible in the position of either an optimal or a suboptimal occlusal adjustment. The variations in the postural activity of the lateral pterygoid and in the iterative activity of the temporomeniscocondylar frenum (retrodiscal pad) will modulate (i.e., stimulate or restrain) the condylar cartilage growth rate and modify the condyle growth direction, producing a more *anterior* or more *posterior* growth rotation of the mandible.

Such possibility for the lower jaw to adjust in length to the upper jaw during growth certainly favored the genetic variations that led to posteroanterior facial shortening, molarization of the postcanine teeth, and, subsequently, mastication. Needless to emphasize, in the absence of adjustment of mandibular teeth to maxillary teeth, the forces of occlusion would expose the periodontal structures to repeated traumas that would result in the loss of the teeth. The responsiveness of the condylar cartilage growth to local factors opens up the possibility of mastication and, in this way, facilitates a high basic metabolism and the maintenance of a constant body temperature (i.e., makes possible a steady high level of activity).

How can we conceive growth mechanisms of the mammalian mandible, including the human mandible? Our research investigations led us to the following theorizations:

A relatively stable *periosteal* contribution exists that is subordinated both to orders affecting the whole organism and to local control factors represented primarily, but not solely, by muscular contractions. Thus, by the very nature of bone growth and remodeling (i.e., by surface apposition and resorption), the periosteal growth of the mandible is *commanded* rather than regulated. The mechanisms involved are necessarily slow and rough.

A *cartilaginous* contribution (condylar, coronoid, and angular) exists that is more easily modifiable and more subject to local control systems through feedback loops. Integrated within the local regulative loop, the cartilaginous contribution to mandibular growth is more rapidly brought into play and is intended for fine growth adjustment ensuring an efficient occlusion. Viewed from this standpoint, the growth of the condylar cartilage is seen as a mechanism that at *each moment* depends on messages of local origin. Thus it is the expression of a regional structural homeostasis that enables the coordinated growth of the masticatory apparatus. This is not to say that periosteal deposition of bone is only an accessory mechanism; the consequences of condylectomy and acromegaly bear witness to the contrary. However, since in both these situations the increase in size of the mandible is more subject to an overall command than to local regulation, mandibular overgrowth from

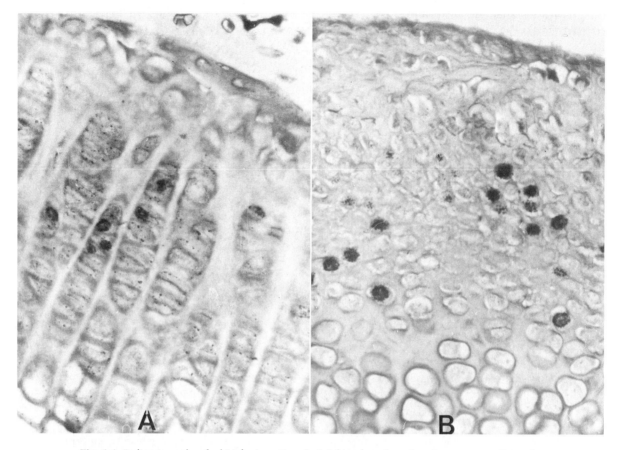

Fig. 1-1. Radioautographs of a histologic section. **A,** Epiphyseal cartilage. In primary-type cartilages the chondroblasts divide and synthesize intercellular matrix. **B,** Condylar cartilage of the mandible. In secondary-type cartilages the cells that divide the prechondroblasts are not yet surrounded by cartilaginous matrix.

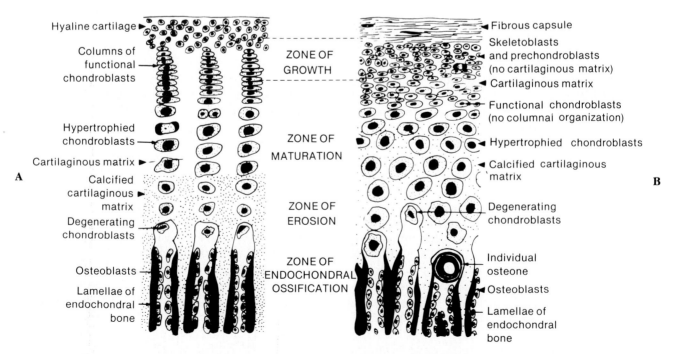

Fig. 1-2. Histologic structure of a primary-type, **A,** and secondary-type, **B,** cartilage.

an intense and perpetuated subperiosteal ossification alone may well lead to occlusal disharmony.

Stutzmann (1976) places emphasis on the following fact: *primary* cartilages exist in the axial skeleton, the skull base, and the limbs; the dividing cells, differentiated chondroblasts, are surrounded by cartilaginous matrix, which isolates them from local factors able to restrain or stimulate cartilaginous growth. *Secondary* cartilages (Figs. 1-1 and 1-2) exist in condylar and coronoid (and, in small mammals, in angular) processes and sometimes in sutures; the dividing cells, prechondroblasts, are not surrounded by cartilaginous matrix (i.e., are *not* isolated from local factor influence). This is an attempt to make intelligible the difference between *primary* and *secondary* cartilages, even if evolutionary mechanisms escape (at the present time) unequivocal rationalization.

In conclusion, our findings regarding the singular biologic behavior of the condylar cartilage help to explain the evolutionary supremacy of the new joint between the skull and the lower jaw—namely that it characterizes all mammals as well as allows the phylogenetic success of mammals.

Another osteologic character of mammals should be pointed out: there is a so-called secondary bony palate separating the nasal cavity from the oral cavity. This

structure also facilitates mastication. Such a phylogenetic origin of the human bony palate helps to explain biologic and pathologic peculiarities of the midpalatal suture.

Cybernetic features

Craniofacial growth is an extremely complex process. When we want to account for scientific findings relative to its mechanisms and to the modus operandi of orthopedic and orthodontic appliances, nowadays a set of approaches exists for us to utilize:

1. We may relate our discoveries by just placing the observations next to each other. This manner of working has been and sometimes is quite common but is to some extent outdated if not obsolete.
2. We may construct diagrams (Figs. 1-3 and 1-4) displaying the qualitative relations between observations. This procedure, the first step toward modelization, is not only directly more helpful but also operationally more heuristic and of more new fact–finding potential.
3. We may improve the diagrams by making the relationships related by the model either continuous or discontinuous. This line of action is much more time consuming, and hence unpopular, especially for a busy professional.

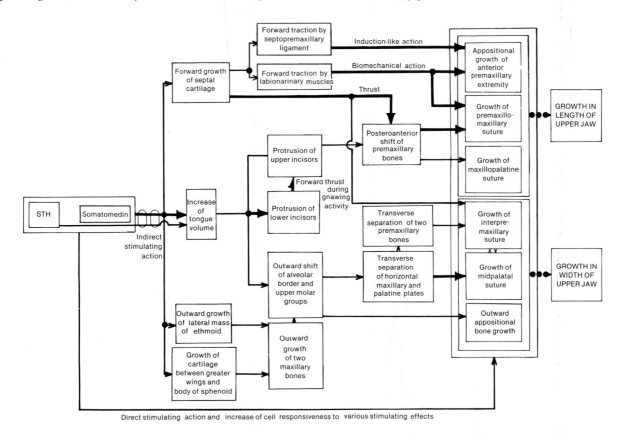

Fig. 1-3. Functional diagram for the sequential analysis of upper jaw growth control by STH-somatomedin.

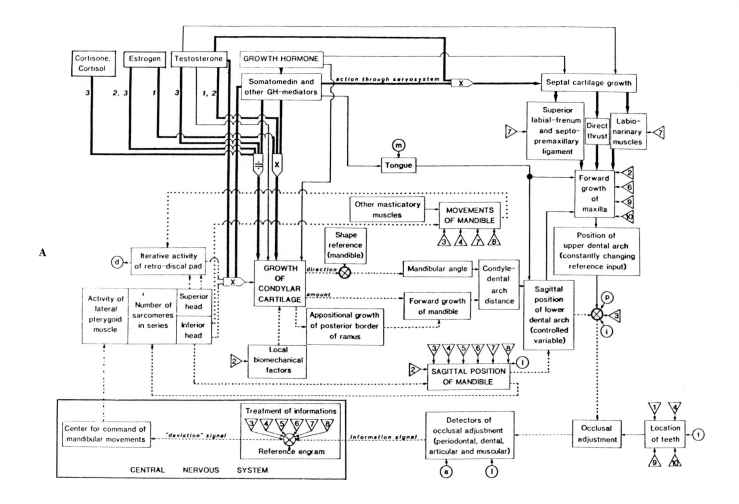

A

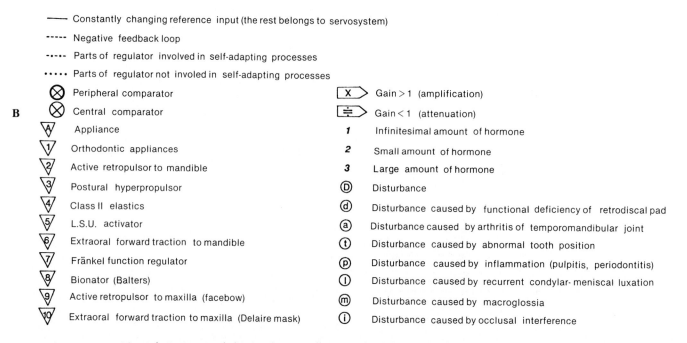

B

Constantly changing reference input (the rest belongs to servosystem)

Negative feedback loop

Parts of regulator involved in self-adapting processes

Parts of regulator not involed in self-adapting processes

⊗ Peripheral comparator
⊗ Central comparator

A Appliance
1 Orthodontic appliances
2 Active retropulsor to mandible
3 Postural hyperpropulsor
4 Class II elastics
5 L.S.U. activator
6 Extraoral forward traction to mandible
7 Fränkel function regulator
8 Bionator (Balters)
9 Active retropulsor to maxilla (facebow)
10 Extraoral forward traction to maxilla (Delaire mask)

X⟩ Gain > 1 (amplification)
÷⟩ Gain < 1 (attenuation)

1 Infinitesimal amount of hormone
2 Small amount of hormone
3 Large amount of hormone
Ⓓ Disturbance
ⓓ Disturbance caused by functional deficiency of retrodiscal pad
ⓐ Disturbance caused by arthritis of temporomandibular joint
ⓣ Disturbance caused by abnormal tooth position
ⓟ Disturbance caused by inflammation (pulpitis, periodontitis)
Ⓛ Disturbance caused by recurrent condylar-meniscal luxation
ⓜ Disturbance caused by macroglossia
ⓘ Disturbance caused by occlusal interference

Fig. 1-4. A, Functional diagram for controlling growth of the mandibular condylar cartilage. **B,** Key. (Compare with Fig. 2-16.)

C

ROTATION GROUP	OCCLUSAL RELATIONSHIP	COMPARATOR	SUGGESTED TREATMENT	EXTRACTION	COMMENTS
P2 DOB / P2 DN	I / c/c / II	M / M / M	/ 9 / 9	+(0) / ++ / ++	
R2 DN / R2 DOB	I / c/c / II	M * / M * / M *	/ 9+1 / 9	/ ++ / ++	First molar relationship is occlusion-determinative
R2 DDB	II	M *	9	++	
A2 DN / A2 DDB	II	I / I or P	9 / 9	++ / ++	
P1 MOB / P1 MN	III	M	2		Long-lasting mandibular growth
P1 NOB / P1 NN	1 / c/c / III	M / M / M	/ 2 / 2		
R1 NN / R1 NOB / R1 NDB	I / c/c / II	M * / M * / M *	/ 9+1 / 9+1	/ ++ / ++	
A1 DDB	II	I or P	5,7,8,(4),(6)	+(0)	
A1 DN	1I / c/c / I	I / I / I	5,7,8,(4),(6)	+(0) / +(0)	
A1 NN	I / c/c / II	I / I / I	/ 1 / 5,7,8,(4),(6)	++ / +(0)	
A1 NDB	I / c/c / II	I or P / I or P / I or P	/ 5,7,8,(4),(6) / 5,7,8,(4),(6)	- / - / -	
A3 MN / A3 MDB	I / III	I / I	10		Surgery indicated
R3 MDB / R3 MN / R3 MOB	I / III	M / M / M	/ 10+1 / 10+1		
P3 MN / P3 MOB	III	M	2+10		Surgery indicated

Fig. 1-4, cont'd. C, Clinical effectiveness of orthopedic, functional, and orthodontic appliances as related to facial growth rotation groups. (According to Lavergne and Petrovic.)

Mandibular rotation—*A,* anterior; *R,*neutral; *P,* posterior

Basal growth inequality—*1,* mandible = maxilla; *2,* mandible < maxilla; *3,* mandible > maxilla

Posteroanterior state—*N,* normal; *D,* distal; *M,* mesial

Vertical state—*OB,* open bite; *N,* normal; *DB,* deep bite

For example, *R1 NN* means: *R,* neutral mandibular growth rotation; *1,* small basal growth difference; *N,* neutral basal posteroanterior relationship; and *N,* neutral basal vertical relationship.

4. We may further improve the diagrams by using matrices in mathematical language—tabular lines and arrays (generally of numbers)—to describe the interactions among parts of the morphophysiologic system.

   In these models the output appears usually proportional to the input(s); in other words, we are making use of linear differential equations.

   Such an image implies a proper research approach, which is often difficult to put into practice but is indisputably rewarding for both the medical biologist and the clinician.

5. We may also take advantage of cybernetics based on communication and information theory, particularly on feedback control systems.

   Cybernetics has brought to biologic and biomedical sciences some new and advantageous concepts—e.g., negative and positive feedback, self-regulation, reference input, open and closed loop, regulation versus servosystem, gain (amplification of attenuation), and systems and circuit analysis.

   In this situation also, linear differential equations are put into operation almost exclusively. A relevant and well-chosen investigatory strategy is implicated from both a conceptual and a methodologic point of view. Often disregarded as a pointless sophistication in accounting for biologic and biomedical findings, the cybernetic approach is, in fact, a major breakthrough in scientific and clinical orthodontics and dentofacial orthopedics, especially in the decision making process and problem solving (Milhorn, 1966; Petrovic, 1977).

6. We may, finally, turn to the so-called catastrophe theory, a topologic concept designed to describe discontinuities (Fig. 1-5). In the framework of cybernetic models, discontinuities correspond to sudden changes from one reference of the control system to another. Because the bifurcation-type situation is rather frequent during ontogenesis, catastrophe theory enables one to relate faithfully, either qualitatively or quantitatively, many nonlinear relationships that would be, to a great degree, difficult to describe by just manipulating classical differential equations (p. 56).

   When one associates cybernetics with the catastrophe theory, it becomes obvious that the biologic and biomedical representation of the craniofacial growth mechanisms as well as the modus operandi of orthodontic and orthopedic appliances has made significant progress. It is needless to add that only accurate knowledge can teach the clinician what to do: modern decision making in orthodontics and dentofacial orthopedics is grounded on a highly sophisticated portrayal of the biologic and biomedical reality.

It would be superfluous to stress the obstacles and handicaps at this level of investigation, as well as the frustration of the researcher in facing a paucity of results. Furthermore, there is sometimes a painful experience for the potential user. Despite these drawbacks, however, the impending future must turn to this approach.

A rational, intellectually consistent, and inter-individual vision of dentofacial malrelations is still far from supplanting the unshaken self-confidence–based doctrinal statements of some brillant clinicians. Indeed, many controversies in the contemporary history of orthodontics and dentofacial orthopedics are more a matter of conflicts between individuals or "chapels" than confrontations between theories and concepts!

One reason for this state of affairs lies in the frequently encountered, ambiguous, and inarticulate account for the orthodontist's assumed position and reasoning. Yet the epistemologic consistency of any newly formulated theory or concept cannot be legitimately established and evaluated without expressing unequivocally the principles of reasoning put into operation throughout the course of the research investigation. There can be no sound research achievement leaving out a circumspect and well-advised epistemologic and methologic inquiry into the theoretical basis and structure of a discipline like orthodontics. Otherwise, professional intercommunication remains difficult if not impossible. To be sure, the rationalization of orthodontic diagnostic and treatment procedures in toto is a difficult task with ordinary language, especially when the problems of immediate clinical effectiveness outweigh the conceptual coherence. Still, in the long run, there can be no efficient clinical activity in orthodontics and dentofacial orthopedics without the realization that dentofacial malrelations are part of an indivisible reality even when we are dealing with different diagnostic and treatment approaches.

Cybernetics and the theory of control are, in this respect, a new and powerful tool. They are coping, in a rigorous way, with the study of communications, control mechanisms, and finalized organizations in both living and technologic systems. In other words, they are the language of a combined analysis and systemic approach to biology and biomedical sciences. They make it possible to account for the properties of a normal or pathologic system as emerging from the organization of connectivity relations. Willingly or reluctantly the modern orthodontist must become acquainted with the cybernetic language, among other reasons because the cybernetic thinking is the main way to data processing and computerizing.

A cybernetically organized system operates through signals transmitting information. A physiologic signal may be of physical, chemical, or electromagnetic nature.

Usually it is of very low energy. Craniofacial growth and development are an information-processing phenomenon that includes production, perception, transmission, and storage of information. Petrovic (1977, 1982) was the first to set forth a cybernetic model accounting for the physiologic phenomena involved in facial growth and the modus operandi of orthodontic and functional appliances (Fig. 1-4); but it should be immediately emphasized that this model is only one of several possible rational descriptions of the reality. There is no reason to give preference to one research approach for its presumably uppermost heuristic value. In the same way, according to Popperian epistemologic precepts, there is no cybernetic model and no set of equations that can describe craniofacial growth and the modus operandi of orthodontic and functional appliances in an exclusive and definitive manner. Petrovic (1982) has pointed out that cybernetics is definitely a part of orthodontics but *his own* cybernetic model is not.

The formation and renewal of the craniofacial skeleton are a many-faceted phenomenon. It is the connections between constituents that are complex, however, and not the constituents themselves. In other words, the complexity results from the organization, the structured whole being infinitely more complex than the simple sum of its constituents. This means that the physiologic properties of the craniofacial skeleton are not simply related to the cells and intercellular substances or to elementary intercellular actions but originate from the tissue and organ system as a whole with all its interactions and feedbacks. The identification and analysis of feedback loops (i.e., the regulation processes) are one of the main tasks of the Strasbourg laboratory in the field of craniofacial growth. So far, only the cybernetic language may accurately render the intricacy and complexity of the craniofacial morphogenesis and the means to influence it.

The study of a morphophysiologic system consists of describing its properties. Usually the researcher is measuring, simultaneously, either the spontaneous or the experimentally and therapeutically induced variations of a parameter chosen as the stimulus (input) and the

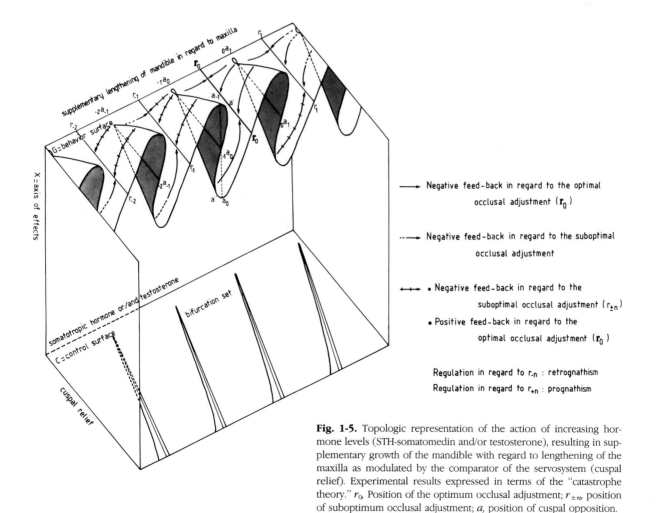

Fig. 1-5. Topologic representation of the action of increasing hormone levels (STH-somatomedin and/or testosterone), resulting in supplementary growth of the mandible with regard to lengthening of the maxilla as modulated by the comparator of the servosystem (cuspal relief). Experimental results expressed in terms of the "catastrophe theory." r_0, Position of the optimum occlusal adjustment; $r_{\pm n}$ position of suboptimum occlusal adjustment; a, position of cuspal opposition.

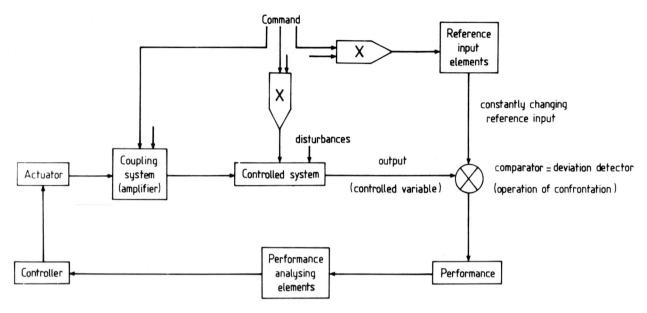

Fig. 1-6. Elements and organization of a servosystem.

variations of one or several parameters chosen as the response (output). The output is related to the input by a so-called transfer function that characterizes the system under investigation. In other words, the system is described as a function of changes affecting the various parameters.

Specifying some details may be useful.

The input and the output are generally represented by arrows. In dealing with time-dependent phenomena each arrow represents a signal, and in the frame of an entity the signal may become a message. The percentage of what is not directly indispensable to the message but may contribute to the reliability of the message transmission is considered to be the redundancy. The translation of a message from one language into another is called *transcodage*.

A given physiologic system under investigation is represented by a black box. The "content" of the black box is usually unknown.

When a physiologic system is designed for maintaining, in spite of disturbances, a specific correspondence between the "output" and the "input," it is a closed loop control system. The closed loop system is characterized by the presence of a feedback loop and a comparator. The so-called open loop system has no feedback loop and no comparator.

The closed loop control system has two variations:

1. *The regulator.* In this case the main input is a constant. The comparator detects the disturbances or the effects of the disturbances. The regulator is a negative feedback system; this means that a distur-

bance causes a change which tends to restore the state of the disturbed system to the initial conditions.

2. *The servosystem or follow-up system* (Fig. 1-6). In this case the main input is not a constant but displays variations as a function of time.

• • •

The control theory is becoming the common language of science and technology. The definitions may vary with disciplines and authors, so it is imperative to recall the basic definitions of concepts and terms as prescribed by Petrovic and Stutzmann (1977, 1982) in the field of craniofacial growth and the modus operandi of orthodontic and functional appliances.

The command. The command is a signal established independently of the feedback system under scrutiny. It affects the behavior of the control system without being affected by the consequences of this behavior. For instance, to the best of our knowledge, the secretion rate of growth hormone–somatomedin, testosterone, and estrogen does not seem to be modulated by the variations of craniofacial growth.

Reference input elements. Reference input elements establish the relationship between the command (e.g., growth hormone–somatomedin) and the reference input (the sagittal position of the upper dental arch). They include the septal cartilage, the septopremaxillary frenum, the labionarinary muscles, and the premaxillary and maxillary bones.

Reference input. The reference input is a signal established as a standard of comparison (i.e., it is located ahead of the comparator). Ideally it should be totally independent of the feedback.

The controller. The controller is located between the deviation signal and the actuating signal.

Actuating signal. The actuating signal corresponds to the output signal of the controller (i.e., to the input signal of the controlled system). The activity of the lateral pterygoid muscle and the retrodiscal pad corresponds to the actuating signal.

Controlled system. The system that is controlled is a part of the control system located between the actuating signal and the directly controlled variable. A good example would be the growth of condylar cartilage.

Controlled variable. This is the output signal of the system. The best example would be the sagittal position of the mandible (i.e., of the lower dental arch).

The gain. The gain of a system is the output divided by the input. When it is greater than 1, amplification is present; when inferior to 1, attenuation. The pterygocondylar coupling is an example of gain. According to Petrovic's investigation, the basic value of the gain is determined genetically but it may be amplified by growth hormone–somatomedin and by testosterone or attenuated by estrogen.

Feedback signal. The feedback signal is the function of the controlled variable that is compared to the reference input. In a regulator or servosystem it is negative.

The disturbance. Any input other than the reference chosen by the researcher as the main input signal is considered to be a disturbance. The disturbance is responsible for deviation of the output signal. It may act on any element of the regulating system. The concept of disturbance is sometimes difficult to grasp. For instance, the supplementary lengthening caused by growth hormone–somatomedin is greater for the mandible than for the maxilla. This implies that the increase in hormone level probably has a disturbing effect on occlusal adjustment.

The attractor. This is the final structurally stable steady state in a dynamic system. An example would be the full interdigitation type of occlusal relationship (full Class I, but to a certain degree also full Class II or full Class III).

The repeller. This is the set of all unstable equilibrium states, including their limit points. An example would be the cusp-to-cusp type of occlusal relationship.

The fractal. The mathematician Mandelbrot coined the neologism "fractal" from the Latin adjective *fractus* corresponding to the verb *frangere* (which means to break creating irregular fragments). So fractal means both "fragmented" and "irregular." One may say that the fractal approach to form goes beyond the topologic approach, the fractal and topologic features being complementary.

The interdental relationship represents a natural shape that may be represented by fractal geometry as developed by Mandelbrot in 1982. Our semiquantitative evaluation of electromyographic records is also based on an analysis using fractal geometry.

Fractal curve. This is the curve for which the fractal dimension exceeds the topologic dimension.

The noise. This is chance fluctuations of a signal and the manifestations thereof. The weaker the signal, the greater will be the relative weight of the noise.

Scaling fractals. The word *fractals* points to a disorder and concerns cases of intractable irregularity whereas the term *scaling* points to a sort of order. Indeed, according to Mandelbrot (1982), most fractals are invariables under certain transformations of scale.

Final methodologic comments

The cybernetic theory of craniofacial growth mechanisms is based on both analytic and synthetic approaches. The proposed functional diagrams (Figs. 1-3 and 1-4) are not static conceptual viewpoints but dynamic representations of experimental findings concerning the thus-far detected and investigated phenomena of growth and growth determinism in the postnatal period. Such cybernetic models have, above all, a heuristic value: they open new perspectives and provide a new working hypothesis to be tested. It is inherent in the methodology of scientific investigation that the construction of a *general* model (i.e., the true discovery) precede any long experimental work designed to refute or corroborate the working hypothesis resulting from the model. Cybernetic models, which are continuously revised to conform to new findings, offer a general overview while also enabling such close critical scrutiny to be performed as to leave no opportunity for confusion.

In methodology, animal experimentation is designed to detect *causal* relationships. In clinical research, conditions are not always set up to establish that a phenomenon is actually produced orthodontically or orthopedically. For instance, selecting a given parameter of facial growth and comparing an individual to a population is not an ideal procedure for evidencing therapeutically produced variations. Also, failing to detect the effect of a functional appliance does not allow one to conclude that the given parameter is "genetically determined"! Last but not least, one must take into account the existence of the temporal organization of tissue growth (Oudet and Petrovic, 1978a, 1982; Petrovic et al., 1981ce, 1982b, 1984; Oudet et al., 1984).

In connection with the last, indeed, the condylar cartilage and alveolar bone of growing children exhibit a higher percentage of cells in the DNA-synthesis phase during the night than during the day. In other words, the first sleeping hours are the most favorable moment for triggering therapeutically an increased number of cell divisions in both condylar cartilage and alveolar bone. Logically, the mitosis rate itself will be highest during the "breakfast time." Also the growth in length of the masticatory muscles, especially the lateral pterygoids, appears to be more important during the night than during the day. In fact, the L.S.U. activator and similar appliances are most efficient when worn during the night (Petrovic et al., 1981d, 1982b; Oudet et al., 1984).

These general methodologic considerations will enable one to take a valid approach to the problems concerning the biologic mechanisms of facial growth and the modus operandi of functional appliances (Petrovic, 1974, 1983, 1984b; Linge, 1977; Petrovic and Stutzmann, 1981).

CHAPTER 2

RESEARCH FINDINGS IN CRANIOFACIAL GROWTH AND THE MODUS OPERANDI OF FUNCTIONAL APPLIANCES

There is no universal agreement concerning the mechanisms of craniofacial skeletal growth. Nevertheless, the various theoretical explanations can be tentatively categorized.

Genetic control theory

The genetic control theory stipulates that the genotype supplies all the information required for the phenotypic expression (i.e., that craniofacial growth is genetically predetermined). However, although the basic role of genes is widely acknowledged, the problem is to know whether and how some general, regional, and local factors actually *modulate* the gene expression.

Cartilage-directed growth theory

According to Scott (1953, 1954, 1967), cartilages are the primary factor in craniofacial growth control (i.e., the synchondrosis, nasal septum, mandibular condyle, etc. are the actual growth centers). Sutural growth should be considered as only compensatory.

Functional matrix theory

According to the functional matrix theory (M.L. Moss, 1960, 1962) regional and local factors do play a role in craniofacial morphogenesis. The growth of cartilage and bone appears to be a compensatory response to functional matrix growth (the functional matrix includes muscles, nerves, glands, teeth). In fact, there are two types of functional matrix (Moss and Salentijn, 1969): periosteal (including, for instance, muscles) and capsular (including, for instance, neurocranial fossa as well as nasal, orbital, oral, and pharyngeal cavities). The growth of the functional matrix is *primary,* that of a skeletal unit *secondary* (i.e., craniofacial growth represents, at a given instant, the outcome of functional demands). The functional matrix working hypothesis has initiated many experimental and clinical investigations but also has given rise to fruitful controversy (Johnston, 1976).

Servosystem theory

A further step in understanding the mechanisms of craniofacial growth was made when Charlier and Pe-

trovic (1967) and Stutzmann and Petrovic (1970) detected in organ culture, in both transplantation and in situ investigations, the following basic dissimilarities relative to different growth cartilages:

When the growth results from cell division of differentiated chondroblasts (epiphyseal cartilages of the long bones and cartilages of the synchondroses of the cranial base and of the nasal septum, all stemming from the *primary* cartilaginous skeleton of the organism), it appears to be subject to *general* extrinsic factors and more specifically to somatotrophic hormone–somatomedin, sexual hormones, thyroxine, etc. In this case the effect of local biomechanical factors is reduced to modulation of the *direction* of growth (with no effect whatsoever on the *amount* of growth).

When growth results from cell divisions of *pre*chondroblasts (condylar, coronoid, and angular cartilages of the mandible, the midpalatal suture cartilage, and all the secondary formation during phylogenesis and ontogenesis), it is subject, to some extent, to local extrinsic factors. In this case the growth *amount* can be modulated (increased or decreased) by the appropriate orthopedic devices.

Further research based on factorial quantitative analysis has led to a servosystem theory of the processes controlling postnatal craniofacial growth (Petrovic and Stutzmann, 1980b). According to this concept, the influence of the STH-somatomedin complex on the *growth of the primary cartilages* (epiphyseal cartilages of the long bones, cartilages of the nasal septum and sphenoccipital synchondrosis, lateral cartilaginous masses of the ethmoid, cartilage between the body and greater wings of the sphenoid, etc.) has the cybernetic form of a "command" (i.e., does not include any so far detected local feedback loops). Quite the contrary, the influence of the STH-somatomedin complex on the *growth of the secondary cartilages* (condylar, coronoid, and angular cartilages of the mandible, cartilages of the midpalatal suture, some other craniofacial sutures, and the provisional callus during bone fracture repair, and to some extent [but to some extent only] rib growth cartilages) comprises not only a *direct* but also some *indirect* effects on cell multiplication. With condylar, coronoid, and angular cartilages the indirect effects correspond to *regional* and *local* factors involving primarily neuro-muscular mechanisms relative to postural occlusal adjustment (Fig. 1-4).

Defects in mandibular growth resulting from condylectomy and resection of the pterygoid and masseter muscles were extensively investigated. A summary of this controversial question may be found in Petrovic et al. (1982b).

The sagittal growth rates of the maxilla and mandible are represented as a function of the STH-somatomedin and testosterone levels. For each level of activity of the lateral pterygoid muscle, the slope of the straight line for condylar cartilage growth and mandible lengthening is greater than that for maxillary growth (except after resection of the lateral pterygoid). In the case of the

usual contractile activity of the lateral pterygoid muscle, and for the *normal* STH-somatomedin level, the straight lines for maxillary and condylar cartilage growth cross at M. When the testosterone level varies from T_2 to T_3, the growth rate of the condylar cartilage will vary from C_2 to C_3, partly as a result of the regulatory functioning of the servosystem. When the STH-somatomedin or testosterone level is higher than T_3, the prognathism will not be corrected any more because the activity of the lateral pterygoid muscle is already at its minimum. On the contrary, when the STH-somatomedin or testosterone level is lower than T_2, the retrognathism will not be corrected any more because the activity of the lateral pterygoid cannot exceed its maximum (Fig. 2-1).

In the case of the condylar cartilage, several components in the servosystem are essential: the so-called pe-

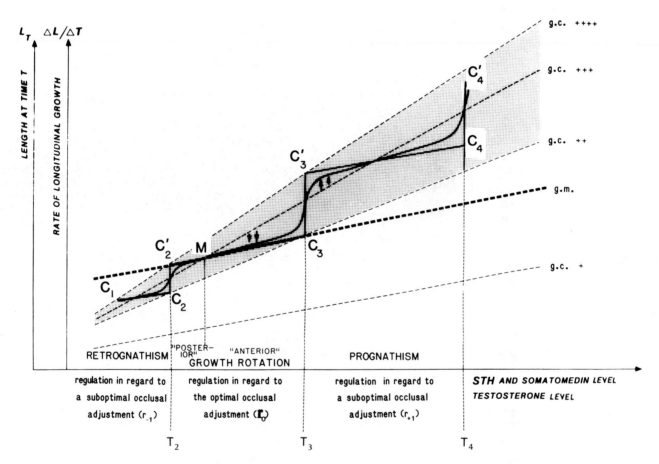

Fig. 2-1. Semihypothetical diagram of the multiplicative interaction between growth hormone and somatomedin or testosterone secretion rates and lateral pterygoid muscle activity on the condylar cartilage growth rate. A comparison with the action of the same hormones on septal cartilage and maxillary growth rates (bidimensional presentation of a phenomenon with three variables). *g.m.,* Lengthening of the maxilla (correlates directly with lengthening of the septal cartilage); *g.c.* +, growth of the condylar cartilage when the lateral pterygoid muscle is removed; *g.c.* ++, growth of the condylar cartilage for minimal contractile activity of the lateral pterygoid muscle; *g.c.* +++, growth of the condylar cartilage for mean contractile activity of the lateral pterygoid; *g.c.* ++++, growth of the condylar cartilage for maximal contractile activity of the lateral pterygoid; ⌐ , position of cuspal opposition; ⌒ , actual growth of the condylar cartilage.

ripheral comparator represented by the operation of confrontation between the respective positions of the upper and lower dental arches and the output (i.e., the rate and the direction of condylar cartilage growth). The upper dental arch is the constantly changing reference input, and the lower arch the controlled variable. The gain of the servosystem corresponds roughly to the coupling between the lateral pterygoid activity and the iterative activity of the temporomeniscocondylar frenum (better known as the retrodiscal pad), on one side, and the rate and orientation of the cell multiplication in the condylar cartilage, on the other side.

BIOLOGIC FEATURES OF PRIMARY AND SECONDARY-TYPE CARTILAGES

In primary cartilages (epiphyseal, sphenoccipital synchondrosis, nasal septal, etc.) the chondroblasts divide and synthesize intercellular matrix (Figs. 1-1 and 1-2). In secondary-type cartilages (condylar, coronoid, angular, and those in some craniofacial sutures), the cells that divide (i.e., the prechondroblasts) are not yet surrounded by cartilaginous matrix (Figs. 1-1 and 1-2). When the secondary-type prechondroblast begins synthesizing the specific cartilaginous matrix, it usually stops dividing. Emphasis is placed on the following point: in primary cartilages the cartilaginous matrix seems to isolate the dividing chondroblasts from local factors able to restrain or stimulate the cartilage growth rate whereas in secondary-type cartilages the dividing cells are not surrounded by the cartilaginous matrix and are *not* isolated from the influence of local factors. In other words, local extrinsic factors *may* modulate (stimulate or restrain) the growth rate of secondary-type cartilage. The experiments carried out in this laboratory since 1968 have demonstrated that some masticatory muscles and appropriate orthopedic appliances can modify the rate and amount of condylar cartilage growth. Experiments performed on the young rat were later confirmed by Stöckli and Willert (1971), McNamara

et al. (1975), L. Graber (1975), Demner and Nassibulin (1977), Komposch and Hockenjos (1977), and Komposch (1978) on the monkey. Accordingly, because of its particular biologic features, the secondary-type prechondroblast presents similarities to the preosteoblast. Indeed, both the prechondroblast Type II and the preosteoblast are able to divide. Neither the prechondroblast Type II nor the preosteoblast is surrounded by specific intercellular matrix (cartilage or bone). When either starts to synthesize the specific intercellular matrix, both cell varieties stop dividing and become respectively chondroblast Type II or osteoblast. The multiplication rate of both the prechondroblast Type II and the preosteoblast can be modulated (either increased or decreased) by intrinsic as well as local extrinsic factors.

Nature of cells belonging to the mitotic compartment of secondary-type cartilage

According to experiments carried out by Stutzmann and Petrovic (1976, 1982) in vivo, in cell culture, and in transplantation, the mitotic compartment of secondary-type cartilage contains two cell varieties. The first is the *skeletoblast,* a fibroblast-like pluripotential stem cell, originating from the embryonic mesenchymal cell. In cell culture, migrating skeletoblasts form a loose arrangement. Their intermitotic interval is relatively long (Fig. 2-2). The maximum number of cell divisions may reach 60. Spontaneously, the skeletoblast usually differentiates into a preosteoblast, but under specific conditions it may differentiate into a secondary-type prechondroblast as well as into an osteoclast (by fusion). The second is the *prechondroblast,* a round cell originating from the skeletoblast. In cell culture, migrating prechondroblasts form a compact arrangement. Their intermitotic interval is relatively short (Fig. 2-2). The pre-

		cell cycle time (Tc)	observed maximal number of cell generations (nG)
flattened stem cell	SKELETOBLAST	5 to 10 days	>30
globular cell	PREOSTEOBLAST or PRECHONDROBLAST TYPE II	1 to 2 days	< 10

Fig. 2-2. The mitotic compartment of secondary-type cartilage contains two cell varieties: There is a fibroblast-like pluripotential *stem* cell, the skeletoblast. In cell culture the cell cycle time *(Tc)* of this type is relatively long (5 to 10 days). The maximum number of cell generations *(nG)* seen is over 30. There is also a *globular* cell, the preosteoblast or prechondroblast Type II. In cell culture the cell cycle time of this type is relatively short (1 to 2 days) and the maximum number of cell generations is less than 10.

chondroblast is a differentiated cell; it matures into only a secondary-type chondroblast. The maximum number of cell divisions is less than 10. Prechondroblast multiplication is controlled by general and local extrinsic or intrinsic factors. The cytoplasmic Ca^{++} concentration is lower, and the Na^+ higher, in prechondroblasts (and preosteoblasts) than in skeletoblasts.

The previous investigations have shown that there is a continuing need for the prechondroblast to perceive its environment, to monitor the requirements of mass tissue in relation to those of whole condylar cartilage. When some part of the chondroblast mass is lost by resection or by hypertrophy and death, an increased multiplication of prechondroblasts occurs. Clearly, in such a case, there are signals that respond to sensing of the volume of the chondroblastic zone. Short-range interactions were detected biologically, but no regulator action could be identified (Stutzmann and Petrovic, 1982.)

Condylar cartilage before and after resection of the lateral pterygoid muscle

In the normal condylar cartilage of growing individuals, skeletoblasts multiply and some differentiate into prechondroblasts. The resection of the lateral pterygoid muscle brings about a significant slowing down of the condylar cartilage growth rate (Stutzmann and Petrovic, 1974ab). The skeletoblasts no longer differentiate into prechondroblasts. Consequently the percentage of skeletoblasts increases, to the detriment of prechondroblasts. When the maximum number of the prechondroblast cell divisions is about 8 to 10, the stock of prechondroblasts progressively decreases. When the stock is completely exhausted, and only from this moment on, skeletoblasts start differentiating into preosteoblasts and then osteoblasts. The condyle then increases further in size through periosteal-type growth. It is as if the prechondroblasts had an inhibiting effect on the differentiation of skeletoblasts into preosteoblasts (Stutzmann and Petrovic, 1982) (Fig. 2-3).

Since these findings have elicited controversy and some misunderstanding, it is appropriate to try to interpret why. One major factor would be the interruption of the circulatory (i.e., nutritional) dependence on the blood supply originating directly from the lateral pterygoid muscle and indirectly through the retrodiscal pad.

Condylar cartilage after homoplastic transplantation into the rat testis or anterior chamber of the eye

After intratesticular or intraocular transplantation the condyle undergoes histologic modifications similar to those observed after resection of the lateral pterygoid muscle (Fig. 2-3). Three weeks after transplantation the mitotic compartment contains mostly skeletoblasts. A few prechondroblasts continue to divide before becoming chondroblasts. Here and there, skeletoblasts start differentiating into osteoblasts. Five weeks after transplantation the mitotic compartment consists of only skeletoblasts, which later differentiate exclusively into preosteoblasts and osteoblasts.

Development of the rat midpalatal suture

The double differentiating potentiality of the skeletoblast also has been evidenced clearly in the rat midpalatal suture. The intermaxillary portion of the fast-growing midpalatal suture includes a secondary-type cartilage. During this period the skeletoblast differentiates exclusively into a prechondroblast; but from the age of 37 to 40 days, when the growth rate slows, the skeletoblast begins to differentiate into a preosteoblast. Accordingly, the cartilaginous suture becomes a bony-type suture, like the other craniofacial sutures. When growth at the midpalatal suture is restrained experimentally before the age of 37 to 40 days by either local mechanical constraint or resection of the primary cartilages between the body and greater wings of the sphenoid and the lateral cartilaginous masses of the ethmoid, skeletoblasts (instead of differentiating into prechondroblasts) differentiate into preosteoblasts (Stutzmann and Petrovic, 1976, 1982).

Homology between the preosteoblastic layer of the mandibular periosteum and the prechondroblastic layer of the condylar cartilage

At the boundary between the condylar cartilage and the condylar periosteum, skeletoblasts stop differentiating into *prechondroblasts* belonging to the mitotic compartment of the condylar cartilage and begin to differentiate into preosteoblasts belonging to the subperiosteal layer of the condyle. What happens in the growing rat after resection of the condylar cartilage, superior head of the lateral pterygoid muscle, disc, and retrodiscal pad with the condylar bone remaining intact? Initially skeletoblasts originating from the subperiosteal layer multiply, migrate, and finally completely cover the resected surface. Then, if no inflammation has occurred and if mandibular mobility is maintained, the newly formed skeletoblasts differentiate locally into secondary cartilage. To some extent this newly formed condylar cartilage corresponds exactly to the cartilage observed temporarily during fracture repair.

Growth hormone and its mediators—mode of action on different varieties of cartilage

Investigations carried out in the Strasbourg laboratory since 1967 have demonstrated the following:
1. The growth of epiphyseal cartilages of the long bones, cartilage of the sphenoccipital synchondroses, lateral cartilaginous masses of the ethmoid, and cartilage between the body and greater wings

of the sphenoid (all stemming from the primary cartilaginous skeleton of the organism) is subject to *general* extrinsic factors and more specifically to growth hormone (STH) and somatomedin. In this case orthopedic devices can modulate the *direction* but not the *amount* of growth (Charlier and Petrovic, 1967; Petrovic et al., 1975b).

2. The growth of condylar, coronoid, and angular cartilages of the mandible, cartilage in some cranial sutures, and cartilage in the postfracture callus (all of secondary formation during phylogenesis and ontogenesis) is subject to *local* extrinsic factors as

well as to growth hormone and somatomedin. In this case appropriate orthopedic devices may modulate both the direction and the amount of growth.

Intrinsic regulation of the condylar cartilage growth rate

Experimental results have shown the existence of an *intrinsic* regulatory mechanism of the condylar cartilage growth rate. The variations of cell density as such cannot account, at least not completely, for this finding. In other words, there is a "negative feedback signal" originating from the proximal part of the chondroblastic

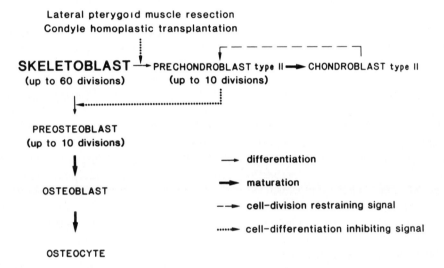

Fig. 2-3. Double differentiating potential of skeletoblasts. According to local and biologic conditions these cells may differentiate into a prechondroblast Type II or a preosteoblast.

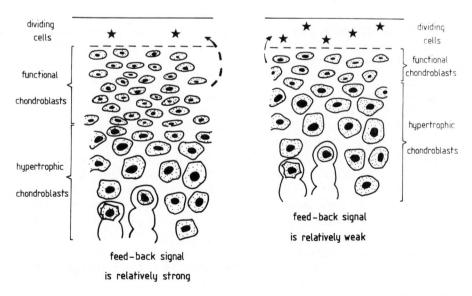

Fig. 2-4. Intrinsic regulation of the condylar cartilage growth rate: variations in the rate of chondroblastic hypertrophy and subsequent variations of the prechondroblastic multiplication restraining signal (the "feedback" signal).

zone and exerting a restraining effect on the prechondroblastic multiplication rate (Fig. 2-4). The concept of an intrinsic regulation of the condylar cartilage growth rate can help explain the effects of some orthopedic or orthodontic appliances as well as of a hormone such as thyroxine: the earlier commencement of chondroblastic hypertrophy and the subsequent decrease in the prechondroblast division–restraining signal appear to be an important intermediary step in the growth-stimulating effect of the mandibular postural hyperpropulsor and similar appliances, as well as of Class II elastics. The acceleration of the chondroblastic maturation rate is, in a similar way, an intermediary step for the growth rate–stimulating effect of thyroxine (Stutzmann and Petrovic, 1975b, 1979).

Osteochondral rib transplant

Is the osteochondral rib transplant an appropriate biologic substitute for condylar cartilage in the surgical treatment of temporomandibular ankylosis? The human rib cartilage is composed, in the portion close to the sternum, of cells designated precursor chondroblasts (Petrovic, 1984a) (Fig. 2-5, A). In the postnatal period these cells become quiescent; mitoses are infrequent. Nevertheless, in cell culture, each precursor chondroblast may divide 35 to 50 times. During the growth period, a few millimeters ahead of the osteochondral junction area, the precursor chondroblast will differentiate into a cell termed by Petrovic progenitor chondroblast (Fig. 2-5, B). Once fully differentiated each progenitor chondroblast divides no more than 8 to 11 times, but cell division occurs at short intervals. The chondroblasts issuing from a progenitor chondroblast constitute a pyramid-like structure, being a component of what is actually the primary-type growth cartilage of the rib (Fig. 2-5, B to D). The cartilage matrix surrounding the cells issuing from the progenitor chondroblast is biochemically different from the matrix surrounding the precursor chondroblasts.

Using rib cartilage fragments removed during surgery in growing children (2 to 14 years old), Petrovic and Stutzmann recently made several organ culture experiments, with provocative observations. When an osteochondral junction fragment was exposed to light pressure, the cells belonging to the area where precursor chondroblasts differentiate into progenitor chondroblasts, and only in this area, displayed the following variations (in comparison to identical rib fragments cultivated as controls):

1. Intracellular concentration of Na^+ tended to decrease.
2. Intracellular concentrations of Ca^{++} and H^+ tended to increase.

3. Intracellular pH was lowered.
4. Na^+, K^+–ATPase activity was intensified.
5. Ca^{++}, Mg^{++}–ATPase and H^+–ATPase activities were diminished.
6. The numbers of cell divisions declined slightly but significantly demonstrated a slowing down of the growth rate.

When the juvenile human (or rat) condylar cartilage was exposed, in organ culture, to an identical pressure, similar although much more pronounced variations were observed. However, such variations were never detected in growth cartilages of metatarsals, tibia, fibula, radius, and cubitus (Petrovic, 1982, 1984a). In other words, the differentiation rate of the precursor chondroblast into a progenitor chondroblast is submitted not only to the *command* represented by genetic, hormonal, and humoral factors but also to a local *regulation* that includes regional biomechanical factors. This finding implies that an autologous osteochondral rib transplant is to be preferred to a metatarsal cartilage transplant in the treatment of temporomandibular ankylosis and in similar situations (i.e., when one needs a substitute for the condylar cartilage). This finding also implies that the rib transplant must include a sufficient portion of precursor chondroblasts, which are able to divide 35 to 50 times and whose growth rate is modulable by local biomechanical factors at the time the cell reaches the transient stage of differentiation into the progenitor chondroblast.

CONTROL OF MAXILLARY GROWTH

It is known that the increase in *length* of the maxilla in mammals is due to the growth at the premaxillomaxillary and maxillopalatine sutures, as well as to subperiosteal deposition of bone in the anterior region. The premaxillomaxillary suture persists much longer in the young rat and the monkey than in the human. This means that its participation in the forward growth of the upper jaw ceases much later in the rat or the monkey than in the human child. In all cases the stem cell skeletoblast differentiates into a "preosteoblast" and the preosteoblast multiplies and becomes an osteoblast, which after surrounding itself with bone matrix becomes an osteocyte. The increase in *width* of the maxilla is attributed to the growth at the midpalatal suture and to bone deposition along the lateral areas of the alveolar ridge. In the young rapidly growing rat the midpalatal suture is unusual in that it is composed of a secondary type of cartilage on each side of the median line. In this case the skeletoblast differentiates into a prechondroblast, and it is the prechondroblast that divides and matures into a secondary type of chondroblast; the cartilage formed is later replaced by bone.

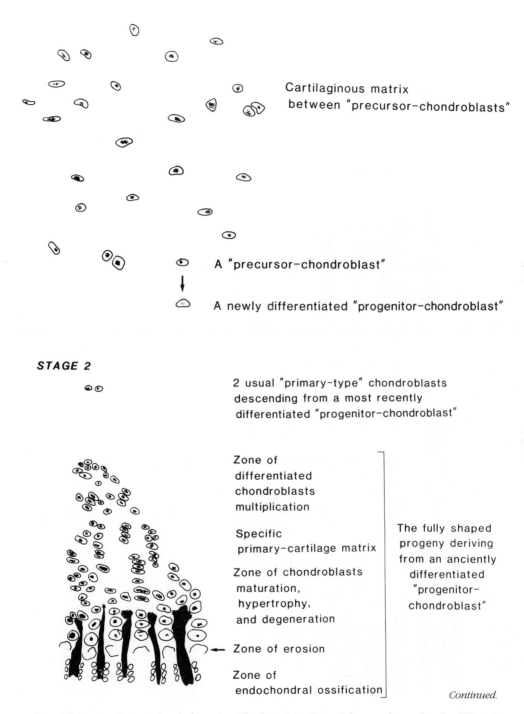

STAGE 1

Cartilaginous matrix
between "precursor-chondroblasts"

A "precursor-chondroblast"

A newly differentiated "progenitor-chondroblast"

STAGE 2

2 usual "primary-type" chondroblasts
descending from a most recently
differentiated "progenitor-chondroblast"

Zone of
differentiated
chondroblasts
multiplication

Specific
primary-cartilage matrix

Zone of chondroblasts
maturation,
hypertrophy,
and degeneration

← Zone of erosion

Zone of
endochondral ossification

The fully shaped
progeny deriving
from an anciently
differentiated
"progenitor-
chondroblast"

Continued.

Fig. 2-5. Human rib osteochondral junction. The four stages *(1 to 4)* that are observed in the differentiation of precursor chondroblast into progenitor chondroblast and its progeny.

STAGE 3

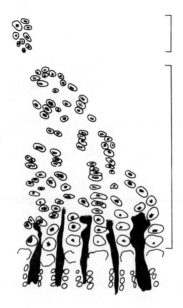

A new-formed progeny originating
from a recently differentiated
"progenitor-chondroblast"

The completed progeny of
an anciently differentiated
"progenitor-chondroblast"

STAGE 4

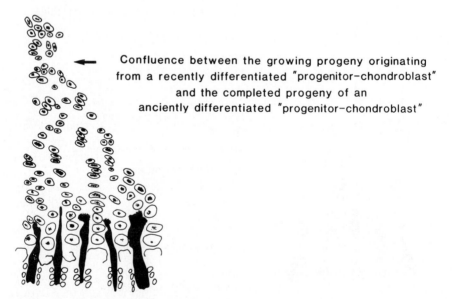

Confluence between the growing progeny originating
from a recently differentiated "progenitor-chondroblast"
and the completed progeny of an
anciently differentiated "progenitor-chondroblast"

Fig. 2-5, cont'd. For legend see p. 25.

The mechanisms controlling the growth of the upper jaw are presently under investigation. Divergence of opinion exists on several points:

1. According to Weinmann and Sicher (1955) and Prahl (1968), sutural tissue has an autonomous growth potential; but according to Scott (1956), M.L. Moss (1962), Petrovic et al. (1969), and Persson (1973), sutural growth is subject to extrinsic factors.

2. According to Scott (1953), Baume (1961), Wexler and Sarnat (1961), Petrovic et al. (1969), Ronning (1971), and Kvinnsland (1974), the growth of the nasal septal cartilage constitutes an important factor in the control mechanisms of vertical and horizontal facial growth, including that of the maxilla. This opinion is not shared by Moss (Moss et al., 1968; Moss, 1976) and Melsen et al. (1981).

3. According to Scott (1967), the cartilage of the midpalatal suture is capable of separating adjacent bones. However, according to Stutzmann and Petrovic (1970), it is the separation of the horizontal processes of the two maxillae that stimulates the growth of this suture.

• • •

As is represented by the functional diagram (Fig. 1-3), growth hormone (STH) and somatomedin as well as testosterone and estrogen are seen to play a primary role in the extrinsic control of postnatal growth of the upper jaw. Their effect is twofold, direct and indirect (Stutzmann and Petrovic, 1976, 1978a).

Direct effect

The direct effect represents almost the entire influence of STH-somatomedin on growth of the sphenoccipital synchondrosis and nasal septal cartilage, the lateral masses of the ethmoid bone, and between the body and greater wings of the sphenoid. Only a minor part of the effect of STH-somatomedin on growth of the cranial and facial sutures is of a direct nature; in these areas STH-somatomedin has a direct effect primarily on the *responsiveness* of the preosteoblasts to regional and local factors, stimulating the skeletal cell multiplication rate. Where there is secondary cartilage, the direct effect of STH-somatomedin is seen also on both the multiplication and the responsiveness of prechondroblasts.

Indirect effect

The indirect effect of STH-somatomedin occurs through a number of intermediaries.

Forward growth of the septal cartilage. The forward growth of the septal cartilage in the rat produces a forward shift of the premaxillary bone that gives rise to an increase in the growth of the premaxillomaxillary suture and, to a lesser extent, the maxillopalatal suture.

It also results in a forward traction by means of the septopremaxillary ligament and the labionarinary muscles on the anterior end of the premaxilla, which results in local stimulation of bone growth.

Thrust effect. The anterior extremity of the nasal septal cartilage spreads laterally on both sides of the median line in an anteroinferior direction to penetrate directly into the premaxillary bone. Such a configuration supports the hypothesis that forward growth of the nasal septal cartilage produces a sufficient thrust on the premaxillary bone to stimulate the growth of the premaxillomaxillary suture and, to a lesser extent, that of the maxillopalatal suture. The thrust effect on the premaxillary bone consists of a histologic *traction component* represented by collagen fibers connecting the cartilage and the bone trabeculae located immediately posterior.

Septopremaxillary ligament traction effect. The study of human fetuses led Latham (1970) to formulate the hypothesis that forward growth of the nasal septal cartilage has a traction effect on the premaxillary bone via the septopremaxillary ligament. According to studies of the septopremaxillary ligament in the young rat (Stutzmann and Petrovic, 1976, 1978a), the number of dividing preosteoblasts and the osteoblastic activity are significantly greater where this ligament contacts the premaxillary bone. In any case, the histologic characteristics of the septopremaxillary ligament imply that this so-called ligament is hardly able to provide necessary traction on the premaxillary bone to give rise to an increased growth at the premaxillomaxillary suture. In other words, histologically it is *misnamed* a ligament.

Findings after resection of the septopremaxillary ligament in the young rat (Stutzmann and Petrovic, 1976, 1978a) clearly show that a stimulating action on the growth at the premaxillomaxillary suture must be excluded. However, the ligament does have a local, induction-like, stimulating effect on subperiosteal growth.

Labionarinary muscle traction effect. The forward growth of the septal cartilage brings about a forward traction on the premaxillary bone via the labionarinary muscles, resulting in a biomechanical promotion of the forward growth of the upper jaw. In humans the absence of labial muscle attachment on the nasal septum in cleft lip could be responsible for bone malformations. The surgical reattachment of the orbicularis oris and alar muscles is an essential part of the repair of cleft lip and palate (Delaire, 1961, 1978; Delaire and Chateau, 1977).

Unilateral resection of the labionarinary muscles in the young rat produces a unilaterally decreased forward growth on the operated side. On the opposite side the outward growth of the premaxilla is slightly increased.

Experimental investigations in young rats on the mechanisms of action of the Fränkel (1973) appliance (Table 2-1) have shown that the superior labial frenum and the labionarinary muscles are the mediators of the

Table 2-1. Effects of FRVS (Fränkel superior retrolabial vestibular shields) on sagittal growth of the rat upper jaw

(A) DIVIDING CELL INDEX, ANTERIOR EXTREMITY OF PREMAXILLARY BONE

	N	*Mean (%)*	*Standard error*
No appliance			
No operation	12	17.04	
Resection of labial frenum	12	15.37	1.3976
Resection of both labial frenum and labionarinary muscles	12	13.68	
Appliance			
No operation	12	29.65	
Resection of labial frenum	12	22.40	1.3976
Resection of both labial frenum and labionarinary muscles	12	14.40	

Analysis of variance

Source of variations	*Sum of squares*	*Degrees of freedom*	*Mean square*	*F ratio**
Resection effect	1038.47	2	519.33	22.15
Shield effect	830.28	1	830.28	35.42
Interaction	424.20	2	212.10	9.05
ERROR	1547.30	66	23.44	
TOTAL VARIATION	3840.25	71		

Smallest significant difference between two means (%)
  5% level: 2.79
  1% level: 3.71
  0.1% level: 4.81

(B) CALCULATED LENGTH OF PREMAXILLOMAXILLARY SUTURE

	N	*Mean (mm)*	*Standard error*
No appliance			
No operation	12	1.30	
Resection of labial frenum	12	1.28	0.0487
Resection of both labial frenum and labionarinary muscles	12	0.90	
Appliance			
No operation	12	1.80	
Resection of labial frenum	12	1.74	0.0487
Resection of both labial frenum and labionarinary muscles	12	0.95	

Analysis of variance

Source of variations	*Sum of squares*	*Degrees of freedom*	*Mean square*	*F ratio*
Resection effect	5.9529	2	2.9764	104.66
Shield effect	2.0503	1	2.0503	72.10
Interaction	0.7608	2	0.3804	13.37
ERROR	1.8769	66	0.02843	
TOTAL VARIATION	10.6409	71		

Smallest significant difference between two means (mm)
  5% level: 0.10
  1% level: 0.13
  0.1% level: 0.17

*The variance ratio. F distribution was discovered by the statistician R.A. Fisher (1924) and named F by L.W. Snedecor. It is a theoretical probability distribution, like the t-distribution in the so-called student test. It is used in the analysis of variance. With it one is evaluating the "null hypothesis" of no difference between two population *variances.*

Table 2-1. Effects of FRVS (Fränkel superior retrolabial vestibular shields) on sagittal growth of the rat upper jaw—cont'd

(C) CALCULATED LENGTH OF MAXILLOPALATAL SUTURE

	N	Mean (mm)	Standard error
No appliance			
No operation	12	0.60	
Resection of labial frenum	12	0.60	0.011
Resection of both labial frenum and labionarinary muscles	12	0.32	
Appliance			
No operation	12	0.79	
Resection of labial frenum	12	0.76	0.011
Resection of both labial frenum and labionarinary muscles	12	0.35	

Analysis of variance

Source of variations	Sum of squares	Degrees of freedom	Mean square	F ratio
Resection effect	1.9996	2	0.9998	649.65
Shield effect	0.2977	1	0.2977	193.45
Interaction	0.0714	2	0.0391	25.38
ERROR	0.1016	66	0.0015	
TOTAL VARIATION	2.4771	71		

Smallest significant difference between two means (mm)
5% level: 0.02
1% level: 0.03
0.1% level: 0.04

(D) LENGTH OF UPPER JAW

	N	Mean (mm)	Standard error
No appliance			
No operation	12	16.66	
Resection of labial frenum	12	16.27	0.0996
Resection of both labial frenum and labionarinary muscles	12	14.74	
Appliance			
No operation	12	18.14	
Resection of labial frenum	12	17.49	0.0996
Resection of both labial frenum and labionarinary muscles	12	14.90	

Analysis of variance

Source of variations	Sum of squares	Degrees of freedom	Mean square	F ratio
Resection effect	89.1268	2	44.5633	373.99
Shield effect	16.3401	1	16.3401	137.99
Interaction	5.9335	2	2.9667	24.89
ERROR	7.8643	66	0.1192	
TOTAL VARIATION	119.2647	71		

Smallest significant difference between two means (mm)
5% level: 0.19
1% level: 0.26
0.1% level: 0.34

so-called superior retrolabial "lip pads" (FRVS) in their stimulating effect on sagittal growth of the maxilla.

Outward growth—effects of the Fränkel lateral vestibular shields on widening of the upper jaw. The outward growth of the lateral cartilaginous masses of the ethmoid and the cartilage between the body and greater wings of the sphenoid brings about a "lateralization" of the alveolar ridges on both the left and the right side and, in turn, stimulates the growth of the midpalatal suture (i.e., the outward growth of the maxilla) (Fig. 1-3).

Experimental findings reported recently by Stutzmann et al. (1983) demonstrate that the lateral vestibular shields (FLVS) bring about an enhanced and supplementary widening of the upper jaw (Table 2-2). The appliance acts essentially by stimulating midpalatal suture growth and, to a lesser extent, increasing bone apposition on the external subperiosteal layer of the maxilla. Another effect of the buccal shields stressed by Fränkel is the influence on the eruptive path of the succedaneous teeth at the critical time in their development. The relief of pressure from the cheeks in the dentoalveolar area seems to allow a more downward and outward eruptive path at a time of maximum viability, permitting horizontal and vertical adjustment of the osseous tissues involved.

It should be mentioned that the stimulating effect on sutural growth is observed even when the cartilaginous-type midpalatal suture has become a bony-type suture (i.e., when it is in a phase of less rapid growth) (Table 2-3). The results are similar in nature but not in extent. Indeed, the effect is proportionally more intense during the period from day 20 to day 48 of rat age, a prepubertal period, when the suture growth is naturally more rapid, than during the period from day 40 to 180, when sutural growth progressively slows down. Extrapolating to the human, this observation would coincide with the transitional period before puberty, when Fränkel feels there is the greatest potential for width increase. In other words, the greatest change is to be seen during the period encompassing the tooth exchange time.

At the end of the experimental period (180 days) when all growth is finished, the width of the upper jaw remains greater in the animals treated with the lateral vestibular shields than in the nontreated ones. The supplementary widening of the upper jaw persists and seems stable when growth is completed.

The results clearly demonstrate that the three investigated factors are differentially involved in the *spontaneous* lateral growth of the upper jaw.

The lateral vestibular sulcus seems to play only a minor role; after bilateral sectioning, lateral growth is only slightly affected. This same observation has been made in the study of *Saimiri scireus* monkeys by Graber

(1983c), in which the vestibular shields initially enhanced proliferation in the sulcus after appliance placement (an adaptation?) but disappeared quickly with less activity subperiosteally than in the alveolar process covering the buccal surfaces of the posterior monkey teeth. Significantly greater proliferation did occur in the experimental animals in this area than in the controls and remained stable as shown in the rat study.

Although indications are that the sulcus area is not a major growth area, regardless of whether there is resection of sulcular tissue little question exists that the cheeks and tongue do influence jaw growth. Under normal conditions, as far as the teeth and investing tissues are concerned, a dynamic balance exists between the restraining buccinator mechanism on the outside (the cheeks) and the tongue on the inside that exerts a positive outward pressure both during rest and during active function. It is quite clear from this research project that any "perturbation" of this balance, produced by either resection of the cheek muscles or a reduced tongue mass, will modify the lateral growth of the upper jaw. Thus the resection of the cheeks favors, first, bone deposition on the external subperiosteal layer of the maxilla and, second, the outward thrust effect of the functioning tongue on the contiguous buccal segments that results in a significant supplemental upper jaw widening. A narrowed or reduced tongue, produced by surgical stenoglossia, no longer exerts a sufficient outward thrust on the adjacent molar segments to maintain the usual growth of the midpalatal suture. The wearing of lingual shields also reduces the outward thrust effect of the tongue, and this may well affect the eruption of the succedaneous teeth since the tendency is to erupt in a more vertical inclination and lingual direction when tongue pressure is reduced or absent.

Nevertheless, the effect produced by surgical narrowing of the tongue on the widening of the upper jaw is less pronounced than that elicited by the wearing of lateral *lingual* shields. Indeed, when the volume of the tongue was experimentally reduced in the growing rat (i.e., when we changed either the longitudinal dimension [partial glossectomy] [Stutzmann and Petrovic, 1976] or the transverse dimension [experimental stenoglossia]), we observed that with time the tongue presented the tendency to recover if not its normal volume at least its usual position. We therefore repeated the partial glossectomy that had been done in previous experiments 2 weeks after the initial operation. For technical reasons the experimental stenoglossia was not redone. So, after several weeks, the increased transverse dimension of the tongue was great enough to exert again an outward thrust on the two molar groups and to stimulate the midpalatal suture growth. This happened even when this suture had become a bony type. Conse-

Table 2-2. Effects of FLVS (Fränkel lateral vestibular shields) and lingual shields from day 20 to 48 on widening of the rat upper jaw (12 male animals in each group)

(A) INDEX OF EXTERNAL MAXILLARY PERIOSTEUM (^{3}H-METHYL-THYMIDINE–LABELED PREOSTEOBLASTS)

		Mean (mm)	Standard error
No operation and no lateral lingual shields	No FLVS	6.20	
	FLVS	11.84	
Section of vestibular sulcus	No FLVS	6.42	
	FLVS	6.82	
Experimental stenoglossia	No FLVS	5.86	
	FLVS	8.37	
			± 0.2602
Resection of buccinators and masseters (anterior portion)	No FLVS	8.40	
	FLVS	8.79	
Lateral lingual shields	No FLVS	4.95	
	FLVS	7.74	
Resection of buccinators and masseters plus lateral lingual shields	No FLVS	5.83	
	FLVS	6.37	

Analysis of variance

Source of variation	Sum of squares	Degrees of freedom	Mean square	F
FLVS effect	150.5734	1	150.5734	185.24
Various experimental procedure effects	179.6325	5	35.9265	44.21
Interaction	128.4122	5	25.6824	
ERROR	107.2767	132	0.8127	
TOTAL	565.8948	143		

Smallest significant difference betwen two means (mm)
5% level: 0.51
2.5% level: 0.59
1% level: 0.68
0.1% level: 0.87

(B) DISTANCE BETWEEN TWO UV-VISIBLE TETRACYCLINE-LABELED SURFACES, ONE ON EACH SIDE OF MIDPALATAL SUTURE

		Mean (mm)	Standard error
No operation and no lateral lingual shields	No FLVS	1.28	
	FLVS	1.71	
Section of vestibular sulcus	No FLVS	1.34	
	FLVS	1.64	
Experimental stenoglossia	No FLVS	1.22	
	FLVS	1.44	
			± 0.039
Resection of buccinators and masseters (anterior portion)	No FLVS	1.63	
	FLVS	1.75	
Lateral lingual shields	No FLVS	1.02	
	FLVS	1.26	
Resection of buccinators and masseters plus lateral lingual shields	No FLVS	1.16	
	FLVS	1.16	

Analysis of variance

Source of variation	Sum of squares	Degrees of freedom	Mean square	F
FLVS effect	1.7667	1	1.7667	96.74
Various experimental procedure effects	5.4758	5	1.0952	59.97
Interaction	0.6559	5	0.1312	7.18
ERROR	2.4106	132	0.0183	
TOTAL	10.3090	143		

Smallest significant difference between two means (mm)
5% level: 0.08
2.5% level: 0.09
1% level: 0.10
0.1% level: 0.13

Continued.

Table 2-2. Effects of FLVS (Fränkel lateral vestibular shields) and lingual shields from day 20 to 48 on widening of the rat upper jaw (12 male animals in each group)—cont'd

(C) DISTANCE BETWEEN LINGUAL SURFACES OF TWO FIRST MOLARS

		Mean (mm)	Standard error
No operation and no lateral lingual shields	No FLVS	4.37	
	FLVS	5.20	
Section of vestibular sulcus	No FLVS	4.36	
	FLVS	4.72	
Experimental stenoglossia	No FLVS	4.14	
	FLVS	4.66	
			± 0.0721
Resection of buccinators and masseters (anterior portion)	No FLVS	4.60	
	FLVS	5.08	
Lateral lingual shields	No FLVS	3.76	
	FLVS	4.26	
Resection of buccinators and masseters plus lateral lingual shields	No FLVS	3.95	
	FLVS	4.08	

Analysis of variance

Source of variations	Sum of squares	Degrees of freedom	Mean square	F
FLVS effect	7.8493	1	7.8493	125.92
Various experimental procedure effects	15.7181	5	3.1436	50.43
Interaction	1.5540	5	0.3108	
ERROR	8.2282	132	0.0623	
TOTAL	33.3497	143		

Smallest significant difference between two means (mm)
5% level: 0.14
2.5% level: 0.16
1% level: 0.19
0.1% level: 0.24

quently, 4 weeks after the operation, there was no longer any difference in the midpalatal suture growth rates between the control group and the stenoglossia group. This finding implies that from a therapeutic point of view the surgical reduction of tongue volume is justified only in the presence of a genuine macroglossia.

The quantitative analysis revealed an amplification type of interaction between the morphologic factors investigated in this research and in the vestibular shield treatment. It should be emphasized again that a quantitative experimentation such as this is less important per se than as a statistical tool for searching out the existence of possible interactions between the different physiologic factors, as well as between these physiologic factors and a specific functional or fixed type of orthodontic appliance (Stutzmann et al., 1983).

These experiments demonstrated beyond any doubt that the effect of the lateral *vestibular* shields on the transverse growth of the maxilla is relayed, partly through passive resistance against the pressure of the buccinators and the anterior portion of the masseters and partly through the tension created in the vestibular sulcus. Clearly, when the pressure of the tongue on the two molar groups is the usual one (i.e., when no stenoglossia has been surgically created and no lingual shields are in place), the end result will be a significantly increased transverse growth of the maxilla.

The quantitative analysis showed that when one of the three factors investigated in this study (tongue, vestibular sulcus, cheek muscles) was modified (either suppressed or just moderated) the appliance-produced effect on the widening of the maxilla was of similar magnitude. However, depending on which factor was experimentally modified, the appliance-produced supplementary widening of the upper jaw resulted either from a supplementary growth of the midpalatal suture only or from both a supplementary growth of the midpalatal suture and a supplementary bone apposition on the lateral vestibular side of the maxilla.

Only when the two opposing factors (pressure of the tongue on one side, pressure of the buccinators and the anterior portion of the masseters on the other) were modified simultaneously did the appliance become ineffective. In this case the tension of the sulcus from the

Table 2-3. Effects of FLVS (Fränkel lateral vestibular shields) from day 40 to 180 on widening of the rat upper jaw (20 male animals in each group)

(A) DISTANCE BETWEEN TWO UV-VISIBLE TETRACYCLINE-LABELED SURFACES, ONE ON EACH SIDE OF MIDPALATAL SUTURE		Width of nonfluorescent bone surface (mm)	
At age 40 days	*From age 40 days to sacrifice (180 days)*	*Mean*	*Standard error*
No operation	No FLVS	1.26	
	FLVS	1.85	
Section of vestibular sulcus	No FLVS	1.20	
	FLVS	1.54	
			0.0392
Experimental stenoglossia	No FLVS	0.57	
	FLVS	0.98	
Section of vestibular sulcus and experimental stenoglossia	No FLVS	0.57	
	FLVS	0.67	

Analysis of variance

Source of variations	*Sum of squares*	*Degrees of freedom*	*Mean square*	*F*
(1) Sulcus effect	1.156	1	1.156	37.65
(2) Stenoglossia effect	23.409	1	23.409	762.51
(3) FLVS effect	5.184	1	5.184	168.86
Interactions				
(1) × (2)	0.009	1	0.009	0.29 NS*
(1) × (3)	0.784	1	0.784	25.53
(2) × (3)	0.441	1	0.441	14.36
(1) × (2) × (3)	0.009	1	0.009	0.29 NS*
ERROR	4.6640	152	0.0307	
TOTAL	35.6560	159		

Smallest significant difference between two means (mm)
    5% level: 0.08
    2.5% level: 0.09
    1% level: 0.10
    0.1% level: 0.13
*Not significant.

Continued.

wearing of vestibular shields was insufficient to stimulate the growth rate of the midpalatal suture and bring about a supplementary widening of the upper jaw.

Another point must be elucidated. In animals in which the buccinators and the anterior portion of the masseters were bilaterally resected, the wearing of the lateral vestibular shields did give rise to a supplementary widening of the upper jaw; yet the sutural contribution appears to have been meager and new bone apposition on the vestibular side of the maxilla hardly different from that observed in the reference animals. This apparent contradiction may be tentatively explained in the following two ways:

1. Since the ^{3}H-methyl-thymidine–labeled preosteoblast index is a "snapshot" only of what is occurring during the hour before sacrifice, we can assume that in this experimental variety the sum of the "snapshots" during the 4 weeks following the onset of the experiment was sufficient to account for the appliance-produced additional widening of the maxilla.

2. We can also assume that the tension effect of the sulcus was more operative immediately after the muscle resection than at the end of the experiment. Indeed, the postoperative edema probably made the sulcus less elastic, and thus its pulling effect would be increased during this transient period.

These two tentative explanations are not mutually exclusive.

Finally, needless to emphasize, this study was certainly *not* an exhaustive one with regard to factors involved in the pathogenicity and correction of the transverse dimension. For instance, previous investiga-

Table 2-3. Effects of FLVS (Fränkel lateral vestibular shields) from day 40 to 180 on widening of the rat upper jaw (20 male animals in each group)—cont'd

(B) DISTANCE BETWEEN LINGUAL SURFACES OF TWO FIRST MOLARS

At age 40 days	From age 40 days to sacrifice (180 days)	Width of maxilla (mm) Mean	Width of maxilla (mm) Standard error
No operation	No FLVS	5.61	
	FLVS	6.57	
Section of vestibular sulcus	No FLVS	5.55	
	FLVS	6.13	
			0.0600
Experimental stenoglossia	No FLVS	4.58	
	FLVS	5.13	
Section of vestibular sulcus and experimental stenoglossia	No FLVS	4.47	
	FLVS	4.78	

Analysis of variance

Source of variations	Sum of squares	Degrees of freedom	Mean square	F
(1) Sulcus effect	2.3353	1	2.3353	32.43
(2) Stenoglossia effect	59.9883	1	59.9883	833.17
(3) FLVS effect	14.3820	1	14.3820	199.75
Interactions				
(1) × (2)	0.0041	1	0.0041	0.06 NS*
(1) × (3)	0.9502	1	0.9502	13.20
(2) × (3)	1.2058	1	1.2058	16.74
(1) × (2) × (3)	0.0413	1	0.0413	0.57 NS*
ERROR	10.9379	152	0.0720	
TOTAL	89.8449	159		

Smallest significant difference between two means (mm)
 5% level: 0.23
 2.5% level: 0.26
 1% level: 0.30
 0.1% level: 0.39
*Not significant.

tions in the growing rat (Petrovic et al., 1969; Stutzmann and Petrovic, 1976) had shown that the number of dividing cells in the midpalatal suture is much higher in the oral region than in the nasal region but that this difference tends to decrease after removal of the nasal septal cartilage. After the cartilage is removed, the transverse growth of the upper jaw is slightly (but still significantly) reduced and even the appositional bone on the oral surface of the palate (as revealed by tetracycline labeling) is slowed. In other words, further investigations on the potential lateral expansion and the mechanical action of the Fränkel appliance should also take into account the role of the septal cartilage.

The reported findings throw new light on the mechanism of maxillary widening produced by the Fränkel appliance. They display the complexity of the appliance action at the tissue level. Above all, they are a conceptual tool for the clinician facing the problem of the narrow maxillary arch.

CONTROL OF MANDIBULAR GROWTH

Growth control involves a multitude of factors. These factors do not form independent causal chains. Rather, there is an interaction among them (Petrovic et al., 1975b) that is often highly important. For this reason, whenever possible, these factors were studied together rather than separately so their possible interactions might be detected.

Any research investigation on the control mechanisms of craniofacial growth should take into account not only *local* and *regional* extrinsic factors (as represented by tissue contacts, muscles, blood supply, nerve signals, etc.) but also *general* factors (growth hormone [STH] and somatomedin, thyroxine, and sex hormones). Moreover, according to previous findings, it is indispensable to study *simultaneously* both the effects of these hormones and the effects due to regional and local extrinsic factors. For instance, the roles of STH-somatomedin and the nasal septal cartilage in the

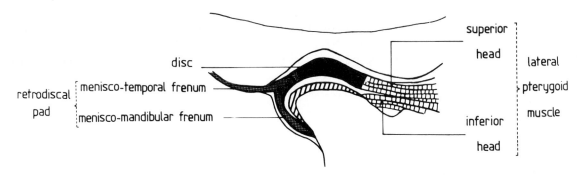

Fig. 2-6. Sagittal section of the temporomandibular joint of the rat.

lengthening of the upper jaw cannot be studied separately; indeed, the effect of STH and somatomedin is relayed and expressed through the forward growth of the nasal septal cartilage (Stutzmann and Petrovic, 1976). In addition, growth hormone–somatomedin and testosterone or estrogen have not only a *direct* effect on the condylar cartilage growth but also an *indirect* one. Indeed, both the magnitude and the direction of condylar growth present quantitative variations in response to the physiologic or to experimentally or therapeutically implanted lip pads that produce changes in the sagittal growth of the maxilla (Fig. 1-4). As long as the growth variations do not exceed a certain limit, no significant alterations in the sagittal relationship of the dental arches occur. Effective operation of the servosystem can take place only through slow gradual changes.

Servosystem theory of facial growth

The variation in direction and magnitude of condylar growth is partly a quantitative response to the experimentally effected changes in the lengthening of the maxilla. Variations in maxillary growth may be induced through resection of the nasal septal cartilage and/or administration of growth hormone (Gasson et al., 1975) or testosterone or by orthopedic appliances. As long as the growth alteration does not exceed a certain limit, no significant changes in the sagittal relationship of the dental arches occur (Fig. 2-1). This action can be considered part of a servosystem in which the upper dental arch is the "constantly changing reference input" and the lower arch the "controlled variable." Effective operation of the servosystem can take place only through *gradual* changes between the dental arches (Petrovic and Stutzmann, 1977).

The "operation of confrontation" between the dental arches elicits in certain cases a deviation signal that modifies the activity of the lateral pterygoid and other muscles of mastication, allowing the mandible to adjust to the optimum occlusal position. This change in lateral pterygoid activity then influences the growth rate of the condylar cartilage. To some extent, experimental de-

vices (e.g., the hyperpropulsor or Class II elastics) can elicit similar condylar responses. The hyperpropulsor acts to position the reference input more anteriorly. After an experimentally induced latent period the growth rate increases relative to the degree of appliance activation. The receptors associated with the deviation signal are therefore involved with the regulation of condylar growth. Although little research has been conducted in this aspect of receptor function, it is clear that the elicited signal not only causes an improvement in masticatory function but also synchronizes the growth between the maxilla and the mandible during the entire developmental period of the facial skeleton.

The physiologic adaptation of mandibular length to maxillary length occurs through a variation in both growth *rate* and growth *direction* of the condylar cartilage. Growth hormone–somatomedin affects the lengthening of the mandible (through condylar growth) to a greater extent than the lengthening of the maxilla (Fig. 2-1). If this hormonal effect remains within physiologic limits, the occlusion will not be significantly altered, since a concomitant *reduction* in the angle between the ramus and the corpus decreases the actual length of the mandible. The explanation of the adjustment mechanism is to be found in the servosystem.

In this connection, another clinically important observation in the growing child should be reported: in *anterior* "growth rotation" both the subperiosteal ossification rate and the alveolar bone turnover are generally increased; in *posterior* growth rotation they are decreased. Because the subperiosteal ossification rate usually parallels the condylar cartilage growth rate, this finding may account for a greater responsiveness to orthopedic and, of course, to orthodontic appliances in the case of anterior growth rotation.

The elastic meniscotemporal frenum with its condylar attachment (retrodiscal pad, Fig. 2-6) is a predominant intermediary between the variations of lateral pterygoid activity and the growth of the condylar cartilage (Fig. 1-4) in the rat (and in humans). When the lateral pterygoid muscle is missing or nonfunctional, direct repetitive stimulation of the frenum itself elicits the same condylar response as if the muscle were intact. However, physiologically, the lateral pterygoid does appear to be essential for *fine* occlusal adjustment. An important aspect of this newly discovered role of the retrodiscal pad is that it helps to explain why Class II elastics increase the condylar cartilage growth rate, provided the mandible is *not* immobilized in the *protruded* position.

The peripheral comparator (Fig. 1-4) serves to adjust the sagittal anterior growth of the facial skeleton so the optimum (or a suboptimum) occlusal relationship will be maintained between the upper and lower incisors, canines, and molar cusps. Such relationships correspond to a stable situation for masticatory function. The transposition from one stable situation to another (i.e., to an "attractor" [p. 17]) is accompanied by a physiologic discontinuity (i.e., to a topologic bifurcation-type instability [Fig. 1-5], whose critical point lies in the edge-to-edge or cusp-to-cusp relationship and which corresponds to the "repeller" [p. 17] [Petrovic and Stutzmann, 1977]). Needless to say, lack of interdental contacts corresponds to the absence of both stable and unstable bifurcation-type situations.

The existence of bifurcation-type situations at the peripheral comparator of the servosystem implies that the facial growth should be accounted for by using unpredetermined and discontinuous models rather than deterministic and continuous ones. This precept applies also to models designed for growth forecasting in orthodontic practice.

The existence of bifurcation-type situations at the peripheral comparator also makes intelligible the evidence that the genome only partially determines the phenome. Indeed, a given genome codes not for a singular phenotype but for a regulatory pattern (i.e., for several possible phenotypes). In other words, at critical moments of facial development very small fluctuations taking place around the bifurcation can give rise to different types of occlusal relationships. This situation is encountered in orthodontic practice mostly in patients between 8 and 10 years of age.

Obviously the cybernetic theory of facial growth and the crucial topologic concept of structural and functional stability and instability (Petrovic et al., 1975b; Petrovic and Stutzmann, 1977) are highly useful in a systematic and computerized approach to clinical situations (Lavergne and Petrovic, 1983).

In addition to the peripheral comparator, a central comparator of the servosystem has also been described (Fig. 1-4). The reference for this is a sensory *engram* for the postural activity of the muscles of mastication corresponding to a habitual anteroposterior mandibular position. This engram develops from repeated mandibular posturing for which the minimal deviation signal of the peripheral receptors results. It might be called the postural rest position. Such an engram allows for the detection and correction of deviations from the optimum or suboptimum occlusal position (Petrovic, 1977).

Postural hyperpropulsor

Appropriate functional appliances placing the rat mandible in a forward postural position increase the condylar cartilage growth rate and growth amount (i.e., the mandible becomes longer than that in control animals). With time, during the growth period, the sagittal deviation produced by the postural hyperpropulsor decreases through the supplementary forward growth of the mandible. This implies that, simultaneously, the deviation signal also decreases; in other words, the *supplementary* growth rate of the condylar cartilage and the *supplementary* lengthening of the mandible also decrease. Periodic increases in the thickness of the postural hyperpropulsor lead to increases in lateral pterygoid muscle activity as recorded electromyographically (and, certainly, increases in the activity of the retrodiscal pad) and these, consequently, bring about a new increase in the rate and amount of condylar cartilage growth. When the appliance is removed after the growth of the animal has been completed, no relapse is observed. When the appliance is removed before growth is completed, no significant relapse is detected if a good intercuspation has been achieved during the experimental phase; but if a good intercuspation has not been achieved, the comparator of the servosystem imposes an increased or decreased condylar growth rate until a state of intercuspal stability is established. Functional maxipropulsion involving periodic forward repositioning appears to the the best procedure for eliciting orthopedically a supplementary lengthening of the mandible. No genetically predetermined final length of the mandible has been detected in these experiments (Petrovic et al., 1981a).

When a young rat is fitted with a postural hyperpropulsor and similar functional appliances for 10 to 12 hours daily, everything occurs as if the upper dental arch (the "constantly changing reference input") were in a more anterior position than is actually the case (Fig. 1-4). The "confrontation" between the dental arches then gives rise to a deviation signal, which is reduced by an appropriate forward positioning of the lower dental arch through the propulsion of the mandible. Needless to say, the increased contractile activity of the lateral pterygoid muscle produces a supplementary growth in the condylar cartilage and thereby a supplementary lengthening of the mandible. With time, this supplementary lengthening will reduce the anatomic repositioning of the mandible and, thus, the intensity of the deviation signal. As a consequence, the increased activity of the lateral pterygoid and the supplementary growth of the condylar cartilage will also tend to diminish (Petrovic and Stutzmann, 1977). When the mandible reaches the length corresponding to the new occlusal relationship imposed by the postural hyperpropulsor, the intensity of the deviation signal in the treated animals will no longer differ significantly from that in untreated animals and, henceforth, the condylar cartilage growth rate in the treated animals will become virtually the same as that in the untreated animals. Nevertheless, as long as the rat is wearing the postural hyperpropulsor, its mandible will be longer than that of the untreated animal.

If, on the other hand, the postural hyperpropulsor is then removed, the "confrontation" between the two dental arches will detect the appliance-produced excessive anterior position of the lower dental arch and will give rise to another deviation signal, which will be reduced by a *diminution* in the contractile activity of the lateral pterygoid muscle and, thereby, through a *reduction* in the condylar cartilage growth rate. The mandible then will tend to reach the length it would have in the absence of treatment with the functional appliance (Table 2-4). Under these conditions, with an animal that is still growing, relapse after removal of the functional appliance appears, in the light of our cybernetic theory, as

the expression of a regulatory mechanism tending to minimize the deviation from the optimum occlusal adjustment.

The angle between the mandibular plane and the main orientation of newly formed endochondral bone trabeculae located under the condylar cartilage ("Stutzmann's angle") increases *at the beginning* of the treatment (Table 2-4, *B*). With time, however, the difference between treated and control animals becomes undetectable. (Tables 2-4, *B* and *C*, and 2-5, *D*). In other words, the opening of Stutzmann's angle is only a *transient* remedial event. Everything happens as if in the regulatory system controlling mandibular morphogenesis, the *shape* (in cybernetic language the "reference input") and the *rate* and *amount* of growth were controlled variables. Indeed, a deviation from the normal shape (e.g., the opening of Stutzmann's angle), occurring as a transient phenomenon in response to the placing of a functional appliance, tends to be reduced and is observed only in the long run, through the appropriate increase in *growth* rate and amount.

These findings imply that the variations in the direction of growth of the condylar cartilage and of the condyle produced by a functional appliance account for only a small part, if any, of the differences observed at the end of growth between treated and untreated indi-

Table 2-4. Forward repositioning of the mandible

Periodic forward repositioning of mandible (12 male rats in each group sacrificed at age 48 or 180 da)

  Example: in experimental group 0_5
  - No treatment was applied from birth to day 20 (0.0)
  - A 2 mm thick postural hyperpropulsor was worn from day 20 to 48 (2.0)
  - A 3 mm thick postural hyperpropulsor was worn from day 48 to 76 (3.0)
  - A 4 mm thick postural hyperpropulsor was worn from day 76 to 120 (4.0)
  - The postural hyperpropulsor was removed at day 120; thus from day 120 to 180 no treatment was applied (0.0)
  - The rat was sacrificed at day 180

Based on the analysis of variance, a standard error was calculated for the whole 48-day-old population curd the whole 180-day-old population. The difference (experimental group 0_5, control group A_5, Table 2-4, *A*) was equal to 3.30 mm (23.35 − 20.05 mm). This difference, which was greater than 0.24 mm, is significant at the 1% level.

(A) NUMBER OF ^{3}H-METHYL-THYMIDINE–LABELED CELLS IN CONDYLAR CARTILAGE

		Age (days)			Mean	Standard error
		0	20	48		
Thickness of postural hyperpropulsor (mm)	A_1	0.0	0.0		878	
	B_1	0.0	0.5		1049	
	C_1	0.0	1.0		1316	40.63
	D_1	0.0	2.0		1499	
	E_1	0.0	3.0		818	

  Smallest significant difference between two means
  5% level: 81
  1% level: 108
  0.1% level: 141

Continued.

Table 2-4. Forward repositioning of the mandible—cont'd

(B) ANGLE BETWEEN GROWTH DIRECTION OF CONDYLE AND MANDIBULAR PLANE

		Age (days)			Mean (degrees)	Standard error
		0	20	48		
Thickness of postural hyperpropulsor (mm)	A_1	0.0	0.0		128.9	
	B_1	0.0	0.5		136.0	
	C_1	0.0	1.0		136.9	0.6880
	D_1	0.0	2.0		140.5	
	E_1	0.0	3.0		129.2	

Smallest significant difference between two means (degrees)
   5% level: 1.4
   1% level: 1.8
   0.1% level: 2.4

Analysis of variance

		Age (days)						Mean (degrees)	Standard error
		0	20	48	76	120	180		
Thickness of postural hyperpropulsor (mm)	A_4	0.0	0.0	0.0	0.0	0.0		131.9	
	B_4	0.0	0.5	0.5	0.5	0.5		131.8	
	C_4	0.0	0.5	0.5	0.5	0.0		132.0	
	D_4	0.0	0.5	0.5	0.0	0.0		132.0	
	E_4	0.0	0.5	0.0	0.0	0.0		132.2	
	F_4	0.0	1.0	1.0	1.0	1.0		133.1	
	G_4	0.0	1.0	2.0	3.0	3.0		134.9	
	H_4	0.0	1.0	2.0	3.0	0.0		133.0	
	I_4	0.0	1.0	1.0	1.0	0.0		132.3	
	J_4	0.0	1.0	1.0	0.0	0.0		131.8	0.4378
	K_4	0.0	1.0	0.0	0.0	0.0		132.0	
	L_4	0.0	2.0	2.0	2.0	2.0		133.9	
	M_4	0.0	2.0	3.0	3.0	3.0		134.7	
	N_4	0.0	2.0	3.0	4.0	4.0		135.9	
	O_4	0.0	2.0	3.0	4.0	0.0		135.0	
	P_4	0.0	2.0	2.0	2.0	0.0		133.3	
	Q_4	0.0	2.0	2.0	0.0	0.0		131.9	
	R_4	0.0	2.0	0.0	0.0	0.0		132.0	

Smallest significant difference between two means (degrees)
   5% level: 0.9
   1% level: 1.1
   0.1% level: 1.5

viduals. No significant effect of the postural hyperpropulsor can be detected histologically in the condyle after the growth is completed.

The mechanisms of action of the Fränkel appliance on the sagittal growth of the mandible are physiologically similar to the mechanism of action of the postural hyperpropulsor.

For a young patient with a retropositioned lower dental arch, the conditions are different, since the fitting of a postural hyperpropulsor is intended precisely to reduce the sagittal malrelation. From these observations we can infer that a rational orthodontic treatment must lead to the minimization of deviation from the optimum occlusal adjustment so the risk of relapse will be decreased.

Class II elastics

Intermaxillary *intra*oral elastics, placed daily for 14 hours in the rat bilaterally, between the first superior molar and the third inferior molar are not only an orthodontic device that is able to move teeth but also a functional appliance capable of stimulating the growth rate

Table 2-4. Forward repositioning of the mandible—cont'd

(C) LENGTH OF MANDIBLE

		Age (days)			Mean (mm)	Standard error
		0	20	48		
Thickness of postural hyperpropulsor (mm)	A_1	0.0	0.0		13.95	
	B_1	0.0	0.5		14.95	
	C_1	0.0	1.0		15.25	0.0754
	D_1	0.0	2.0		15.44	
	E_1	0.0	3.0		13.58	

Smallest significant difference between two means (mm)
　5% level: 0.15
　1% level: 0.20
　0.1% level: 0.26

Analysis of variance

		Age (days)						Mean (mm)	Standard error
		0	20	48	76	120	180		
Thickness of postural hyperpropulsor (mm)	A_4	0.0	0.0	0.0	0.0	0.0		20.05	
	B_4	0.0	0.5	0.5	0.5	0.5		21.12	
	C_4	0.0	0.5	0.5	0.5	0.0		21.06	
	D_4	0.0	0.5	0.5	0.0	0.0		20.50	
	E_4	0.0	0.5	0.0	0.0	0.0		20.15	
	F_4	0.0	1.0	1.0	1.0	1.0		21.62	
	G_4	0.0	1.0	2.0	3.0	3.0		21.93	
	H_4	0.0	1.0	2.0	3.0	0.0		21.91	
	I_4	0.0	1.0	1.0	1.0	0.0		21.48	
	J_4	0.0	1.0	1.0	0.0	0.0		20.65	0.0734
	K_4	0.0	1.0	0.0	0.0	0.0		20.28	
	L_4	0.0	2.0	2.0	2.0	2.0		22.57	
	M_4	0.0	2.0	3.0	3.0	3.0		23.68	
	B_4	0.0	2.0	3.0	4.0	4.0		23.67	
	O_4	0.0	2.0	3.0	4.0	0.0		23.35	
	P_4	0.0	2.0	2.0	2.0	0.0		22.29	
	Q_4	0.0	2.0	2.0	0.0	0.0		22.02	
	R_4	0.0	2.0	0.0	0.0	0.0		21.44	

Smallest significant difference between two means (mm)
　5% level: 0.14
　1% level 0.19
　0.1% level: 0.24

and amount of the condylar cartilage (Table 2-5). One is dealing really with the influence on *growth* of the mandible, because no such effect can be detected once the growth is completed (i.e., in the adult) (Petrovic et al., 1981a).

The postural hyperpropulsor gives rise to a highly significant increase in the contractile activity of the lateral pterygoid muscle, detectable electromyographically; the Class II elastics do not (significantly). The stimulating action of the Class II elastics on the lengthening of the condyle appears to be mediated primarily through the meniscotemporocondylar frenum (retrodiscal pad), a structure that according to previous investigations (Petrovic and Stutzmann, 1979c) also mediates, at least partly, the stimulating effect of the increased contractile activity of the lateral pterygoid muscle on condylar cartilage growth. Indeed, only in the presence of the retrodiscal pad are the Class II elastics able to elicit an earlier start of the chondroblast hypertrophy and an increased growth rate of the condylar cartilage. Our concept of an intrinsic regulation of the prechondroblasts multiplication (Stutzmann and Petrovic, 1975b, 1979) accounts partly for the phenomenon. Only "functional" (i.e., not yet hypertrophied) chondroblasts produce a prechondroblast multiplication restraining signal so that when the number of "functional" chondroblasts decreases, regardless of the primary cause, the magnitude of the negative feedback signal also decreases and, consequently, the prechondroblast multiplication rate *increases*.

The *intra*oral Class II elastics stimulate in a significant manner the growth rate of the condylar cartilage and the lengthening of the mandible (Table 2-5), while the *extra*oral elastics designed to effect active hyperpropulsion of the mandible (Petrovic et al., 1974b) have a very little effect (Table 2-6). In the first case, however, the mandible remains *mobile;* in the second case it is *immobilized.*

The lateral pterygoid muscle appears to be a major intermediary in maintaining the optimum occlusal adjustment during growth as well as in the action of functional appliances (e.g., the postural hyperpropulsor,

Table 2-5. Effects of various functional appliances on growth of the rat mandible (12 animals in each group)

(A) NUMBER OF ³H-METHYL-THYMIDINE–LABELED CELLS IN CONDYLAR CARTILAGE	Mean (degrees)	Standard error
No appliance	859	
Bionator (end to end)	988	
Bionator (1 mm forward)	1199	25.47
Fränkel *superior* retrolabial vestibular shields (lip pads)	1236	

Smallest significant difference between two means (degrees)
  5% level: 51
  1% level: 69
  0.1% level: 90		

No appliance	878	
Postural hyperpropulsor (0.5 mm)	1049	
Postural hyperpropulsor (1 mm)	1316	41.73
Intraoral elastic forces	1336	

Smallest significant difference between two means (degrees)
  5% level: 84
  1% level: 112
  0.1% level: 147		

(B) ANGLE BETWEEN GROWTH DIRECTION OF RAT CONDYLE AND MANDIBULAR PLANE (48 days old)	Mean (degrees)	Standard error
No appliance	126.3	
Bionator ("end to end")	130.5	
Bionator (1 mm forward)	132.9	0.437
Fränkel *superior* retrolabial vestibular shields (lip pads)	131.2	

Smallest significant difference between two means (degrees)
  5% level: 0.9
  1% level: 1.2
  1% level without appliance: 1.5		

No appliance	128.9	
Postural hyperpropulsor (0.5 mm)	136.0	
Postural hyperpropulsor (1 mm)	136.9	0.569
Intraoral elastic forces	137.6	

Smallest significant difference between two means (degrees)
  5% level: 1.1
  1% level: 1.5
  0.1% level: 2.0		

Table 2-5. Effects of various functional appliances on growth of the rat mandible (12 animals in each group)—cont'd

(C) LENGTH OF RAT MANDIBLE (distance between mental foramen and posterior border of condylar cartilage) (48 days old)

	Mean (mm)	Standard error
No appliance	14.24	
Bionator (end to end)	14.67	
Bionator (1 mm forward)	15.29	0.1596
Fränkel *superior* retrolabial vestibular shields (lip pads)	15.22	

Smallest significant difference between two means (mm)
  5% level: 0.32
  1% level: 0.43
  0.1% level: 0.56

	Mean (mm)	Standard error
No appliance	13.95	
Postural hyperpropulsor (0.5 mm)	14.87	
Postural hyperpropulsor (1 mm)	15.25	0.0730
Intraoral elastic forces	15.26	

Smallest significant difference between two means (mm)
  5% level: 0.15
  1% level: 0.20
  0.1% level: 0.26

(D) ANGLE BETWEEN GROWTH DIRECTION OF RAT CONDYLE AND MANDIBULAR PLANE (180 days old)

	Mean (degrees)		Standard error
	Applied from		
	20 to 180 da	120 to 180 da	
No appliance	131.9		
Bionator (end to end)	134.5	132.8	
Bionator (1 mm forward)	132.8		0.555
Postural hyperpropulsor (0.5 mm)	132.1	132.0	
Postural hyperpropulsor (1 mm)	133.1	133.1	
Intraoral elastic forces	133.2	132.7	
Fränkel *superior* retrolabial vestibular shields (lip pads)	132.4	132.4	

Smallest significant differences between two means (degrees)
  5% level: 1.1
  1% level: 1.45
  0.1% level: 1.87

(E) LENGTH OF RAT MANDIBLE (distance between mental foramen and posterior border of condylar cartilage) (180 days old)

	Mean (mm)		Standard error
	Applied from		
	20 to 180 da	120 to 180 da	
No appliance	20.05		
Bionator (end to end)	20.83	20.23	
Bionator (1 mm forward)	21.63		0.2221
Postural hyperpropulsor (0.5 mm)	21.12	20.17	
Postural hyperpropulsor (1 mm)	21.62	20.13	
Intraoral elastic forces	22.93	20.19	
Fränkel *superior* retrolabial vestibular shields (lip pads)	22.94	20.18	

Smallest significant differences between two means (mm)
  5% level: 0.44
  1% level: 0.58
  0.1% level: 0.75

L.S.U. activator, Fränkel appliance). For the stimulating effect of the Class II elastics, however, the biologic "actuator" seems to be the retrodiscal pad.

Herren-type (or L.S.U.-type) activator

The word *activator* is often misleading because it refers to various appliances operating, biologically, in different ways. The Herren activator, or the Louisiana State University modification of it (R. Shaye), is different from a postural hyperpropulsor insofar as it opens the construction bite well beyond postural rest position, similar to that achieved by the Harvold-Woodside activator (Woodside, 1984). Indeed, according to Herren (1953) and Auf der Maur (1978), the wearing of this appliance does *not* bring about any increased activity of the lateral pterygoid muscle.

In our experiments, male rats wore either a Herren-type or an L.S.U.-type activator for 12, 18, or 22½ hours daily. The appliance was fixed to the maxilla. A 2.0 mm forward positioning of the mandible was obtained through the construction bite and the vertical increase in the molar bite was 0.4, 0.8, or 1.8 mm. (For details see tables in Petrovic et al., 1982b). The mobility of the lower jaw was lessened by extending the sides of the appliance lingually as deep as possible toward the bottom of the oral cavity. No free movement of the mandible was possible without a minimal opening of several millimeters. In fact, no actual increase in the electromyographically recorded activity of the lateral pterygoid muscle was detected during the wearing of the Herren-type activator (Fig. 2-7), corroborating the observations of Herren and Auf der Maur.

Nevertheless, both the Herren-type and the L.S.U.-type activator did produce an increased growth rate and amount of the condylar cartilage and a supplementary lengthening of the mandible at the posterior border when the appliance was worn for 12 or 18 hours daily and when the molar bite height was 0.4 or 0.8 mm (Table 2-6). When the vertical dimension of the appliance was increased to 1.8 mm, the condylar cartilage growth and lengthening of the mandible were *not* promoted any more.

The analysis of our experimental findings strongly suggests that the Herren-type and L.S.U.-type activators' actions have a *two*-step effect. Indeed, during the time that the appliance is worn, the more-forward positioning of the mandible is the *cause* of the reduced increase in length of the lateral pterygoid muscle (Table 2-6, *D,* and Fig. 2-8) (Petrovic et al., 1973, 1982b; Oudet and Petrovic, 1978b). At the same time a new sensory engram is formed for the new positioning of the mandible. The corollary to this is that during the period where the activator is not worn, the mandible is functioning in a more forward position so the retrodiscal pad will be *much more* stimulated than in controls. The increased repetitive activity of the pad produces an earlier onset of hypertrophy of the condylar chondroblasts. This earlier commencement, along with the simultaneous decrease in the number of functional (not yet hypertrophied) chondroblasts, implies that the decrease of the

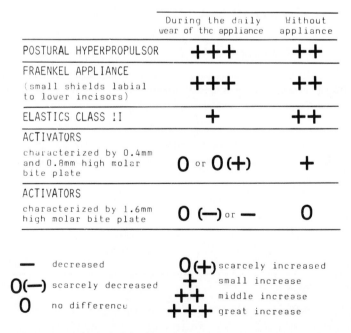

	During the daily wear of the appliance	Without appliance
POSTURAL HYPERPROPULSOR	+++	++
FRAENKEL APPLIANCE (small shields labial to lower incisors)	+++	++
ELASTICS CLASS II	+	++
ACTIVATORS characterized by 0.4mm and 0.8mm high molar bite plate	0 or 0(+)	+
ACTIVATORS characterized by 1.6mm high molar bite plate	0 (−) or −	0

— decreased
0(−) scarcely decreased
0 no difference

0(+) scarcely increased
+ small increase
++ middle increase
+++ great increase

Fig. 2-7. Semiquantitative evaluation of the electromyographic activity in the lateral pterygoid muscle of the young rat during the weeks after beginning treatment.

Table 2-6. L.S.U. activator and extraoral forward traction

(A) GROWTH OF CONDYLAR CARTILAGE (number of ^{3}H-thymidine labeled nuclei)

	Mean	Standard error	$A_{12}^{0.8}$*	$A_{18}^{0.8}$	$A_{22}^{0.8}$	$\overline{LPM}$	$\overline{LPM}$ + $A_{12}^{0.8}$	FT_{12}	FT_{22}	$\overline{LPM}$ + FT_{12}
						Comparisons between means: "t-test" values (15 animals each)				
C	859	14	10.33§	3.54§	0.95 NS	18.93§	10.08§	3.47‡	0.30 NS	15.36§
$A_{12}^{0.8}$	1139	23		7.27§	8.58§			6.07§		
$A_{18}^{0.8}$	933	16			2.11†					
$A_{22}^{0.8}$	881	19							1.26 NS	
$\overline{LPM}$	470	15					2.51†			0.75 NS
$\overline{LPM}$ + $A_{12}^{0.8}$	549	27								1.77*
FT_{12}	947	21							3.75§	15.75§
FT_{22}	851	14								
$\overline{LPM}$ + FT_{12}	489	20								

(B) ANGLE BETWEEN NEWLY FORMED ENDOCHONDRAL BONE TRABECULAE AND MANDIBULAR BONE

	Mean	Standard error	$A_{12}^{0.8}$	$A_{18}^{0.8}$	$A_{22}^{0.8}$	$\overline{LPM}$	$\overline{LPM}$ + $A_{12}^{0.8}$	FT_{12}	FT_{22}	$\overline{LPM}$ + FT_{12}
C	126.3	0.4	12.59§	3.17‡	0.57 NS	23.82§	30.72§	4.38§	0.20 NS	23.43§
$A_{12}^{0.8}$	133.5	0.4		9.70§	12.71§		20.00§	7.28§		
$A_{18}^{0.8}$	128.1	0.4			2.75†					
$A_{22}^{0.8}$	126.6	0.4							0.71 NS	
$\overline{LPM}$	141.8	0.5					4.55§			0.19 NS
$\overline{LPM}$ + $A_{12}^{0.8}$	144.7	0.4								4.23§
FT_{12}	129.1	0.5							4.15§	18.47§
FT_{22}	126.1	0.5								
$\overline{LPM}$ + FT_{12}	141.9	0.5								

C, Controls
$A_{12}^{0.8}$, Activator (sagittal deviation = 2 mm; vertical deviation = 0.8 mm) 12 hours per day
$A_{18}^{0.8}$, Activator (sagittal deviation = 2 mm; vertical deviation = 0.8 mm) 18 hours per day
$A_{22}^{0.8}$, Activator (sagittal deviation = 2 mm; vertical deviation = 0.8 mm) 22½ hours per day
$\overline{LPM}$, Resection of lateral pterygoid muscle
FT_{12}, Forward traction (sagittal deviation = 2 mm) 12 hours per day
FT_{22}, Forward traction (sagittal deviation = 2 mm) 22½ hours per day
Significance:
  *10% level (indicative)
  †5% level
  ‡1% level
  §0.1% level
  NS, Not significant

Continued.

Table 2-6. L.S.U. activator and extraoral forward traction—cont'd

(C) DISTANCE BETWEEN MENTAL FORAMEN AND POSTERIOR BORDER OF CONDYLE

	Mean	Standard error	$A_{12}^{0.8}$*	$A_{18}^{0.8}$	$A_{22}^{0.8}$	LPM	LPM + $A_{12}^{0.8}$	FT_{12}	FT_{22}	LPM + FT_{12}
							Comparisons between means: "t-test" values (15 animals each)			
C	14.21	0.16	7.75§	5.92§	0.11 NS	7.22§	5.45§	2.25†	0.18 NS	6.74§
$A_{12}^{0.8}$	16.05	0.17		1.65 NS	5.71§		13.87§	6.03§		
$A_{18}^{0.8}$	15.64	0.19			4.37§					
$A_{22}^{0.8}$	14.24	0.27							0.24 NS	
LPM	12.54	0.16					2.60†			0.78 NS
LPM + $A_{12}^{0.8}$	13.08	0.13								1.86*
FT_{12}	14.70	0.14							2.14†	10.34§
FT_{22}	14.16	0.20								
LPM + FT_{12}	12.71	0.15								

(D) LATERAL PTERYGOID MUSCLE (number of sarcomeres in series)

	Mean	Standard error	$A_{12}^{0.8}$*	$A_{18}^{0.8}$	$A_{22}^{0.8}$	LPM	LPM + $A_{12}^{0.8}$	FT_{12}	FT_{22}	LPM + FT_{12}
C	2272	22	10.55§	6.03§	8.33§			5.26§	5.35§	
$A_{12}^{0.8}$	1931	24		3.36‡	1.33 NS			4.70‡		
$A_{18}^{0.8}$	2055	28			1.93*					
$A_{22}^{0.8}$	1979	27							2.45†	
FT_{12}	2094	25							0.45 NS	
FT_{22}	2070	29								

C, Controls
$A_{12}^{0.8}$, Activator (sagittal deviation = 2 mm; vertical deviation = 0.8 mm) 12 hours per day
$A_{18}^{0.8}$, Activator (sagittal deviation = 2 mm; vertical deviation = 0.8 mm) 18 hours per day
$A_{22}^{0.8}$, Activator (sagittal deviation = 2 mm; vertical deviation = 0.8 mm) 22½ hours per day
LPM., Resection of lateral pterygoid muscle
FT_{12}, Forward traction (sagittal deviation = 2 mm) 12 hours per day
FT_{22}, Forward traction (sagittal deviation = 2 mm) 22½ hours per day
Significance:
 *10% level (indicative)
 †5% level
 ‡1% level
 §0.1% level
 NS, Not significant

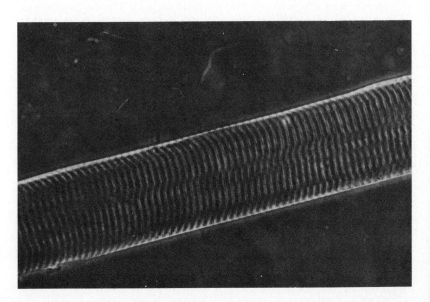

Fig. 2-8. Segment of the isolated muscle fiber from the lateral pterygoid muscle. In phase contrast microscopy the sarcomeres are clearly visible.

negative feedback signal has a restraining effect on the prechondroblast multiplication rate (Stutzmann and Petrovic, 1975b, 1979). Consequently, the growth rate of the condylar cartilage is accelerated. In other words, once more, the lateral pterygoid muscle does mediate *pro parte* the action of the appliance but in the case of the Herren or L.S.U.-type activator the stimulating effect on condylar growth appears to be produced mostly during the time that the appliance is *not* worn. Indeed, when either the Herren-type or the L.S.U.-type activator is worn for 22½ hours daily or almost full time, the length of the lateral pterygoid muscle is decreased but *no* actual stimulating effect on the condylar cartilage growth rate is detected. Furthermore, when the vertical

dimension of the activator used in young rat experiments is opened to 1.8 mm, mandibular lengthening is *not* promoted. In this case the growth of the lateral pterygoid muscle, as estimated by the number of serial sarcomeres, is *not* reduced significantly.

TENTATIVE CAUSAL INTERPRETATION OF THE MODUS OPERANDI OF FUNCTIONAL APPLIANCES

The servosystem concept accounts not only for biologic organization but also for the *mechanisms of action* of appliances used in dentofacial orthopedics. According to our experimental investigations (Petrovic, 1982), functional appliances may be (tentatively) divided into two categories (Fig. 2-9).

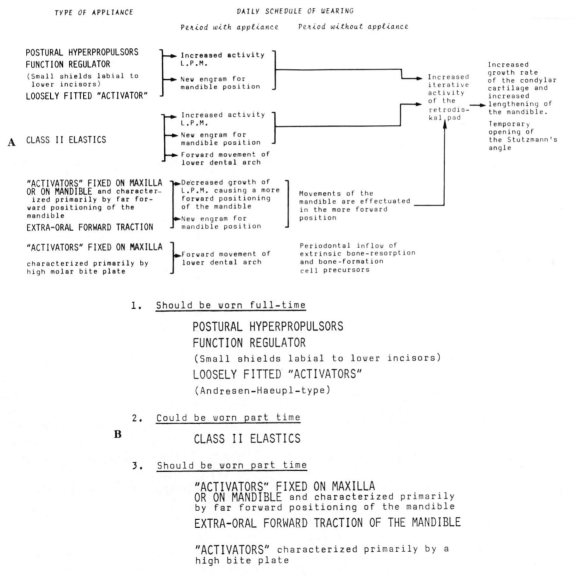

Fig. 2-9. A, Tentative classification of orthopedic appliances according to their effect on condylar growth and mandibular lengthening. **B,** Daily duration of wearing of an orthopedic appliance.

1. The postural hyperpropulsor, the Andresen-Häupl appliance, Class II elastics, the Fränkel appliance (small lip pads labial to the lower incisors), and the Balters Bionator all exert their effects mainly through the *movements* of the mandible. Indeed, their stimulating effect on condylar cartilage growth is produced mainly during the wearing of the appliance.

2. The Herren and L.S.U. activators and, by inference, the Harvold and Hamilton activators as well as extraoral forward traction on the mandible seem to exert their effects mostly through the sagittal *repositioning* of the mandible.

Regardless of these differences in mode of action of the various functional appliances, the following causal chain is involved:

Functional appliance

↓

Increased contractile activity of
lateral pterygoid muscle

↓

Intensification of retrodiscal pad
(bilaminar zone) repetitive activity

↓

Increase in growth-stimulating factors
- Enhancement of local mediators
- Reduction of local regulators (factors having negative feedback effect on cell multiplication rate)

↓

- Additional growth of condylar cartilage
- Additional subperiosteal ossification of posterior border of mandible

↓

Supplementary lengthening of mandible

Investigations underway concerning the signals that locally affect the condylar cartilage–stimulating action of the postural hyperpropulsor, Fränkel appliance, L.S.U. activator, Bionator, and Class II elastics have led to several findings (Petrovic, 1982; Petrovic and Stutzmann, 1982).

1. Electron micrographs of the condylar cartilage show that cell-to-cell cytoplasmic junctions between skeletoblasts become quantitatively reduced. Consequently, possibilities of inhibitory intercellular communications are cut down: the cell division rate increases. Simultaneously, the rate of differentiation of skeletoblasts into prechondroblasts also increases.

2. Characteristic and consistent transmembrane ion flux variations are detected: intracellular Na^+ concentration is raised; intracellular K^+ concentration is lowered; discharge of H^+ from both skeletoblasts and prechon-

droblasts is increased, leading to a rise of intracytoplasmic pH. Intracytoplasmic Ca^{++}, however, is maintained at a lower level.

3. Calmodulin as well as Ca^{++}, Mg^{++}–ATPase and H^+–ATPase activities are promoted whereas cAMP, fibronectin, Na^+, K^+–ATPase activity, cell transglutaminase, heparan sulfate, and other glucosaminoglycan levels are reduced. Nevertheless, first, the antimultiplicative effect of cAMP is not a direct one but results from the amplification of specific growth-regulating signals (detected biologically but not yet identified) and, second, the cell division process is initiated through a momentary surge of cytoplasmic Ca^{++} and endogenous cAMP.

4. The local *coupling* mechanisms include the following:

a. An open loop part of the control system, which has a *stimulating* effect on cell multiplication and consists of growth hormone, testosterone, estrogen (in low doses), insulin, insulin-like substances (including liver-synthesized and locally produced somatomedins), glucagon, parathormone, calcitonin, calmodulin, and prostaglandin $F_2\alpha$. There are also mitogenic peptides that could correspond, operationally, to the fibroblast growth factor, endothelial cell–derived growth factor, platelet-derived growth factor, and monocyte-derived growth factor. Unexpectedly, these growth-promoting factors operate primarily by counteracting or even canceling the effects of agents that amplify the intercellular signal restraining skeletoblast or preosteoblast multiplication. In other words, these mitogenic peptides are not, in the strictest sense, *initiators* of cell division but are, instead, required for the G_1 (or rather G_0) skeletoblast and preosteoblast *either* to become, after an 8-to-10-hour lag time, again responsive to the specific gene-produced messenger initiating a new cell cycle *or* to repress directly the gene that controls the production of the agent amplifying the cell division–restraining signal. Whatever the mechanism involved, the cell will be converted from a quiescent to a new cycle stage.

b. A feedback part of the control system, having an inhibitory effect on cell multiplication and consisting of regulators of *local* origin: skeletoblast or prechondroblast multiplication–restraining signal of unknown nature, contact inhibition–type signal, cAMP, prostaglandin E_2, and a somatostatin-like substance.

5. The intensification of retrodiscal pad activity is associated with an *increase* in blood and lymph flow (i.e., in open loop factors supply) and with a *decrease* in cell catabolite concentration and negative feedback factors. These changes account for the supplementary growth of the condylar cartilage caused by functional appliances.

Table 2-7. Condylar cartilage reaction to retropulsive forces (chin cup type of appliance) in rats

	No. of animals	Mean	Standard error
(A) 48-DAY-OLD ANIMALS			
Number of ^{3}H-methyl-thymidine–labeled cells in condylar cartilage*			
Controls	6	952	51
Treated	12	667	30
Length of mandible (mm)*			
Controls	20	16.15	0.03
Treated	20	15.29	0.06
Number of serial sarcomeres in lateral pterygoid muscle*			
Controls	6	2443	73
Treated	12	2831	38
(B) 180 DAY-OLD ANIMALS			
Angle between growth direction of condyle and mandibular plane*			
Controls	12	131.9	0.38
Treated	12	130.0	0.46
Length of mandible (mm)*			
Controls	12	19.55	0.52
Treated	12	17.65	0.12
Number of serial sarcomeres in lateral pterygoid muscle†			
Controls	12	2226	22
Treated	12	2624	21

*Difference significant at 0.1% level.
†Difference not significant.

Active retropulsion of the mandible. The active retropulsion of the mandible (with chin caps) is considered more orthopedic than functional. However, the position of the condyle in the glenoid fossa is affected in a manner similar to that with the Class III activator and the Fränkel FR III.

When growing rats are subjected to active retropulsion, such as with chin cap therapy, the number of dividing cells in the mandibular condylar cartilage decreases dramatically. The direction of growth becomes more vertical, as evidenced by the closing of the Stutzmann angle, which measures trabecular alignment with the mandibular plane. The length of the mandible decreases markedly. Table 2-7 compares chin cap treated and control animals for both 48-day and 180-day periods of wear. At 48 days the number of labeled cells is greater, the length of the mandible is greater, and the number of serial sarcomeres is greater in the treated group. By 180 days the angle between the trabeculae of the growing condyle and the mandibular plane still shows a difference that is significant at the 0.1% level. Mandibular length is less in the chin cap animals. The serial sarcomere count is still more for the treated animals but is not statistically significant.

It is clear that chin cap therapy performs an orthopedic function, restraining the condylar cartilage growth rate as the condyle grows more in an upward and forward direction (Charlier et al., 1969b; Petrovic et al., 1975b). This research substantiates the experimental and clinical studies by Graber et al. (1967) and Graber (1983c) on squirrel monkeys and on large numbers of young Class III patients.

Last but not least, functional appliances that modulate the growth rate of the condylar cartilage also influence, in the growing rat, bone formation and mineralization in the mandible as a whole (Petrovic et al., 1982d).

SPONTANEOUS AND THERAPEUTICALLY INDUCED VARIATIONS IN HUMAN ALVEOLAR BONE TURNOVER—a quantitative study

Variations in human alveolar bone turnover relative to many physiologic functions can easily be investigated. Understandably, in dealing with human bone, biopsy is done only for compelling medical reasons; in addition, there is a high probability that in such cases one is facing a pathologic state.

There is an exception, however. During tooth extraction it is easy to get alveolar bone fragments. Furthermore, when the tooth is extracted for orthodontic purposes, the alveolar bone is generally normal and the turnover rate superior to that found in other parts in the skeleton. Finally, because alveolar bone fragments are a by-product of tooth extraction, the researcher may use them in any way that is revealing.

We have chosen to investigate alveolar bone turnover by using organ culture and measuring appropriate physiologic parameters. In this discussion only data relative to the first mandibular premolar will be reported.

The literature contains a large number of studies regarding the response of alveolar bone to both physiologic and orthodontically induced tooth movement (Stein and Weinmann, 1925; Reitan, 1947, 1960, 1964, 1974; Macapanpan et al., 1954; Storey, 1955; Graber et al., 1967; Baumrind, 1969, 1970; Gianelly, 1969; Kvam, 1970; Baron, 1973; Rygh, 1973; Markostamou, 1974). These investigations were based mostly on histologic descriptions; only a few were designed to quantify alveolar bone formation and/or resorption (Kingler, 1971; Baron, 1973; Markostamou and Baron, 1973).

Orthodontically induced tooth movement is dependent on bone density, the number of cells involved in bone formation and bone resorption, and the magnitude and timing of the applied force. It also depends, however, on the rate of physiologic bone remodeling activity as well as the possibility of increasing this remodeling orthodontically.

In addition, according to the experiments made in

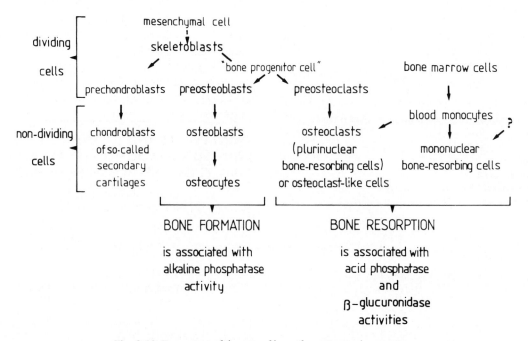

Fig. 2-10. Parameters of the rate of bone formation and resorption.

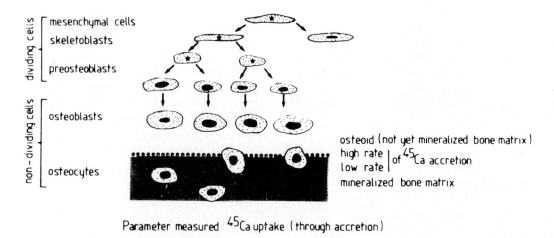

Fig. 2-11. Parameters of the rate of bone mineralization.

our laboratory since 1969 (Lemoine and Petrovic, 1969; Lemoine, 1970; Lemoine et al., 1970; Petrovic, 1970; Stutzmann et al., 1979, 1980b), mononuclear cells of extrinsic origin may also be involved in alveolar bone remodeling activity.

The purpose of the present investigation was as follows:

1. To analyze quantitatively the physiologic alveolar bone turnover rate in 11-to-13-year-old boys as a function of the timing of extraction (morning versus evening), the season (spring versus fall), the growth rotation* of the mandible, and the location of the bone (mesial versus distal) with regard to the extracted premolar

2. To analyze quantitatively the variations of alveolar bone turnover as a function of orthodontic treatment variety (light versus heavy, and intermittent versus continuous, forces).

Choice of parameters in the quantitative evaluation of human alveolar bone turnover

The mitotic index is of little use in evaluating alveolar bone turnover. Indeed, first, it is often impossible to know whether the dividing cell is a preosteoblast or a preosteoclast; and, second, many of the bone forming or bone resorbing cells in alveolar bone are of *extrinsic* origin. (For details see Stutzmann et al., 1979, 1980b, and Stutzmann and Petrovic, 1981.)

Bone formation rate. Alkaline phosphatase activity was used as a parameter of osteoblast activity and ^{45}Ca uptake as a parameter of bone mineralization (Figs. 2-10 and 2-11).

Bone resorption rate. β-Glucuronidase and acid phenylphosphatase activities were used as parameters of bone resorption intensity (Fig. 2-10).

This choice does not imply at all that these two enzymes are involved *directly* in the resorption of bone; but previous experiments (Stutzmann et al., 1979, 1980b) have shown that their activities vary directly with the intensity of bone resorption, whatever the relationship between enzymes activities and bone resorption.† The osteoclast count as such is a poor parameter of bone resorption (Stutzmann et al., 1979, 1980b; Stutzmann and Petrovic, 1981) because some mononuclear cells,

mainly of *extrinsic* origin, also participate in this phenomenon.

Experimental procedure

Human alveolar bone fragments, together with adjacent periodontal tissue, were obtained from 11-to-13-year-old boys during the extraction for orthodontic purposes of mandibular first premolars. The specimens were always taken from both mesial and distal sides relative to the extracted tooth.

First series. In the first experimental series, alveolar bone specimens were removed in the same individual during mandibular first premolar extractions, the initial specimen taken between 10:00 AM and 12:30 PM and the next between 10:00 PM and 12:30 AM or vice versa. Thirty specimens could be obtained each time.

The specimens were immediately placed in organ culture with the apparatus of Petrovic and Heusner (1961; Heusner and Petrovic, 1964) modified by Petrovic, Stutzmann, and Malan (Fig. 2-12). Tissue culture 199 medium was supplemented with 0.15 mg/ml ascorbic acid and 15% calf serum, and 0.05 microcurie of ^{45}Ca was added. After a 3-day organ culture, the following were noted:

- ^{45}Ca uptake (counts per minute, c.p.m.) was measured by the method of Humphrey (1965).
- Alkaline and acid phenylphosphatase activities (enzyme units [e.u.]/g fresh bone) were estimated by the method of Vaes and Jacques (1965) with phenylphosphate as a substrate.
- β-Glucuronidase activity (Fishman units [F.u.]/mg protein) was estimated by the method of Plaice (1961).

Second series. In the second experimental series 150 specimens were removed between April 1 and July 1, and then 80 others between October 15 and January 15.

In the first group (I), 110 alveolar bone specimens were taken from anteriorly "growth rotating" (anteriorly "inclined") mandibles (I_A) and 40 from posteriorly rotating (posteriorly "inclined") mandibles (I_P). In the second group (II), half were taken from anteriorly rotating mandibles and half from posteriorly rotating ones.

The orthodontic treatment consisted of a mesially directed force (Class II elastics) applied for 10 days. Only the individuals in the first group were treated (Fig. 2-13), the experimental design was as follows:

1. Forty individuals in Group I_A and all the individuals in Group I_P—light (50 to 75 g) and intermittent (14 hours daily) forces

2. Twenty five individuals in Group I_A—heavy (175 to 275 g) intermittent (14 hours daily) forces

3. Twenty five individuals in Group I_A—light (50 to 75 g) continuous forces

4. Twenty individuals in Group I_A—heavy (175 to 275 g) continuous forces

---

*In the strictest sense, "growth rotation" refers only to the time-related variations observed during the growth of an individual. When dealing with the basic features of a given individual, one should use "inclination" as more appropriate. In other words, "inclination" is preferable to "growth rotation"; but we have chosen rather to comply with the common usage.

†According to our observations (Stutzmann et al., 1979, 1980), the turnover of bone resorbing cells (osteoclasts as well as mononuclear cells) is significantly accelerated when the bone resorption is stimulated. In other words, the increase in lysosomal enzyme activities can be related to the *shortened* life-span of bone resorbing cells.

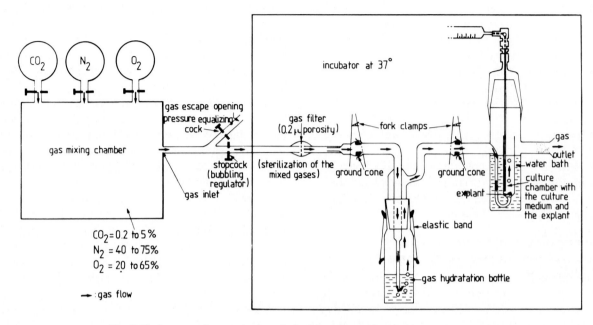

Fig. 2-12. Apparatus for organ culture in liquid nutrient with constant gas renovation.

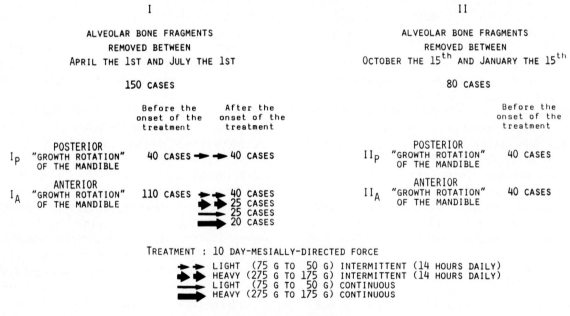

Fig. 2-13. Experimental design.

The methodologic approach was as follows: The mandibular first premolar and the contiguous mesially and distally located alveolar bone fragments were removed on one side (either left or right) *before* the onset of orthodontic treatment. The removed alveolar specimens were immediately organ-cultured for 3 days, and the previously selected parameters measured. Class II elastics were then applied on the contralateral side (either right or left). After 10 days of orthodontic treatment the mandibular first premolar and the contiguous alveolar fragments were removed and studied in organ culture as outlined.

Experimental findings

According to the results of this investigation using the organ culture method, human alveolar bone turnover displays diverse but consistent variations. Some of the factors responsible have been identified; many others have not. For this reason certainly, our experimental data are not distributed normally. Besides, on the basis of prior research (Stutzmann et al., 1979, 1980a), the selected parameters of the alveolar bone turnover rate appear to be preferable to the histomorphometric analysis; however, such a quantitative evaluation certainly needs further improvement.

Significant nyctohemeral variations in bone turnover have been discovered (Table 2-8, *A*) and are important in the biologic understanding of rhythmic fluctuations in human bone turnover as well as in the medical decision concerning the best moment for applying a given therapeutic agent. For instance, if orthodontic forces must be applied only during part of the day, it is advantageous for the practitioner to be able to choose the time when the effect is supposed to be greatest.

Significant seasonal variations in the alveolar bone turnover rate have also been discovered (Table 2-8, *B*) and are of obvious clinical interest. To take an example, when investigating the alveolar bone turnover rate in 20-to-25-year-old male patients, before and after a 21-day orthodontic treatment (Class II elastics), we discovered that the orthodontically induced increase in cell activity was significantly greater in the spring than in the fall.

A puzzling observation was the following (Table 2-8, *C*): In the anteriorly rotating mandible the alveolar bone formation rate was usually notably greater on the mesial side than on the distal and the resorption rate was markedly greater on the distal side. This would imply that in most anteriorly rotating mandibles the first premolar undergoes a physiologic distalization rather than a mesialization during growth. Only in the posteriorly rotating mandible did the parameters of alveolar bone turnover support the classic concept of mesialization during growth.

A strong correlation between the alveolar bone turnover rate and the direction of mandibular growth rotation was detected (Table 2-8, *D*). High bone formation and resorption rates were associated mostly with *anteriorly* rotating mandibles; conversely, low bone formation and resorption rates were generally connected with *posterior* rotation.

How can such a correlation be explained? Previous experiments on young rats (Petrovic and Stutzmann, 1979) have shown that the direction of mandibular growth rotation is related to the magnitude of the mandibular growth rate. In *anterior* growth rotation the response of cells (prechondroblasts of secondary cartilage, subperiosteal and trabecular preosteoblasts of the mandible) to stimulating factors such as growth hormone–somatomedin, testosterone, muscle activity, etc. is higher than when the mandible is of the *posterior* rotational type. This concept is consistent with the clinical observation of a thick, massive, mandible seen in the extreme anterior rotation and a slender, gracile, ramus and corpus seen in the extreme posteriorly rotating jaw (Gasson, 1977ab).

The rate of alveolar bone turnover and the direction of mandibular growth rotation are important to the clinician. Indeed, according to our research investigations (Table 2-9, *A*), the magnitude of an orthodontically induced increase in alveolar bone turnover is statistically greater in the anteriorly rotating mandible than in the jaw with posterior rotation. Furthermore, the magnitude of the increase is greater when the applied forces are light than when they are heavy (Table 2-9, *B* and *C*). In addition, the effectiveness of light forces is enhanced when the forces are applied not continuously but intermittently.

These findings can be interpreted as follows:

1. Light and intermittent forces have a less adverse effect on local periodontal tissue and on local circulatory conditions. Consequently, local cell multiplication and differentiation are less impaired.

2. Previous research (Stutzmann et al., 1979, 1980ab), however, has brought to light another factor: The increased alveolar bone resorption rate on the mesial side as well as the increased alveolar bone formation on the distal side, produced orthodontically by mesially directed forces, involves cells of *extrinsic* origin (circulating monocyte-type cells). This extrinsic contribution of bone resorption and bone formation cell precursors might account, at least partly, for the effectiveness of light over heavy and intermittent over continuous orthodontic forces in tooth movement, since light and intermittent forces have less of an adverse effect on local circulatory conditions.

Table 2-8. Variations in alveolar bone turnover during orthodontic treatment (11-to-13-year-old boys)

	N	Median	Median difference (evening-morning)	Wilcoxon value of Z*
(A) AS FUNCTION OF TIMING OF EXTRACTION (MORNING VERSUS EVENING)				
Alkaline phenylphosphatase activity (enzyme units, e.u.)				
Morning	30	157.5 (117 to 183)	24 (−7 to 87)	− 4.47 (p < 0.001)
Evening	30	183.5 (146 to 227)		
^{45}Ca uptake (counts per minute, c.p.m.)				
Morning	30	12,433 (6871 to 16,550)	646 (−2166 to 3716)	− 1.24 (p = 0.11) (NS)
Evening	30	12,631 (9147 to 15,625)		
β-Glucuronidase activity (Fishman units, F.u.)				
Morning	30	35.17 (22.46 to 42.48)	2.87 (−2.43 to 8.93)	− 4.44 (p < 0.001)
Evening	30	38.25 (22.79 to 46.46)		
Acid phenylphosphatase activity (e.u.)				
Morning	30	14.98 (10.45 to 17.84)	0.51 (−0.89 to 2.16)	− 3.89 (p < 0.001)
Evening	30	16.16 (10.87 to 19.50)		

*Wilcoxon matched-pairs signed-ranks test.
Morning (alveolar bone removed between 10:00 AM and 12:30 PM).
Evening (alveolar bone removed between 10:00 PM and 12:30 AM).

	N	Median	Range	Mann-Whitney U test value of Z
(B) AS FUNCTION OF SEASONS (SPRING VERSUS FALL)				
Alkaline phenylphosphatase activity (e.u.)				
Spring	80	160	128 to 212	9.86
Fall	80	132	120 to 158	(p < 0.001)
^{45}Ca uptake (c.p.m.)				
Spring	80	12,461	4156 to 23,196	4.12
Fall	80	9585	3172 to 18,238	(p < 0.001)
β-Glucuronidase activity (F.u.)				
Spring	80	38.15	20.32 to 54.15	9.10
Fall	80	24.14	12.83 to 37.49	(p < 0.001)
Acid phenylphosphatase activity (e.u.)				
Spring	80	15.66	7.09 to 25.93	4.69
Fall	80	12.38	6.42 to 21.72	(p < 0.001)

Spring (alveolar bone removed between April 1 and July 1).
Fall (alveolar bone removed between October 15 and January 15).

Table 2-8. Variations in alveolar bone turnover during orthodontic treatment (11-to-13-year-old boys)—cont'd

		N	Median		Median of differences (distal-mesial)		Wilcoxon value of Z*
(C) AS FUNCTION OF LOCATION (MESIAL VERSUS DISTAL) OF EXTRACTED MANDIBULAR PREMOLAR							
Alkaline phenylphosphatase activity (enzyme units, e.u.)							
Anterior	Distal	40	169	(136 to 214)	-14.5	$(-39$ to $34)$	-2.56 (p = 0.005)
	Mesial	40	176	(135 to 232)			
Posterior	Distal	40	166	(134 to 191)	26	$(-37$ to $53)$	-3.92 (p < 0.001)
	Mesial	40	138	(119 to 189)			
^{45}Ca uptake (counts per minute, c.p.m.)							
Anterior	Distal	40	13647	(5016 to 21,355)	-716	$(-7818$ to $1542)$	-2.85 (p = 0.002)
	Mesial	40	14,564	(5843 to 25,037)			
Posterior	Distal	40	10,942	(4392 to 17,939)	1378	$(-3552$ to $4222)$	-2.84 (p = 0.002)
	Mesial	40	9623	(3920 to 20,648)			
β-Glucuronidase activity (Fishman units, F.u.)							
Anterior	Distal	40	44.06	(22.70 to 57.56)	3.16	$(-4.70$ to $8.32)$	-3.24 (p = 0.001)
	Mesial	40	42.47	(23.71 to 53.91)			
Posterior	Distal	40	30.17	(17.83 to 48.82)	-4.99	$(-13.74$ to $13.11)$	-2.19 (p = 0.014)
	Mesial	40	35.33	(22.82 to 45.63)			
Acid phenylphosphatase activity (e.u.)							
Anterior	Distal	40	16.66	(6.94 to 28.40)	2.10	$(-5.74$ to $9.21)$	-3.06 (p = 0.001)
	Mesial	40	13.82	(7.39 to 26.91)			
Posterior	Distal	40	12.34	(3.61 to 25.69)	-5.37	$(-11.09$ to $8.09)$	-2.85 (p = 0.002)
	Mesial	40	16.04	(9.63 to 25.17)			

*Wilcoxon matched-pairs signed-ranks test.
Anterior (anterior growth rotation of the mandible).
Posterior (posterior growth rotation of the mandible).

	N	Median	Range	Mann-Whitney U test value of Z
(D) AS FUNCTION OF GROWTH ROTATION OF MANDIBLE (ANTERIOR VERSUS POSTERIOR)				
Alkaline phenylphosphatase activity (e.u.)				
Anterior	80	152	123 to 212	5.04 (p < 0.001)
Posterior	80	134	120 to 173	
Uptake of ^{45}Ca (c.p.m.)				
Anterior	80	12,795	4738 to 23,196	6.65 (p < 0.001)
Posterior	80	8233	3172 to 19,293	
β-Glucuronidase activity (F.u.)				
Anterior	80	32.34	17.82 to 54.15	4.72 (p < 0.001)
Posterior	80	25.74	12.83 to 42.65	
Acid phenylphosphatase activity (e.u.)				
Anterior	80	14.27	6.42 to 25.93	1.83 (p = 0.034)
Posterior	80	13.09	6.83 to 22.28	

Note: the Wilcoxon test is used for *matched* pairs (e.g., morning versus evening) whereas the Mann-Whitney test is used for *independent* samples (e.g., spring versus fall).

Table 2-9. Variations in alveolar bone turnover during orthodontic treatment (11-to-13-year-old boys)

(A) LIGHT INTERMITTENT MESIALLY DIRECTED FORCES

Growth rotation *Distal side: formation*	N	Median difference before and after treatment		Mann-Whitney U test value of Z
Alkaline phenylphosphatase activity (enzyme units, e.u.)				
Anterior	40	1062	(334 to 1410)	5.96
Posterior	40	387	(93 to 1151)	(p < 0.001)
^{45}Ca uptake (counts per minute, c.p.m.)				
Anterior	40	51,377	(14,709 to 85,480)	6.77
Posterior	40	15,121	(2297 to 44,004)	(p < 0.001)
Mesial side: resorption				
β-Glucuronidase activity (Fishman units, F.u.)				
Anterior	40	306.27	(100.55 to 418.64)	5.01
Posterior	40	147.45	(47.50 to 304.72)	(p < 0.001)
Acid phenylphosphatase activity (e.u.)				
Anterior	40	131.85	(45.87 to 170.46)	7.27
Posterior	40	39.95	(19.71 to 88.50)	(p < 0.001)

(B) AS FUNCTION OF INTENSITY AND DURATION OF APPLIED FORCES

Forces (mesially directed) *Distal side: formation*	N	Median difference (before and after treatment)		Mann-Whitney U test value of Z		
				H.I.	L.C.	H.C.
Alkaline phenylphosphatase activity (e.u.)						
Light intermittent (L.I.)	40	1062	(334 to 1410)	1.80 (p=0.04)	5.65 (p<0.001)	5.88 (p<0.001)
Heavy intermittent (H.I.)	25	885	(285 to 1360)		3.95 (p<0.001)	4.82 (p<0.001)
Light continuous (L.C.)	25	436	(231 to 962)			2.54 (p=0.005)
Heavy continuous (H.C.)	20	322	(127 to 743)			
^{45}Ca uptake (c.p.m.)						
L.I.	40	51,377	(14,709 to 85,480)	1.79 (p=0.04)	5.92 (p<0.001)	5.96 (p<0.001)
H.I.	25	42,703	(12,412 to 74,386)		4.82 (p<0.001)	5.57 (p<0.001)
L.C.	25	22,781	(4349 to 40,307)			3.68 (p<0.001)
H.C.	20	8065	(1684 to 27,544)			
Mesial side: resorption						
β-Glucuronidase activity (F.u.)						
L.I.	40	306.27	(100.55 to 418.64)	2.56 (p=0.005)	5.25 (p<0.001)	5.23 (p<0.001)
H.I.	25	191.00	(103.10 to 398.33)		2.86 (p=0.002)	5.28 (p<0.001)
L.C.	25	158.26	(71.66 to 205.28)			4.59 (p<0.001)
H.C.	20	68.80	(16.17 to 173.90)			
Acid phenylphosphatase activity (e.u.)						
L.I.	40	131.85	(45.87 to 170.46)	4.30 (p<0.001)	6.45 (<0.001)	6.26 (p<0.001)
H.I.	25	83.29	(40.10 to 120.88)		5.25 (p<0.001)	5.60 (p<0.001)
L.C.	25	37.68	(22.47 to 72.15)			3.79 (p=0.001)
H.C.	20	24.86	(5.55 to 47.48)			

3. Research now in progress (Stutzmann and Petrovic, 1984) indicates that variations in the magnitude and duration of force may affect the type of collagen in the periodontal ligament (Fig. 2-14). With light forces, only collagen I is detected. This corresponds to the normal nonorthodontic situation. With heavy continuous forces, not only collagen I but also collagen III is found. Collagen III is usually associated with tissue repair.

Do the findings reported by Stutzmann and Petrovic relative to alveolar bone turnover correspond to clinical observations? Orthodontists who treated patients in whom the alveolar bone had been investigated were asked to evaluate semiquantitatively *for each individual* the clinical effectiveness (0 to +4) of the treatment 1 year later. In this way it was possible to compare statistically the clinical effectiveness of the treatment with the findings relative to alveolar bone turnover (Table 2-10). There was strong agreement that the higher the alveolar bone turnover rate the faster was the movement of teeth and the shorter the duration of the treatment.

This last point (duration) is of paramount importance, for it means that, independent of the variety and modality of an orthodontic treatment, the rapidity and duration of the treatment are dependent on the basic alveolar bone turnover rate (which characterizes a given individual, of a given sex and at a given age). It is now up to clinical orthodontic investigation to test further the validity and the applicability of these conclusions based on the physiologic findings relative to human alveolar bone turnover *before* and *after* an orthodontic treatment.

Generally the high turnover rate of mandibular alveolar bone is associated with *anterior* growth rotation, the standard turnover rate with *neutral* growth rotation, and the low turnover rate with *posterior* growth rotation. These findings are confirmed in 11-to-13-year-old boys who have undergone (surgical treatment of mandibular fractures (in the area of the ramus): In anterior growth rotation the subperiosteal ossification was significantly higher than in posterior growth rotation (Table 2-11) (Petrovic and Stutzmann, 1982).

The reported investigations of alveolar bone turnover before and 10 days after the onset of orthodontic treatment elucidate greater clinical effectiveness in patients whose mandible presents an *anterior* rather than a *posterior* growth rotation (Fig. 2-15). Still, the clinical situation is always more complex than the general biomedical and orthodontic rules suggest. Indeed, according to Stutzmann and Petrovic (1984), about 20% of 11-to-13-year-old boys with a high turnover rate of the mandibular alveolar bone displayed not an "anterior" but a "posterior" growth rotation. Interestingly, in about two thirds of such cases the children suffered from respiratory or allergic problems.

Once more, a better knowledge of underlying physiologic and pathophysiologic mechanisms should lead to a better use of therapeutic armamentaria. To have orthodontic control of biologic laws implies an accurate and detailed understanding of the normal order of living matter.

Finally, an organ culture study of human alveolar bone turnover rate has been designed that will test whether the Fränkel appliance effect results in forward movement of the mandibular premolars (Petrovic et al.,

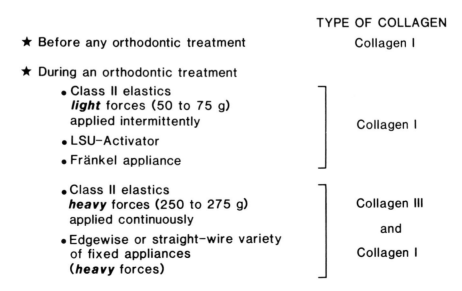

Fig. 2-14. Type of collagen in the periodontal ligament as a function of orthodontic treatment.

Table 2-10. Human alveolar bone turnover as a function of the clinical effectiveness of orthodontic treatment

Origin: Mandibular first premolar alveolar bone removed from 11-to-13-year-old boys and organ-cultured for 3 days
Treatment: Light intermittent mesially directed forces. Daily duration: approximately 16 hours. Mandible in anterior growth rotation

Effectiveness of orthodontic treatment	Observations	Median	Range	Effectiveness of orthodontic treatment	Observations	Median	Range
(A) ALKALINE PHOSPHATASE ACTIVITY (enzyme units, e.u.)				**(E) ALKALINE PHOSPHATASE ACTIVITY (e.u.)**			
0	—			0	—		
0 +	—			0 +	3	131	128 to 134
+	1	152		+	20	152	135 to 164
+ +	5	152	148 to 179	+ +	10	157	152 to 163
+ + +	12	165	150 to 185	+ + +	7	166	157 to 173
+ + + +	22	182.5	160 to 212	+ + + +	—		
(B) ⁴⁵Ca UPTAKE (counts per minute, c.p.m.)				**(F) ⁴⁵Ca UPTAKE (c.p.m.)**			
0	—			0	—		
0 +	—			0 +	3	5984	5532 to 6471
+	1	6154		+	20	8669	4156 to 13,080
+ +	5	10,373	5429 to 12,954	+ +	10	12,310	9705 to 14,242
+ + +	12	13,152	7538 to 17,346	+ + +	7	15,958	11,723 to 19,293
+ + + +	22	15,806	11,963 to 23,196	+ + + +	—		
(C) ACID PHENYLPHOSPHATASE ACTIVITY (e.u.)				**(G) ACID PHENYLPHOSPHATASE ACTIVITY (e.u.)**			
0	—			0	—		
0 +	—			0 +	3	7.56	7.09 to 8.31
+	1	7.16		+	20	12.86	8.13 to 16.24
+ +	5	12.49	8.27 to 14.84	+ +	10	18.30	15.58 to 20.81
+ + +	12	14.78	10.31 to 20.18	+ + +	7	21.16	15.87 to 22.58
+ + + +	22	17.63	13.06 to 25.93	+ + + +	—		
(D) β-GLUCURONIDASE ACTIVITY (Fishman units, F.u.)				**(H) β-GLUCURONIDASE ACTIVITY (F.u.)**			
0	—			0	—		
0 +	—			0 +	3	25.48	24.63 to 27.01
+	1	23.20		+	20	30.45	20.32 to 35.24
+ +	5	32.31	25.23 to 44.86	+ +	10	37.03	32.98 to 41.84
+ + +	12	42.92	30.64 to 49.86	+ + +	7	39.32	35.52 to 42.65
+ + + +	22	45.86	38.47 to 54.15	+ + + +	—		

Table 2-11. Quantitative estimation of ³H-thymidine–labeled cells in the mandibular subperiosteal layer (11-to-13-year-old boys)

Growth rotation of the mandible	N	Median (%)	Range (%)	Median test (×2)
Anterior	65	7.5	0.4 to 14.5	
				24.81 (p<0.001)
Posterior	64	4.1	0.2 to 14.9	

1982f). According to these findings, the therapeutic effect of the Fränkel Function Regulator is certainly not a result of dentoalveolar changes in the mandible. An orthopedically elicited *supplement* of mandibular growth is postulated and has already been demonstrated in the growing rat.

BIFURCATION TYPE OF SITUATION DURING FACIAL GROWTH—its meaning in the pathogenesis of malocclusion and in treatment planning

Every orthodontic treatment plan involves, to a great degree, growth prediction. Amazingly, most of the growth prediction methods implicitly take as a precondition the continuity of facial development. Experimen-

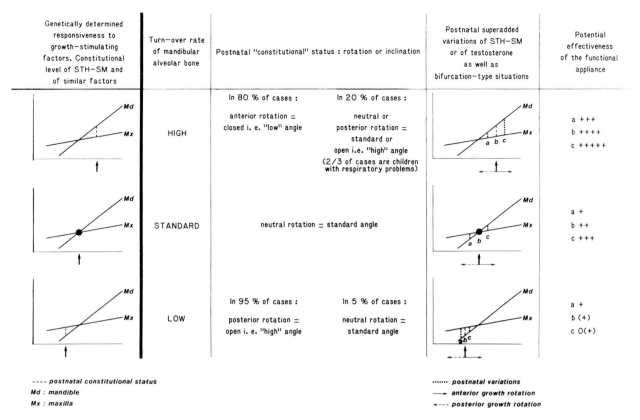

---- *postnatal constitutional status*
Md : mandible
Mx : maxilla

······ *postnatal variations*
⟶ *anterior growth rotation*
◀--- *posterior growth rotation*

Fig. 2-15. Tentative matching of findings in humans (turnover rate of mandibular alveolar bone, postnatal constitutional inclination and rotation, effectiveness of various functional appliances) with experimental findings in the rat (postnatal superadded variations of STH-somatomedin and/or testosterone as well as "bifurcation-type" situations of incisors). Positive correlation between the turnover rate of mandibular alveolar bone as estimated *before* treatment and the effectiveness of functional appliances as estimated by the clinician 1 year *after* the onset of the treatment. In our samples, when the alveolar bone turnover rate was high, only children with respiratory and/or allergy problems displayed a neutral or even posterior growth rotation sometimes associated with a deep bite.

tal investigations have detected the existence of nonlinear and unanticipated variations in the growth rate and direction of the mandible resulting from bifurcation-type alterations of the intercuspal relationship (Petrovic et al., 1975b; Petrovic and Stutzmann, 1977). The experimental and cybernetic approach to this finding has revealed, furthermore, that among all the conceivable occlusion-forming patterns, only a limited number of occurrences are within the realm of biologic possibility and just a few are commonly realized during the process of postnatal facial growth and development (Petrovic and Stutzmann, 1977). In addition, recent clinical findings (Lavergne and Gasson, 1977, 1982) have led to a morphogenetic classification of human facial development that presupposes the existence of some kind of biologic *discontinuities*.

Moss and Salentijn (1970) have described a logarithmic growth of the human mandible, and there is no major reason to "refute" (in the Popperian sense) such a statement. However, this affirmation, based on using just three reference points, is poorly substantiated as yet.

Todd et al. (1980) and Todd and Mark (1981ab) have published a topologic method aiming at the description of facial development by using a transformation equation (cardioidal strain) between two stages of facial development. This method, although conceptually productive, has raised controversy (Bookstein, 1981; Todd and Mark, 1981ab) and reconsideration (Moiroud, 1981).

Cardioidal strain
$$\theta' = \theta$$
$$R' = R(1 + k(1 - \cos \theta))$$

As a point of special interest: according to Todd and Mark (1981ab), this method reflects the "global regularity of the biologic mechanisms that control growth."

The same cardioidal strain transformation equation has been used by Lavergne and Petrovic (1983), less to describe the facial development than to test precisely the actuality of a "global regularity" during postnatal craniofacial skeleton growth in the child.

Experimental investigations have demonstrated beyond any doubt that the occlusal relationship plays a significant role in the processes controlling facial growth. According to the servosystem theory (Petrovic et al., 1975b; Petrovic and Stutzmann, 1977), the growth of the mandible is subject to the modulating effects of regional and local factors including mechanisms that regulate the occlusal relationship. The so-called peripheral comparator of the servosystem is represented by the operation of "confrontation" between the upper and lower dental arches (Fig. 1-4). The peripheral comparator has several stable positions, each corresponding to some type of Class I, II, or III intercuspation. Any given occlusal relationship is stable with respect to limited fluctuations and disturbances. The stable positions are separated by unbalanced states corresponding generally (but not specifically) to cuspal occlusion. Each cusp-to-cusp unstable position corresponds to a functional discontinuity (i.e., to a topologic "bifurcation"-type instability as described by Thom [1972] and Zeeman [1976]). Lack of interdental contacts corresponds to the absence of both stable and "bifurcation" situations.

The topologic concept of discontinuity connotes that at critical points the servosystem behavior goes through some basic switch, implying continuous quantitative variations that still appear qualitative in nature (Petrovic and Stutzmann, 1977).

The values of the coefficient K have been calculated by Lavergne and Petrovic (1983) from cephalometric measurements. Careful analysis of the transformation coefficient K led to a major result: as long as there is no change in the molar relationship, the value of the coefficient K does not vary significantly from one reference point to another on the bony profile; but as soon as there is a shift in the molar relationship, the coefficient value will not be the same anymore for points located on the mandible and on the midface and skull. This finding brings to light the existence of discontinuities during postnatal facial growth in the child. It also strongly suggests the existence of a correlation, and even of a causal dependence, between the occlusal relationship and the growth of the facial skeleton, especially the mandible.

The occlusal development appears to involve *two* phases (Lavergne and Petrovic, 1983):

1. The first consists of all the morphogenetic processes that lead to a stable occlusion. During this phase different parts of the servosystem are already existent and functional, but the stage of a stable occlusal development capable of serving as a peripheral "comparator" is not yet achieved; and without an operational peripheral comparator having for reference a stable position between the lower and upper dental arches, the creation of an *engram** for the adequate postural activity of the masticatory muscles is not possible. The engram will serve as a reference for the central comparator. In other words, during the first phase the mandibular morphogenesis cannot be *regulated* through information originating from the occlusal relationships.

2. The beginning of the second phase coincides with the setting up of a stable occlusion, which serves as a peripheral comparator and which, in turn, is required for the formation of the central comparator reference (engram). (See Fig. 1-4.) From now on, the morphogenesis of the face will be regulated to minimize possible deviations from the achieved stable occlusal adjustment, regardless of whether this occlusal relationship corresponds to a Class I, Class II, or Class III intercuspation.

From the clinical viewpoint there is a matter of concern: The duration of the first phase may vary; short in some children, it may be long in others and even permanent in those in whom an actual peripheral comparator is never established.

Depending on the relationship between the maxilla and the mandible, the denture as a whole or only one group of teeth may be operating as a peripheral comparator of the servosystem. In the latter case, recent findings (Lavergne and Petrovic, 1983) show the existence of a clinically interesting consistency: the peripheral comparator may be located in the area of the molars or near the incisors or sometimes the canines.

The problem is not just an academic one. In the *posteriorly* rotating mandible special therapeutic attention should be given to the molar group whereas in the *anterior* rotation major consideration should be assigned to the incisor and canine group. Indeed, the action of the peripheral comparator is an important part of both orthodontic and orthopedic treatment. It is obvious that whenever, in a growing child, a curative measure alters the position of the group of teeth operating as a part of the peripheral comparator (incisor-canine group in anteriorly rotating mandibles, molar group in posteriorly rotating mandibles, or denture as a whole in many cases) we are dealing not only with an orthodontic treatment (moving the teeth) but also with a functional or orthopedic one (modulating the rate, amount, and direction of growth in the facial skeleton).

---

*According to Petrovic and Stutzmann (1977), this engram is developed through the repeated sagittal positioning of the mandible that is coincident with the minimization of "deviation signals" originating from the occlusal adjustment. Deviation is detected by appropriate periodontal, dental, muscular, and temporomandibular joint capsule receptors. Such minimization is achieved in a stable, either optimal (Class I) or suboptimal (full Class II or full Class III), occlusal relationship.

According to the concept developed by Lavergne and Petrovic (1983), the pathogenesis of many interjaw malrelations is to be looked for in the malfunctioning of the servosystem. Although there are several alternatives, so far just two basic situations have been distinguished:

1. The malfunctioning of the servosystem appears to involve mainly the peripheral comparator.
   a. It may be morphologically defective (e.g., multiple caries, extreme bruxism).
   b. It may be morphologically acceptable but its reference inadequate (e.g., an anteriorly rotating mandible associated with a distal basal interjaw relationship, a posteriorly rotating mandible associated with a mesial basal interjaw relationship).
2. The malfunctioning of the growth process control appears to result mainly from the shortcoming of the servosystem. Basically the control system operates faultlessly, but it is unable fully to correct the discrepancy between growth rates of the upper and lower jaws.
   a. This may be observed in an anteriorly rotating mandible associated with a mesial basal interjaw relationship (Class III).
   b. It may also be seen in a posteriorly rotating mandible associated with a distal basal interjaw relationship (Class II).

Needless to say, the no. 2 situation may be coupled with either 1a or 1b.

What should the orthodontist keep in mind from all these developments?

The cybernetic theory of facial growth and the crucial topologic concept of structural and functional stability and instability (Petrovic et al., 1975b; Petrovic and Stutzmann, 1977) are useful tools in a systematic and computerized approach to clinical situations with regard to diagnosis, prognosis, and therapeutics (Lavergne, 1982; Lavergne and Gasson, 1982).

The existence of discontinuities in the functioning of the peripheral comparator of the servosystem controlling the growth of the facial skeleton is unquestionably a salient point in growth prediction as well as in treatment planning and decision making. The first of these statements implies that what may appear during the growth period as an *invariant* is, in fact, the result of a physiologic *regulation;* for a given occlusal relationship, random (purposeless but not causeless) growth fluctuations are detected and counterbalanced. It also implies that the final pattern of occlusal relationships emerges in a series of bifurcations having, to some extent (but to some extent only), a random character. Indeed, a given occlusal pattern (Class I or Class II or Class III) may have been initiated by nonessential or fortuitous influences; but, once it is formed, it remains relatively unaltered because random growth fluctuations are neutralized by means of regulatory mechanisms and local optimization processes. In other words, a full Class II, with a stable occlusal relationship; will but rarely grow into a Class I; only an appropriate orthodontic or orthopedic treatment may successfully achieve such a conversion.

The existence of discontinuities (i.e., of bifurcation-type situations at the peripheral comparator of the servosystem) implies that facial growth can be accounted for by taking advantage of stochastic discrete models rather than making use of deterministic continuous ones. This statement also bears on models designed for growth forecasting in the orthodontic treatment program and follow-up.

Along these lines, the existence of discontinuities at the peripheral comparator also makes intelligible the fact that the genotype only partially determines the phenotype. Indeed, a specific genome is encoded for an overall regulatory pattern not for a singular phenotype (i.e., for an inventory of possible stable situations). Under such conditions, at crucial moments of facial development, *very small* fluctuations taking place around the bifurcation can lead to two very different types of occlusal relationships. A case in point is the ultimate status of the occlusion resulting from a flush terminal plane occlusal relationship. Depending on a number of local factors, this bifurcation-type condition can lead to a Class I, a Class II, or a Class III malocclusion.

CLINICAL MEANING OF EXPERIMENTAL FINDINGS RELATIVE TO CRANIOFACIAL GROWTH MECHANISMS—and to the modus operandi of functional appliances

The question often arises "What is the interest, for the clinician, of concepts based on experimental research findings?" The answer is rather simple. Animal experimentation takes aim at the formulation of biologic and biomedical laws and at the *explanation* of biologic mechanisms underlying specific pathologic states. This does not imply endorsement of extrapolation-type statements that apply to what might occur in humans in a specific situation, either normal or pathologic (Petrovic, 1972; Petrovic et al., 1975b; Petrovic and Stutzmann, 1980a). However, if no significant morphologic difference can be detected between specific mammalian species for a given entity of the tissue cell or molecular level, then rejection of biologic similarity is unscientific and methodologically unsound. A specific example is the condylar cartilage. Some clinicians even make a more serious methodologic error. They seem to disregard the well-grounded fact that, biologically, the behavior of the condylar cartilage is strikingly different from the behavior of primary-type cartilages.

The most remarkable observations, in this respect, were made recently at the molecular biology level (Petrovic, 1982; Stutzmann and Petrovic, 1982) and can be summarized as follows:

1. In growing rats *and* children the cytosolic level of Na^+ is higher in secondary-type cartilage prechondroblasts and in primary-type chondroblasts than in secondary-type chondroblasts. Lower cytosolic levels of Na^+ account, to a large extent, for the repression of mitogenesis-specific genes in secondary-type chondroblasts (i.e., for the loss of their ability to divide).

2. In growing rats *and* children the cytosolic Ca^{++} concentration is basically lower in preosteoblasts and secondary-type prechondroblasts (globular cells, high rate of multiplication) than in skeletoblasts (flattened cells, low rate of multiplication).

3. In growing rats *and* children the cytosolic level of Ca^{++} is lower in actively dividing secondary-type prechondroblasts than in prechondroblasts about to mature into secondary-type chondroblasts.

4. In growing rats *and* children an appropriate force applied to the condylar cartilage in organ culture experiments produces a significant decrease of cytosolic Na^+ concentration in condylar cartilage prechondroblasts. Compressive forces of similar or higher magnitude do *not* produce detectable changes of cytosolic Na^+ concentration in metatarsal growth cartilage or in the epiphyseal plate chondroblasts of the tibia, fibula, and radius.

5. In growing rats *and* children the osteochondral zone of the rib displays a biologic peculiarity. The area where the precursor chondroblast differentiates into the progenitor chondroblast (see p. 24) *(and this area exclusively)* is responsive to local biomechanical factors. Indeed, in organ culture experiments, when appropriate pressure was applied to the rib fragment, a decrease in both the number of mitoses and the corresponding variations in ionic fluxes was observed in the area of differentiation of precursor into progenitor chondroblasts. The biomechanically caused modifiability of the rat and infant osteochondral rib zone is certainly of less magnitude than that detected in the condylar cartilage. Nevertheless, such a biomechanically induced modifiability appears to be totally lacking in the metatarsal growth cartilage as well as in other so-called primary cartilages.

In organ culture experiments therefore *each variety* of rat and human cartilage can be said to display a similar responsiveness to biomechanical factors, especially evident at the molecular biology level. Accordingly, in growing rats, when the postural hyperpropulsor, Fränkel appliance, L.S.U. activator, Bionator, and even Class II elastics all produce a significant decrease of cytosolic Ca^{++} concentration in skeletoblasts and prechondroblasts as well as a significant increase of cytosolic Na^+ concentration in condylar cartilage prechondroblasts, and when tensile forces of similar or higher magnitude do not produce detectable changes of cytosolic Na^+ concentration in metatarsal growth cartilage and in the tibia, fibula, and radius epiphyseal plate chondroblasts, then there is no valid reason to discount the ability of functional appliances to modulate (stimulate or restrain) the growth rate of the human condylar cartilage and, secondarily, of the subperiosteal ossification rate at the posterior border of the mandible.

A provocative counterpart of the viewpoint concerning the biologic similarity or dissimilarity at the tissue and cell level is represented by the mode of lengthening of the maxilla. In both the rat and the monkey, as well as in almost all other mammals, the premaxillomaxillary suture contributes substantially to the sagittal growth of the maxilla during the major part of the postnatal period; yet in the human the premaxillomaxillary suture cannot be considered at all as contributing to the lengthening of the maxilla (Stutzmann and Petrovic, 1976, 1978a).

In other words, the interspecies validity of experimental findings depends not so much on the zoologic or evolutionary relationship between two mammals as on the *morphophysiologic similarity between the tissues and cells* under scrutiny. However, even in the case of biologic similarity, experimental findings are merely powerful *conceptual tools* in clinical investigations; indeed, the methodologically valid corroboration of a working hypothesis formulated from animal experimentation can be gathered only in the human species itself, and then only in specific and appropriate observational conditions. Even when a structure such as the condylar cartilage or a process such as subperiosteal ossification is almost identical in various mammals, there are still some *quantitative* differences in the relative cell and tissue amounts as well as in the responsiveness to various factors exerting, actually or potentially, an influence on the structure under scrutiny. In addition, future research investigations may always yield new information implicating the existence of some differences between two mammals. Finally, it should never be forgotten that even in the human species itself significant differences may exist *between individuals*. For instance, between individuals with an anteriorly rotating mandible (highly responsive to functional appliances) and individuals with a posteriorly rotating mandible (much less responsive to functional appliances), a marked variability in response can be seen.

The quantitative aspects of comparing the effects of a factor in two different mammals should be elaborated.

In their experimental and clinical investigations relative to the sodium fluoride (NaF) dose administered and to the bone turnover rate, Petrovic and Shambaugh (1966, 1968) made a very interesting observation. They were able to determine which daily dose of NaF stimulated *optimally* and *safely* bone formation and mineralization in the rat and the human. The question then arose: "Taking into account the difference in body size between the rat and the human, which parameter should be selected *as the reference* for the quantitative comparison of the optimum doses as empirically detected?"

• The body weight? In this case the optimum daily dose of NaF is relatively much lower in the human than in the rat. So, with the body weight as reference, the dose determined to be optimal in rats would be toxic in humans.

• The body surface? In this case, the optimum daily dose of NaF appears to be about the same in rats and in humans. This finding is, in fact, perfectly logical: mathematically, the metabolic rate is a function of the body surface; and it is physiologically and pharmacologically legitimate and plausible that the action of NaF would depend on the metabolic rate.

It follows from this example that the effect of a factor in two animal species (rat and human) may be compared not only qualitatively but also quantitatively, provided the mechanism of action is known and, accordingly, the proper reference of quantitative comparison is selected.

BIOLOGIC PECULIARITIES OF THE MANDIBLE—
occlusal pattern and cephalometric findings

In light of our research investigations in the rat (Petrovic, 1982; Petrovic et al., 1982b) and the human (Lavergne and Petrovic, 1983), how can we describe the functional relationships between tissue and cell determinants of the growing mandible, on the one side, and general extrinsic factors (e.g., hormones) and local extrinsic factors (biomechanical agents), on the other?

This is definitely a crucial problem in clinical orthodontics. Indeed, the orthodontist may alter the local biomechanical situation; but so far it has not been possible to modulate specific tissue and cell characteristics, since they seem to be determined genetically. Nevertheless, there is a salient point: inability to modify specific features of the mandibular tissues does not bestow the right to ignore them. On the contrary, the orthodontist must make a special effort to be acquainted with the distinctive features of the facial skeleton so their existence will be recognized and their involvement in the treatment effect considered. The reasons are obvious: first, a better knowledge and understanding of mandibular tissue behavior and responsiveness to intrinsic and extrinsic factors make the diagnosis of a skeletal malre-

lation or malocclusion more accurate; second, the choice of the most appropriate therapeutic procedure depends primarily on the biologic responsiveness of the involved tissues. The difficult problem is deciding how the orthodontist can acquire information about the biologic peculiarities of the facial skeleton tissues in an individual patient.

Several approaches to this problem have been described and widely discussed in the orthodontic community. In this section a new approach, founded on cephalometric analysis, will be presented and compared point by point with animal experiments as well as with cell and molecular biology findings in different mammals, including humans (Lavergne and Petrovic, 1983 and unpublished data).

Previous investigations have shown that there is a new way of categorizing children that takes into consideration both the mandible and the maxilla, directing attention to individuals who are morphogenetically and morphologically alike and who grow and respond alike to a given type of orthopedic or functional treatment (for details see Lavergne, 1982; Lavergne and Gasson, 1982; Lavergne and Petrovic, 1983). This systematization has recently been further elaborated (Lavergne and Petrovic, 1985), presently taking the form of a three-level arborization (Fig. 2-16):

1. The first level, based on the quantitative determination of the difference between maxillary and mandibular sagittal growth (Lavergne and Gasson, 1977; Lavergne and Petrovic, 1985), likewise has three main branches.

   a. In about 70% of the children in the Strasbourg sample, sagittal growth of the mandible and the maxilla remained quantitatively in the same range. Any tendency toward sagittal deviation from the normal occlusal relationship during growth was either physiologically corrected through the "peripheral comparator" of the servosystem as described by Petrovic (1974) or orthopedically curable (by appropriate functional appliances).

   b. In about 3% of the children, sagittal growth of the mandible was by far superior to that of the maxilla.

   c. In about 25% of the children, sagittal growth of the mandible was by far inferior to that of the maxilla.

   In the two last situations (i.e., b and c) the spontaneous servosystem correction of the discrepancy was moderate (clinically insufficient). Even an orthopedic treatment using a functional appliance is usually *not fully* efficient.

   Cell and organ culture investigations strongly suggest that the first-level trifurcation results

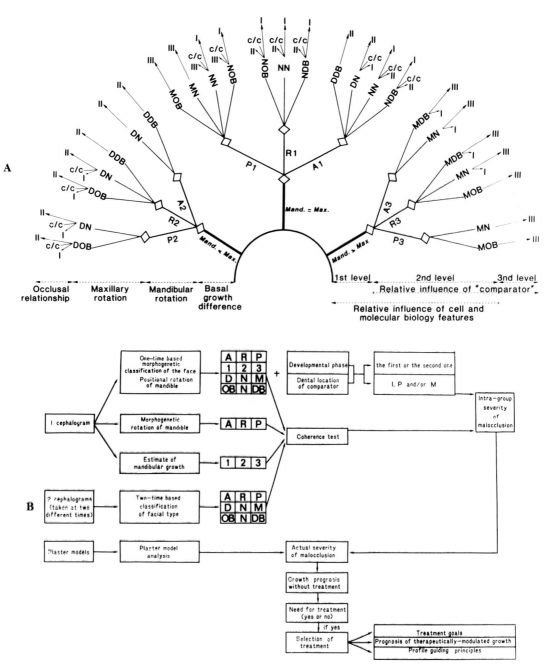

Fig. 2-16. Morphogenetic classification of human facial development according to Lavergne and Petrovic (1983).

A, Three-level arborization. *I, II,* and *III,* First molar occlusal relationships (stable); *c/c,* cusp-to-cusp molar relationships (unstable); *long straight arrow,* main outcome; *short arrow,* less frequent outcome; *straight line,* unachieved outcome.

B, Flow diagram of orthodontic planning. Only 25 of the 33 outcomes at the second level are represented; 8 outcomes (constituting 3% of the population studied) are omitted. *A, R,* and *P,* Anterior, neutral, and posterior mandibular rotation; *1, 2,* and *3,* mandible equal to, less than, or greater than maxilla; *D, N,* and *M,* posteroanterior state distal, normal, or mesial; *OB, N,* and *DB,* openbite, normal, and deep bite. For example, *R1NN* means neutral mandibular growth rotation, small basal growth difference, normal basal posteroanterior relationship, and normal basal vertical relationship.

C, Sequence for identifying **(C₁)** growth rotation group, **(C₂)** morphogenetic rotation of the mandible, **(C₃)** growth of the mandible, and **(C₄)** location of the comparator. Each group consists of patients who are morphogenetically and morphologically similar, which means they grow and respond to a particular type of treatment in almost the same way.

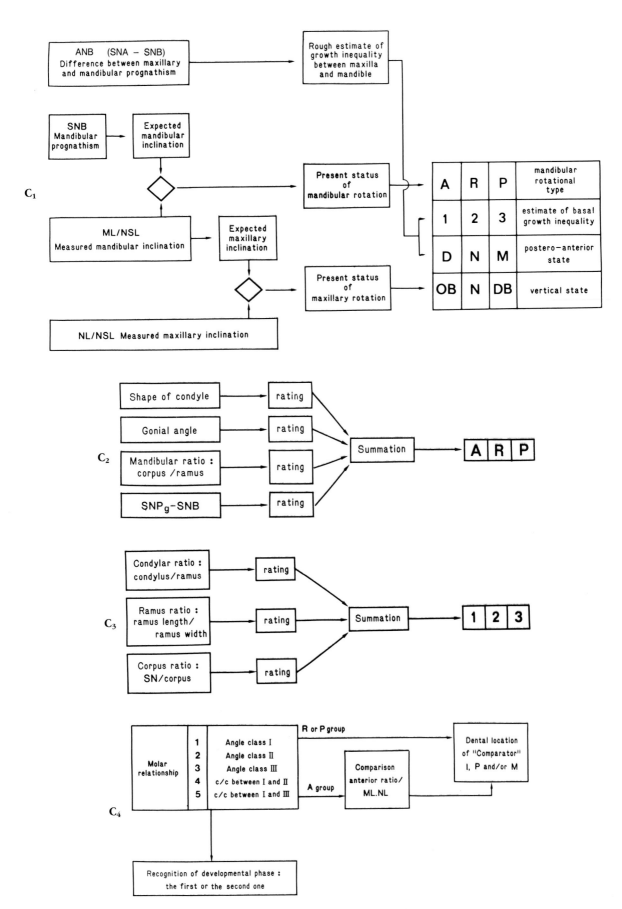

Fig. 2-16, cont'd. For legend see opposite page.

from quantitative differences at the cell and molecular biology level. Indeed, to take an example (Petrovic, 1982), changes in ionic (Na^+, Ca^{++}, H^+) flux rates and in the percentage of mitoses in human condylar cartilage under the influence of hormones (STH-somatomedin, insulin) and local biomechanical factors is by far smaller in the c. branch than in the a. branch. Furthermore, the mitotic index in the mandibular subperiosteal layer and the turnover rate of the alveolar bone are also smaller in the c. branch (Stutzmann and Petrovic, 1984).

2. The second level, based on the variations in direction of mandibular and maxillary growth, leads to ramifications overlying each of the three main branches. It relates to what is called "growth inclination" and "growth rotation" of both the mandible and the maxilla. The variations observed at this ramification level depend at least partly on respiration, phonation, and deglutition (normal or abnormal) factors. The occlusal relationship functioning as the peripheral comparator of the physiologic servosystem that regulates the growth rate of the mandible plays a rather subordinant role; however, in some clinical situations it can markedly modulate the *direction* of growth of the condyle and even of the ramus.

3. The third level, based on the occlusal relationship functioning as the peripheral comparator of the servosystem, has subdivisions that may represent either an aggravation or a melioration of the malocclusion resulting from the first two arborizational levels. Both full Class I and full Class II intercuspations correspond to a stable occlusal situation; they are separated by unstable occlusions (cusp-to-cusp), which represent functional "discontinuities." A stable occlusion coincides with a well-established "comparator reference" functioning cybernetically as an "attractor" (p. 17); that is, any tendency toward sagittal deviation from the stable occlusion will be detected by the peripheral comparator and, consequently, reduced or even canceled through the servosystem. From this point of view, the sagittal deviation appears to be the *first cause* initiating regulatory physiologic processes and a stable occlusion (either Class I or Class II) is the *ultimate outcome*. Logically a full Class II with a stable occlusal relationship will seldom if ever be allowed to grow spontaneously into a Class I.

Topologically an unstable occlusal relationship corresponds to a bifurcation type of situation and acts as a "repeller." For example, there is in the second-level arborization a group in which 50% of the children have, at the time of permanent first molar eruption, an unstable (i.e., bifur-

cation-type) situation. Later on, in half these children the occlusal relationship will develop into a Class I, and in the other half into a Class II. A salient point is as follows: in the unstable occlusal situation (the "repeller"), a minimal fluctuation in molar position can lead to one or another stable situation; in other words, it can be the source of two types of occlusal relationship. This minimal fluctuation can be either "spontaneous" (dental disharmonies, e.g., variations in tooth size and form, caries, early loss of teeth) or therapeutically induced (i.e., facebow, the appliance indicated in this specific example) (Lavergne and Petrovic, 1983).

This new way of reasoning in dentofacial orthopedics leads to a number of conclusions (Fig. 2-17):

1. The occlusal situation, including skeletal and dental malrelations, is determined by morphophysiologic characteristics (represented formally by the three-level arborization). In shifting from the first to the third level, the proportion of basic tissue and cell peculiarities decreases whereas the proportion of the interdental relation pattern increases. Because of "vertical" feedback connections among the three levels of the arborization, any appropriate physiologic or orthopedic operation that puts to use the comparator and the servosystem and aims at modulating the occlusal adjustment will exert a mild regulating effect on the growth amount and have a powerful regulating effect on the morphogenetic rotation of the mandible (Lavergne and Gasson, 1977). Accordingly, treatment of skeletal malrelations could be greatly facilitated if therapeutic agents were able to amplify the mandibular tissue and cell responsiveness to functional appliances. Needless to say, such amplifying agents remain to be discovered and carefully investigated.

2. A Class I or Class II occlusal situation may have been initiated by casual fluctuations at the peripheral comparator of the servosystem; but, once established, a given occlusal pattern will remain basically unaltered. Indeed, random growth fluctuations are constantly regulated by regional and local feedback mechanisms and local optimization processes (Petrovic, 1974, 1977, 1982).

CONCLUSION

The treatment of dentofacial malrelations implies a considerable insight into the modalities of craniofacial growth. In addition, this growth cannot be adequately understood without a knowledge of the mechanisms controlling it and of the essential role played by hormones (e.g., STH and somatomedin, sexual hormones, thyroxine) as well as the role of the lateral pterygoid muscle, retrodiscal pad (meniscotemporocondylar frenum), and local mediator-type and regulator-type chemical factors.

This is why research has concentrated on the *simultaneous* study of the effects of hormones and orthopedic and functional appliances on craniofacial growth. Results have demonstrated that the interaction

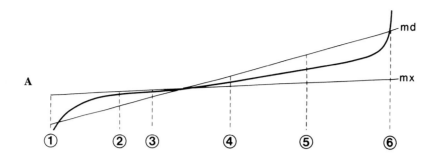

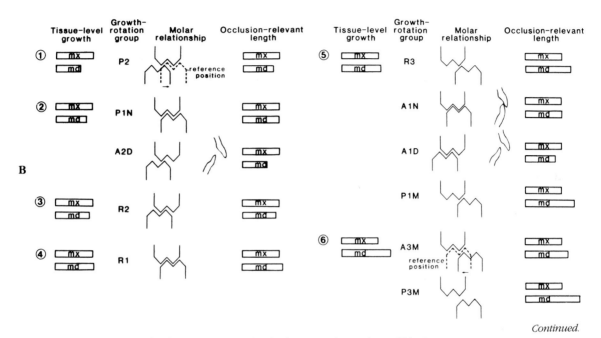

Continued.

Fig. 2-17. Tissue-level growth concept for the human and animal mandible (rat, guinea pig, mouse, rabbit, squirrel, monkey) based on the correlation between alveolar bone turnover rate and condylar cartilage growth and responsiveness to functional appliances. Indeed, the mean alveolar bone turnover rate for each parameter of the distal and mesial sides is an expression of the tissue-level growth rate (basically constitutional but to some extent modulated by hormones and other factors controlling skeletal growth).

The difference between the distal and mesial sides for the two parameters of alveolar bone formation (alkaline phosphatase, ^{45}Ca uptake) and the two parameters of alveolar bone resorption (β-glucuronidase, acid phosphatase) allows us to estimate the direction and magnitude of spontaneous posteroanterior movement of the first premolar (i.e., before any orthodontic movement).

Eleven individual cases (representing 11 growth rotation groups according to the classification of Lavergne and Petrovic, see Fig. 2-16) are arranged in order of increasing mean values of tissue-level growth rate. Based on the mean values of alveolar turnover, these 11 rotational group cases actually fall into 6 categories, each corresponding to a specific situation as represented in Fig. 2-16 and accounting for the forward growth of the mandible in relation to the forward growth of the maxilla.

A and **B**, Tissue-level growth, growth rotation, and occlusion-relevant mandibular length as a frame of reference for the treatment decision. **C** and **D**, Tissue-level growth rate and posteroanterior movement of the first premolar as estimated from the alveolar bone turnover rate in boys 10 to 12 years of age.

The main findings are as follows:
1. The higher the mean value of the alveolar bone turnover rate, the greater will be the mandibular growth at the tissue level.
2. However, bifurcation-type events at the peripheral comparator of the servosystem (Lavergne and Petrovic, 1983) appear to be responsible, on their own, for the differences in occlusion-relevant length of the mandible and for the variations in the growth rotation types. Indeed, the growth rotation groups *P1N* and *A2D* belong to tissue level growth category 2; *R3, A1N, A1D,* and *P1M* belong to category 5; and *A3M* and *P3M* belong to category 6.

C

Category	Alveolar bone turnover rate "Growth rotation" group	Alkaline Phosphatase Activity				^{45}Ca uptake			
		distal side	MEAN VALUE	difference distal minus mesial	mesial side	distal side	MEAN VALUE	difference distal minus mesial	mesial side
1	P2	92	75	34	58	6583	5981	1204	5379
2	P1 N	123	107	32	91	10852	8879	3946	6906
	A2 D	118	115	5	113	9255	9114	281	8974
3	R2	130	129	2	128	9007	8804	405	8602
4	R1	162	154	15	147	9847	9482	729	9118
5	R3	185	164	41	144	15628	12242	6772	8856
	A1 N	154	158	- 8	162	11426	12081	- 1311	12737
	A1 D	142	159	- 34	176	9805	12027	- 4445	14250
	P1 M	187	161	52	135	15434	11963	6942	8492
6	A3 M	168	213	- 91	259	10512	16242	- 11460	21972
	P3 M	181	192	- 22	203	13603	14966	- 2726	16329

D

β-glucuronidase Activity				Acid Phosphatase Activity				Alveolar bone turnover rate level	Direction of premolar movement
distal side	MEAN VALUE	difference distal minus mesial	mesial side	distal side	MEAN VALUE	difference distal minus mesial	mesial side		
12.03	14.92	- 5.78	17.81	7.84	9.80	- 3.92	11.76	+	mesial
16.95	23.05	- 12.21	29.16	13.29	16.41	- 6.24	19.53	++	mesial
22.86	22.94	- 0.16	23.02	15.91	16.18	- 0.54	16.45	++	?
25.90	27.67	- 3.54	29.44	19.18	19.59	- 0.83	20.01	++	?
25.86	32.32	- 12.92	38.78	19.64	21.16	- 3.05	22.69	++	mesial
38.55	44.80	- 12.51	51.06	26.95	28.73	- 3.57	30.52	+++	mesial
49.02	45.91	6.21	42.81	31.25	29.68	3.14	28.11	+++	distal
51.33	44.43	13.80	37.53	32.56	28.41	8.30	24.26	+++	distal
37.25	45.68	- 16.87	54.12	22.47	28.02	- 11.10	33.57	+++	mesial
43.60	67.56	- 47.92	91.52	28.76	42.62	- 27.72	56.48	++++	distal
51.28	56.66	- 10.77	62.05	38.52	41.30	- 5.57	44.09	++++	distal

Fig. 2-17, cont'd. For legend see p. 65.

between functional or orthodontic appliances and certain hormones governing craniofacial skeletal growth is such that no rational planning of therapy is possible without taking this interaction into account.

According to experimental investigations in the rat and other laboratory animals, appropriate functional appliances, placing the mandible in a forward postural position, increase the condylar cartilage growth rate and, secondarily, the subperiosteal ossification rate at the posterior border of the mandible. Consequently, the mandible becomes longer than in control animals.

With time, during the growth period the sagittal deviation produced by the postural hyperpropulsor will decrease through the supplementary forward growth of the mandible. This implies that, simultaneously, the deviation signal will also decrease (i.e., the supplementary growth rate of the condylar cartilage *and* the supplementary lengthening rate of the mandible).

Recurrent reactivation (increasing the thickness) of the postural hyperpropulsor involves a new increase in lateral pterygoid activity as recorded electromyographically (and, certainly, a new increase in retrodiscal pad activity) and, consequently, will bring about a new increase in the rate and amount of condylar cartilage and mandibular growth. In other words, functional maxipropulsion involving *periodic* forward repositioning appears to be the best procedure for eliciting orthopedic mandibular lengthening.

When the appliance (postural hyperpropulsor, L.S.U. activator, Fränkel Function Regulator, Bionator, Class II elastics) is removed after the growth of the animal is completed, no relapse is observed. When the appliance is removed before growth is completed no significant relapse is detected *if* a good intercuspation has been achieved during the experimental phase; if a good intercuspation has *not* been achieved, the comparator of the servosystem imposes either an increased or a decreased condylar growth rate until a given state of intercuspal stability is established.

No genetically predetermined final length of the mandible was detected in these experiments. Functional and orthopedic appliances may be the cause of an increased or a decreased final length of the mandible. However, there is a genetically determined responsiveness of various growth sites to growth-stimulating or growth-inhibiting factors (Fig. 2-9):

As for the functional appliances, Petrovic's experimental research investigations lead to the following tentative clinical implications:

- The postural hyperpropulsor, Andresen-Häupl activator, Fränkel appliance, Bionator, and Class II elastics all exert their action mainly through the *movements* of the mandible. Their stimulating effect on condylar cartilage growth is produced chiefly *during* the wearing of the appliance.
- The Herren-type or L.S.U.-type activator and extraoral forward traction exert their action mainly through the sagittal repositioning of the mandible. This kind of functional appliance seems to have a two-step effect: during the time of wearing the appliance, the more forward positioning of the mandible is the cause of reduced growth of the lateral pterygoid muscle; simultaneously a new sensory engram is formed for the new positioning of the lower jaw. During the time that the activator is *not* worn, the mandible is functioning in the more forward position in such a way that the retrodiscal pad will be much more stimulated than in the controls. The increased repetitive activity of the retrodiscal pad produces an earlier beginning of the condylar chondroblast hypertrophy and, consequently, an increased growth rate of the condylar cartilage. In other words, the lateral pterygoid muscle does mediate the action of the activator but the stimulating effect on condylar growth appears to be produced almost exclusively during the time when the appliance is *not* worn.

CLOSING COMMENTS—the changing scene

A new technique is available for obtaining three-dimensional cross-sectional pictures of thin slices through the human head: nuclear-magnetic resonance imaging or NMR spectroscopy. In the ordinary procedure only the resonance of hydrogen nuclei is employed, yielding images of internal structure without the use of x-rays. In the future the administration of NMR "tracers" (short-lived radioactive phosphorus, carbon, sodium, manganese, etc.) will provide information on dynamic biochemical phenomena. In other words, the orthodontist will be able to analyze the functioning of some human tissue in situ, without biopsy. Many problems we are encountering today in animals will be investigated directly in human patients, without exposure to any real danger.

The image-processing by computer (CAT scan) is a new approach in craniofacial growth investigation. Automatic extraction of information provided by a different kind of image from that used in clinical orthodontics is becoming useful in daily practice with the development of new computer programs for pattern recognition.

It is a sad fact of life, however, that decision making is not always a completely rational process. Modern psychology of individual preferences has shown that such deviations from "pure" discursive reasoning often follow regular patterns, which should be investigated so that discrepancies between what is subjective and what is objective in clinical decisions can be discerned. Everyone knows that "risk quest" or "risk reluctance" (sometimes based on possible lawsuit!) may influence a surgical decision. Nevertheless, the orthodontist should be better aware of the rules of cognitive operations by which alternative realities are "fabricated" to be able to bring to light the biases that may misrepresent a set of clinical data and pervert his judgment and therapeutic choice.

The treatment decision as related to growth rotational categorization of the face according to Lavergne and Petrovic (Fig. 1-4, *C*) will become an assistive conceptual tool in orthodontic practice.

CHAPTER 3

PRINCIPLES OF
FUNCTIONAL APPLIANCES

Functional appliances are considered by many authorities to be orthopedic in nature, influencing the facial skeleton of the growing child in the condylar and sutural areas. This is not the only attribute of functional appliances, however, since they also exert an orthodontic effect on the dentoalveolar area. The uniqueness of functional appliances is their mode of force application. They do not act on the teeth like conventional appliances, using mechanical elements such as springs, elastics, or ligatures, but rather transmit, eliminate, or guide natural forces (e.g., muscle activity, growth, or tooth eruption).

The influences of natural forces and the functional stimulation on form were first reported by Roux in 1883 as a result of studies on the tail fin of a dolphin. He described the characteristics of functional stimuli as they build up, mold, remold, and preserve tissue. His working hypothesis became the background of both general orthopedic and functional dental orthopedic procedures.

Häupl saw the potential of the Roux hypothesis and applied his concepts to the correction of jaw and dental arch deformities, utilizing functional stimuli. Actually the clinical aspects had already been put into use by Andresen, and the results of the appliances were already apparent; but Häupl was able to explain how functional appliances worked through the activity of the orofacial muscles. Function is inherent in all cells, tissues, and organs. It influences the medium in which it works, literally as a functional stimulus. The goal of functional dental orthopedics is to utilize this functional stimulus, channeling it as far as the tissues, jaws, condyles, and teeth will allow. The mode of transmission is "passive" in the sense that mechanical force-producing elements are unnecessary. The forces that arise are purely functional and are intermittent in nature. According to Häupl, this is the only mode of force application that can build up tissue, since with continuous active forces bone remodeling cannot take place. Because of the ability of the passive appliance to transfer muscle forces from one area to another, functional orthopedic appliances were considered to be a "transformator."

As biologic as this approach seemed, the principles of Häupl and their application with activator therapy had some detrimental consequences for the development of orthodontics in Europe. Many orthodontists were convinced that only tissue preserving treatment, as exemplified by the activator, should be used. The application of mechanical force was considered unbiologic and a technical error.

The convictions of European orthodontists were enhanced by the research of Oppenheim, who published his investigations under the title "Crisis in orthodontics." He showed the potential tissue damaging side effects of heavy orthodontic forces. This strengthened the working hypothesis of Häupl, who decried the use of artificial mechanically produced forces on the tissues. For many schools throughout Europe the activator became the only, the universal, appliance. Too often, however, its widespread use was without differential diagnosis and correct application. Some European orthodontists even considered active removable appliances with screws and springs to be dangerous to the teeth and investing tissues.

Schwarz (1952) pointed out that the activators worked not only by transmitting functional force stimuli on an intermittent basis but also with light compressive forces like the removable active plates. Reitan, in his doctoral thesis in 1952, showed that no special histologic picture evolved from the use of functional appliances; and he questioned the Roux "shaking of the bones" hypothesis, terming it speculative. Subsequent research by Benninghoff and Pauwels in general orthopedics, and many investigators such as Sicher and Weinmann, Moss, Petrovic, Moyers, McNamara, and Sander, supported the Reitan attack on the "special quality of efficiency" claimed for activators by Häupl. Thus it has now been shown rather conclusively that each force application, whether induced by muscles or by mechanical elements, alters the equilibrium of the tissues, even as the normal growth processes do, and produces a strain in the tissues that can be considered a mechanical phenomenon.

The results of the foregoing research make an alteration in the original treatment concepts necessary. The clinician must combine various therapeutic methods either consecutively or simultaneously. None of these methods has the ability to produce a uniquely different quality of reaction. As Reitan has shown, even the lightest of forces produces hyalinization changes in bone, despite the claims of the light wire fixed appliance proponents. Each appliance has the ability, assuming its correct application, to work with optimal forces or traumatic forces. All functional appliances take advantage of the interaction between mechanical function and morphologic design, utilizing the common mechanisms of bone turnover rhythm, activation, resorption, and bone formation.

Forces. The types of force employed in orthodontic and orthopedic procedures are compressive, tensile, or shearing (Fig. 3-1). Mechanical appliances work mostly by compressive forces and pressure strain. In functional appliances tensile forces also cause stress or strain. With each force application, both external (primary) and internal (secondary) forces can be observed.

The *external* forces are the primary motivating influences developed by the appliance. They are the various forces acting on the dentition, such as the occlusal and muscle forces (from the tongue, lips, and cheeks). A prime objective of functional appliances is to take advantage of these natural forces and transmit them to the selected area for the desired change.

The *internal* secondary forces are the reactions of tissues to the primary forces. They produce strain in the contiguous tissues, which leads to the formation of an osteogenic guiding structure (i.e., deformation and bracing of the alveolar process). This reaction is important for secondary tissue adaptation. The strain and deformation of the tissues result in remodeling, displacement, and all the alterations that can be achieved by orthodontic therapy. The deformation of osseous tissues with removable functional appliances is advantageous for two reasons: (1) With these appliances it is possible to load both the teeth and the alveolar process. (2) It is also possible to perform the treatment in the mixed or transitional dentition, when the bony structures have a good fibroblast turnover and bioelasticity.

Differences. There are quantitative differences in force application, depending on the parameter and the kind of application. A force can produce the desired orthodontic effect only if it has a certain duration, direction, and magnitude.

1. The duration of force in functional appliance treatment is interrupted, because the appliance is not usually worn constantly but only for 12 to 16 hours per day.

2. The direction of force for the movement of teeth should be consistent, whether a stress or strain. With functional forces it is possible to stimulate tooth movement in one direction and then, while the appliance is not being worn, to drive the teeth in the opposite direction by the forces of intercuspation and occlusion. (Such "jiggling" effects should be avoided, however, and eliminated if possible.)

3. The magnitude of force is low in functional appliance therapy. If the induced strain is too high, the patient has difficulty wearing the appliance. Application of heavy forces (e.g., headgear therapy) is not feasible when applied directly to a pure functional appliance. The combination is useful, however.

Treatment principles. The applied force is compressive or tensile. Depending on the type applied, two treatment principles can be differentiated: force application and force elimination.

1. In force application, compressive stress and strain act on the structures involved and the result is a primary alteration in form with a secondary adaptation in function. All active fixed or removable appliances work according to this principle.

2. In force elimination the abnormal and restrictive environmental influences are eliminated, allowing op-

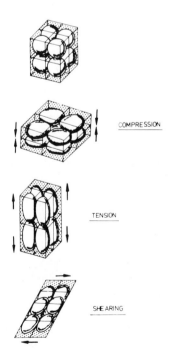

Fig. 3-1. Various types of force. Each force application means a deformation and strain in the tissues. The individual types have different modes of deformation as a consequence.

timal development. Primarily function is rehabilitated and is followed by a secondary adaptation in form.

a. During the elimination of pressure a tensile strain can arise as a result of the viscoelastic displacement of periosteum and the bone forming response in affected areas. Tension can be even more effective than pressure, because the bony structures are made to resist pressure but not tension.

The oral and vestibular screening appliances work by eliminating pressure. The shields and pads of the Fränkel appliance, however, also have as a primary objective the development of periosteal pull, or tension, to enhance osteogenic response in the affected area.

By the use of either of these principles, it is possible to perform tooth movement. The teeth will move if the balance of the forces acting on them (e.g., occlusal forces plus lip, cheek, and tongue forces) are altered. The alveolar bone is pure membranous bone that by its nature is responsive to the slightest change in balance. This balance can be altered by the application of a complementary artificial force of muscular or mechanical origin (the force application principle); or when one of the components of the total force acting on the teeth in three planes is eliminated, the teeth will respond to the reduced force by setting up a new balance (the force elimination principle) (Fig. 3-2).

Application. With both of these fundamental treatment approaches it is possible to alter the strain distribution in the bone and induce bone remodeling and tooth movement.

Together with this physical force effect, functional appliances can incite a sensory stimulation that will trigger

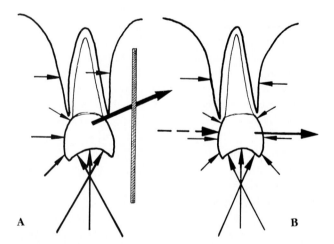

Fig. 3-2. Various possibilities for tooth movement. Natural forces are effective on the teeth from all directions. To achieve tooth movements, one of these force components can be eliminated, **A,** or an additional force can be used, **B.**

a neuromuscular response. When the posture of the mandible is altered, as by the new construction bite of a functional appliance, the nueromuscular adaptability to the new spatial skeletal relationship is possible only with the help of sensory input. Petrovic et al. have already shown the adaptive response of muscle to hyperpropulsion of the mandible in rats by means of foreshortening the lateral pterygoid muscle to hold the forward posture. McNamara has described the reaction of condylar structures to muscle strain and the compensatory adaptability and reestablishment of the original muscle activity. This reactive process not only is biomechanical but can equally be considered a neurotrophic response, as described by Moss.

Neuromuscular response. The success of functional appliance therapy is dependent on the neuromuscular response. Children with neuromuscular diseases such as poliomyelitis or cerebral palsy dysplasia cannot be treated successfully with functional appliance therapy.

The functional methods apply mechanical forces and get reactive muscle compensation. They also take advantage of the existing growth and developmental processes going on at the time of treatment, including osseous formation and tooth eruption. *Biologic treatment,* in its strictest sense, works by guiding or controlling natural processes and forces. In many cases functional appliances can be considered biologic by virtue of their force elimination and growth guidance functions. In addition to the advantage of tissue kindness, or a tissue conserving attribute, they also are more prone to achieve stability of treatment result as perverted perioral muscle function is rehabilitated. The retention requirements are often minimal. Even when there is a relapse after treatment, it is usually not as severe as when fixed appliances and heavy forces are used to shift the teeth to a predetermined ideal occlusion, an occlusion that may be dentally perfect but is out of balance with the environmental forces.

Functional appliance results are subject to the same problems of pubertal and postpubertal growth, with the mandible outgrowing the maxilla. When the direction of growth is horizontal or there is an upward and forward rotational pattern of mandibular growth, posttreatment stability in the lower anterior segment is under attack regardless of the appliance used. The treatment concept is that functional appliance therapy, in addition to eliminating functional disturbances, should work with growth and development as much as possible. An orthodontic maxim also applies to functional appliances, "to treat in the malposed area, at the right time with the right force." In many cases the implementation of this concept requires more than one method—functional and fixed together—to attain the achievable optimum. This is the goal of modern orthodontics, to make the appliances subservient to the achievable goals.

• • •

As has been stressed, there are two major principles applied in the use of functional appliances: force elimination and force application. These will be discussed separately. First, for the balance of this chapter, the force elimination principle and its application will be described. In Chapter 6, force application via the activator will be taken up.

FUNCTIONAL THERAPY BY FORCE ELIMINATION—SCREENING THERAPY

There are a number of appliances that primarily influence the lip, cheek, and tongue muscles. They can guide the stomatognathic function (as the functional regulator of Fränkel does) or can work solely by eliminating unwanted muscle influence to permit undisturbed development of the dentition (e.g., the vestibular screens designed by Kraus). The pure screening appliances are primarily designed not so much to change the form of the dental arches as to eliminate abnormal perioral muscle functional effects on the developing dentoalveolar area. Unfavorable environmental influences are considered to be a barrier to normal development. Acting over a long period, they can cause adaptation of orofacial structures and create a true developmental malocclusion; hence the need for early interceptive therapy.

The primary objective of putting a protective barrier or screen in the path of abnormal muscle forces has also been called *inhibitory treatment,* for the purpose is to inhibit the deformation of the dentition by altering the functional balance. Screening therapy will not work, of course, in morphogenetic pattern–type deformities. The principle is interaction between form and function and is based on the recognition that function does influence structure to a significant degree and that even the growth process is dependent to a certain extent on function. A basic tenet of this approach is that normal function leads to normal structure and proportions whereas abnormal function leads to malformation and malocclusion. A change in function will cause a change in structure. If there has already been adverse reaction of the dentoalveolar area when the patient is first seen, then the objective of the screening therapy is to reestablish normal function of the molding lip, cheek, and tongue muscles with the expectation that subsequent development will take care of the transient environmental assault on the integrity of the dentition. Some clinicians like to explain the use of the vestibular screen using the functional matrix concepts of Moss. The screen extends the capsular matrix to a more normal space, thus allowing the musculature to function over an artificial normal dentoalveolar shell until it can do so without the prosthetic replication. Meanwhile, the screen removes untoward deforming forces from the developing dentition, allowing the teeth and alveolar processes to move downward and outward to approximate the matrix that has been provided by the acrylic screen. Proper morphology and proper function then team up to ensure stability of the acquired relationship.

The reestablishment of normal growth and development after the elimination of unfavorable environmental influences can be achieved through the common characteristics shared by the processes of metabolism and biologic functions (i.e., the ability to follow nature's "game plan," by maintaining the developmental rhythm and pattern as controlled by phylogenetic factors). The disturbing environmental influences are opposed by heredity. Thus a normal stomatognathic system exists only when there is normal expression of the hereditary pattern, untrammelled by environmental exigencies. However, to complete the rationale, to give a normal hereditary pattern the best chance to express itself, or to correct the effects of the perverse environmental assault, interceptive therapy must start early so it will have the greatest adaptive opportunity and the most amount of growth to work with. Beside the clinical examination, the functional and cephalometric analyses indicate to the perceptive clinician the ground rules for planning, treating, and retaining the correction.

Appliances for this kind of treatment are not likely to produce iatrogenic damage since the elimination of dysfunction removes a roadblock to normal physiology. The therapeutic measures interrupt the abnormal reflex pattern and reestablish normal exteroceptive and proprioceptive engrams to ensure the inherently normal developmental pattern.

For example, in cases of habitual mouthbreathing, it can be noted that both the anterior and the posterior oral seals are not closed, the tongue is flat, and the contact of the tongue with the upper posterior teeth and palatal tissue is missing. Treating this nonphysiologic reflex pattern of habitual mouthbreathing with the help of a vestibular screen, we provide a substitute for the anterior lip seal and subsequently establish the anterior lip seal with our therapy. By eliminating the nonphysiologic reflex pattern, we also derive the added benefit of an improved posterior oral seal.

APPLIANCE CONSTRUCTION— THE VESTIBULAR SCREEN

The basic appliance for screening therapy is the vestibular screen (Fig. 3-3). The most common modifications are the lower lip shield, the tongue crib, the combination vestibular screen and tongue crib, and the vestibular screen with breathing holes.

The effectiveness of this simple appliance is based on its correct construction. Made properly, it can be quite effective in eliminating dysfunction of the orofacial muscles; but it must be made properly to achieve the maximum correction. Models that have been mounted on a straight line articulator are used, along with a proper construction bite. Unlike the construction bite for an activator, however, this one is always made the same way. An edge-to-edge bite is taken, without consideration of the facial pattern. In activator therapy the mandible is guided into a predetermined position by the construction bite, with exact planning required to achieve this relationship. In contrast, the construction bite for screening treatment does not predetermine a precise mandibular forward posturing but requires only that the mandible be moved forward to the edge-to-edge relationship. After elimination of abnormal perioral muscle function, the mandible should retract into its normal centric-relation balanced posture since the shield does not interfere with this process. A shield made with the teeth in habitual occlusion would interfere with normal function. Of course, in open bite cases there is a space between the incisal edges vertically but the sagittal relationship approximates an end-on contact. After the wax construction bite has been taken, it is chilled and replaced on the casts to be checked for accuracy. The casts must reproduce the depths of the vestibular sulcus and labial fold for proper fabrication of the screen, similar to what is required for a Fränkel Function Regulator. Either a thermoplastic custom tray or a regular tray with peripheral wax buildup will work quite well. The casts are then inserted in the wax bite and mounted on a straight line fixator before being sent to the laboratory for fabrication (Fig 3-4).

The vestibular shield extends into the vestibular sulcus to the point where the mucosal tissue reflects outward (the labial fold). Care must be taken not to impinge on muscle attachments, the frenum, etc. It is wise to outline the desired extension of the screen in pencil on the models. This should approximate the configuration of a full denture periphery. Vertically the appliance extends from the upper to the lower labial fold, and distally as far as the distal margin of the last erupted molar. If the acrylic is overextended, it will be uncomfortable to the patient when attempting to close the lips, impinging on the mucosa. Lip seal with comfort is very important. However, if the screen is too short, it will be inadequately anchored in the soft tissue and will tip, causing uncontrolled loading and movement of the upper incisors.

When the shield is in the mouth, not only the mandible but also the alveolar process and teeth should be relieved. *The appliance should not interfere with the mandible's returning to its centric relation.* Some clinicians believe that the vestibular screen is contraindi-

A

B

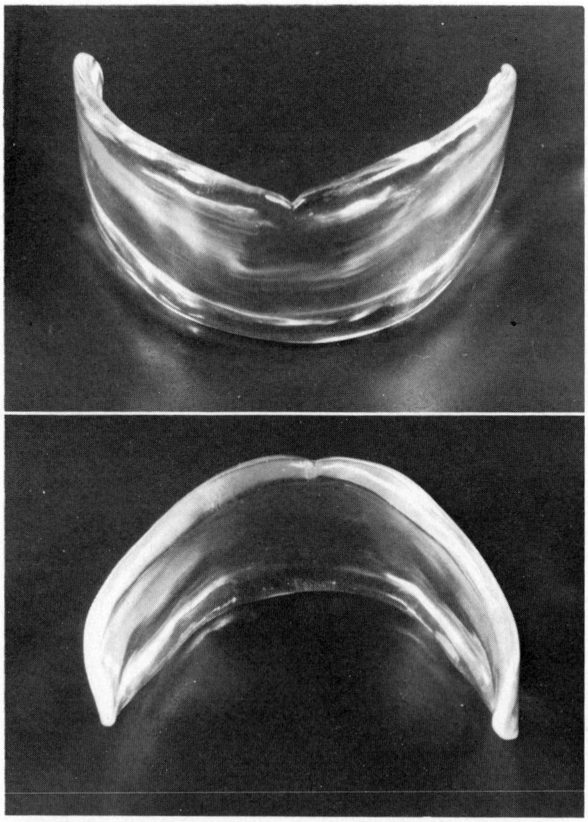

Fig. 3-3. Vestibular screen. **A,** Labial and, **B,** lingual views.

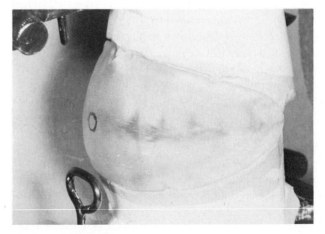

Fig. 3-4. Vestibular screen in construction bite on the articulator.

cated in Class II, Division 1, malocclusions with a deep overbite because of the tendency to tip the maxillary incisors lingually, deepening the bite and trapping the mandible in a retruded position. This is true if in the construction of the appliance its role in inhibitory treatment is not considered. If the screen is fabricated in the proper forward construction bite, the mandible can move only anteriorly from its retruded position. Lingual tipping of the teeth can be prevented if there is no contact between the shield and the incisor teeth.

To ensure that unwanted pressures are not created, the articulated models are covered with 2 to 3 mm of wax over the labial surfaces of the teeth (Fig. 3-5). If one dental arch is crowded and the other is relatively normal, the layer of wax on the crowded arch should be thicker. If expansion procedures have been performed prior to placement of the vestibular shield (as for a functional cross-bite), the shield is constructed following the same principles. The teeth and alveolar process are covered with wax and then the shield is fabricated

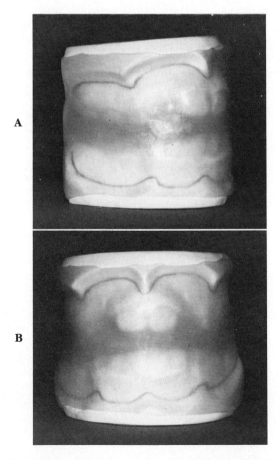

Fig. 3-5. Casts in construction bite prepared for fabrication of a vestibular screen with wax layer. The extent of the appliance is marked. **A,** Lateral and, **B,** frontal views.

in self-curing acrylic over the wax relief. The completed vestibular shield should be in contact only with the upper and lower labial folds (sulci terminali) during the anterior positioning of the mandible. It is fabricated without a holding ring, as used by some operators, since this might interfere with the desired lip seal.

The appliance should be worn at night, and 2 to 3 hours per day, when the child is not in school. During TV time it is not difficult to get the patient to adjust to the bulk. Lip exercises can make the appliance a potent tool, for the patient learns the importance of lip seal. Holding a piece of paper between the lips while wearing the vestibular shield assists in this process.

Properly made and worn, the appliance is effective in eliminating abnormal sucking habits and lip dysfunction. It helps to establish a proper lip seal and indirectly influences the posture of the tongue. The shield interrupts the contact of the tip of the tongue and lower lip, a vestige of the infantile suckling pattern. This leads to maturation of the deglutitional cycle, with the creation of a somatic swallowing pattern. In most of the patients the vestibular screen can remove the maturation roadblock and establish normal tongue posture. Some patients, however, persist in thrusting the tongue, even with the screen in place. This can be seen by the clinician since the acrylic is clear and the tip of the tongue shoves against the lingual surface of the screen. In such instances a lingual restricting tongue screen is also needed and can be added to the vestibular screen with through-the-bite wire support. In most instances, as the abnormal peroral muscle function is eliminated, there is autonomous self-improvement of the malocclusion, especially the dentoalveolar relationships.

The management of the appliance is simple. During the first few days the patient may show some irritation in the vestibular sulcus or around the labial frenum. The acrylic is carefully reduced and polished in these areas—care being taken not to remove too much material, as in fitting a full denture. When there is a confirmed mouthbreathing habit with allergies present, some patients have difficulty sleeping with the appliance. In these cases breathing holes can be made in the anterior part of the screen at the interincisal level.

As the patient wears the shield and shows progress, holding the appliance well in the vestibule, the acrylic periphery can be reduced. The lower margin can also be trimmed 2 to 3 mm, which will enable a better lip seal to be achieved. Lip seal exercises should continue. They are a "must" during TV time. As one clinician tells his patients, "No tickie, no Tellie—and you know what the tickie is!"

It should be remembered that the appliance only eliminates pressure. It cannot create a tensional effect on the vestibular periosteum, as claimed by Fränkel for the Function Regulator, to enhance bone formation in this region. The important thing is to have a soft-tissue seal of the screen in the peripheral portions with no strain.

There are many variations of the basic screen. The shield can be modified to specific needs and morphology, eliminating pressure in particular areas, but all such constructions should follow the same principles just elucidated.

Lower lip shield

The lower lip shield is really just the lower half of a full vestibular shield (Fig. 3-6). It is extended into the vestibular sulcus to the depths of the labial fold and as far as the distal margin of the last molar. It is fabricated on a lower cast in which the wax relief has been placed as with a full screen. The shield makes contact only in the depths of the lower vestibular sulcus. Although the appliance is made on the lower cast only, the occlusal relationship should be considered. It extends superiorly to the incisal third of the lower teeth. However, if this disturbs the occlusion, the margin must be reduced.

There should be no contact between the shield and either the upper or the lower incisor teeth, even in habitual occlusion (Fig. 3-7). Patients can wear the shield without difficulty, but anchorage can be improved after eruption of the permanent first molars by adding reverse Adams-type clasps to these teeth (wire framework on the lingual, the clasps anchored in buccal acrylic) (Fig. 3-8). The lower lip shield has the added advantage of being wearable during the day, both at school and at home. Talking can be quite normal after some practice.

The purpose of the lower shield is to eliminate the persistent and pernicious hyperactivity of the mentalis muscle, with its forcing of the lower lip into the overjet

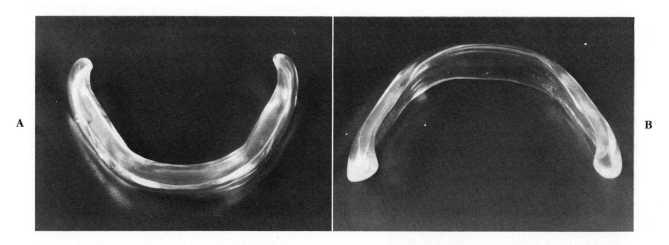

Fig. 3-6. Lower lip shield. **A,** Labial and, **B,** lingual views.

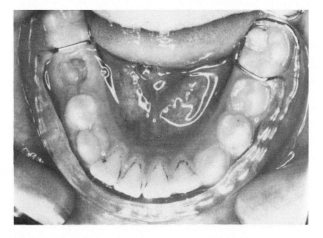

Fig. 3-7. Lower lip screen in the mouth. Note that it stands away from the teeth.

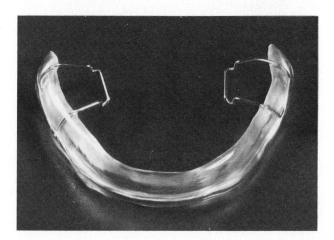

Fig. 3-8. Lower lip screen with Adams clasps to enhance stability.

space. The cardinal sign of a crinkling chin ("golfball chin") is indicative of the need for some screening device to prevent this malfunction from forcing the lower incisors lingually while increasing the protrusion of the upper incisors. Again, the lip pads of the Fränkel appliance perform the same function. By guiding the lower lip into a more forward position, eliminating the lip trap, they enable dentoalveolar development to follow a normal pattern. The only indication for this type of appliance is the elimination of perverted lower lip function in Class II, Division I, malocclusions (or in Class I flush terminal plane situations with a large overjet that has already trapped the lip and in which the lower incisors are already lingualized and crowded—often with denudation of the labial mucosa). As soon as the overjet

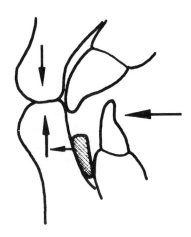

Fig. 3-9. Effectiveness of the lower lip screen in the presence of labial movement. Lip seal is reestablished and the contact between tongue tip and lower lip interrupted without interference from anterior positioning of the tongue.

diminishes and normal lip seal is established, which can happen quickly, even with potentially incompetent lips, use of the shield is discontinued; but if a residual hyperactivity of the mentalis muscle remains, the shield should be worn until this extraoral manifestation of abnormal function is eliminated. The clinician will observe a spontaneous uprighting of the lower incisors in many of these cases, with resultant decrowding. If some distal driving of the lower molars is needed to gain a minor degree of space, a lip bumper is indicated with muscle anchorage.

As has been stressed, the shield alters the functional equilibrium of the orofacial musculature, moving the lower lip anteriorly and letting the lower incisors assume their normal unrestrained position. The tip of the tongue follows this movement and supports the newer, more normal, labial position. Indeed, it is probably a primary motivating factor in tipping the lower incisors to a more desired labial position. However, if the incisors are tipped labially before treatment, such tongue activity can create further procumbency, which is undesirable. The tongue action has been seen with palatographic registration checks after lower screen insertion. There is a definite anterior posturing in many cases (Figs. 3-9 and 3-10). Thus the lower vestibular shield is contraindicated in patients in whom an already excessive labial tipping of the lower incisors exists.

Tongue crib (oral shield)

If the patient thrusts the tongue interdentally in either the anterior or posterior regions of the dental arches, a malocclusion can result. However, a tongue crib (Fig. 3-11) with a removable or fixed appliance can inhibit this abnormal function.

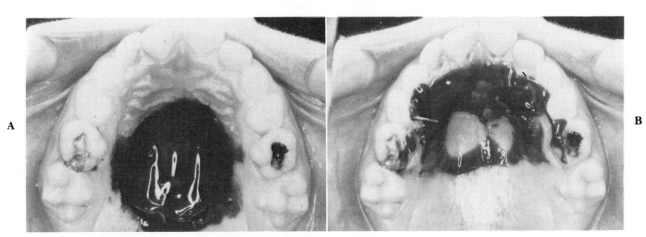

Fig. 3-10. Side effect of the lower lip screen on tongue position. **A,** Palatogram without the appliance. **B,** Palatogram with the appliance in position. The dark field indicates contact of the tongue with the hard palate during swallowing.

With a removable appliance the crib for an anterior open bite consists of a palatal plate with a horseshoe-shaped wire crib. The plate can be anchored, depending on the state of dental development, with arrowhead or Adams clasps. The malocclusion and the age of the patient determine the crib length (6 to 12 mm) and its distance from the lingual surfaces of the upper incisors (3 or 4 mm). The crib is placed in the area of the local tongue dysfunction and resultant malocclusion. It should neither touch the teeth nor disturb the occlusion. It can be made out of 0.8 mm wire or formed of acrylic. It acts as an inhibitory appliance only, so the acrylic construction should not interfere with the autonomous improvement of the open bite.

The tongue crib is not exclusively a screening device. Some elements of the appliance incorporate features of the active plate. The labial bow not only helps retention but also can tip the upper incisors lingually. If the crib is placed at the gingival third, a proper adjustment can stimulate the eruption of these teeth, a movement needed in open bite problems. The acrylic can also be interposed between the teeth, covering the occlusal sur-

faces of the upper molars, to prevent eruption of these teeth while enhancing anchorage of the plate. This is especially beneficial in open bite problems (Fig. 3-12). The bite blocking here can be 3 to 4 mm, which is usually beyond the postural vertical dimension in open bite patients. In such cases a stretch reflex is elicited from the closing muscles that enhances the depressing action on the buccal segments and helps in closing down the anterior open bite. Also the appliance can incorporate

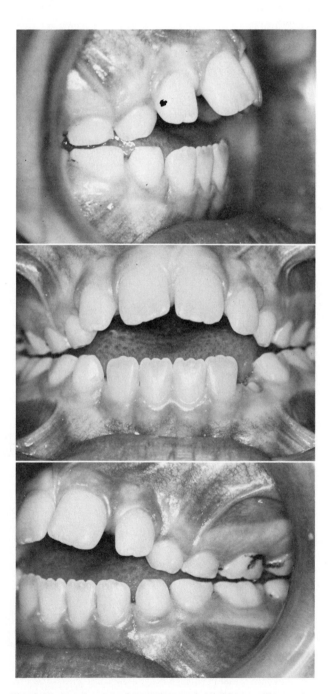

Fig. 3-13. Anterior open bite with crowding of the maxillary arch in a 9-year-old patient (A.B.).

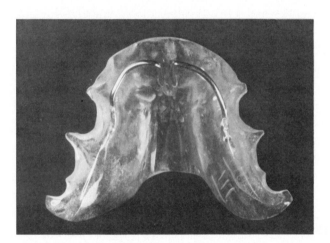

Fig. 3-11. Tongue screen with a wire crib.

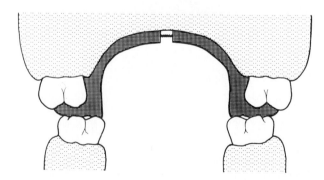

Fig. 3-12. Acrylic plate extended occlusally to inhibit eruption of the posterior teeth.

an expansion screw, since many open bite problems also have a narrow upper arch.

Thus the appliance combines inhibitory action via the screen and mechanical action via the jackscrew, labial bow, etc. (Figs. 3-13 and 3-14).

The tongue crib can also be used with fixed appliances, with the specific aim of eliminating tongue dysfunction. Circumferential clasps that snap above the molar buccal tubes can enhance anchorage of the removable palatal tongue crib. In addition, the crib can be combined with the vestibular shield, with through-the-bite supporting and connecting wires.

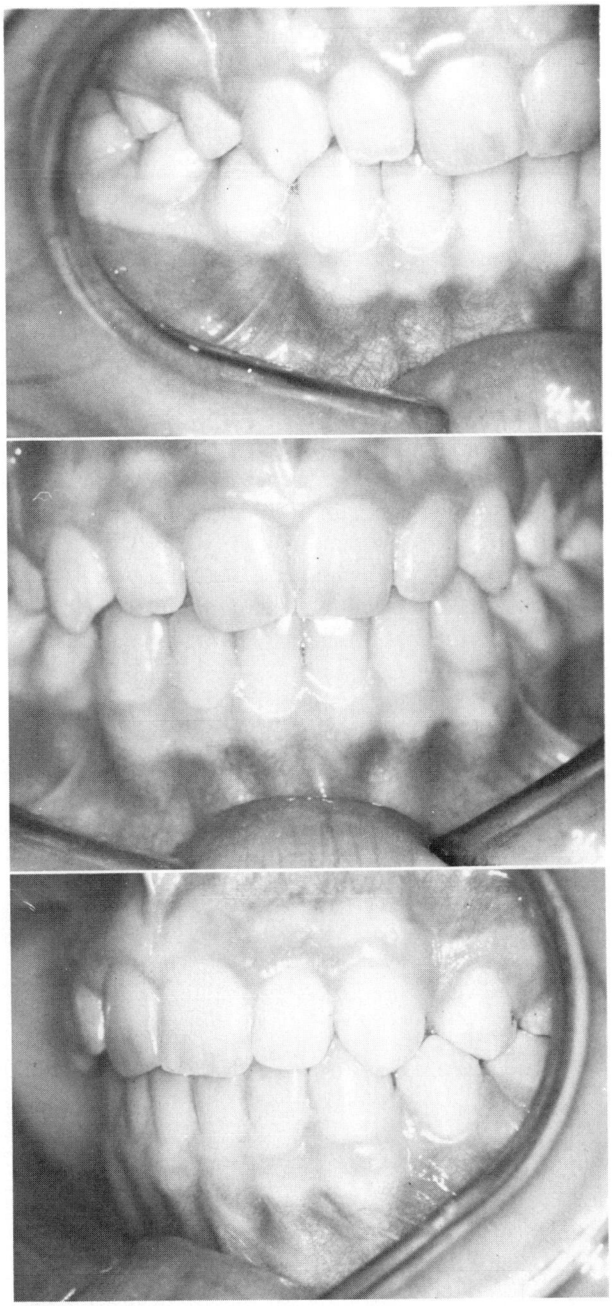

Posterior tongue crib. Appliances such as a posterior tongue crib are used in cases of unilateral or bilateral open bite and true deep overbite (with infraclusion of molar segments). The posterior appliance consists of a plate attached to the teeth with clasps and supported by a labial bow. (Fig. 3-15). Multiple arrowhead clasps provide good retention. The plate is in contact with all the teeth and is trimmed in the area of the open bite to allow extrusion of the teeth. This means that the only contact with the teeth is above the greatest convexity of the lingual tooth surfaces. In the area of the open bite there is a crib to intercept the thrusting tongue. The wire framework extends below the occlusal surface sufficiently to prevent the tongue from inserting into the interocclusal space during postural rest position (Fig. 3-16). Because the crib is 2 to 3 mm away from the teeth,

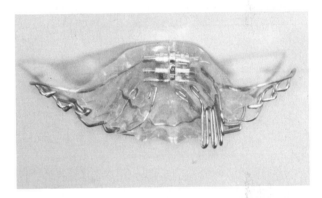

Fig. 3-15. Palatal plate with a lateral tongue crib.

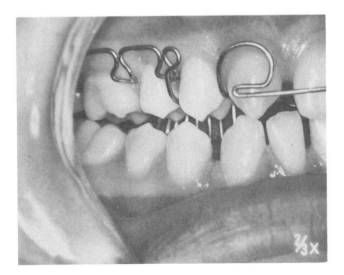

Fig. 3-16. Palatal plate with lateral tongue crib in the mouth.

Fig. 3-14. After orthodontic treatment and eruption of the permanent teeth.

it does not contact them. This type of plate can also be worn during the daytime, and it can be used in combination with the vestibular screen. When used with the screen, it needs no palatal acrylic but only the restricting crib construction formed from the through-the-bite wire elements.

Combination vestibular screen and tongue crib

A tongue crib or oral screen can be attached to the vestibular screen in several ways.

A crib of wire or acrylic can be placed in the area of the open bite (Fig. 3-17) and attached to the vestibular screen by a wire that extends around the last molar tooth; or it may be passed through the interocclusal space in the region of the canine and first premolar. In either instance it should not touch the teeth, even in occlusion.

A crib can also be attached to the vestibular shield

when tongue thrusting persists during wearing of the vestibular shield alone (Fig. 3-18). This appliance is worn at night and for 1 to 2 hours during the day. If a tongue crib is used, the vestibular shield can be left open in the anterior region since the tongue action is being controlled by the oral portion of the appliance. The advantage is that the appliance can then be worn during the day, prolonging its wearing time and potential effectiveness.

Vestibular screen with breathing holes

The use of three small holes at the interincisal level in the anterior portion of the vestibular shield enhances wear for patients who have difficulty breathing through their nose (Fig. 3-19). Habitual mouthbreathers adjust better with this modification, though part of the adjustment is probably psychologic, since the vestibular shield does not stop oral respiration. These holes can be gradually reduced after the patient becomes accustomed to the appliance, which will stimulate nasal breathing. A basic requirement of such control is the elimination of any structural barriers to normal nasal breathing—enlarged tonsils and adenoids, enlarged turbinates, etc. This requires otolaryngologic teamwork. The mere removal of occluding epipharyngeal tissue does not ensure nasal breathing. Many children continue as mouthbreathers through force of habit. In some cases the adenoids proliferate again. Thus the oral screen can assist in conversion of a mouthbreather to a nasal breather at a critical time, preventing the need for another bout with the surgeon at a later date. Lip seal exercises in conjunction with vestibular screen wear are again very important.

INDICATIONS FOR SCREENING THERAPY

These appliances are to be used only in the deciduous and mixed dentitions.

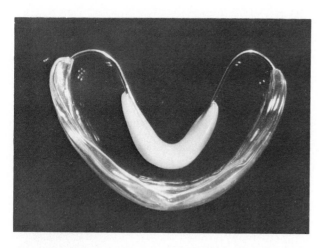

Fig. 3-17. Combined vestibular screen with an acrylic tongue crib.

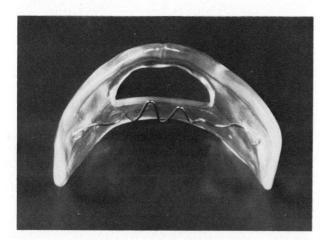

Fig. 3-18. Combined vestibular screen, open anteriorly, and a wire tongue crib.

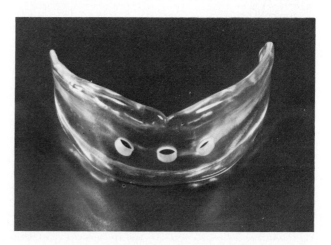

Fig. 3-19. Vestibular screen with holes.

Deciduous dentition indication

The screening type of appliance is indicated to intercept and eliminate all abnormal perioral muscle function in all acquired malocclusions that have resulted from abnormal habits, mouthbreathing, nasal blockage, etc. The creation of open bite, narrow maxillary arch, or overjet problems is a consequence of prolongation of these habits. Nothing is gained by waiting in such cases. Open bites created by fingersucking and retained visceral deglutitional pattern tongue function can be helped with a vestibular screen. Self-correction of the malocclusion is frequently possible, as shown in Fig. 3-20. In this 4-year-old girl with a fingersucking habit, a vestibular screen was placed. The habit was stopped by her wearing the appliance at night and for 2 to 3 hours per day. The improvement in the open bite occurred in 3 months.

Often, because of a lower tongue position and unopposed muscle forces of the buccinator mechanism on the maxillary buccal segments, a child's abnormal sucking habits will cause not only an open bite but also an excessive overjet and a bilateral narrowing of the max-

illary arch. This three-dimensional deformation disorients the proprioceptive and exteroceptive stimuli emanating from the normal occlusal relationship. The child tries to seek the best possible position for the teeth to chew. With a narrow arch the result is often a convenience shift to one side or the other as the mandible swings anterolaterally, with the condyle coming forward on the noncrossbite side. Initially the crossbite can be on one side or the other until one becomes preferred. This kind of functional aberration is often revealed by occlusal wear patterns of the deciduous teeth, particularly the canines. In severe accommodative bites of this type the first step in treatment is an expansion plate. After correction of the crossbite the remaining open bite and dysfunction can be treated with a vestibular screen.

Another instance of screening appliances being used in the deciduous dentition is when the vestibular screen serves as a pretreatment device. In this case the plan is to use an activator or an active plate later on. The first assault on the malocclusion with a simple appliance conditions the young patient and usually has some benefit in reducing the severity of the malocclusion by screening the developing dentition from abnormal perioral muscle function.

In hyperkinetic or potential behavior problem children with persistent fingersucking and concomitant tongue thrust, the use of a vestibular shield first is more likely to be successful and produce less psychologic trauma. An example is a 3-year-old boy with a severe open bite malocclusion and a bilaterally compressed upper arch (Fig. 3-21). An older sister had also had an open bite malocclusion with a vertical growth pattern, which had required extensive treatment at a later age. Because the patient evidenced an intensive fingersucking habit and a crossbite in addition to the open bite and because of the unfavorable family history, treatment was done at this early age. The unusual amount of anxiety in this patient necessitated reversing treatment objectives, and the neuromuscular dysfunction was corrected first. The patient stopped the fingersucking on his own. The open bite and arch form improved within 5 months, but the crossbite persisted. Expansion treatment could then be carried out.

A final indication for the vestibular screen in the deciduous dentition is the patient with nasorespiratory problems. Using a vestibular screen with breathing holes can help reestablish normal nasal breathing in these cases.

Mixed dentition indication

Unlike the deciduous dentition, the mixed dentition is more limited in the ways a screen can be used. Usually a combination-type screen with some other method of therapy is necessary. In only a few malocclusion

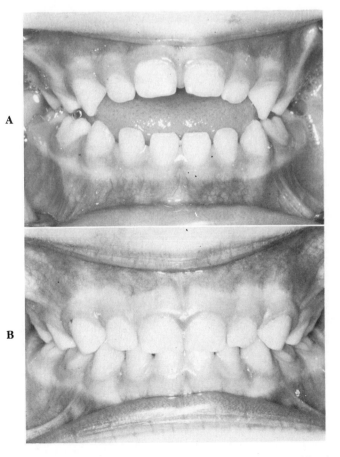

Fig. 3-20. A, Anterior open bite and dysfunction in a 4-year-old girl. **B,** After 3 months of treatment with a vestibular screen.

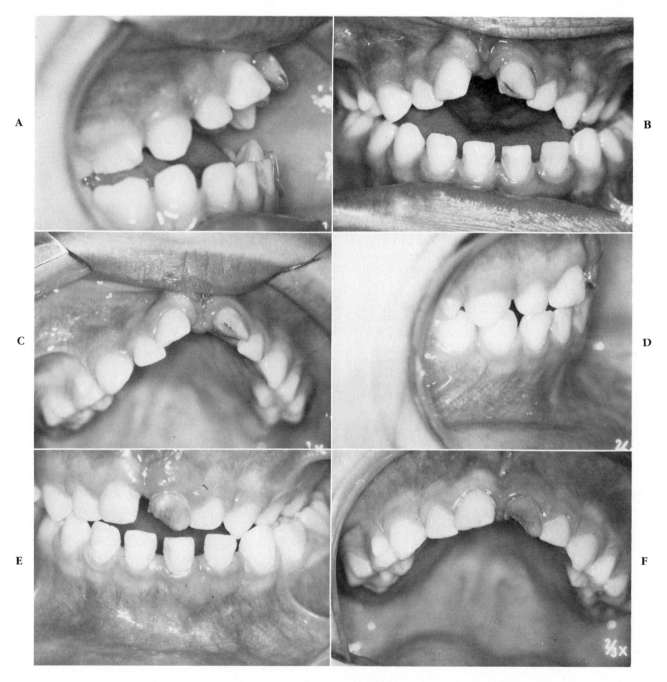

Fig. 3-21. A to **C,** Open bite malocclusion with lateral cross-bite in a 3-year-old boy. **D** to **F,** After 5 months of treatment with a vestibular screen. The open bite improved, but the cross-bite persisted.

problems is it possible to use the screening appliance as the sole form of treatment. These are recently acquired malocclusions resulting from local environmental factors whose only symptoms are due to abnormal perioral muscle function. Treatment in these cases aims at the elimination of deforming muscle habit patterns, permitting normal development and eruption of the teeth. Thus screening therapy is causal and physiologic and the improvement of the malocclusion is due to autonomous self-adjustment.

It is not difficult to use screening therapy for this age group; however, success is dependent on establishing a proper differential diagnosis. The correct functional and skeletal assessment criteria must be used. Postural rest position of the mandible is not influenced by such treatment, but in recently acquired malocclusions this is not a therapeutic objective. The appliance is indicated in so-called functional retrusion cases, in which there is an anterior postural rest position with the mandible closing upward and backward into occlusion under forced guid-

ance by the teeth. Usually there is also an excessive overbite in these cases.

An example of the type of case amenable to successful treatment is a 9-year-old girl with an open bite, a tongue postural and sucking habit, and persistent mouthbreathing (Fig. 3-22). The growth direction was average, not markedly vertical or horizontal. The abnormal function was eliminated after 1 year of vestibular screen therapy. In addition, the bite was closed, the gingival tissue inflammation was improved, and the mouthbreathing was greatly reduced. The dentition was controlled until eruption of the permanent teeth, and the result was stable without any form of retention.

Skeletal discrepancies cannot be altered by screening appliances alone. If the morphogenetic pattern and growth direction are abnormal, therapeutic alteration of the local environmental conditions cannot prevent the expression of a dysplastic endogenous pattern. Screening therapy is probably contraindicated in such cases, or it can be used only in conjunction with other methods. Indeed, screening therapy in the mixed dentition can often be used with other forms of treatment, even when the correction cannot be achieved by the screen alone. The elimination of abnormal environmental pressures is a proper treatment objective in a majority of cases in the mixed dentition. Thus the screen can be used in pretreatment instances, during treatment with other appliances, or as a posttreatment retention adjunct.

Indications for pretreatment use of screening therapy. As in the deciduous dentition, screening appliances in the mixed dentition can be used to eliminate abnormal perioral muscle functional influences before some other form of treatment is started. Rapid improvement can usually be seen in the initial stages of treatment; but as treatment progresses and improvement is minimal despite the elimination of abnormal perioral muscle function, the etiologic basis of the malocclusion is due to other nonenvironmental factors that need different approaches to treatment. A case in point is the following illustration:

An 8-year-old boy (Fig. 3-23) with an anterior open bite and abnormal tongue posture and function presented for treatment. The growth pattern was horizontal. As is often the case, the dentition was biprotrusive. The mandible was orthognathic but the maxilla was prognathic with a long base and slight upward and forward inclination. Screening therapy was instituted; and the open bite and axial inclination of the incisor teeth improved, although the uprighting of the lower incisors was insufficient. The mandible grew 3.5 mm and the angle S-N-B increased. A retroinclination of the maxillary base that diminished the prognathic profile could be seen, but no reduction in the A-N-B angle was evident (Fig. 3-24). No further improvement could be achieved

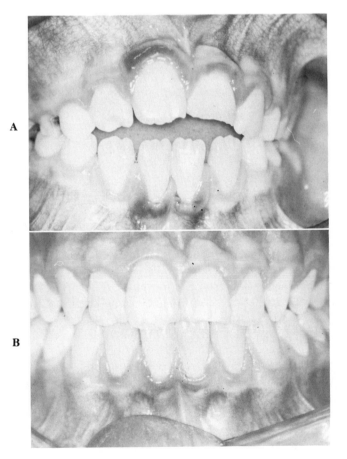

A,

B,

Fig. 3-22. A, Dysfunction, disturbed nasal respiration, and open bite malocclusion in a 9-year-old girl. **B,** After screening therapy and eruption of the permanent teeth.

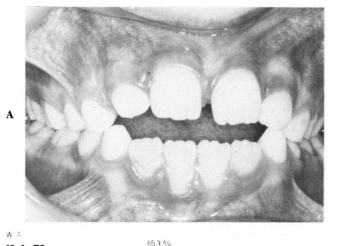

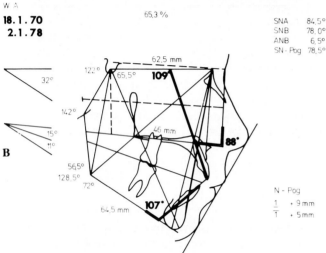

Fig. 3-23. A, Open bite malocclusion and horizontal growth pattern in an 8-year-old patient (W.A.). **B,** Cephalometric tracing.

Fig. 3-24. A, After 15 months of screening therapy (W.A.). **B,** Cephalometric tracing.

using the inhibitory type of treatment, however. Indicated therapy was the uprighting of lower incisors with fixed tooth control mechanics.

As in the deciduous dentition, habitual mouthbreathing in the mixed dentition can be treated by using a vestibular shield with breathing holes. Before the screen is placed, however, the posture of the tongue should be examined. If the tongue is retracted with a humped up dorsum but flat surface (as is common in Class II malocclusions), screening appliances can be used; but if there is a flat anteriorly postured tongue, the screen is contraindicated because of the Class III tendency. The screen could actually make the anterior posturing of the tongue more severe.

Indications for combination with other appliances. Some appliances (e.g., the activator) have shortcomings because of their limited wearing time during the day. With confirmed abnormal habit patterns (partic-

ularly tongue and lip problems) nocturnal wear may not be enough to eliminate abnormal pressures, with the result that treatment response is slowed. For tongue thrust problems in patients wearing activators, a plate with a tongue crib can be worn during the day to offset the deleterious effects of tongue thrust. Then the activator is worn at night.

In patients with perverted lip habits in which the lower lip is cushioned to the lingual of the upper incisors during the day, the same problem exists—offsetting this deforming action with only part-time activator wear. In such instances a lower lip screen can be worn during the day, with the activator at night. As soon as the sagittal relationship is improved and the lower lip is no longer trapped between the upper and lower incisors during function, the screen can be discontinued and therapy completed with the activator only.

A 10-year-old boy with a Class II, Division I, malocclu-

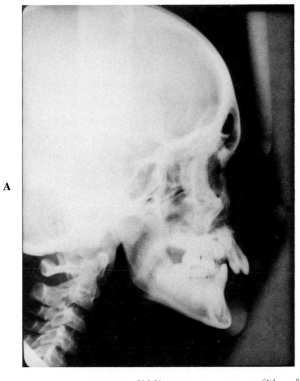

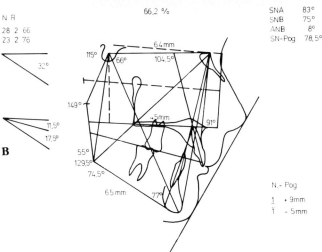

Fig. 3-25. A, Lower lip dysfunction in an 11-year-old patient (N.R.). **B,** Cephalometric tracing.

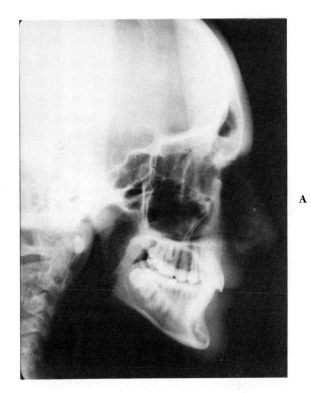

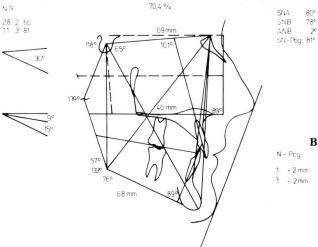

Fig. 3-26. A, After treatment with a lower lip screen and activator and following eruption of the permanent teeth (N.R.). **B,** Cephalometric tracing 5 years later.

sion and associated lower lip habit is shown in Fig. 3-25. His growth pattern was horizontal, the mandibular ramus was long and the body small and retrognathic, and the maxillary base was average and tipped upward and forward (which exaggerated the discrepancy). The lower incisors were markedly tipped to the lingual as a result of the hyperactive mentalis muscle function. In this case, as just recommended, the patient wore an activator at night and a lower lip shield during the day.

The activator promoted the horizontal growth while exerting an inhibiting influence on the maxilla. The lower incisors were tipped labially. The lower lip screen eliminated the lip trap during the day and indirectly contributed to the labial tipping of the lower incisors. Fig. 3-26 shows the case after eruption of the permanent teeth and 1 year after retention, with a balanced relationship.

Simultaneous use of two screening appliances. Fig. 3-27 shows a 9-year-old girl with an anterior open bite associated with a tongue posture and thrust habit, plus lip sucking. The growth pattern was vertical and was partially compensated by a slight downward and backward inclination of the maxilla, which was of average size and orthognathic. The mandible had a short ramus and body. Both upper and lower incisors were tipped slightly to the lingual. Because of the combined lip and tongue dysfunction, a double shield (a vestibular screen

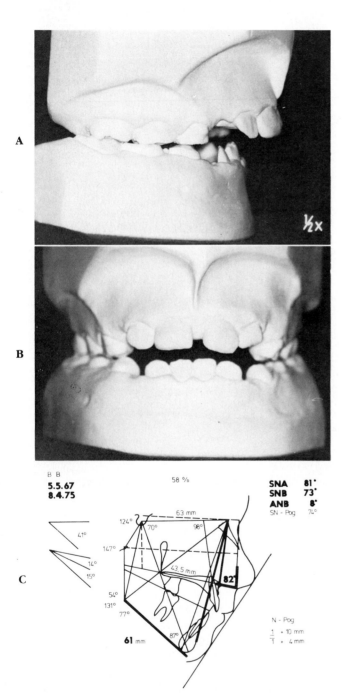

Fig. 3-27. A and **B,** Combined treatment with a vestibular shield and lower lip screen in a 9-year-old girl (B.B.). **C,** Cephalometric tracing.

with an oral tongue screen) was used during the night and a lower lip screen during the day. A high mandibular growth increment was observed during treatment, with a reduction in the A-N-B angle caused partially by a decrease in the S-N-A angle. The vertical growth direction persisted. In spite of this unfavorable pattern, treatment with the combined screens was possible because of the retroclination of the maxilla, which offset the vertical inclination of the mandible (Fig. 3-28).

Even in extraction cases in which abnormal perioral muscle function is present, treatment may be started using a vestibular screen. Such a case is shown in Fig. 3-29, *A,* a 7-year-old girl with an open bite and generalized crowding along with abnormal muscle activity. There was a slight vertical growth tendency; the mandibular ramus and body were both short. The lower incisors were labially tipped. A program of serial extraction was initiated, together with the wearing of a vestibular screen. The open bite closed after 1 year of treatment. Both the mandibular retrognathism and the lower incisor inclination improved. Treatment was completed with an activator after removal of the four first premolars, since it was possible to close the spaces under activator influence by guiding the eruption of the remaining posterior teeth and canines. The abnormal functional pattern did not reappear (Fig. 3-29, *C*).

Assessment of the indications for screening therapy. As stated earlier, the construction of the various types of screens is simple but they are effective only if used properly, with a correct diagnosis as a prerequisite. In determining the correct indications, one should have, besides the general clinical examination, both a functional and a cephalometric analysis.

Cases with functional retrusion–type Class II relationships and functionally deep overbite problems. It is often possible to treat these patients in the early mixed dentition period with screening appliances. When the mandible is guided upward and backward from postural rest to habitual occlusion, they have an excellent prognosis because of the neuromuscular etiology and local tooth guidance factors. They frequently have associated hyperactive mentalis muscle malfunction. In many an original flush terminal plane relationship of the molars has been converted into a Class II intercuspation by the overclosure and tooth guidance, exacerbated by the lower lip trap. In combined tongue and lip dysfunction it is necessary to assess the relationship of the dysfunction to the malocclusion. Screening therapy is successful only when the abnormal perioral muscle function is a primary etiologic factor in the malocclusion. It usually requires a cephalometric analysis to confirm this information.

Need for cephalometric analysis to augment a functional analysis. In skeletal dysplasia, screening therapy alone is inadequate and can be used only in combina-

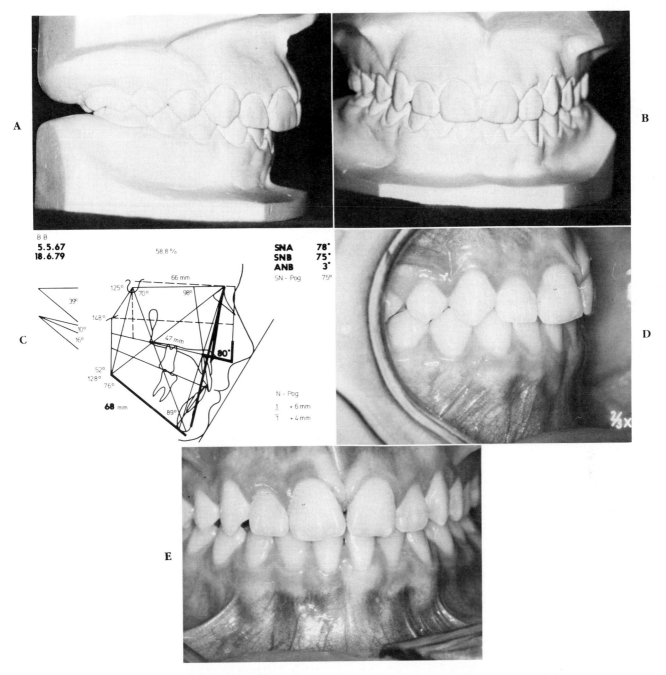

Fig. 3-28. A and **B,** Four years after treatment and eruption of the permanent teeth (B.B.). **C,** Cephalometric tracing. **D** and **E,** Three years out of retention.

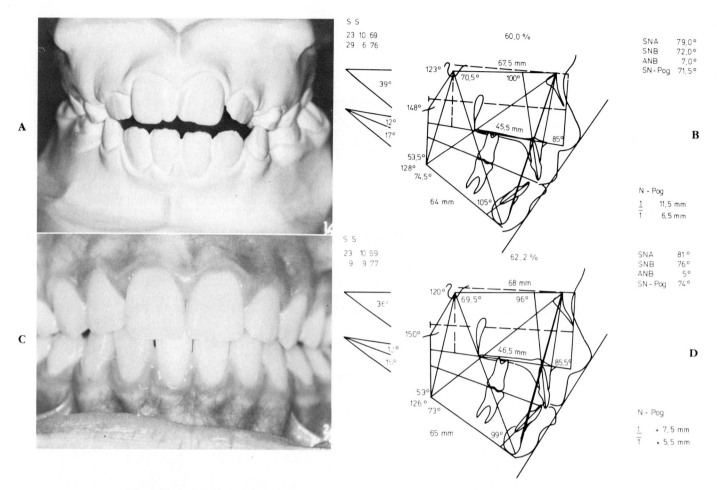

Fig. 3-29. A, Open bite malocclusion and crowding in the upper and lower dental arch in a 7-year-old patient (S.S.). **B,** Cephalometric tracing. **C,** After serial extraction, screening combined with activator therapy, and eruption of the permanent teeth. **D,** Tracing after the screening therapy.

tion with other methods of treatment. The combined modalities eliminate one associated, adaptive, compensatory factor that is not decisive by itself. It is necessary to identify the malocclusion as skeletal before a differential diagnosis can be made.

Differential diagnosis between primary and secondary functional behavior. With a primary tongue dysfunction the malocclusion can be localized in the dentoalveolar region. Early treatment with screening therapy is indicated. In secondary tongue dysfunctions the abnormality also involves the skeletal structures, making screening therapy inadequate. Depending on the severity of the skeletal dysplasia, screening therapy can be combined with other functional and fixed appliance methods. In very severe cases, however, even this combination is contraindicated. In secondary (compensatory-type) tongue dysfunctions, as in skeletal open bite malocclusions, the growth pattern is usually vertical. This unfavorable growth vector can be partially compen-

sated by a downward and backward tipping of the maxillary base. The adaptation of the maxilla to a retroclined mandible can be therapeutically enhanced. On the other hand, the upward and forward inclination of the maxillary base can enhance the severity of the malocclusion. In such cases, with divergent rotation of the skeletal bases, the ultimate problem (as shown by Lavergne and Gasson) can be quite severe. Prognosis for any form of therapy is poor, and surgical intervention may be the only way to correct the problems after the completion of growth. Unfortunately, too many such cases have been treated with ineffective functional and fixed appliances for many years, with only partial correction and with iatrogenic damage in the form of apical resorption, elongated teeth, and sheared alveolar crests. In some cases a dentoalveolar compensation is feasible, with combined extraction of first premolars and multiattachment fixed appliances giving the precise control needed. A careful cephalometric analysis will usually

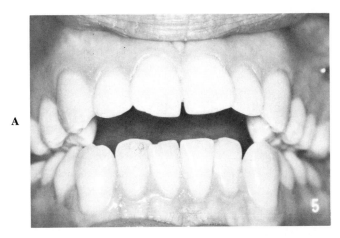

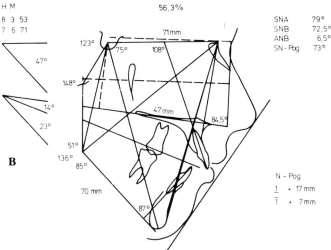

Fig. 3-30. **A,** Skeletal open bite and crowding in an 18-year-old patient (H.M.). **B,** Cephalometric tracing.

Fig. 3-31. **A,** After four–first premolar extraction and active therapy (H.M.). **B,** Cephalometric tracing.

separate these cases and determine which are amenable to orthodontic treatment and which may need combined orthodontic and orthognathic surgical assistance.

Three cases are presented to demonstrate the limitations of functional appliance therapy in the treatment of open bite malocclusions because the correct diagnosis was not made beforehand.

The first patient, H.M. (Fig. 3-30), an 18-year-old girl with an open bite, a vertical growth pattern, and crowding in both upper and lower arches, was treated for many years with functional appliances. The author first saw her at 18 years and recommended removal of the four first premolars with insertion of full fixed appliances. The compensation of the vertical discrepancy was possible because only the mandible and not the maxilla was unfavorably inclined (Fig. 3-31).

In the second patient, a 14-year-old boy (Figs. 3-32 and 3-33), there was a similar malocclusion, but dentoalveolar compensation was more difficult because of the upward and forward inclination of the maxillary base combined with a down-

wardly and backwardly inclined mandibular base. The open bite could not be completely closed by orthodontic means alone, despite combined extraction and fixed appliances, because of the significant divergency of apical bases.

The third patient, R.A. (Fig. 3-34), was a 14-year-old girl also with an open bite but with a horizontal growth pattern. Four first premolars were removed and functional appliance treatment was initiated but was unsuccessful. The reasons for this are the following: Both jaws were prognathic, the upper more than the lower. After the premolar extraction the general dentist, instead of closing spaces above by anchorage control and distalizing the maxillary teeth, moved the prognathic mandible anteriorly with the functional appliance to adapt it to the prognathic maxilla. The bite was later closed with full multibanded fixed appliance therapy, since it was too late for functional treatment (Fig 3-35).

Differential diagnosis of overjet caused by skeletal or functional disturbances. An excessive overjet can be the consequence of abnormal perioral muscle function or a

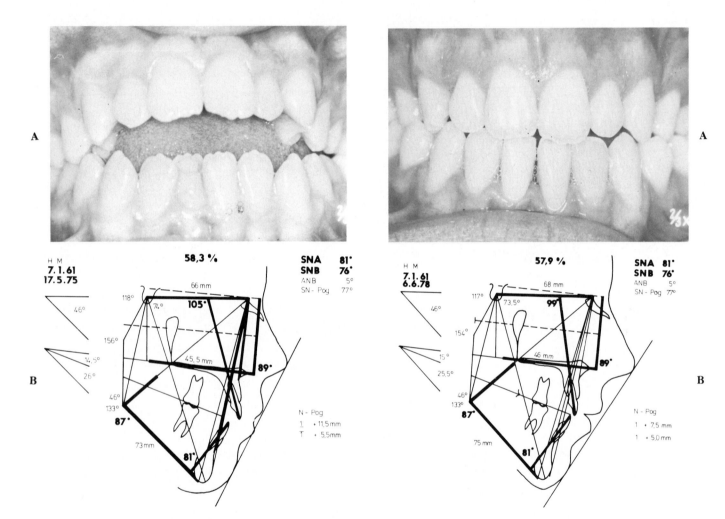

Fig. 3-32. A, Skeletal open bite and crowding in a 14-year-old patient (H.M.). **B,** Cephalometric tracing. Note the vertical growth pattern with forward inclination of the maxillary base.

Fig. 3-33. A, After four-premolar extraction and active therapy (H.M.). **B,** Cephalometric tracing. There were difficulties in therapy because of the divergent growth rotations of the jaw bases.

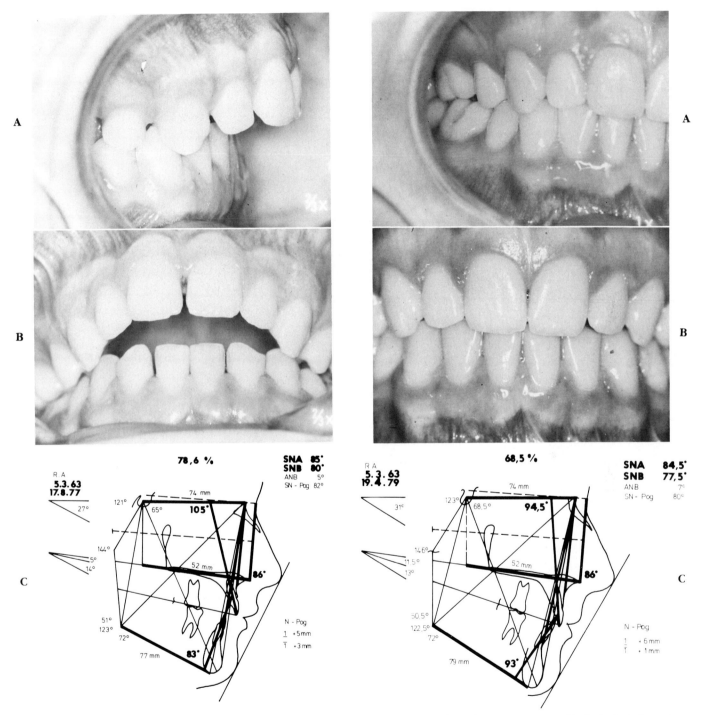

Fig. 3-34. A and **B,** Open bite malocclusion and horizontal growth pattern in a 14-year-old patient (R.A.). **C,** Cephalometric tracing.

Fig. 3-35. A and **B,** After active treatment (R.A.). **C,** Cephalometric tracing.

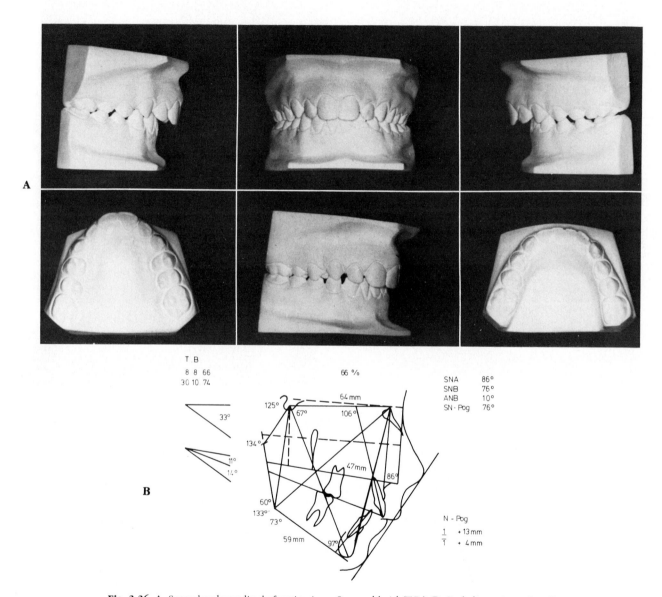

Fig. 3-36. A, Secondary lower lip dysfunction in an 8-year-old girl (T.B.). **B,** Cephalometric tracing. Note the skeletal discrepancy, with an A-N-B of 10°.

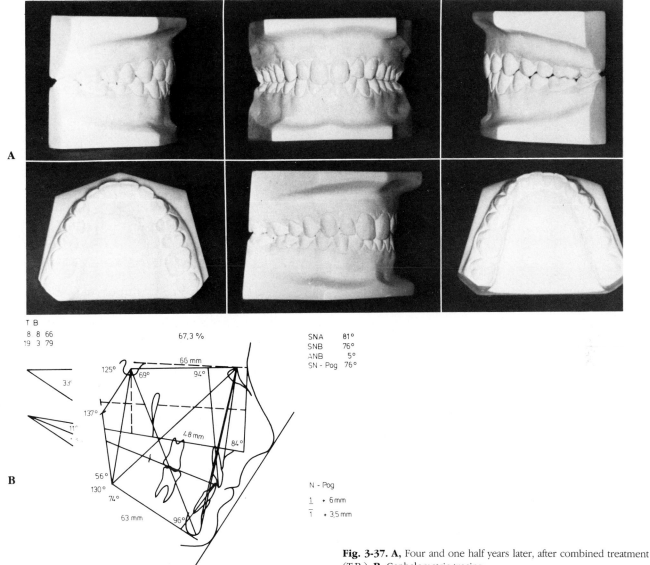

T B
8 8 66
19 3 79

67,3 %

125°   69°   94°
66 mm
137°
4.8 mm   84°
56°
130°
74°
63 mm   96°

3.5°

110

SNA   81°
SNB   76°
ANB   5°
SN - Pog 76°

N - Pog

1 ▸ 6 mm
1 ▸ 3,5 mm

A

B

Fig. 3-37. A, Four and one half years later, after combined treatment (T.B.). **B,** Cephalometric tracing.

skeletal dysplasia. As indicated before, with lip dysfunction the malocclusion is localized in the dentoalveolar region. In cases of skeletal discrepancies the malocclusion is of a skeletal pattern–type origin, with a retrognathic mandible and/or a prognathic maxilla. Screening therapy is successful only in cases of dentoalveolar disharmony. Cephalometric analysis enables one to make the proper differential diagnosis. A case in point follows:

An 8-year-old girl (Fig. 3-36) is shown with an A-N-B angle of 10° and a Class II malocclusion. The maxilla was prognatic, and the mandible small and retrognathic. The upper incisors were tipped slightly labially and the lower incisors were more proclined. In spite of the lip dysfunction, the overjet could not be influenced by a screening appliance because the malocclusion was due to a skeletal disharmony. Not even the use of conventional functional appliances promised success because,

in addition to the retrognathic mandible, the prognathic maxilla had to be influenced by therapy.

This is a good example of a case that would benefit from combined extraoral force on the upper arch and a functional appliance. As shown in Fig. 3-37, the combined approach was successful. There are many of these cases in which combined headgear-activator therapy can produce successful results that are not possible with functional appliances or headgear alone. Thus it is apparent that the screening appliances can be combined with other methods by building some screening elements into the other appliances. The activator can have additional appurtenances (e.g., lip pads or buccal shields) as Fränkel uses in his Function Regulator (Fig. 10-2), although other principles are involved in pure FR therapy.

CHAPTER 4

CEPHALOMETRIC DIAGNOSIS FOR FUNCTIONAL APPLIANCE THERAPY

It is no less important to determine skeletodental relationships for functional appliances than it is to do so for fixed appliances. Proper pretreatment assessment can mean the difference between successful and unsuccessful treatment. This involves a number of diagnostic criteria, but radiographic cephalometrics is an essential component of the diagnostic mosaic. Cephalometrics has been used, and misused, so much, however, that the editor of the *American Journal of Orthodontics* once remarked, as he pondered over a stack of manuscripts that had been submitted for publication, "We are surfeitted with cephalometrics. It is like Dukas' *Sorcerer's Apprentice:* The more I reject, the more the tide increases. Now I know what they mean by a numbers racket." This was a bit facetious, of course, but more than a kernel of truth exists.

Even as cliques and cults have developed in mechanotherapy, so they have in cephalometric diagnosis. A preselected and preprinted group of arbitrary measurements on a two-dimensional lateral head film could be a Steiner analysis, a Tweed analysis, a Holdaway analysis, a Schwarz analysis, a Bimler analysis, a Jarabak analysis, or a Ricketts analysis, to mention just a few of the more popular combinations that have been used routinely by orthodontists in the past 35 years. Treatment decisions have been and continue to be made on "current and choice" cephalometric criteria. The sad fact, however, is that significant information is missing from many cephalometric analyses. Feeding inadequate data into a computer may enhance the glamor in the eyes of the patient, but it does not lend any more credibility to the lines, angles, and linear measurements arbitrarily chosen. The well-known computer acronym *G-I-G-O* applies (i.e., "Garbage In, Garbage Out.").

This chapter is based largely on Chapter 5 in *Removable Orthodontic Appliances* by T.M. Graber and Bedrich Neumann, Philadelphia, 1984, W.B. Saunders Co.

It is the purpose of this chapter to separate the wheat from the chaff and to present and develop a cephalometric analysis that will furnish the most valuable information for functional appliance use without becoming so complicated and lengthy as to discourage clinicians attempting to use it.

An Atlas and Manual of Cephalometric Radiography has recently been published by the author (Rakosi) and gives a general and detailed discussion of the use of cephalometrics in all phases of orthodontics. The most important cephalometric measurements have been chosen so they will specifically assist the clinician in making his diagnosis for functional appliances. Equally important is the fact that this book is a practical tool which permits the assessment of ongoing treatment results, aiding in therapeutic modifiability and attainment of the best possible treatment goals.

Since most functional appliance therapy is instituted in the mixed or transitional dentition stage (or at 8 to 9 years of age), the special criteria chosen are adapted to this age period. However, they can be used equally well in following the progress of each patient into the adult dentition.

There are four major areas of emphasis in the cephalometric diagnostic assessment for functional appliance or functional appliance-headgear orthopedic patients.

1. *Accomplishment of growth increments and the direction or vector of growth.* These vary not only from individual to individual but within the same individual. Longitudinal studies by Graber show that there is often a change in the direction of growth, particularly during the prepubertal period. Although the vector will occasionally become more vertical, it usually becomes more horizontal, giving the impression of following a logarithmic spiral (as has been noted by Moss). Yet there are certain facial pattern characteristics that permit prediction of growth direction probabilities for a particular time frame. The mor-

phologic specifics, particularly of the mandible (where the greatest growth occurs), are of paramount importance for functional orthopedic patients.

2. *Assessment of the magnitude of growth change.* This is as important as determining the direction of growth of the dentofacial complex. Growth amounts can be small, average, or high. They can exhibit spurts (as Woodside has shown) in at least 50% of the cases during the mixed dentition period. Since functional appliances are essentially a deficiency appliance, finding their greatest use in Class II, Division 1, malocclusions with underdeveloped mandibles, the greater the amount of growth that occurs the more favorable is the therapeutic prognosis. In addition to the static linear and angular cephalometric criteria, postural and functional assessment of the mandible is of vital importance.

3. *Inclination and position of the upper and lower incisors.* When evaluating these, it is most beneficial to be able to forecast the probable reciprocal growth increments of the jaw bases. The stability of the cephalometric criteria and derived measure points must be good and the measurements must be reproducible on a longitudinal and interobserver basis.

The orientation of the incisors to the constructed facial plane can be validly assessed only if the plane is assumed to remain identifiable and stable during therapy. If mandibular basal growth exceeds that of the maxilla (as is the case in most patterns) or if the upper terminus, nasion, moves forward less than the mandibular symphysis, then the plane angulation will change. Also the plane moves anteriorly with growth, and this can alter the linear measurements to the upper incisors without any appliance effect on these teeth. The clinician must know the probabilities of growth direction, growth direction change, and growth increments in three dimensions in various parts of the face before he projects his treatment procedures and consequences for the patient. The changes just mentioned obviously create different therapeutic objectives for the upper and lower incisors.

4. *Radiographic cephalometrics.* This allows the identification and localization of the apparent anomaly or abnormality of size, shape, or spatial relationship. It provides a differentiation between skeletal and dentoalveolar malocclusions (or gives information on the combination of factors involved from both areas). This differentiation is important for many reasons.

a. Consideration of the etiology. The consequences of abnormal perioral muscle function can be localized in the dentoalveolar region. An open bite, for example, with a primarily dentoalveolar manifestation is usually the consequence of a neuromuscular dysfunction. If it is combined with a vertical growth pattern, excessive anterior face height, or short posterior face height, then the morphogenetic pattern is the probable primary causative factor.

b. To determine the therapeutic possibilities, it should be known that in dentoalveolar malocclusions caused by neuromuscular dysfunction, a causal form of treatment is possible and is likely to be successful by eliminating the abnormal environmental factors. In skeletally derived malocclusions, a causal type of treatment is possible only by channeling basal growth patterns to provide the morphologic and functional changes needed to establish a normal structural and functional continuum.

If it is not possible to influence the growth processes in a skeletal type of malocclusion, only a compensatory form of therapy can be performed, which usually means adjusting the skeletal dysplasia by making dentoalveolar compromises (e.g., extraction, specific anchorage control, orthognathic surgery) in the most severely dysplastic jaw relationships.

To obtain this vital information before instituting a treatment regimen, whether for fixed or removable appliances or for functional or nonfunctional armamentaria, we must turn to a comprehensive cephalometric analysis.

REFERENCE POINTS, LINES, ANGLES, AND METHODS OF EVALUATION

A large number of cephalometric "packages" are available, from many clinicians and researchers around the world. Since the introduction of cephalometrics as a clinical orthodontic tool some 50 years ago, more articles have appeared on this subject than on any other in the periodical literature; and cephalometrics has played a dominant role in the many thousands of theses written by orthodontic graduate students. To select from this formidable array would be difficult for the uninitiated clinician. However, in a separate book by the author (*Cephalometric Radiography,* Wolfe Medical Publications, 1982) the method that has proved most valuable for the mixed dentition and for planning functional appliance therapy is comprehensively described.

Reference points. This chapter elucidates only some of the measurements that are of special interest, together with their interpretation and application to functional appliance treatment. The following list of definitions of reference points is based on the one in Rakosi's book (see Fig. 4-1):

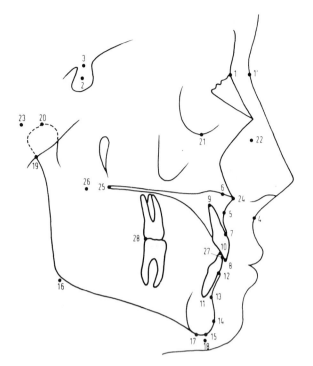

Fig. 4-1. Reference points used in the functional cephalometric analysis. (From Rakosi, T.: An atlas and manual of cephalometric radiography, Philadelphia, 1982, Lea & Febiger.)

Code	Definition
1. N	*Nasion:* most anterior point of the nasofrontal suture in median plane; skin nasion (N′) is located at point of maximum convexity between the nose and forehead
2. S	*Sella:* midpoint of the sella (S), hypophysis cerebri (sella turcica); also midpoint of entrance to the sella; defined as midpoint of the hypophyseal fossa, a constructed (radiologic) point in the median plane
3. Se	*Midpoint of entrance to the sella* (after A.M. Schwarz): at level of the jugum sphenoidale, independent of depth of the sella, it is the midpoint of the line connecting the posterior clinoid process and anterior opening of the sella turcica
4. Sn	*Subnasale:* skin point where the nasal septum merges inferiorly with integument of the upper lip
5. A	*Point A, subspinale:* deepest midline point in curved bony outline from base to alveolar process of the maxilla (i.e., at the deepest point between ANS and Pr); in anthropology it is known as subspinale
6. APMax	*Anteriorly derived landmark for determining length of maxilla:* constructed by dropping a perpendicular from point A to the palatal plane
7. Pr	*Prosthion:* alveolar rim of the maxilla; lowest and most anterior point on alveolar portion of the premaxilla, in median plane, between the upper central incisors

Code	Definition
8. Is (or $\underline{1}$)	*Incisor superius:* incisal edge of the maxillary central incisor
9. Ap $\underline{1}$	*Apicale $\underline{1}$:* apex of the maxillary central incisor
10. Ii (or $\overline{1}$)	*Incisor inferius:* incisal edge of the mandibular central incisor
11. Ap $\overline{1}$	*Apicale $\overline{1}$:* apex of the mandibular central incisor
12. Id	*Infradentale:* alveolar rim of the mandible; highest and most anterior point on the alveolar process, in median plane, between the lower central incisors
13. B	*Point B, supramentale:* most anterior part of the mandibular base; most posterior point in outer contour of the mandibular alveolar process, in median plane; in anthropology it is known as supramentale, between infradentale and pogonion
14. Pog	*Pogonion:* most anterior point of the bony chin (symphysis), in median plane
15. Gn	*Gnathion:* several definitions: according to Martin and Saller (1956), it is located in median plane of the mandible, where anterior curve in outline of the chin merges into body of the mandible; many authors locate it between most anterior and most inferior points of the chin; Craig defines it as the point of intersection of the facial and mandibular planes. For functional appliance analysis, it is the most anterior and inferior point of the bony chin—constructed by intersection of a perpendicular dropped from Me-Pog to the bony outline
16. Go	*Gonion:* constructed point, intersection of the lines tangent to posterior margin of the ascending ramus and the mandibular base
17. Me	*Menton:* according to Krogman and Sassouni, the most caudal point in outline of the symphysis; the lowest point of the mandible (corresponds to anthropologic gnathion)
18. APMan	*Anterior landmark for determining length of mandible:* constructed by dropping a perpendicular from Pog to the mandibular plane
19. Ar	*Articulare:* intersection of dorsal contours of the processus articularis mandibulae and inferior surface of the temporal bone as seen in lateral cephalometric projection; introduced by Björk (1947), it provides radiologic orientation
20. Cd	*Condylion:* most superior point on head of the condyle
21. Or	*Orbitale:* Lowest point on radiograph of the orbit
22. Pn/2	*Constructed point* obtained by bisecting the Pn vertical (dropped from Se-N at N′)
23. FH–R asc	*Intersection* of Frankfort horizontal and posterior margin of the ascending ramus

Code	Definition
24. ANS	*Anterior nasal spine:* pointed tip of the anterior nasal crest in median plane (corresponds to anthropologic acanthion)
25. PNS	*Posterior nasal spine:* constructed radiologic point, intersection of the anterior wall of pterygopalatine fossa and floor of the nose; it marks dorsal limit of the maxilla
26. S′	*Constructed point for assessing length of maxillary base:* in posterior section a perpendicular dropped from Se to the palatal plane
27. APOcc	*Anteriorly derived point for determining occlusal plane:* middle of the incisor overbite in occlusion
28. PPOcc	*Posterior point for determining occlusal plane:* the most distal contact between the posteriormost molars in occlusion
29. Ba	*Basion:* lowest point on anterior margin of the foramen magnum, in median plane
30. Ptm	*Pterygomaxillary fissure:* projection onto the palatal plane; anterior wall represents the maxillary tuberosity outline, posterior wall the anterior curve of the pterygoid process (corresponds to PNS)

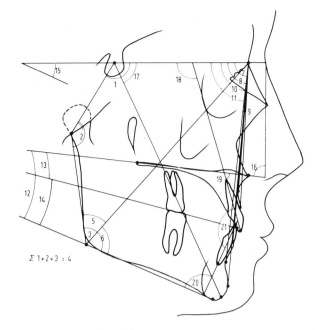

Fig. 4-2. The most valid and frequently used angular measurements. (From Rakosi, T.: An atlas and manual of cephalometric radiography, Philadelphia, 1982, Lea & Febiger.)

Angular measurements. Reference lines enable us to make angular measurements on the radiograph. The following angles are determined routinely (Fig. 4-2):

	Definition	Mean value (degrees)
1. N-S-Ar	Saddle angle	123 ± 5
2. S-Ar-Go	Articular angle	143 ± 6
3. Ar-Go-Me	Gonial angle	128 ± 7
4. Sum	Sum of saddle, articular, and gonial angles	394
5. Ar-Go-N	Go 1, upper gonial angle	52 to 55
6. N-Go-Me	Go 2, lower gonial angle	70 to 75
7. S-N-A	Anteroposterior position of maxilla	81
8. S-N-B	Anteroposterior position of mandible	79
9. A-N-B	Difference between S-N-A and S-N-B	2
10. S-N-Pr	Anteroposterior position of alveolar part of premaxilla (prosthion)	84
11. S-N-Id	Anteroposterior position of alveolar part of mandible (infradentale)	81
12. Pal-MP	Angle between palatal and mandibular planes	25

	Definition	Mean value (degrees)
13. Pal-Occ	Upper occlusal plane angle	11
14. MP-Occ	Lower occlusal plane angle	14
15. S-N-MP	Angle between S-N and mandibular plane	32
16. Pn-Pal	Angle of inclination (∠) between the perpendicular dropped from Se-N at N′ and the palatal plane (after A.M. Schwarz)	85
17. N-S-Gn	(Y-axis) Angle between S-N and S-Gn anteriorly	66
18. 1̲-SN	Angle between upper incisor axis and S-N posteriorly	102
19. 1̲-Pal	Angle between upper incisor axis and palatal plane anteriorly	70 ± 5
20. 1̄-MP	Angle between lower incisor axis and mandibular plane posteriorly	90 ± 3
21. ii angle	Interincisal angle, between upper and lower central incisor axes posteriorly	135

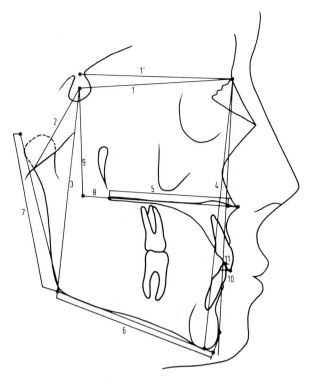

Fig. 4-3. Linear measurements. (From Rakosi, T.: An atlas and manual of cephalometric radiography, Philadelphia, 1982, Lea & Febiger.)

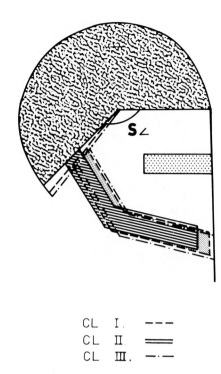

CL I. – – –
CL II. ═══
CL III. –·–

Fig. 4-4. The saddle angle *(S)* is generally large in the retrognathic face but small in the prognathic face.

Linear measurements. Reference lines also enable us to determine linear dimensions on the radiograph (Fig. 4-3):

	Definition	*Mean value (mm)*
1. S-N	(Se-N) Anteroposterior extent of anterior cranial base	71
2. S-Ar	Extent of lateral cranial base	32 to 35
3. S-Go	Posterior face height	
4. N-Me	Anterior face height	
5. MaxBase	Extent of maxillary base correlated with Se-N	
6. ManBase	Extent of mandibular base correlated with Se-N	
7. R asc	Extent of ascending ramus correlated with Se-N	
8. S'-F Ptp	Distance from S' to projection of anterior wall of pterygopalatine fossa on palatal plane; an expression for anteroposterior displacement of the maxillary base	
9. S-S'	Deflection of maxillary base	42 to 57
10. 1̲ to N-Pog	Distance from incisal edge of upper incisor to N-Pog	
11. 1̄ to N-Pog	Distance from incisal edge of lower incisor to N-Pog	

CEPHALOMETRIC ANALYSES

The various cephalometric evaluations can be divided into three groups:
 Facial skeleton
 Jaw bases
 Dentoalveolar relationships

Analysis of the facial skeleton

The first cephalometric analysis includes three angular measurements (saddle angle, articular angle, gonial angle) and four linear measurements (anterior and posterior face height, anterior and posterior cranial base length).

Saddle angle (N-S-Ar). The angle formed by joining these three points is an assessment of the relationship between anterior and posterolateral cranial bases. The position of sella turcica, which is the midpoint of the angle, is determined partly by growth changes in the area. This means that a large saddle angle usually signifies a posterior condylar position and a mandible that is posteriorly positioned with respect to the cranial base and maxilla—that is, unless the deviation in position of the fossa is compensated by angular (e.g., articular angle) and linear (e.g., ramal length) relationships. A noncompensated posterior positioning of the mandible, caused by a large saddle angle, is very difficult to influence with functional appliance therapy (Fig. 4-4).

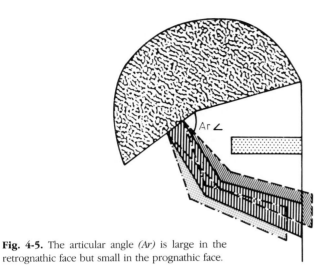

Fig. 4-5. The articular angle *(Ar)* is large in the retrognathic face but small in the prognathic face.

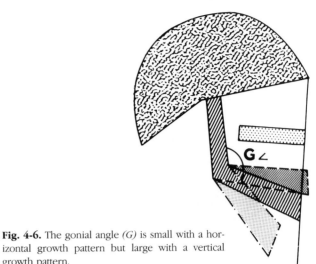

Fig. 4-6. The gonial angle *(G)* is small with a horizontal growth pattern but large with a vertical growth pattern.

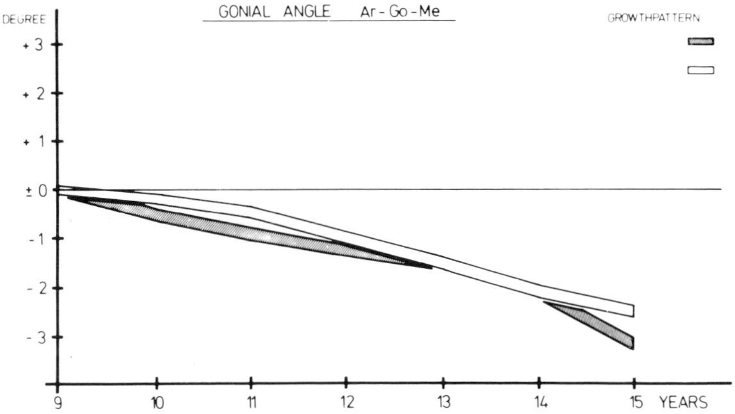

Fig. 4-7. Growth increments of the gonial angle in the horizontal and vertical growth patterns between the ninth and fifteenth years.

Articular angle (S-Ar-Go). The articular angle is a constructed angle between the upper and lower parts of the posterior contours of the facial skeleton. Its size depends on the position of the mandible: large when the mandible is retrognathic, small when the mandible is prognathic. It can be influenced during orthopedic (orthodontic) therapy—decreasing with anterior positioning of the mandible, with closing of the bite, or with mesial migration of the posterior segment teeth; increasing with posterior relocation of the mandible, opening of the bite, or distal driving of the posterior teeth.

An alteration of this angle can be seen in some activator treatment results (Fig. 4-5). In a study of 9-year-old children with horizontal growth patterns, the angle was slightly smaller (on average 139.5°) than in patients with a vertical growth direction (142.4°). The growth increments between 9 and 15 years were −2.89° with the horizontal growth pattern and −2.49° with the vertical growth vector.

Gonial angle (Ar-Go-Me). The angle formed by tangents to the body of the mandible and posterior border of the ramus is of special interest because it not only expresses the form of the mandible but also gives information on mandibular growth direction. If this angle is acute or small, especially in its lower component (the lower Go angle of Jarabak), then the direction of growth is horizontal. This is a favorable condition for anterior positioning of the mandible with an activator.

In patients with a large angle, activator treatment is contraindicated or the appliance must be constructed by taking into account the growth pattern (Fig. 4-6). In 9-year-old mixed dentition children showing a horizontal growth pattern, the average angle is 125.5° (the lower angle being 69.5°). In vertical growth patterns the angle increases to 133.4° (with a larger lower angle of 78.3°).

Between the ninth and eleventh year of growth in this longitudinal study, the growth increment was −2.89° with the horizontal pattern and −2.42° with the vertical pattern (Fig. 4-7).

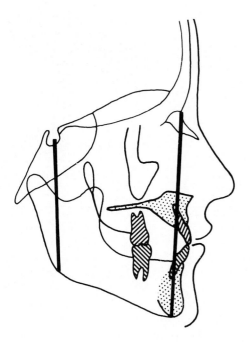

Fig. 4-8. Posterior and anterior face height measurements. A ratio is established between these dimensions that assists in projecting sagittal growth direction probabilities.

Anterior and posterior face height. This measurement is a linear millimetric assessment. The posterior face height (S-Go) and the anterior face height (N-Me) are measured on the lateral cephalogram with the teeth in habitual occlusion (Fig. 4-8).

The posterior face height in the longitudinal study of 9-year-old children with a horizontal growth pattern was longer on the average (69.5 mm) than in children with a vertical growth pattern (64.1 mm). The growth increment with the horizontal growth pattern between 9 and 15 years of age was 11.05 mm, and 10.8 mm in the vertically growing group. The reverse ratio was true of anterior face height. In the horizontal pattern the average was 103 mm with a growth increment of 12.18 mm as opposed to the vertical measurements of 106.6 mm between nasion and menton with a total growth increment of 12.71 mm (Figs. 4-9 and 4-10).

To estimate the direction of growth that is so important in activator treatment, we can compare anterior and posterior face height and set up a ratio, according to the recommendations of Jarabak:

$$\frac{\text{Posterior face height} \times 100}{\text{Anterior face height}}$$

A ratio under 62% expresses a vertical growth pattern whereas over 65% the likelihood is for a horizontal vector. At 9 years of age the average in the horizontally

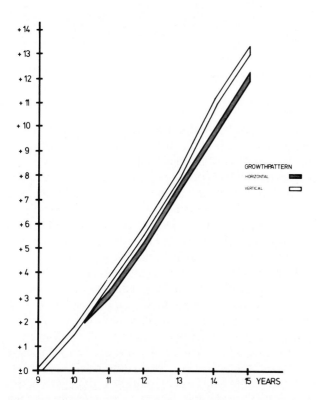

Fig. 4-9. Growth increments of anterior face height (N-Me). Note the difference between horizontally and vertically growing faces.

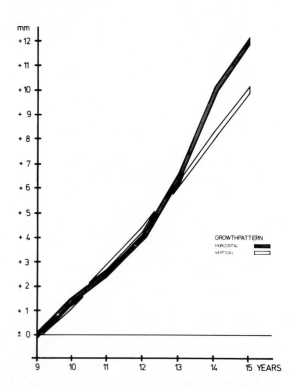

Fig. 4-10. Growth increments of the posterior face height (S-Go). Note that the increments are larger in horizontally growing faces after 13 years of age.

growing group was 67.5%, increasing to 69.9% by 15 years of age. In the vertically growing group the posterior to anterior face height ratio was 60.1% at 9 years, increasing to 62.7% by 15 years. All the measurements showed a general trend toward a more horizontal growth pattern.

Growth forecasting for early mixed dentition treatment with an activator should be done by comparing angular and linear measurements and morphologic characteristics of the mandible (see "Analysis of the jaw bases"). The assessment of growth direction is very important in functional appliance therapy, for determining both whether it should be used and then the construction details, type of construction bite, etc.

Anterior cranial base length (Se-N). The measurement of the anterior cranial base (Fig. 4-11) can also use the center of the superior entrance to sella turcica as a reference point instead of the center of the sella turcica fossa outline as is usually done for cranial base establishment. The correlation of this criterion with the length of the jaw bases enables assessment of the proportional averages of these bases to be made.

In the longitudinal study group the 9-year-old average length of anterior cranial base was 68.8 mm for horizontal growth patterns and 63.8 mm in children with a vertical growth vector. The incremental change between 9 and 15 years was 4.46 mm in the horizontal and 3.52 in the vertical pattern.

Posterior (lateral) cranial base length (S-Ar). The magnitude of this dimension is dependent on the posterior face height and position of the fossa (see Fig. 4-11). A short posterior cranial base occurs in vertical

growth patterns or skeletal open bites, which gives a poor prognosis for functional appliance therapy. In 9-year-old children with a horizontal growth pattern the average length was 32.2 mm, with an increment of 9.16 mm in the following 6 years, as opposed to 30 mm with an increment of 4.47 mm in the vertical pattern.

Analysis of the jaw bases

The angles between the vertical reference lines represent the sagittal relationship of parts (e.g., S-N-A, S-N-B) whereas those between the horizontal lines assist in evaluating the vertical relationship (e.g., base plane angle, inclination angle). The linear measurements give an indication of the length of the maxillary and mandibular bases as well as the ascending ramus. A morphologic assessment, particularly of the mandible, is also important in forecasting the growth direction. Only selected measurements are described in this overview, because of their application in treatment planning for functional appliances.

S-N-A (Fig. 4-12). The angle S-N-A expresses the sagittal relationship of the anterior limit of the maxillary apical base* (point A) as related to the anterior cranial base. It is large in a prognathic maxilla and small in a retruded maxilla. In Class II, Division 1, malocclusions (caused by a prognathic maxilla) with a larger than normal S-N-A, the use of an activator is contraindicated.

McNamara points out in his study that S-N-A does not vary much among the different types of malocclusions nor does it change much with functional appliance treatment. The growth increments are small for this criterion, and the difference between growth direction types is insignificant (Fig. 4-13).

*Axel Lundström's term (1923) for the junction of alveolar bone and basal bone.

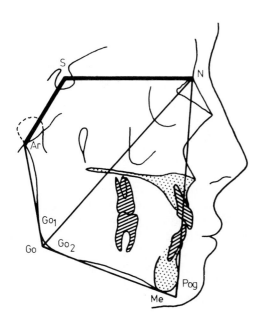

Fig. 4-11. Measurements for the anteroposterior cranial base length (*N-S* and *S-Ar*).

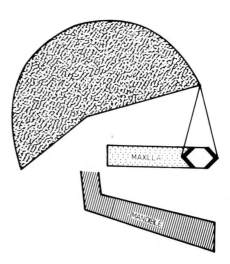

Fig. 4-12. The S-N-A angle expresses horizontal position of the maxillary base in relation to the cranial base.

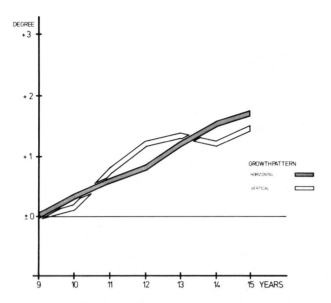

Fig. 4-13. Growth increments of the S-N-A. Terminal growth is greater in horizontally growing patterns.

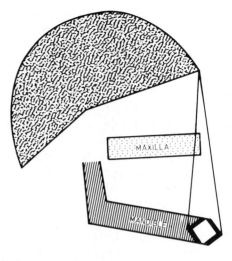

Fig. 4-14. The S-N-B angle expresses horizontal position of the mandibular base in relation to the cranial base.

| | S-N-A (degrees) | |
	9 years	15 years
Average	79.5	81.28
Horizontal	79.73	81.57
Vertical	79.0	80.57

A moderate decrease of this angle is possible by means of conventional activator therapy. A larger decrease is possible with special activator construction.

S-N-B (Fig. 4-14). The angle S-N-B expresses the sagittal relationship between the anterior extent of the mandibular apical base and the anterior cranial base. With a prognathic mandible it is large, with a retrognathic mandible small. Functional appliance treatment is indicated if the mandible is retrognathic, with a small S-N-B. It should be remembered that this angle provides information only on the anteroposterior position of the mandible, not its morphology or growth direction. A posteriorly located mandible can be large or small; if small, the prognosis for anterior posturing in the mixed dentition is good since a larger growth increment can usually be expected.

The average angle and growth increments in the horizontal face type are much larger (77.2° at 9 years and 80.5° at 15 years) than in the vertical growth pattern (74.3° at 9 years and 75.9° at 15 years) (Fig. 4-15). Together with the favorable growth direction, the greater increments of the mandible in the horizontal pattern make successful treatment of these patients possible by anterior posturing of the mandible in functional appliance therapy.

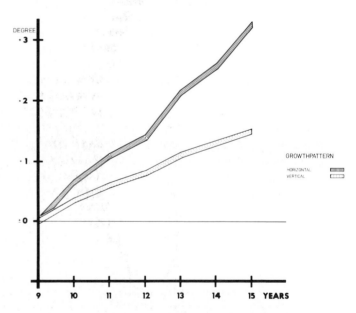

Fig. 4-15. Growth increments of the S-N-B. The greatest divergence in growth accomplishment is apparent here as the mandible grows and is translated more anteriorly in horizontal growth patterns.

Base plane angle (Pal-MP) (Fig. 4-16). The base plane angle, between the maxillary and mandibular jaw bases, is also used to determine the inclination of the mandibular plane itself. In the horizontal growth pattern this angle is small (23.4° at 9 years and 20.5° at 15 years) whereas in the vertical growth group it is larger (32.9° at 9 years and 30.9° at 15 years). The age-dependent decrease in this angle corresponds to the general trend toward a more horizontal growth pattern and expresses

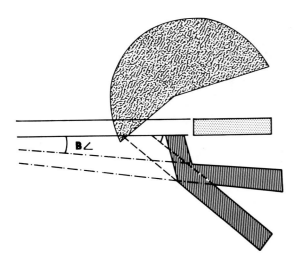

Fig. 4-16. The base plane angle is small with a horizontal growth pattern but large with a vertical (maxillary versus mandibular planes).

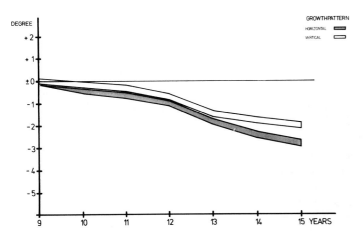

Fig. 4-17. Growth increments of the base plane angle. Note that the angle decreases more in horizontally growing faces.

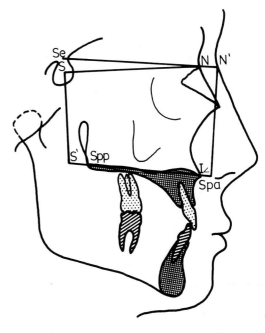

Fig. 4-18. Inclination angle (perpendicular to the maxillary base plane from *N-Se* at *N'*) (I∠).

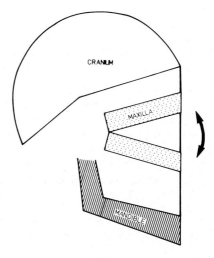

Fig. 4-19. Retroclination and anteclination of the maxillary base. A broad range is possible.

the logarithmic spiral type of growth described by Moss, Graber, and others (Fig. 4-17).

Inclination angle (Fig. 4-18). The inclination angle gives an assessment of the inclination of the maxillary base. It is the angle formed by the Pn line (a perpendicular dropped from N-Se at N') and the palatal plane. A large angle expresses upward and forward inclination whereas a small angle indicates downward and backward tipping of the anterior end of the palatal plane or maxillary base (Fig. 4-19). This angle is not correlated with the growth pattern or facial type. Functional or therapeutic influences can alter the inclination of the maxillary base, however (Fig. 4-20).

Rotation of the jaw bases. The two previous measurements (base plane angle and inclination angle) are used to evaluate the rotation of the upper and lower jaw bases. These rotations are of special interest in treatment with functional appliances since they show whether such appliances are indicated and the criteria in appliance construction.

The rotation of the mandible is growth conditioned and dependent on the direction and mutual relations of growth increments in the posterior (condylar) and anterior (sutural and alveolar) facial skeleton. If condylar growth (plus minimal increments of temporal fossa

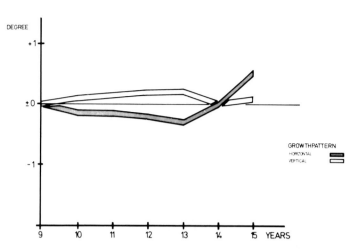

Fig. 4-20. Growth increments of the inclination angle. In horizontally growing faces, terminal growth appears to increase this angle whereas in vertical patterns it remains constant.

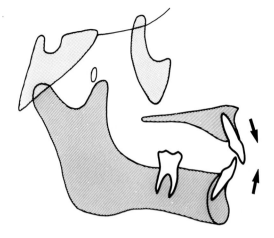

Fig. 4-21. Convergent rotation of the jaw bases (closing down of maxillomandibular basal angles).

growth) proceeds at a higher rate, it results in horizontal rotation. If growth increments are balanced, parallel growth down the Y-axis occurs.

Björk differentiates the two processes involved in rotational growth of the mandible.

1. Remodeling of the mandible in the symphyseal and gonial areas. This is called *intermatrix rotation.* It is a function of the periosteal matrix (Moss), and it often results in a subsequent rotation. More apposition in the gonial area and resorption in the symphyseal area lead to a horizontal rotation. Greater apposition in the symphyseal area with resorption in the gonial region causes a vertical rotation.

2. Vertical or horizontal rotation of the mandible in its neuromuscular envelope. This is *matrix rotation* or a relocation of the functional matrix of Moss. That seen cephalometrically is *total rotation,* consisting of both intermatrix and matrix rotation.

Rotation of the mandible is due to both growth-dependent and functional influences. Functional orthodontic (orthopedic) methods alter the function and guide the growth process. For this reason it is possible to influence therapeutically to a moderate degree the rotation of the mandible.

The pattern of rotation of the maxillary base can be observed by sequential measurements of the inclination angle. Generally the inclination of the maxillary base is stable and no growth-dependent changes are seen. Environmental influences such as neuromuscular dysfunction, occlusal forces, gravity, and nasorespiratory malfunction (according to Linder-Aronson) can modify this inclination. An upward and forward tipping of the anterior part of the maxilla is often seen in confirmed mouthbreathers. A downward and backward tipping of the anterior part of the maxillary base is seen as a natural compensation in patients with vertically growing

faces. The inclination can be influenced by both fixed orthopedic and functional therapeutic techniques.

Mutual relationship of the rotating jaw bases. Rotation of the mandible can be decisive in establishing the vertical proportions of the facial skeleton. In a horizontal rotation the anterior face profile is short whereas in a vertically rotating mandibular pattern it is long. A horizontal rotation means that there is a predisposition toward a deep overbite; an excessively vertical rotation means a tendency toward an open bite. The inclination of the maxillary base is also important to the occlusal relationship. The resultant dentoalveolar malocclusion depends on the combination of these rotations. We can differentiate the following types of rotations as shown by Lavergne and Gasson in human implant studies:

1. Convergent rotation of the jaw bases. This creates a severely deep overbite, which is difficult to manage using functional methods (Fig. 4-21).

2. Divergent rotation of the jaw bases. This can cause marked open bite problems. In severe cases orthognathic surgery is required for the correction (Fig. 4-22).

3. Cranial rotation of both bases. In this horizontal growth pattern there is a relatively harmonious rotation of both jaws in an upward and forward direction. The upward and forward rotation of the maxilla compensates for the upward and forward mandibular rotation, offsetting what could be a deep bite. The result is a normal overbite (Fig. 4-23).

4. Caudal or downward and backward rotation of both bases in a relatively harmonious manner. The downward and backward maxillary rotation offsets what could be an open bite created by the downward and backward mandibular rotation (Fig. 4-24).

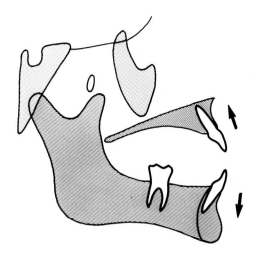

Fig. 4-22. Divergent rotation of the jaw bases (opening up of the base angle).

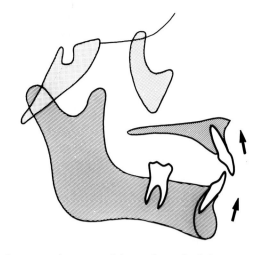

Fig. 4-23. Cranial rotation of the jaw bases (both bases rotating upward and forward).

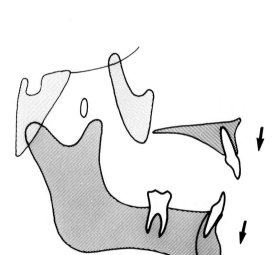

Fig. 4-24. Caudal rotation of the jaw bases (downward and backward).

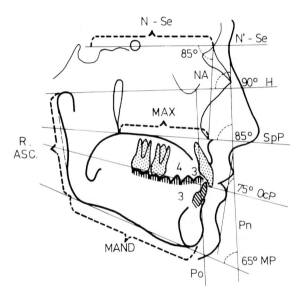

Fig. 4-25. Proportional measurements of the jaw bases and the ascending ramus (after Schwarz).

The therapeutic control of the vertical dimension is usually more difficult than of the sagittal dimension. If a causal therapeutic skeletal reconstruction is not possible, some compensatory form of treatment is indicated. This means, for example, that if the vertical morphogenetic pattern cannot be altered an occlusal adjustment must be achieved by retroclination of the maxillary base, often with tooth sacrifice. Again, orthognathic surgery is the ultimate corrective procedure if the magnitude of the malrelationship transcends orthodontic or orthopedic growth guidance procedures.

Linear measurement of the jaw bases. When the indications for functional appliance therapy are being determined, not only the position but also the length of the jaw bases must be assessed. If the mandible is retrognathic, the question arises whether its size is relatively small or large. This is important in considering the etiology and therapy for each patient. The length of the maxillary and mandibular bases, and of the ascending ramus, is measured relative to Se-N. The measurements used are the ones proposed by Schwarz in his "roentgenostatic analysis" (Fig. 4-25). The ideal dimension relative to Se-N is calculated by using the following formula:

N-Se : ManBase	20 : 21
Ascending ramus : ManBase	5 : 7
MaxBase : ManBase	2 : 3

The evaluations result in two "ideal" dimensions, one related to the length of Se-N and the other to the mandibular base. Table 4-1 has been compiled to simplify the calculations.

Extent of the mandibular base. This is determined by measuring the distance gonion-pogonion (projected perpendicular to the mandibular plane) (Fig. 4-26). Ideally the mandibular base should be 3 mm longer than Se-N up to the twelfth year and 3.5 mm longer after the twelfth year. As much as 5 mm less than this average is considered to be within the norm up to 7 years of age, however, and as much as 5 mm more is normal up to 15 years of age.

In the longitudinal study of children referred to earlier, the length of the base and the growth increments were both higher in the horizontal than in the vertical growth pattern. In the horizontal pattern at 9 years of age the average length was 67.59 mm, increasing to 77.35 mm at 15 years. In the vertical pattern the length in 9-year-olds was 65.23 mm, increasing to 73.5 mm in the 15-year-old sample (Fig. 4-27).

Extent of the maxillary base. This is determined by measuring the distance between the posterior nasal spine and point A projected perpendicularly onto the palatal plane. There are two "ideal" measurements for the evaluation of this dimension: one related to N-Se and the other to the length of the mandibular base.

The difference in lengths of the maxillary base between the two growth patterns studied was slight and the growth increment lower than those of the mandibular base. As Johnston points out, the mandible outgrows the maxilla. In the horizontal pattern group the average length was 44.65 mm in the 9-year-old sample and 48.6 mm in the 15-year-old sample. In the vertical

pattern group the average length was 44.0 mm at 9 years and 47.16 mm at 15 years of age (Fig. 4-28).

Since the growth potential of the mandibular base is greater than that of the maxillary base, the angle S-N-B increases and A-N-B thus decreases. This corroborates the impression of many clinicians that the mandible is less retrognathic after 12 years of age. The growth advantage, with the mandible outgrowing the maxilla by as much as 5 mm, is of special value to functional appliance proponents and, of course, to the Class II patients being treated.

Length of the ascending ramus. This measurement is made by calculating the distance between gonion and condylion. To simplify the location of condylion, a Frankfort horizontal is constructed and is intersected by a tangent to the ramus. The point of intersection represents constructed condylion (Fig. 4-29).

The Frankfort horizontal plane is constructed as follows: the distance between soft tissue nasion (N′) and the palatal plane is bisected along the Pn line; from the point thus created a straight line (H-line) is drawn parallel to the Se-N plane; this becomes the ideal Frankfort horizontal.

The length of the ramus is important in determining posterior face height and subsequent relation to anterior face height. The ramus tends to be longer in horizontally growing patterns, with an average length of 48.9 mm in 9-year-olds and 58.67 mm in 15-year-olds, and it is shorter in vertical patterns, measuring on the average of 44.47 mm in 9-year-olds and 51.7 mm in 15-year-olds (Fig. 4-30).

Evaluation of the length of the jaw bases

Mandibular base. If the length of the mandibular base corresponds to the distance N-Se (ManBase:N-Se + 3

Table 4-1. Linear measurements (mm) of the maxillary and mandibular bases and ascending ramus

Mandible	Maxilla	Ascending ramus	Ramus	Mandible	Maxilla	Ascending ramus	Ramus
56	37	40	22	71	47	50.5	28
57	38	40.5	22.5	72	48	51	29
58	39	41	23	73	48.5	52	29
59	39	42	23.5	74	49	53	29.5
60	40	43	24	75	50	53.5	30
61	40.5	43.5	24	76	50.5	54	30
62	41	44	24.5	77	51	55	31
63	42	45	25	78	52	55.5	31
64	42.5	45.5	25.5	79	52.5	56	31.5
65	43	46	26	80	53	57	32
66	44	47	26	81	54	58	32
67	44.5	47.5	27	82	54.5	58.5	32.5
68	45	48	27	83	55	59	33
69	46	49	27.5	84	56	60	33.5
70	46.5	50	28	85	57	60.5	34

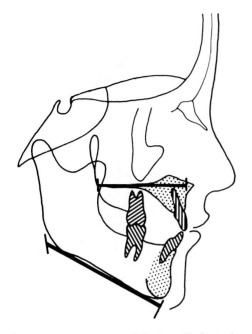

Fig. 4-26. Length measurements of the mandibular and maxillary bases.

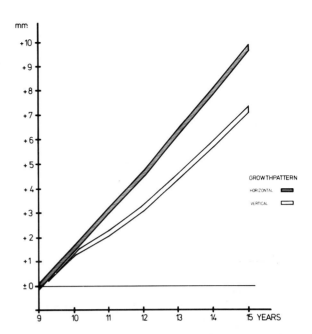

Fig. 4-27. Growth increments of the mandibular base. Note that the increments are greater for horizontal growth patterns.

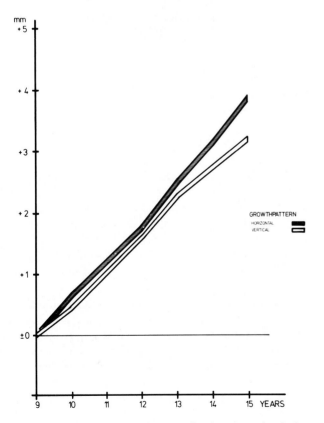

Fig. 4-28. Growth increments of the maxillary base. Note that the base length is greater in horizontally growing faces.

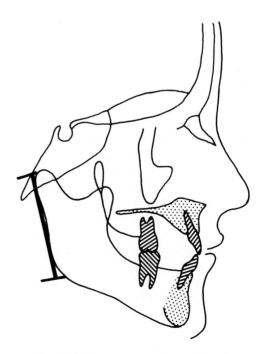

Fig. 4-29. Measurements of the ramal length.

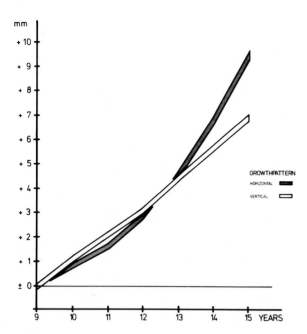

Fig. 4-30. Growth increments of the ramus ascendens (condylion to constructed gonion). Again, greater growth increments are seen in horizontally growing faces.

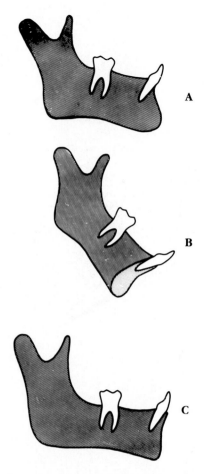

Fig. 4-31. Morphogenetic types of mandible. **A,** Orthognathic. **B,** Retrognathic. **C,** Prognathic.

mm), then this expresses an age-related normal mandibular length and we can expect an average growth increment. If the base is shorter, the growth increment will probably be larger. If it is longer, the growth increment may well be smaller. This forecasting can be made more exact by using two additional measurements, the lengths of both the maxillary base and ascending ramus.

The correlation between length and position of the mandibular base should also be examined. A retrognathic mandible may have either a short or a long base. If the base is short, the cause of the retrognathism is probably a growth deficiency. With a favorable growth direction the prognosis for activator therapy is good. There are two possibilities that can result in a mandibular base that is both long and retrognathic:

1. The mandible is in a functionally retruded (forced) position because of overclosure and occlusal guidance. In postural rest position it is anterior to habitual occlusion. The treatment is simple, eliminating the forced guidance and upward and backward path of closure, in either the mixed or the permanent dentition.
2. The mandible is morphogenetically "built" into the facial skeleton in a posterior position. The temporal fossa itself is posterior and superior. This discrepancy is not compensated, despite the long mandibular base. The prognosis for functional appliance therapy in these cases is poor.

Maxillary base. There are two ideal values for assessing the length of the maxillary base: one related to the

distance N-Se, the other to the length of the mandibular base. A deviation from the mandibular base–related norm means that the maxillary base is too long or too short. If the maxillary base corresponds to the mandibular base–related norm, then the facial skeleton is proportionally developed, particularly if the ramus length also corresponds to these values. If the N-Se length does not relate to these three proportionate measurements, then the facial skeleton is proportionate but either too large or too small.

Ascending ramus. The evaluation of ramus length is performed in a similar manner. If the ramus is too short in relation to the other proportions, a large amount of growth can be expected under the supposition that the growth pattern is not vertical. In the vertical type the ramus remains short. To enhance the differential diagnosis, the morphologic characteristics of the mandible should also be studied.

Morphology of the mandible. The various facial types (orthognathic, retrognathic, prognathic) also reflect to some degree the morphology of the mandible (Fig. 4-31).

In the orthognathic type of face the ramus and body of the mandible are fully developed and the width of the ascending ramus is equal to the height of the body of the mandible, including the height of the alveolar process and the incisors. The condylar and coronoid processes are almost on the same plane, and the symphysis is well developed.

In the prognathic type the corpus is well developed and is wide in the molar region. The symphysis is wider in the sagittal plane. The ramus is wide and long, and the gonial angle is acute or small.

In the retrognathic facial type the corpus is narrow, particularly in the molar region. The symphysis is narrow and long. The ramus is narrow and short. The coronoid process is shorter than the condylar process, and the gonial angle is obtuse or large.

The prognathic type of mandible grows horizontally. Even if there is an average or slightly vertical growth direction in the mixed dentition, shift of the mandible to a horizontal growth direction can be expected in the prognathic type of mandible in the following years. In a retrognathic type of mandible, shift of the growth pattern in the opposite direction is less likely and with much less expressivity.

Analysis of the dentoalveolar relationships

An important part of determining the indications for and construction and management of functional appliances is the assessment of the inclination and position of the incisors with respect to the anterior cranial base, their apical bases, and each other.

Axial inclination of the incisors (Fig. 4-32)

Upper incisors. The long axis of the maxillary incisors, as viewed on the lateral cephalogram, is extended to intersect the S-N line and the posterior angle is measured. Up to the seventh year this angle averages 94° to 100°. One or two years after eruption the inclination increases to an average 102.0°. Larger angles are indicative of incisor procumbency or labial crown tipping for a Caucasian or Oriental sample. Incisor protrusion requires lingual tipping, a therapeutic objective that can be performed quite successfully with removable appliances, if there is adequate space. However, before a decision on the mode of movement of these teeth can be made, an assessment of their position is necessary.

Lower incisors. The posterior angle between the long axis of the lower incisors and the mandibular plane is the classic method of assessing axial inclination of these teeth. The average value often given is 90°, although in most studies of heterogeneous samples it is 4° to 5° more. Between the sixth and twelfth years of life it increases from 88° for the relatively upright deciduous incisors to 94°, on the average, in a normal straight-faced sample.

A smaller angle may be indicative of lingual tipping of

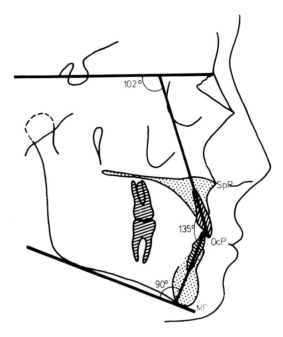

Fig. 4-32. Axial inclination of the upper and lower incisors. (Few normal groups have a 90° inclination of the lower incisors to the mandibular plane, however.)

the incisors, which is advantageous for functional appliance treatment. The activator is most effective in the sagittal plane and tips the lower incisors labially.

If the lower incisors are already labially tipped, then activator treatment is more difficult. It is necessary to reposition the mandible anteriorly and at the same time upright the lower incisors, if possible, by moving them in the opposite direction. To achieve this requires the use of a special appliance design in the lower anterior segment.

Position of the incisors. Linear measurements serve best to assess the position of the incisors with respect to the profile. The most common method is to measure the distance of the incisal edges to the line N-Pog or so-called facial plane (Fig. 4-33).

The average position of the maxillary incisors is 2 to 4 mm anterior to the N-Pog line. The lower incisors vary from 2 mm posterior to 2 mm anterior to this line. The aim of orthodontic treatment is to achieve a similar relationship to this normal guideline. Uprighting of incisors that are tipped too far labially with respect to the N-Pog line is possible with removable appliances. However, space is a consideration. Also, if the labially malpositioned incisor has a good axial inclination already, then bodily movement is required, and this is possible only with fixed appliances and root torque.

The relationship of the lower incisors to the N-Pog line also assists in determining the sagittal discrepancy (Fig. 4-34). Incisors that are behind this line can be moved labially, since space is available. Incisors anterior

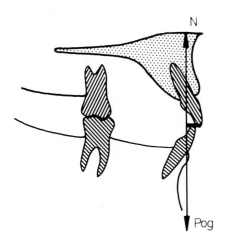

Fig. 4-33. Linear measurements to assess the horizontal position of the upper incisors (with reference to the facial plane).

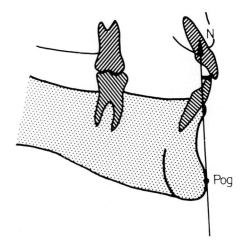

Fig. 4-34. Linear measurements to assess the horizontal position of the lower incisors.

Table 4-2. Linear measurements with growth increments between the ninth and fifteenth years differentiated according to the growth pattern

Age (yr)	Growth pattern	S-N	S-Gn	S-Go	N-Me	ManBase	MaxBase	Ramus
9	Average	64.4	108.6	66.8	104.5	66.5	44.9	46.6
	Horizontal	64.8	108.8	69.5	103.0	67.6	45.7	48.9
	Vertical	63.8	108.5	64.1	106.7	65.2	44.0	44.5
10	Average	64.9	110.8	68.2	106.3	67.9	45.4	47.5
	Horizontal	65.3	111.0	70.9	104.8	69.2	46.3	49.7
	Vertical	64.5	110.5	65.5	108.4	66.5	44.5	45.6
11	Average	65.4	113.0	70.1	108.2	69.2	46.0	48.5
	Horizontal	65.7	113.2	72.1	106.2	70.7	46.9	50.5
	Vertical	65.3	112.5	67.0	110.4	67.4	45.1	46.6
12	Average	66.1	115.3	71.8	110.4	70.4	46.7	49.8
	Horizontal	66.5	115.5	73.7	108.3	72.2	47.8	51.8
	Vertical	65.8	114.8	68.9	112.5	68.5	45.8	47.6
13	Average	66.8	118.0	74.0	112.7	72.0	47.4	51.4
	Horizontal	67.4	118.4	76.1	110.6	73.8	48.3	53.6
	Vertical	66.3	117.4	71.0	114.8	69.9	46.3	49.1
14	Average	67.5	120.5	76.1	115.0	73.4	48.0	53.3
	Horizontal	68.4	121.3	78.5	112.9	75.5	48.9	55.8
	Vertical	66.7	119.8	73.1	117.3	71.2	46.8	50.4
15	Average	68.2	123.3	78.0	117.6	75.1	48.6	55.3
	Horizontal	69.3	124.4	80.6	115.2	77.3	49.6	58.7
	Vertical	67.3	122.3	75.0	119.4	72.6	47.2	51.7

to the facial plane that must be moved lingually need space, which may be obtained only by extraction procedures. Of course, not only the sagittal discrepancy but also the dental discrepancy (crowding) must be considered. Such decisions are important in the treatment plan and can be made only under the assumption that the reference line remains relatively stable. During the mixed dentition, however, with its relatively greater mandibular growth increments, the lower terminus of the reference line drifts forward. This alters the relationship of the facial plane to the incisors, particularly the upper incisors, which appear closer to N-Pog by this differential growth phenomenon. Thus the amount and direction of the growth spurt should be considered in the mixed dentition when the "ought-to-be" position of the incisors is being planned at the end of treatment.

Summary. We can summarize the salient points of the cephalometric analysis for the use of functional appliance therapy as follows:

Cephalometrics enables the anomaly to be located and a differentiation made between skeletal and dentoalveolar malocclusions. If the problem has components from both skeletal and dentoalveolar areas, the cephalometric assessment helps determine the primary and secondary dysplastic structures and possible autonomous compensatory response before treatment. It is possible to determine whether the jaw bases are anteriorly or posteriorly positioned and whether short or long. In the vertical plane the possible rotations of the maxillary and mandibular bases can be observed and the growth pattern delineated. When the biomechanical factors of planned therapy are being considered, the position and inclination of the upper and lower incisors are important from both a functional and an esthetic point of view.

Cephalometrics enhances the assessment of the influences of neuromuscular dysfunction on the dentition. This is vital for diagnosis and treatment planning with functional appliances.

CEPHALOMETRIC EVALUATION OF TREATMENT PROGRESS IN THE MIXED DENTITION

One of the most important tasks of roentgenographic cephalometrics is to help make an objective assessment of the changes induced by therapy, combined with growth and development, as treatment progresses. This should be done periodically. Even the best-developed treatment plan must be altered frequently, and therapeutic diagnosis is the definitive approach. Growth increments and direction, patient cooperation, and unto-

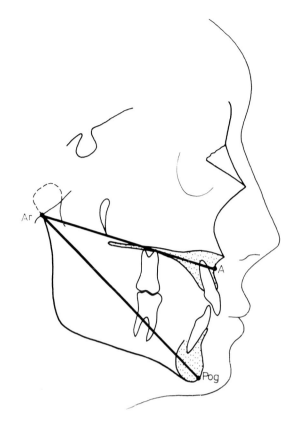

Fig. 4-35. Measurements for evaluating treatment progress in activator cases (maxillary versus mandibular base horizontal change). (Modified after Harvold.)

ward treatment response are difficult factors to control. A change in treatment plan early may make the difference between success and failure. In addition to the cephalometric criteria described at the beginning of this chapter, some complementary measurements can be used both during and after active treatment. There are seven linear measurements that express the growth increments (Table 4-2). It is then possible to compare the measured growth with the average values differentiated according to the morphogenetic pattern. This assists in determining whether the growth increments and direction at that point in treatment are high or low, favorable or unfavorable, in the skeletal areas of greatest concern.

Along with these seven measurements there is a special evaluation in activator cases. The distance Ar-Pog is measured and Ar–Point A is subtracted from it (Fig. 4-35). If the mandible is postured anteriorly, this coefficient increases.

Table 4-3 shows the mode of evaluating growth increments during treatment.

Table 4-3. Mode of evaluation of growth increments during treatment*

Name: I.J.
Age: 8 yr
Treatment: 2 yr
Growth pattern: Vertical

	Before treatment			Growth increment		
	Observed	Average	Difference	Observed	Average	Difference
S-N	63	63.8	−0.8	0	1.5	−1.6
S-Gn	101	108.5	−7.5	5	4.5	+0.5
S-Go	60	64.1	−4.1	4	2.9	+1.1
N-Me	104	106.7	−2.7	6	3.1	+2.9
ManBase	64	65.2	−1.2	3	2.2	+0.8
MaxBase	44	44	0	1	1.2	−0.2
Ramus	36	44.5	−8.5	2	2.1	−0.1
Ar-A to Ar-Pog	10			14		

*The single measurements are compared with the average values from Table 4-2.

CHAPTER 5

FUNCTIONAL ANALYSIS

A major reason for developing functional appliances was the recognition that function per se had an effect on the ultimate morphologic status of the dentofacial complex. The work of Wolf on form and function provided a major stimulus to the nature versus nurture and heredity versus environment controversies. Koch's work on stress trajectories in the head of the femur was emulated by Benninghof's study of stress trajectories in the midface. Both studies clearly demonstrated the response of bone to functional forces. Controversy still surrounds the exact contribution of function as far as size and shape are concerned, but there is no question that function plays an important role. In the craniofacial area particularly, where we are dealing largely with membranous bone, which is much more responsive to functional forces, it is imperative that we understand the actual and potential effects of these forces on the accomplishment of pattern. The alveolar bone is even more responsive to extraneous forces than are basal membranous structures.

When Petrovic was studying otospongeosis with Shambaugh at Northwestern University Medical School some years ago, he turned to the alveolar bone in his research for just this reason; and as the world of orthodontic research knows, this responsiveness so fascinated him that he switched from otolaryngology to orthodontics, providing us with a veritable gold mine of information on the effect of function and malfunction on the dentofacial complex. (See Chapters 1 and 2.)

MANIFOLD DEMANDS OF THE FUNCTIONAL ANALYSIS

It is thus abundantly clear that an appraisal of the functional status of each patient is a no. 1 priority before any form of orthodontic therapy is instituted. Since there are many functions occurring in the stomatognathic system, this means a multiple assessment as we analyze mastication, deglutition, respiration, speech, and posture and the status of each component involved in accomplishing that particular functional activity. Much can be done with a proper clinical examination. This is important not only for determining the current relationship of and past effects of each function on structure but also for understanding the role that this function or group of functions can reasonably be expected to play in the future. If the particular function is abnormal, can or should it be altered? Can the change in forces produced be used to help solve the orthodontic problems? If we change one function (e.g., mastication), what is the potential effect on other functions, which may then exert different forces on the dentofacial skeleton? Clinical study is subjective to a considerable degree, however, and more exacting and reproducible objective criteria must be employed to provide data that are recordable and open to discretionary analysis by qualified observers as well as the patient. So part of the functional analysis should involve cephalometric, myometric, and dentitional mensuration from study models, etc. Most observers think of cephalometric and plaster cast records as static reproductions, but both have functional analysis potential if used correctly. Much can be learned about the dynamics of the stomatognathic system.

Thus, of equal importance to the usual clinical examination and static, cephalometric, and study model analyses is the functional analysis. It is of special significance in treatment with functional appliances because of the dynamic basis of therapy. The role of normal function for optimum growth and development of the orofacial complex has been demonstrated in many laboratory and clinical studies, even as the role of dysfunction in the etiology of malocclusions is well established.

Adaptability and homeostasis—fundamental physiologic phenomena

A good example of the adaptive capability and the interrelationship between function and form is seen in Fig. 5-1. A 5-year-old girl had a fractured mandible that was not mobilized sufficiently. The posterior condylar

This chapter is based largely on Chapter 5 in *Removable Orthodontic Appliances* by T.M. Graber and Bedrich Neumann, Philadelphia, 1984, W.B. Saunders Co.

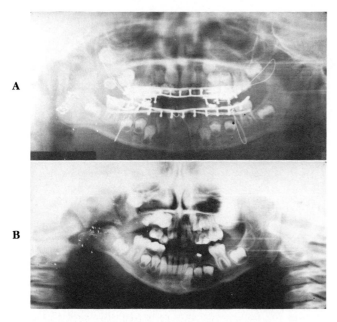

Fig. 5-1. A, Fracture of the ascending ramus insufficiently immobilized. The result was dislocation of the right condyle. **B,** Two years later. Fibrous articulation (pseudarthrosis) in the ascending ramus at the site of the original fracture.

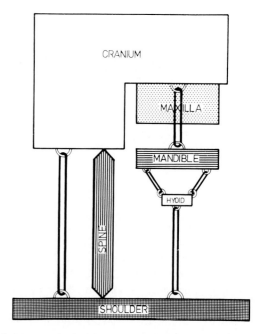

Fig. 5-2. Prevertebral and postvertebral muscle chains. Each neuromuscular component is interactive with the other muscle groups, balancing and stabilizing the head. (After Brodie.)

fragment became ankylosed. Nevertheless, a fibrous joint was formed between the fragments (pseudarthrosis) that permitted functional movement of the mandible. Since function was maintained, there was adaptive remodeling of the structural form in this functioning area.

The adaptability of the condyle to various topographic and functional relationships during the growth period, which has been demonstrated by Petrovic and his associates and is reported in Chapter 2, is one of the basic principles of functional jaw orthopedics. Function is, indeed, the common denominator that joins the individual parts of the orofacial system into a dynamic integrated purposive system. Disturbances in one part of this system do not remain isolated but affect the equilibrium of the whole system (Fig. 5-2). This unique quality is important not only in etiologic considerations but also in assessing the effectiveness and the various side effects of different orthodontic appliances. For example, our own observation shows that appliances which directly influence the muscles of the lips and cheeks (e.g., the inner bow of a headgear facebow) actually have an indirect influence on the position of the tongue.

DIAGNOSTIC EXERCISES

Three diagnostic functional exercises are recommended for the mixed dentition period that are of spe-

cial interest in treatment with functional appliances. The dynamic assessments can be divided as follows:

1. Determination of the postural rest position of the mandible and the interposed freeway space or interocclusal clearance
2. Examination of temporomandibular joint function or dysfunction and condylar movement in carrying out the stomatognathic system tasks (p. 121)
3. Assessment of the functional status of the lips, cheeks, and tongue, with particular reference to any role they might play in dentofacial abnormalities (p. 125)

Determination of the postural rest position and interocclusal clearance

The prime initial task of the functional analysis lies in the assessment of mandibular position as determined by the musculature. This basic position in the adult dentition is centric relation, which can be registered by a variety of gnathologic techniques. Gnathologic principles cannot be applied in the deciduous or mixed dentition, however, because the occlusion is in a transitional stage and the growing condylar structures have not as yet reached their adult form. Since a major determinant of the adult shape is the functional pattern (which originates from the postural resting position of the mandible), registration of this relatively inviolate neuromuscularly derived relationship is a no. 1 priority. It is more likely to be normal and less likely to be affected by skel-

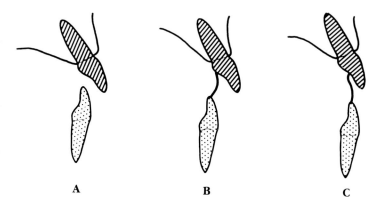

Fig. 5-3. During closing from the rest position, **A,** into the occlusal position there can be a normal arc, **B,** in which the condylar action is primarily rotary, or an abnormal and posteriorly deviated path, **C,** with translatory condylar movement.

etal abnormalities and neuromuscular compensations. In postural resting position the synergistic and antagonistic muscular components are in dynamic equilibrium; their balance is maintained with a basic muscle tonus. The rest position is the result of a myostatic antistretch reflex, responsive only to the permanent exogenous force affecting the orofacial system (i,e., gravity). As a consequence the rest position is dependent on, and alters with, the position of the head.

The movement of the mandible from postural rest position into habitual occlusion is of special interest for all functional analyses. It consists of two components: hinge or rotary action and translatory or sliding movement. The objective of our examination is to assess not only the magnitude and direction of these movements but also the extent of action of each hinge or sliding component. During the closing maneuver from rest position, two phases of the movement can be observed (Fig. 5-3)—the free phase (from postural rest to the point of initial or premature contact) and the articular phase (from initial contact to the central or habitual occlusion position).

Functional patterns without an articular phase, a really free movement from rest position to full occlusal contact, are seen in only a few completely balanced occlusions. A slight sliding component (up to 2 mm), particularly in the transitional dentition, is a normal phenomenon.

If the pattern is abnormal, the sliding can be due to neuromuscular abnormalities, to a disturbance in the tooth-to-tooth interrelationship, or to compensation of a skeletal discrepancy. The net result may combine components from one or more of these potential sources. A differential diagnosis is of great importance for treatment planning.

The regimen for the examination is as follows:
1. Determination of the postural rest position
2. Registration and measurement of the postural rest position
3. Evaluation of the relationship of rest position to occlusal position in the following:

a. Sagittal dimension
b. Vertical dimension
c. Transverse dimension

Assessment of the postural rest position. The rest position of the mandible is dependent on the head and body posture, under the influence of gravity. For this reason it must be determined from a standardized position of the head. The patient is seated upright, preferably with the back unsupported. The head is oriented by having the patient look straight ahead at eye level. Looking directly into a mirror will help establish the optimum head posture, which can be replicated fairly easily. If this seems too variable or if the patient is not relaxed, then the head can be positioned with the eye-ear plane (Frankfort) horizontal.

Several methods are available for determining postural resting position of the mandible, separately or in combination:

Phonetic exercises
Command methods
Noncommand methods
Combined method

Phonetic exercises. The patient, assuming a relaxed upright body posture and looking straight ahead, not at the clinician, is requested to repeat selected consonants. The letter "M" is generally used to start and is repeated five to ten times. "C" also can be used. Repeating the word "Mississippi," or spelling it out, also is a good exercise. After the phonetic exercise the mandible usually returns to postural rest. The patient is instructed not to move the lips or tongue at this time, even when the dentist gently parts the lips to see the interocclusal space and tongue position. This method is common in prosthetic dentistry but less satisfactory for children. In the mixed dentition, language habits are more variant and not yet stabilized. For this reason, phonetic exercises are used less often as the prime determinant, or only as a check on other methods.

Command methods. The patient is asked to perform selected functions, after which the mandible returns to postural resting position. Usually, having the patient lick his lips first and then swallow produces the desired relationship since the mandible returns to postural rest within 2 seconds after the exercise. Phonetic exercises really are a command method, in the strictest sense, and can serve as a double determinant after the licking of lips and swallowing technique.

Noncommand methods. In this case the patient has no idea of what is being examined. Careful observations are made as the patient voluntarily talks and swallows or turns his head while being interrogated on a number of unrelated subjects.

Combined method. To get the best reproduction of the postural resting position in the mixed dentition, the combined method is usually best. The patient first executes a prescribed function (e.g., swallowing) and then relaxes. Then with instructions not to move, the submental muscles can be gently palpated to see whether they are relaxed. Tone is increased in opening or closing maneuvers.

The patient is asked to lick his lips and swallow and then not to move. The intraoral check is done by gently parting the lips and observing the relationship of the canines. Normally the lower canine should be 3 mm below the upper in comparison to the occlusal position. An interocclusal space of 4 mm may still be normal.

Registration of the postural rest position of the mandible. Various methods are recommended for producing the best record.

Direct intraoral procedure
Direct extraoral procedure
Indirect extraoral procedure

Direct intraoral method. In addition to the visual observation just described, when gently parting the lips the clinician can implement a direct intraoral procedure by using a plaster core registration as is sometimes done in prosthodontics. This is not feasible for children in the mixed dentition, however. Mensuration is also difficult, although a millimetric caliper can be used to record the interocclusal space in the canine or incisor area.

Direct extraoral method. Direct caliper measurements can be made on the patient's profile. It is possible to measure the distance from soft tissue nasion (at the bridge of the nose) to menton (on the lowest curvature of the chin). This is done in both postural rest and habitual occlusion. The difference between the two measurements constitutes the interocclusal clearance (Fig. 5-4). The disadvantages with this procedure are that the soft tissue reduces reliability and there is no record of the sagittal relationship.

Indirect extraoral method. This is most commonly used, and various techniques are available: roentgeno-

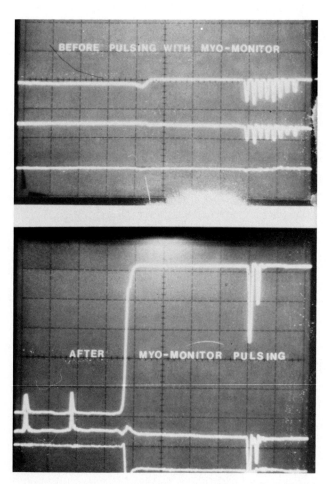

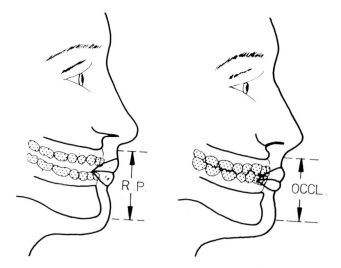

Fig. 5-4. One direct extraoral method of assessment enables the examiner to measure the difference between rest position *(RP)* and occlusal position *(OCCL)* using the lower face height, from subnasale to gnathion or menton, whichever is preferred.

Fig. 5-5. Kinesiographic registration of mandibular movements enables the examiner to make a registration of the rest position of the jaw. (After Jankelson.)

graphic cephalometric, electromyographic, cinefluorographic, kinesiographic (Fig. 5-5).

The cephalometric registration offers the most uniformly successful results. Two or three lateral cephalograms are made under identical exposure and patient positioning conditions: the first in postural rest, the second in initial contact, and the third in full habitual occlusion (Fig. 5-6). Two measurements can be performed on each head film. One records the hinge movement of the condyle, in the vertical plane. The second assesses the sliding or translatory action, in the sagittal plane. Comparison of the single movements permits an assessment of the path of closure of the mandible, which must be determined from rest to initial contact and from initial contact to full occlusion. If there is a significant sliding component from initial contact to occlusion, the abnormality must be recognized and recorded (Fig. 5-7). It should be emphasized again that, normally, condylar movement is both translatory and rotary beyond rest position but from postural rest to habitual occlusion it should show little translation, and primarily a rotary action (as the work of Blume and Boman has demonstrated). In contrast to the records seen when there is functional equilibrium and normal occlusion, a different set of values prevails and frequently a different path of closure for Class II and Class III malocclusions (Figs. 5-8 and 5-9).

The electromyographic, cinefluorographic, and kinesiographic techniques of registering postural rest position require special equipment and are not necessary in routine private practice. They are largely confirmatory of the cephalometric registration.

Evaluation of the path of closure from postural rest to occlusion in the sagittal plane. The condylar movement from postural rest position to occlusion can

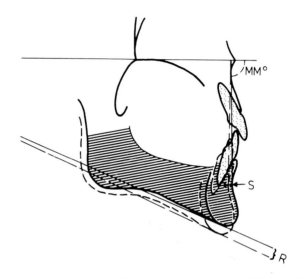

Fig. 5-7. Comparison of occlusal and rest positions. The difference *(R)* represents the rotary movement. In a similar manner the *MM* angle at rest and in occlusion can express the sliding or translatory component *(S).*

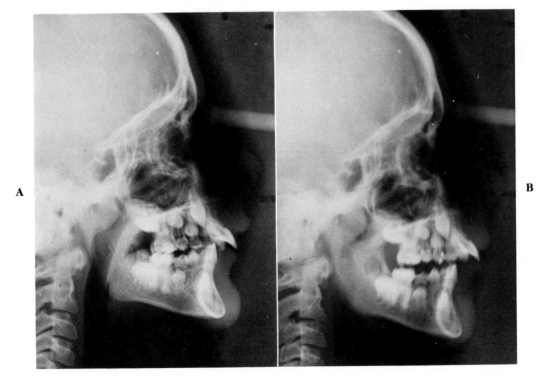

Fig. 5-6. Cephalometric registration of the occlusal, **A**, and rest, **B**, positions.

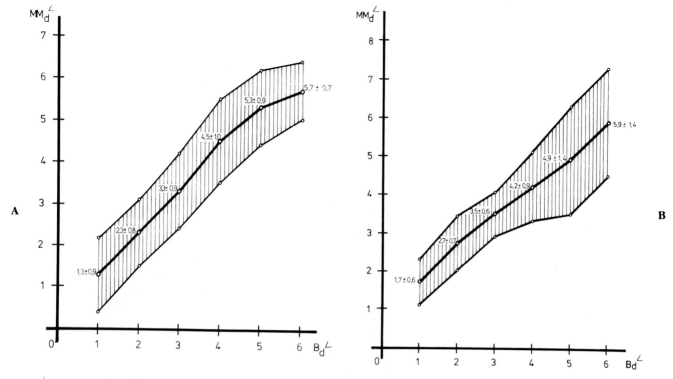

Fig. 5-8. A, Average values of the rotary *(B_d)* and sliding *(MM_d)* components of movement from rest position to occlusion in functionally correct or true Class II malocclusions. **B,** Same relationship in true Class III malocclusions.

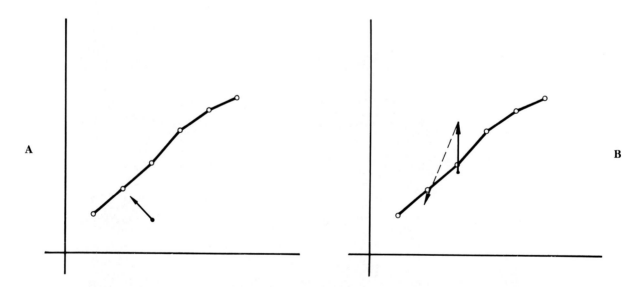

Fig. 5-9. Average curve of the functional relationships and the possible alteration of these relationships during treatment. **A,** In an abnormal path of closure the arrow moves in the direction of the curve after the functional disturbance has been eliminated. **B,** In a malocclusion with abnormal path of closure during treatment a functional disturbance arises because, after improvement of the morphologic relationships, the rest position is not altered (arrow moves away from the curve). In the second phase of treatment or retention (when the functional relationships are stabilized), a new rest position is established (arrow moves in the direction of the curve).

be pure hinge movement, partly hinge and partly anterior translatory displacement, or partly hinge and part posterior superior translatory displacement.

Class II malocclusions. Treatment prognosis for functional appliance therapy is dependent on the analysis of the relationships and the determination of path of closure category.

1. In Class II malocclusions without functional disturbance the path of closure from rest to occlusion is straight upward and forward, with a hinge movement of the condyle in the fossa. This is a true Class II malocclusion (Fig. 5-10).

2. In Class II malocclusions with functional disturbances there is a rotary action of the condyle in the fossa from postural rest to occlusion. From initial contact to full occlusion, condylar action is both rotary and translatory upward and backward (a posterior shift). Thus the movement is combined rotary and sliding (Fig. 5-11). As Boman and Blume showed in their research, this type of activity is the most common, particularly where there is excessive overbite. This functional type of Class II malocclusion appears more severe than it actually is, sagittally.

3. In Class II malocclusions with functional disturbances in which the path of closure is upward and forward from rest to initial contact, usually in the molar region, from initial contact it is possible also for the mandible to be anteriorly displaced as the cusps guide the mandible into a forward position, with translatory movement of the condyle down-

ward and forward on the posterior slope of the articular eminence. The path of closure appears more upward and forward than it would be without tooth interference. This type of problem has been shown by Woodside in his research (Figs. 5-12). The malocclusion is actually more severe than it appears with the teeth in occlusion. This variation of path of closure is least frequent for Class II malocclusions.

In functional Class II malocclusions the elimination of functional retrusion or protrusion leads to an improvement in the sagittal malrelationship. This is a change in the spatial interrelation of parts and is not due to growth and development. In Class II malocclusions with a normal path of closure the intermaxillary relationships still must be altered but this requires both a morphologic and a functional change to produce the desired sagittal correction. The original rotary condylar action from rest to occlusion is not changed, and the ultimate condyle-eminence relationship is the same. However, the clinician hopes for dentoalveolar adjustment as well as optimum horizontal growth of the mandible, under the influence of the activator. He must assess the growth pattern by cephalometrics to be able to project a likely growth direction and the probable incremental needs. In cases with a posterior displacement combined with a projected horizontal growth direction, the prognosis for Class II treatment is very good. When there is an anterior displacement and a vertical growth vector, the prognosis is quite poor. Other combinations are possible—e.g., an anterior displacement and horizontal growth di-

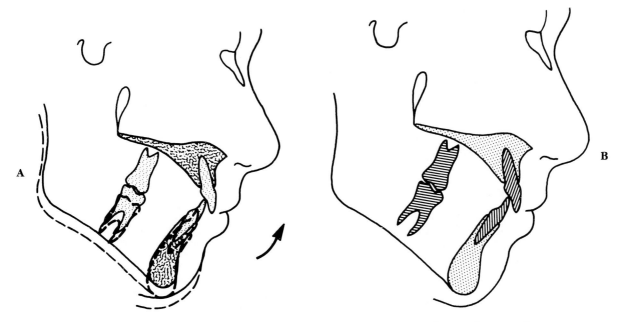

Fig. 5-10. Hinge movement from the rest, **A,** to the occlusal, **B,** position in a functionally correct Class II relationship (with a normal path of closure).

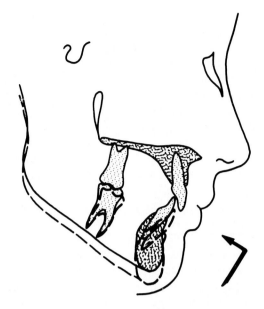

Fig. 5-11. Posterior translation or sliding into the occlusal position in an abnormal functional pattern (with a deviated path of closure).

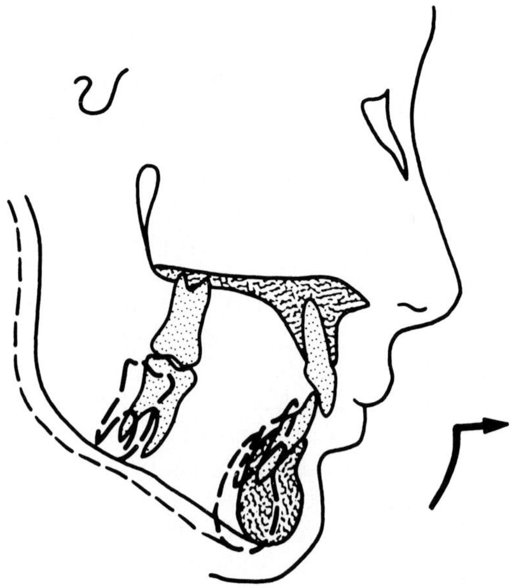

Fig. 5-12. Anterior translation or sliding into the occlusal position in a severe Class II malocclusion.

rection or a posterior condylar displacement with a vertical growth direction. In these last two combinations the prognosis is not as good but can be improved or made worse depending on the age of the patient and the specifics of the facial pattern.

Class III malocclusions (Fig. 5-13). A hinge-type condylar function is often associated with Class III malocclusions with a straight path of closure.

The possibility of successful functional appliance treatment of these problems exists only if the magnitude of the sagittal dysplasia is not too great and if therapy is begun in the early mixed dentition.

When the path of closure is up and back (an anterior postural resting position), the prognosis is even poorer.

In Class III malocclusions with an anterior displacement, creating an upward and forward path of closure with combined rotary and translatory action of the condyle from postural rest to habitual occlusion, the prognosis is much better and treatment success is possible, even in the permanent dentition.

The functional therapy is the most efficient mode of treatment in the mixed dentition. It should be emphasized that a functional analysis alone is not sufficient to determine the prognosis because not every Class III malocclusion with an anterior path of closure is a mandibular displacement with a good prognosis. Sometimes a skeletal Class III relationship is partially compensated by labial tipping of the maxillary and lingual tipping of the mandibular incisors. Because of the extreme tipping possible, there can be an anterior sliding movement into occlusion. Uprighting the incisors into their proper

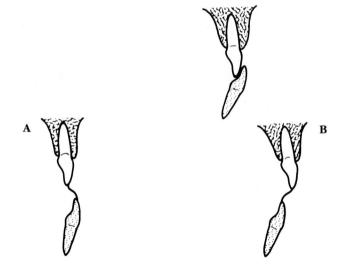

Fig. 5-13. Various functional relationships in the Class III malocclusions. **A,** Anterior rest position in a severe Class III malocclusion. **B,** Posterior rest position in a forced bite type of Class III malocclusion (i.e., pseudo–Class III).

axial inclination results in a severe Class III sagittal tooth relationship. Treatment of this type of malocclusion by orthodontic means is difficult because dentoalveolar compensation is not possible; the incisors are already overcompensated before treatment. Orthognathic surgery at a later date should be considered and pointed out to the patient. This type of malocclusion is referred to as a pseudo–forced bite or displacement (Fig. 5-14). The differentiation of the forced bite from the pseudo–

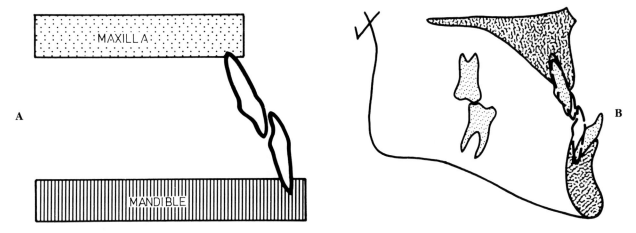

Fig. 5-14. A, Pseudo–forced bite relationship with labial tipping of the upper incisors and lingual tipping of the lower. In reality this is a true Class III problem with a marked basal sagittal malrelationship. **B,** After uprighting of the incisors the real severity of the Class III relationship is quite evident.

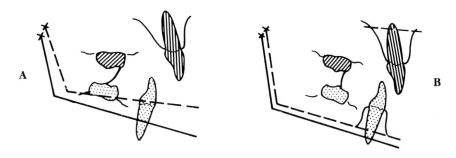

Fig. 5-15. A, True deep overbite with a wide freeway space. **B,** Pseudo–deep overbite with a small freeway space. (After Hotz.)

forced bite problem is usually possible only with the help of a cephalometric analysis.

Evaluation of the path of closure from postural rest to habitual occlusion in the vertical plane. This evaluation is of special interest in the assessment of therapeutic potential in deep overbite cases. It is possible to differentiate two different types of deep overbite (Fig. 5-15).

1. The true deep overbite, with a large interocclusal clearance, is caused by infraclusion of the posterior segments. It is often the result of a lateral tongue posture or tongue thrust. Some Class II, Division 2, malocclusions with adequate lip line relationships are good examples. Treatment in the mixed dentition period requires the elimination of environmental factors that are inhibiting eruption of the posterior teeth. This is a valid and quite attainable functional appliance treatment objective.

2. The pseudo–deep overbite problem, with a small interocclusal space, already has normal eruption of the posterior segment teeth. Further extrusion is possible only to a moderate extent. The deep overbite is combined with overeruption of the incisors. Some Class II, Division 2, malocclusions with a "gummy" smile and a poor lip line relation can fall into this category. The amount of interocclusal clearance can be a distinguishing criterion. The possibility of intruding incisors using functional methods is questionable. To control the vertical dimension, it is usually necessary to drive the maxillary molars distally. Some extrusion is possible, resulting in an increased anterior face height and reduced incisor overbite. All possible intrusive mechanics on the incisor teeth with fixed appliances is usually indicated. Cephalometric analysis is essential to disclose the morphogenetic pattern, growth direction, and precise areas of abnormal tooth position requiring therapeutic guidance.

The prognosis is good in a true deep overbite problem if there is a vertical growth pattern (Fig. 5-16). In

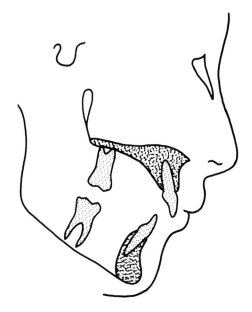

Fig. 5-16. True deep overbite with a vertical growth pattern. The prognosis for treatment of this overbite is good.

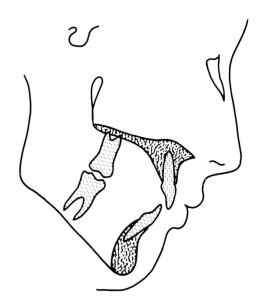

Fig. 5-17. Pseudo–deep overbite with a horizontal growth pattern. The prognosis for treatment is poor.

pseudo–deep overbite problems with a horizontal growth pattern the possibilities of correction with functional appliances are limited (Fig. 5-17).

In combined cases with a true deep overbite and a horizontal growth pattern, or a pseudo–deep bite with a vertical growth pattern, some limited success can be expected (Fig. 5-18).

In Class II malocclusions with deep overbite, the use of functional treatment is sometimes advantageous for improving the sagittal relationship but not for controlling of the vertical dysplasia, and vice-versa. Eight functional combinations between the vertical and sagittal relationship can be categorized (Table 5-1).

Generally, in functional Class II problems with posterior displacement and in functional deep overbite problems with a large interocclusal space, functional appliances have a good prognosis for successful therapy. The basic principle for this treatment is the elimination of disturbing environmental factors and the promotion of optimum growth. In nonfunctional true Class II malocclusions and psuedo–deep overbite problems, therapy is more difficult, regardless of the appliance used, because of multisystem involvement and the need for neuromotor alteration.

Evaluation of the path of closure from postural rest to habitual occlusion in the transverse plane. The clinical examination of the transverse functional relationships is easy to perform. It consists of observing the behavior of the midline of the mandible as the teeth are brought together from rest position to habitual occlusion. In cross-bite cases with a lateral shift of the

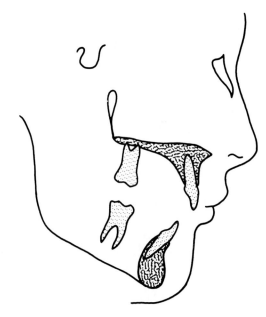

Fig. 5-18. True deep overbite with a horizontal growth pattern. The prognosis for treatment is fair.

mandibular midline, two types can be differentiated (Fig. 5-19).

1. Cases in which the midline shift of the mandible can be observed only in the occlusal position. In postural rest the midlines are coincident and well centered. The mandible slides laterally from rest position into a cross-bite in occlusion. This is called a lateroclusion or pseudo–cross-bite and is

Table 5-1. Correlations between sagittal and vertical relationships for the prognosis of functional therapy

Overbite	Displacement	Growth pattern	Improvement in	
			Deep bite	Sagittal relations
True	Posterior	Horizontal	+	+ +
True	Posterior	Vertical	+ +	+
True	Anterior	Horizontal	+	+
True	Anterior	Vertical	+ +	−
Pseudo	Posterior	Horizontal	−	+ +
Pseudo	Posterior	Vertical	+	+
Pseudo	Anterior	Horizontal	−	+
Pseudo	Anterior	Vertical	−	−

Functional appliance prognosis: + + good, + moderate, − poor.

due to tooth guidance. Treatment requires eliminating the disturbance in the intercuspation. This often is done by merely widening the narrowed maxillary arch (Fig. 5-20). Function is thus rehabilitated and the procedure can be done in the permanent dentition also, although there is some evidence that a prolonged cross-bite relationship can lead to asymmetric jaw growth if allowed to continue for a number of years during the growing period.

2. Cases in which the midline shift is present in both occlusion and postural resting position (e.g., a true asymmetric facial skeleton). This is sometimes referred to as laterognathy (Fig. 5-21). Successful functional appliance treatment is not possible in such cases, and in severe problems surgery is the only alternative.

This first phase of the functional examination thus provides significant information concerning the indications or contraindications for functional appliance treatment.

Examination of the temporomandibular joint and condylar movement

The objective of this aspect of the functional examination is to check whether incipient symptoms of TMJ dysfunction are present. The examination is not as extensive as for patients with frank TMJ problems. However, some initial TMJ symptoms are present in many children with various types of malocclusions in the 8-to-14-year age range. In a study of 232 children in this age group, 41% had various TMJ symptoms.

These symptoms are important for two reasons:

1. By means of early elimination of functional disturbances, some incipient TMJ problems can be prevented or eliminated. This is an indication for early orthodontic treatment.

2. During activator therapy the condyle is displaced or dislocated to achieve a remodeling of the TMJ struc-

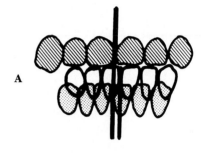

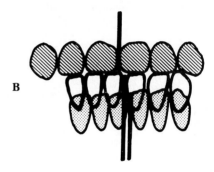

Fig. 5-19. Two functional types of cross-bite. **A,** Midline shift only in full occlusion. In rest position the midlines are well centered. There is a good prognosis for functional appliance therapy. This is called lateroclusion. **B,** Persistence of the midline shift in rest position. The prognosis for treatment is poor. This is termed laterognathy (in rest as well as in occlusion).

tures as well as a change in muscle function. If the temporomandibular structures are not normal at the start and if there is hypersensitivity, the possibility of exacerbating the objective symptoms exists. Fortunately, this seldom happens; and functional appliances themselves often eliminate the unfavorable sensory reactions in the process of posturing the mandible forward. This is a prime requisite for the treatment of many adult TMJ cases. Where TMJ problems are present in the decidu-

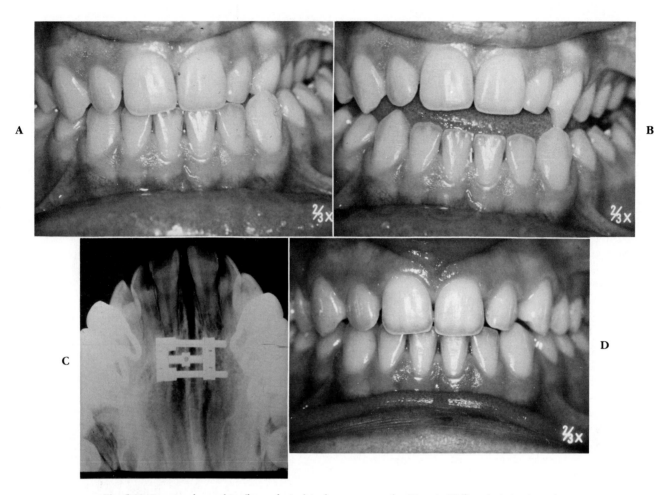

Fig. 5-20. Functional cross-bite (lateroclusion) in the permanent dentition. **A,** Midline deviation in occlusion. **B,** Well-centered midline in rest position. **C,** Palatal expansion or splitting. **D,** Improvement of the cross-bite. There is still a slight midline shift after palatal expansion.

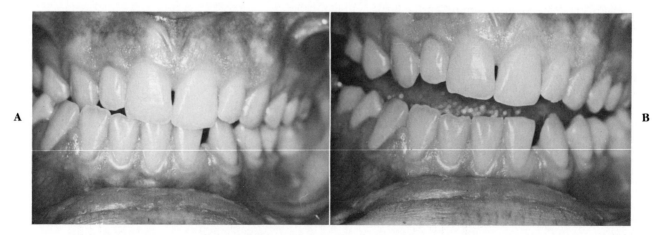

Fig. 5-21. Laterognathy. **A,** Slight midline deviation in occlusion. **B,** Worse in the rest position.

ous dentition, the forward posturing may be better done in a staged progression—step by step.

Early symptoms of TMJ problems are as follows:

Clicking or crepitus
Sensitivity of the condylar region or masticatory muscles
Functional disturbances (e.g., hypermobility, limitation of movement, deviation)
Radiographic evidence of morphologic or positional abnormalities

There is seldom clicking at the initial examination. Crepitus can sometimes be observed during the opening movement (initial, intermediate, or terminal). More frequently there is a terminal clicking or crepitation, because of hypermobility or opening too widely. Terminal crepitus is usually a sign of peripheral irregularity of the articular disk or unevenness of the condylar surface and is amenable to correction. Crepitation during chewing may been seen especially in children with deep overbite. Similarly crepitus can be observed in the closing maneuver in pseudo–anterior crossbite patients or in anterior functional displacement. In 51.5% of patients with initial TMJ symptoms there is recognizable crepitus.

Tenderness to palpation of the condylar region could be found in only 5.3% of the cases reported in the study previously mentioned. The most characteristic symptom for an initial functional disturbance of the TMJ is the palpatory tenderness of the lateral pterygoid muscle. In the referred to study, 52% reported tenderness in the right pterygoid and 59% in the left.

In addition, the other possible TMJ abnormalities in this age group include hypermobility. By this is meant an opening of more than 45 mm in 6 to 8-year-old children and 49 mm in 10 to 12-year-old children. The problem is mostly habitual, but it could mean a predisposition to later TMJ dysfunction. In the study 50.5% showed hypermobility. In 22% there was even an anterior displacement of the condyle over the articular tubercle. Other symptoms include limited movement be-

cause of muscle spasm. This is seen in isolated cases and is not a major concern. Deviation of the opening or closing movement, sagittally or transversely, can be seen in 24% of the cases studied in which there were TMJ symptoms. In 11.5% there was an **S** type of opening as the condyles moved forward or backward unevenly in the functional maneuvers. Deviation was most frequently accompanied by crepitus, or even clicking. Condylar dislocation was seen mostly with some form of functional deviation. In 36% of the cases of dislocation there was also condylar deviation during opening and closing.

Neuromuscular involvement in TMJ problems was also seen in the lip and tongue areas. Whereas in children without TMJ dysfunction 20.5% of the sample showed abnormal perioral activity, the percentages were significantly higher in children with TMJ symptoms (43%). Tongue dysfunction was seen in 12.4% of the non-TMJ sample as opposed to 21% in the TMJ problem group.

Radiographic evidence of structural abnormality in the temporomandibular joint in children is relatively rare. However, morphology is difficult to interpret with even the best laminagraphs, so the claims by some clinicians that flattening of the condylar surface and eminence occurs frequently are hard to verify. The relationship of the condyle to the fossa structures can be abnormal because of anterior or posterior displacement, as discussed earlier (Fig. 5-22).

The greatest frequency of the various TMJ symptoms was seen in Class II malocclusions: 53% had some TMJ symptoms whereas 68% had abnormal perioral muscle function. In addition, the TMJ cases usually had a deep bite, together with a horizontal growth direction of the mandible. This study confirms the observations made by Graber (1984) in his study of 374 TMJ patients. In the Rakosi TMJ study the frequency of TMJ symptoms was also high in Class III malocclusions with anterior displacements, cross-bite conditions, or tongue dysfunction.

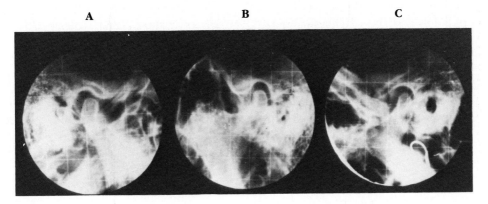

A   B   C

Fig. 5-22. Three radiographic condylar findings. **A,** Anterior dislocation (right condyle). **B,** Eucentricity (left condyle). **C,** Posterior dislocation (left condyle).

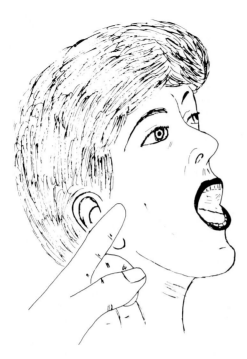

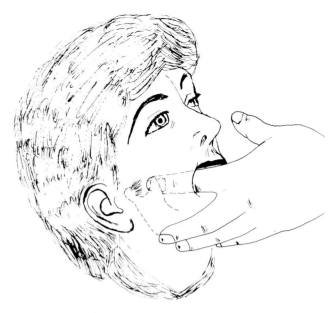

Fig. 5-24. Palpation of the lateral pterygoid muscle area.

Fig. 5-23. Checking the temporomandibular joint. Palpation of the condyle with the index finger during opening and closing movement.

Clinical functional examination for the TMJ area. The simplified clinical examination consists of three steps:

1. Auscultation
2. Palpation
3. Functional analysis

Auscultation. To check for signs of clicking or crepitus, a stethoscope is used. Actually a stereostethoscope, as designed by Watt, is better than the conventional instrument since it allows the operator to determine the magnitude and timing of abnormal sounds for each joint simultaneously.

The examination is performed by having the patient open and close into full occlusion. If there is clicking or crepitus the patient is instructed to bite forward into incision and to repeat the opening and closing movements. These are checked for any sounds with the stethoscope. Most often, sounds disappear in the protruded position.

Palpation. The condyle and fossa are palpated with the index finger during opening and closing maneuvers (Fig. 5-23). The posterior surface can be palpated by inserting the little finger in the external auditory meatus. Besides tenderness, the condyles can thus be checked for synchrony of action and coordination of relative position in the fossae.

Palpation of the associated musculature is an important part of the examination. In TMJ patients it is essen-

tial to palpate the muscles of the face, head, and neck. Experience has shown that children with incipient TMJ symptoms almost always demonstrate some tenderness in the lateral pterygoid muscle. Palpation of this muscle is difficult but can be approximated by placing the forefinger behind the maxillary tuberosity, right above the occlusal plane, with the palmar surface of the finger directed medially toward the pterygoid hamulus (Fig. 5-24).

In patients with early TMJ symptoms there is commonly a unilateral tenderness, left or right side. If hypersensitivity or pain is present on both sides, the condition is more protracted and palpation of other associated muscles is indicated. The tenderness of the superior head of the lateral pterygoid muscle is an important diagnostic clue because it may well indicate abnormal functional loading of the joint itself. This requires further study for possible etiologic factors.

Functional analysis. A dislocation of the condyles or discoordination of the movements is an early symptom of functional disturbance. Palpation and inspection usually enable the clinician to make the necessary determination. In severe cases or in patients with TMJ disease, a gnathologic registration may be of benefit. Myographic recordings will also assist in this functional analysis (i.e., myomonitoring). Simple electronic devices also help measure the silent period of muscular contraction—a cardinal sign of dysfunction in many cases.

Functional movements of the mandible and condyles are carefully assessed. The extent of maximum opening is measured between the upper and lower incisors with a Boley gauge (Fig. 5-25). In overbite cases this amount

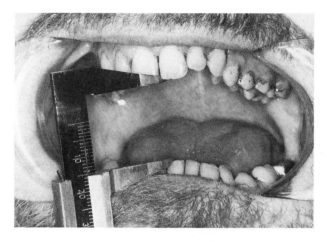

Fig. 5-25. Measuring the amount of mandibular opening. A Boley gauge may be used. Normally the distance is between 40 and 65 mm.

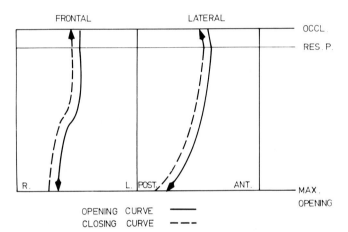

Fig. 5-26. Closing and opening curves of the mandible, frontal and lateral views.

must be added to the measurement, whereas in open bite the amount that separates the incisors on full occlusion must be subtracted. The direction of the opening and closing movements should be registered graphically with curves (Fig. 5-26). Premature contacts and deviations in sagittal and transverse directions are assessed.

Further dysfunction signs are sought in the lips, tongue, etc. As has been pointed out in the study of 232 children, lip dysfunction coexists significantly with incipient TMJ symptoms. Perioral neuromuscular abnormalities, together with crepitus and tenderness of the lateral pterygoid muscle, are the most important signs of early TMJ dysfunction. As a rule of thumb the diagnosis of an incipient TMJ problem can be made when two of the three signs mentioned are present.

There are some specific measures that can be employed to prevent these functional TMJ disturbances:

1. Early care of deciduous teeth for caries, interferences, etc., especially the deciduous molars
2. Elimination of tooth guidance cross-bites and unwanted translatory condylar movement in the deciduous dentition
3. Elimination of neuromuscular dysfunctions, especially involving the lips, and habits that force the mouth open

If incipient TMJ signs already exist at the time of the first examination of the patient, then early orthodontic treatment is recommended, especially in (1) Class II malocclusions with excessive overjet, horizontal growth pattern, and lower lip cushioning to the lingual of the upper incisors (lip trap); (2) deep overbite problems; (3) anterior open bite, with associated abnormal lip, tongue, and finger habits; and (4) crossbite conditions.

In patients with clicking and functional disturbances, muscle exercises are recommended, along with interceptive appliance guidance (e.g., bite planes, the Bionator).

This approach is beneficial with patients who already have TMJ problems and thus require special examination and care.

Assessment of stomatognathic dysfunction

Before functional appliance treatment is instituted, a thorough analysis of all possible dysfunctions is necessary. A dysfunction can be a primary etiologic factor in a malocclusion. Many dysfunctions are acquired in the early stages of development. Neonates are capable of performing some vital functions—suckling, swallowing, and breathing—that are unconditioned reflex actions. Many functions that are learned during the first months or years of life—chewing, phonation, mimicry—are conditioned reflex actions developed from the unconditioned ones. Together with the normal physiologic reflex activities, certain unphysiologic reflex actions develop concurrently. These include the dysfunctions mouth breathing and bruxism. Some children seem to show a predisposition toward certain dysfunctions— they copy their peers or parents. Children with psychologic or adjustment problems often use certain dysfunctions as an escape mechanism or an attention-getting mechanism. When these parafunctional habits are prolonged, there is the potential for the dysfunction to cause a malocclusion. The deformation of structures is such that the adaptive functional activity persists after the disappearance of the original inciting factor (e.g., thumb sucking and fingersucking). The adaptive dysfunction exacerbates the malrelationship that already exists. Not all thumb, finger, tongue, and lip dysfunctions produce sufficient deformation of the teeth and supporting tissue to persist after cessation of the habit. In these cases autonomous adjustment restores the normal overbite and overjet. When there is already a pattern-type predilection toward an abnormal sagittal or transverse malrelationship, the likelihood of persistence of dysfunctions is enhanced by the deforming and adaptive perioral malfunction. In a study of over 2000 pre–school-aged children there was confirmation of this observation: 79% of children with Class II malocclusions had abnormal perioral habits; in Class III the percentage was 64%; in Class II, Division 2, 43%; in open bite problems, 91%; in cross-bite, 77%. However, 54% of the children in the sample without malocclusion had what was considered to be bad habits (Fig. 5-27).

Malocclusions that are acquired as a result of dysfunctions can usually be treated simply by elimination of the disturbing environmental influences, which will foster normal development. Functional appliances serve well in this respect. In developmental malocclusions or those attributable to a morphogenetic basis, a causal functional rehabilitation is not possible. Other means of therapy must be enlisted in such cases. In planning treatment with the help of functional analysis, it is important to know this ahead of time.

The functional examination to ascertain the dysfunctional aspects requires an assessment of the tongue, lips, cheeks, and hyoid musculature. Examination of the swallowing function usually involves all areas, though each muscle group can be studied separately. The primary means of examination are clinical observation and functional testing, supported by cephalometric analysis. More sophisticated techniques of functional analysis are helpful (e.g., electromyography, cinefluorography, kinesiology), but these are not usually available in private practice.

Evaluation of the swallowing function. The first and most obvious step is to study the deglutitional cycle.

In neonates the tongue seems relatively large and in the forward suckling postural position for nursing. The tip actually inserts through the anterior gum pads and takes part in the anterior lip seal. This tongue position and the coincident swallowing are termed infantile or *visceral.*

With eruption of the incisors (e.g., about 6 months of age), the tongue position starts to retract. Over a period of 12 to 18 months, as proprioception causes tongue postural and functional changes, there is a transitional period. Between 2 and 4 years of age the functionally balanced or mature *somatic* swallow is seen in normal developmental patterns (Fig. 5-28). The visceral type of swallowing can persist well after the fourth year of life, however, and is then considered a dysfunction or abnormal because of its association with certain malocclusion characteristics.

Several factors can account for the persistence of infantile swallowing patterns. Separately or in combination they may be due to fingersucking, bottle-feeding, mouthbreathing, tongue sucking, or central nervous system type of developmental retardation.

The symptoms of a retained visceral swallowing pattern usually include a forward tongue posture and tongue thrusting during swallowing, contraction of the perioral muscles (hyperactive mentalis and orbicularis oris contraction), often excessive buccinator hyperactivity, and swallowing without the momentary tooth contact normally required. When all these symptoms are present, the pattern is often called a *complex tongue thrusting problem.* A variety of malocclusions may accompany the group dysfunctions. Open bite conditions often exist in both anterior and posterior regions. Elimination of the problem is usually more difficult in a complex tongue thrust, and a long period of retention

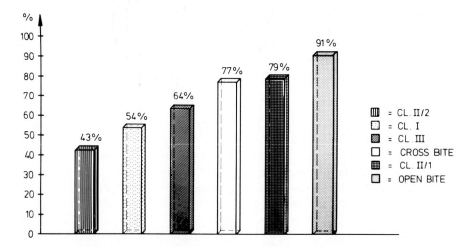

Fig. 5-27. Frequency of abnormal sucking habits and perioral function in various malocclusions and in the normal (Class I) occlusion.

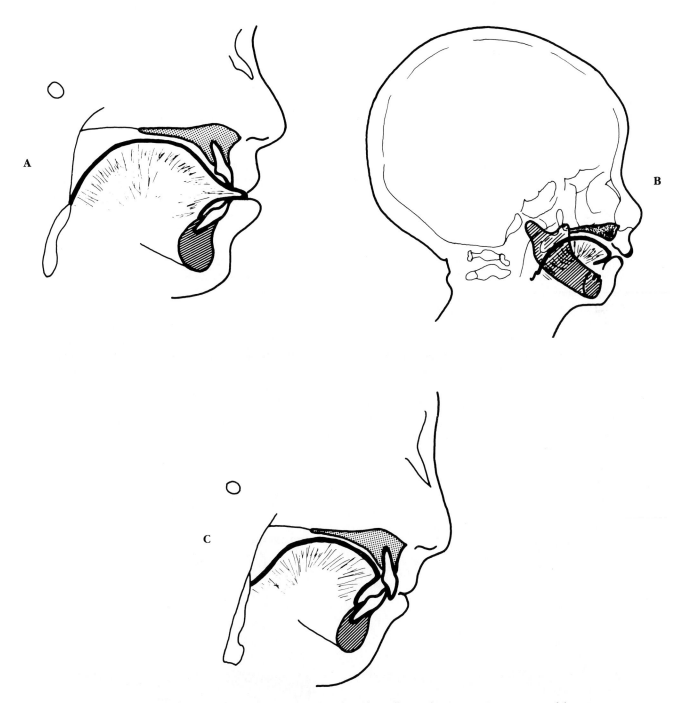

Fig. 5-28. Various deglutitional patterns. **A,** Visceral suckle-swallow in the neonate. **B,** Persistence of the infantile type of swallowing. **C,** Somatic or mature type of swallowing.

is necessary to prevent the return of the visceral swallowing pattern, if, indeed, it has been eliminated in the first place.

More amenable to interception is the *simple tongue thrust*. This is largely a localized anterior tongue posturing forward during rest and active function with localized anterior open bite. Attendant muscle abnormalities are of more an adaptive than a primary nature in such cases. The prognosis for functional therapy is usually good, and autonomous improvement can often be seen.

Normal deglutition. In the normal mature swallow there is no tongue thrust or constant forward posture. The tip of the tongue is supported on the lingual of the dentoalveolar area; the contraction of perioral muscles is slight during deglutition, and the teeth are in momentary contact during the swallowing cycle. The objective of functional appliance therapy is to establish this type of pattern for dysfunction patients.

Various means, using more sophisticated armamentaria, have been devised to analyze tongue function. On the bases of original work by Gwynne-Evans, Ballard, and Björk, it is possible to divide the deglutitional cycle into four stages (Fig. 5-29):

Stage 1. The anterior third of the superior surface of the tongue is flat or retracted. The food bolus is collected on the flat anterior part of the tongue or in the sublingual area in front of the retracted tongue. The posterior arched part of the dorsum is in contact with the soft palate. This indicates that the posterior seal is closed; swallowing cannot yet take place. The teeth and lips are not in contact.

Stage 2. The soft palate moves in a cranial and posterior direction. The palatolingual and palatopharyngeal seals are now open. The tip of the tongue moves upward while the dorsum drops, creating a groove or depression in the middle third and permitting posterior transport of the bolus. Simultaneously there is a slight contraction of the lip muscles while the lips are in contact and the anterior teeth approximate at the end of this stage. The symptoms of tongue thrust syndrome, if they exist, can be observed during this stage.

Stage 3. The superior constrictor muscle ring in the epipharyngeal wall (known as Passavant's pad) starts to constrict. It can be seen on the lateral cephalogram or by cinefluorography as a bulge in the posterior wall. The soft palate assumes a triangular form; and both tissues together form the palatopharyngeal seal, often referred to as the velopharyngeal seal. With closing off of the nasopharynx the posterior part of the dorsum of the tongue drops more; this allows the bolus of food to pass through the isthmus faucium. Simultaneously the anterior part of the tongue is pressed against the hard palate, which helps manipulate the bolus in a posterior direction. The teeth are in contact (usually slightly forward of full contact) and the lips are together. If tongue thrusting is present, the tongue has not retracted but has narrowed with the tip pressed forward to help in the anterior lip seal. It is at this time that a momentary negative atmospheric pressure is created.

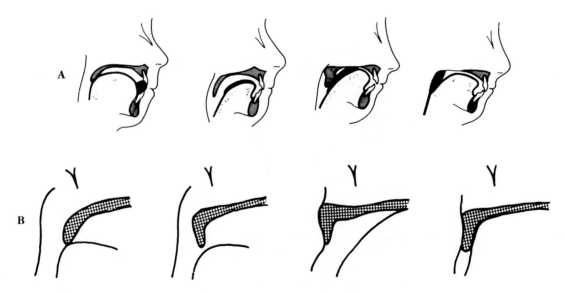

Fig. 5-29. A, Four stages of the oral phase of swallowing. Note the change in tongue position as the food bolus is transported into the oropharynx during the deglutitional cycle. **B,** Function of the posterior seal in the four stages (velopharyngeal valving).

Stage 4. The dorsum of the tongue now moves posteriorly and superiorly as the palatopharyngeal tissues move downward and forward. The tongue thus pushes against the tensed soft palate, squeezing the residual food bolus out of the oropharyngeal area. The terminal action is likened to squeezing a tube of toothpaste.

This basic deglutitional cycle can be seen only in normal functional patterns with normal occlusions. During cinefluorographic examinations by the author many variations have been observed.

In the first stage the bolus of food was collected not only in front of the retracted tongue tip but sometimes also on the back of the protruded flat tongue. Such a variation has been seen in the visceral type of swallowing and in Class III malocclusions, in which the tongue position is habitually low. In the second stage the transfer of the food bolus can be performed by peristaltic-like movements of the tongue along its dorsum or by shovellike movements of the tip of the tongue (Fig. 5-30).

Cinefluorographic pictures also showed that the basic position of the tongue was different in different malocclusions. The basic position was high or flat. In the flat posture the functional pattern was more extensive, because a longer path was necessary to achieve palatolingual seal.

Of the four stages studied, the second stage has shown the greatest intraindividual variations. The iden-

tical pattern in the second stage could be reproduced only if the examination was performed under the same conditions.

The type of therapy indicated depends on the problem. Usually the sequelae of an abnormal swallowing pattern can be treated with an oral screen type of appliance. The treatment of a simple tongue thrust is causal and usually successful. In the more complex type of problem, commonly referred to as a tongue thrust syndrome, treatment can lead to an improved morphologic relationship; but the atypical functional pattern often persists, making it necessary to resort to prolonged retention.

The use of myofunctional therapy is beneficial in helping to eliminate residual perioral muscle abnormalities. Lip exercises can improve lip seal—e.g., holding a sheet of paper between the lips (Fränkel) (Fig. 5-31). This is repeated several times a day. Children in school are asked to hold the lips together while in class, practicing with a small piece of paper. It is admittedly difficult to influence unconscious functions with conscious exercises.

Because of the diversity of tongue function during swallowing, no tongue exercises are recommended before or during treatment. During active treatment, tongue posture and function are controlled by the appliance. With an improved morphologic relationship the prognosis for establishing of normal function is improved. If spaces are present, the tongue tends to seek

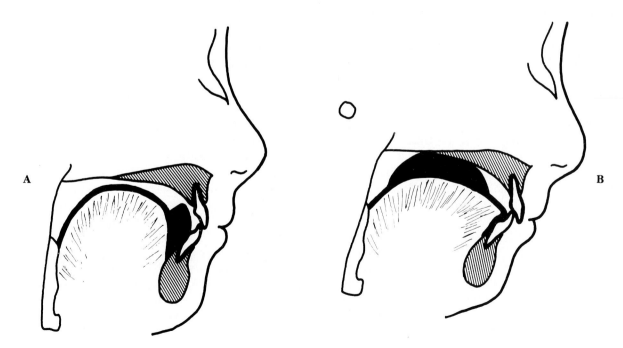

Fig. 5-30. Variations in the first phase of swallowing. **A,** Collecting phase in front of the tongue tip. This is encountered more frequently. **B,** Collecting phase on the dorsum of the tongue. This is frequently due to different consistencies of food.

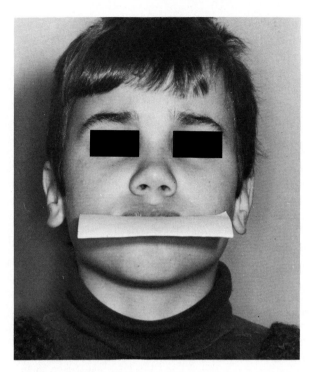

Fig. 5-31. Lip exercises with a small piece of cardboard or paper. (After Fränkel.)

them out and press into them; hence anterior space closure is advisable. If the visceral deglutitional pattern persists in the retention phase, there are supportive exercises that can be prescribed to assist in establishing the somatic swallowing pattern.

Examination of the tongue. As already indicated not only the function but also the posture, size, and shape of the tongue are significant. Such potential etiologic factors should be considered before any form of therapy is prescribed. Even in malocclusions with a morphogenetic component, the growth, posture, and function of the tongue are important. The flat, low-lying, anteriorly postured tongue is a factor in the development of Class III malocclusions. Since similar tongue problems can occur within one family, it can be difficult to determine the precise roles of heredity and imitation; yet the role of tongue dysfunctions is well documented in various types of malocclusion. As pointed out earlier, the nursing mode can be critical. The nonphysiologic design of the nipple on the baby bottle can force the tongue (and cheeks) to perform atypical and compensatory functions to extract the milk, with subsequent adaptive responses of the associated dentoalveolar tissues leading to characteristic malocclusions (Fig. 5-32).

The work of Moyers and Linder-Aronson points up the possible role of nasal and pharyngeal blockage and the compensatory tongue posture. Allergies may be a potent factor in their situation. With excessive epipharyngeal lymphoid tissue the tongue naturally postures forward to maintain an open airway. If the nasal passages are closed, this means mouth breathing, with its attendant drop in mandibular (and tongue) posture. In the literature the term "adenoidal facies" is often used. This is only one possible adaptive response to respiratory difficulty, but it should be recognized.

Although the connection between speech disorders and malocclusions has not been determined exactly, the tongue does play a central role in phonation. Palatographic examinations by the author have shown compensations in articulation associated with severe malocclusions. Speech disorders are also observed in conjunction with less severe malocclusions. When good compensation is possible, the prognosis for functional therapy is also good.

Tongue function. The significance of so-called tongue thrust has been evaluated by a number of authors with regard to its role in the etiology of malocclusion. According to one school of thought (Ballard, Tulley, Cleall, Milne and Cleall, Fränkel, Subtelny and Sakuda), tongue thrust is the consequence of an abnormal morphologic relationship, an adaptive phenomenon. Other investigators (Andrew, Hopkin, McEwan, Jann and Jann, Baker, Pensa, Kortsch) consider the tongue a primary etiologic factor. The experience of the authors is that abnormal tongue posture and function can be a primary factor, as a consequence of retained infantile deglutitional patterns or other abnormal oral habits, but it may also be strictly secondary or adaptive to the unfavorable morphologic pattern. Functional appliance therapy is indicated when there is reason to believe that the role of tongue malfunction is primary. However, when tongue function is adaptive to morphologic aberrations, its secondary or subordinate role does not make it the no. 1 priority. A correction of the basal dysplasia of skeletal parts will often result in the establishment of a normal tongue function. It is obvious that the object of the tongue function assessment is to make a differential diagnosis and determine which role the tongue plays.

Tongue posture. It is the considered opinion of some investigators that tongue posture is more important than tongue function (Mason and Proffit). The posture and shape can be flat or arched, protracted or retracted, narrowed and long, spread laterally and shortened, etc. Tongue posture is examined clinically with the mandible itself in postural rest position. A sagittal cephalometric registration of this relationship is also possible.

In a series of studies by the author, tongue posture was compared at rest position and in habitual occlusion. From the basic tongue posture at rest position an assessment of three regions—the root, the dorsum, and the tip—was made which disclosed the following:

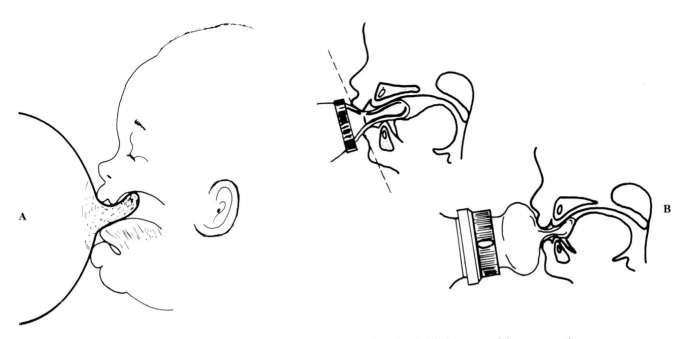

Fig. 5-32. A, Normal position of the tongue in breast-feeding. **B,** Modified position of the tongue with various nipples in bottle-feeding. The lower jaw is usually forced open to a greater degree, increasing the buccinator pressure particularly on the posterior segments of the maxillary arch. The normal plunger effect of the tongue in the natural nursing exercise is not possible.

That the root is usually flat in cases of mouth breathing and deep overbite (caused by a small tongue) and in all other cases there is usually a slight contact of the tongue with the soft palate.

That in Class II, Division 1, malocclusions and deep overbite the dorsum of the tongue is arched and high whereas in all other malocclusions there is a tendency for the tongue to flatten out in accordance with the length of the interocclusal space.

That the tip of the tongue is usually retracted in Class II, Division 1, malocclusions but in other malocclusion categories a slight anterior gliding of the tongue tip occurs while the mandible is moving into postural rest position.

It may be logically assumed that the changes in position of the tongue tip relate directly to mandibular malformations.

CEPHALOMETRIC EVALUATION OF TONGUE POSTURE. The clinical examination of the tongue and associated structures enables one to make only a subjective evaluation of its status. However, further complementary, exact, and reproducible study techniques are needed if important decisions such as a glossectomy are to be made. The cephalometric analysis is exacting, reproducible, and simple and can be employed in private practice.

The assessment is made from a lateral cephalogram taken in postural rest and habitual occlusion. Exposure is adjusted to reveal the soft tissue. The size of the tongue can be measured on the occlusal film. A successful analysis depends on the proper utilization of correct mensurational data. A baseline or reference line for measurement should satisfy the following criteria:

1. The greatest possible area of the tongue should lie above the reference line, since the two-dimensional radiograph does not show the anatomic borders of the tongue and the transverse dimensions.
2. The baseline should be independent of variations in skeletal structures.
3. The relation of the baseline to the tongue should not change with changes in mandibular position.
4. The baseline should remain constant with changes in tongue position.
5. The anatomic and functional properties of the tongue should relate to the baseline.
6. The measurement should be easy to make and replicate.

Fig. 5-33 shows the reference points and lines. *Is1* is the incisal margin of the lower incisors; *V,* the most caudal point on the shadow of the soft palate or its projection onto the reference line; *Mc,* the tip of the distobuccal cusp of the lower first molar. *Is1* and *Mc* are connected by a straight line extended to *V* to form the reference line. It has the following features: (1) A relatively large part of the tongue as seen on the cephalo-

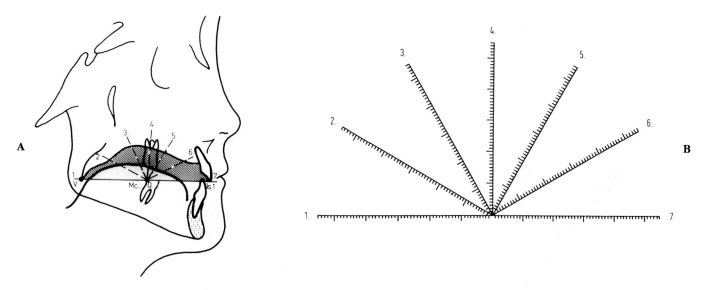

Fig. 5-33. A, Means of assessing tongue position and morphology on the cephalogram. **B,** Template for the assessment.

gram normally lies superior to it. (2) Skeletal relationships do not affect it. (3) Changes in tongue position do not influence it.

After the line is constructed, it is bisected between *Is1* and *V*. This point is called *0,* and a perpendicular is constructed from it to the palatal contour. A transparent template has been developed to make the necessary measurements. The baseline of the template coincides with the constructed reference line, and the vertical line intersects the reference line at *0.* From point *0,* where three lines now meet, four more lines are constructed as shown by the illustration of the template. These seven lines form six angles of 30° each. The lines can be marked in millimeters. Placing the template over the constructed lines permits reading off the exact measurements.

Assessment of tongue size from the occlusal cephalogram requires measurement of the distance between the superior tongue surface and the roof of the mouth. This is done along the seven constructed lines. The measurements give the relative size of the tongue (i.e., the size in relation to the oral cavity). Only when the entire oral cavity is filled can a diagnosis of macroglossia be made. This, of course, must be supported by clinical evidence.

The measurements made from the tongue template can be expressed by graphs (Fig. 5-34). The palatal vault may be represented by a horizontal line, and the seven single measurements by a curve. The distances between the reference line and the seven points on the constructed curve will graph the relationships of the superior surface of the tongue to the palatal vault and the soft palate to the tip of the uvula.

The posture of the tongue can be similarly evaluated by measurements taken on the postural rest position lateral cephalogram. To assess the posture and mobility of the tongue, one can calculate the differences between rest and occlusal positions. The occlusal position is taken as zero, with changes in rest position given as positive or negative figures (i.e., positive if the tongue is higher in rest position, negative if lower).

Changes in tongue position are reflected mainly by the position of the tip of the tongue. The positions of the other parts of the tongue also are subject to change, although not relative to the mandible but in conjunction with it. The changes in tongue tip position relate closely to the different types of malocclusion. In Class II the tip of the tongue is more retruded in rest position; in Class III it lies further forward in rest position (Fig. 5-35). It may be assumed that changes in tongue tip position relate to mandibular malformation tendencies.

Tongue size. The size and shape of the tongue show many variations—bulky and short, narrow and long, even wide and long. There are numerous clinical methods of assessing tongue size. The most common is to check whether the patient can touch his chin with his tongue tip. A "positive" result from this test is considered an indication of macroglossia. The recommendation of a glossectomy has actually been made on the basis of such an overly simplistic test. Both macroglossia (enlarged tongue) and microglossia (small tongue) are correlated with certain symptoms in the dentoalveolar area and the skeletal pattern that should be considered in the evaluation.

In macroglossia the oral cavity is filled by the tongue

PALATAL VAULT

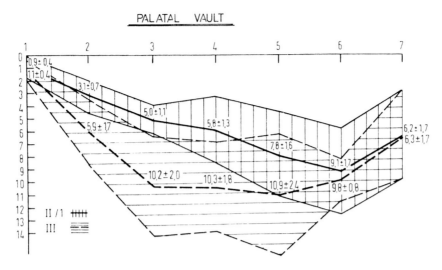

Fig. 5-34. Average tongue position values with standard deviations in Class II and Class III malocclusions. Note the lower tongue position in Class III cases.

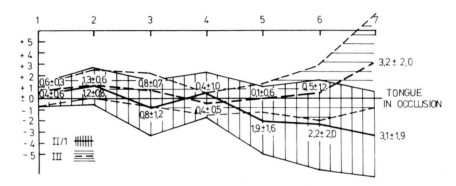

Fig. 5-35. Average tongue mobility values with standard deviations in Class II and Class III malocclusions.

mass. There does not seem to be enough space in the mouth, and the epipharynx is narrow. Indentations are evident on the tongue periphery and spaces exist between the incisors, which are procumbent. The tongue is protruded, and usually there is an open bite. A true macroglossia often occurs with certain pathologic conditions such as myxedema, cretinism, Down's syndrome, and hypophyseal gigantism. However, in children with the problem the definitive diagnosis of macroglossia cannot be made without a cephalometric analysis. A skeletal open bite with a tongue thrust can be mistaken clinically for a case of macroglossia. An example of the problems that can be encountered is the 5-year-old girl in Fig. 5-36, who has a Class III relationship, vertical growth pattern, and open bite. A glossectomy had been performed at 2 years of age and again at 4 years. Despite this, her tongue thrust and open bite persisted.

The obvious characteristic of microglossia or hypoglossia is a very small tongue. The protruded tongue tip reaches the lower incisors at best, and the floor of the mouth is elevated and visible on each side of the diminutive tongue. The dental arch reflects the small tongue size and is collapsed and reduced, with extreme crowding in the premolar area. There is usually a severe Class II relationship. Third molars are usually impacted at the angle of the jaw. In these cases of microglossia or aglossia (congenital absence of the tongue) severe functional disturbances are also present. The centrifugal force of the tongue is minimal or absent (Fig. 5-37). These cases provide an excellent example of the dynamics of muscle balance, or imbalance. The localized effects are extreme. In some cases teeth from the posterior segments are tipped so markedly to the lingual as to touch each other in the midline. Despite this deformity and the dysfunc-

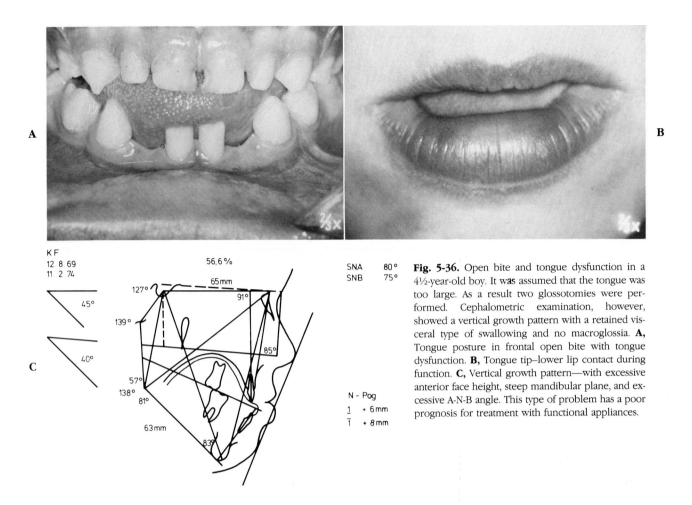

Fig. 5-36. Open bite and tongue dysfunction in a 4½-year-old boy. It was assumed that the tongue was too large. As a result two glossotomies were performed. Cephalometric examination, however, showed a vertical growth pattern with a retained visceral type of swallowing and no macroglossia. **A,** Tongue posture in frontal open bite with tongue dysfunction. **B,** Tongue tip–lower lip contact during function. **C,** Vertical growth pattern—with excessive anterior face height, steep mandibular plane, and excessive A-N-B angle. This type of problem has a poor prognosis for treatment with functional appliances.

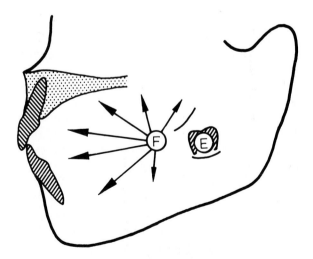

Fig. 5-37. The centrifugal force of the tongue *(F)* and eruption potential of the teeth *(E)* are important natural forces that can be influenced and guided with functional appliances.

tion, all evidence points to a relatively localized insult, with the effects limited mostly to the dentoalveolar area. An example of hypoglossia is the 35-year-old man in Fig. 5-38, who has a severe malocclusion associated with the deformity. Cephalometric analysis revealed a horizontal growth pattern, small gonial angle, and normally developed maxillary and mandibular bases. The bizarre dentoalveolar manifestations are evident from the anteriorly malposed and labially tipped upper incisors, together with the extreme retropositioning and lingual tipping of the lower incisors.

The implications in this circumstance are of interest not only for determining etiology but also for assessing the potential role of functional appliances that can screen, shield, or relieve, the teeth and investing tissues from functional forces. The pathologic teaches us much about the physiologic. In this case the functional abnormality affects the dentoalveolar region primarily, not the basal skeletal structure. Oral and vestibular screens that are incorporated into functional appliances have similar capabilities. It is a well-known fact that fixed appliances also have a localized effect primarily, which is why it is so important to locate the malocclusion and correct the

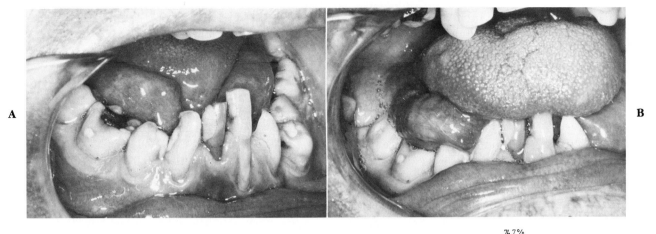

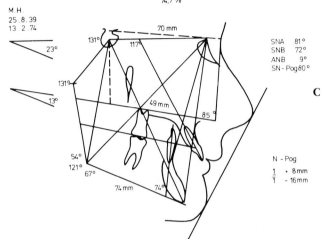

Fig. 5-38. Hypoglossia in a 35-year-old man. **A,** The tongue is habitually in the floor of the mouth. **B,** Even with the tongue maximally protracted, it barely clears the lingually tipped lower incisors. **C,** Dentoalveolar localization of the malocclusion in congenital hypoglossia. Both the tongue and the adaptive lower lip malfunction combine to retract the lower incisors and tip the maxillary incisors labially.

sagittal dysplasia before applying even simple inhibitory therapy.

Tongue dysfunction. The most common tongue dysfunctions are those involving selective outer pressure (pressing) and tongue biting. Tongue thrusting can be anterior, posterior, or combined. The consequences of the localization of aberrant pressures depend on the area of applied pressure:

1. Anterior open bite—anterior tongue thrust (and posture)
2. Lateral open bite or deep overbite—the result of lateral tongue thrust or postural spread that causes infraclusion of the posterior teeth
3. Edge-to-edge incisal and cuspal relationship of the teeth in the buccal segments—may mean a combined thrust, anterior and posterior open bite occurring from what is called a complex tongue thrust

The recognition of areas of excessive tongue pressure is important not only for determining the etiology of the associated malocclusion but also for providing information needed in fabrication of the screening appliance. As

has been pointed out, depending on the dentcalveolar and skeletal relationships, abnormal tongue function and posture can be a primary etiologic factor, usually with an anteriorly relocated flat tongue or a secondary adaptive and compensatory function and position resulting from a skeletal dysplasia. In either case the tongue dysfunction provides the anterior seal of the oral cavity.

The dentoalveolar anterior and posterior open bite problems are usually attributable to abnormal tongue posture and function and usually respond successfully to functional appliance intervention in the mixed dentition. This is also true for cases of deep overbite, in which lateral tongue spread during function and posture has led to infraclusion of the posterior teeth. The space is maintained by invagination of the peripheral portions of the tongue into the interocclusal space while the mandible is in the postural resting position. In such cases there is a large freeway space and the deep overbite is functional.

A second type of overbite (called a functional pseudo-overbite) is caused by supraclusion of the incisors. In this case there is a small freeway space. Functional appliance intervention, particularly when there are developmental disturbances, is not indicated. Fixed appliances and orthopedic guidance are more likely to correct the problem.

In skeletal open bite problems there is a genetically determined vertical growth pattern, often associated with marked antegonial notching. This type of case does not offer a favorable prognosis for orthodontic therapy. The inclination of the maxillary base should also be considered in the evaluation of these open bite problems. An upward and forward inclination enhances the open bite relationship, whereas a maxillary base that is tipped down anteriorly compensates for it. The inclination of the maxillary base can be influenced both by functional factors and by habits, good and bad.

The consequence of tongue posture and function abnormalities in the dentoalveolar region also depends on the skeletal pattern. In a horizontal growth pattern the forward tongue thrust or posture can result in a bimaxillary protrusion. With the tongue pressing against the lingual surfaces of both upper and lower incisors simul-

taneously, there is often spacing in the incisor segments (Fig. 5-39). In a vertical growth pattern, the tongue thrust can open the bite and the lower incisors may be tipped lingually. During the abnormal functional and postural forward positioning, the tip of the tongue lies between the dental arches, in contact with the lower lip, which the patient constantly sucks. Thus the incisors are tipped lingually (Fig. 5-40).

PALATOGRAPHIC EXAMINATION OF TONGUE DYSFUNCTION. A complementary evaluation of tongue function is possible using the palatographic technique, which permits tongue function to be observed during swallowing and speaking and also allows the influence of various functional orthodontic appliances on the tongue to be evaluated. Originally palatographic procedures were used only for speech disorders. There is a direct and indirect method.

In the *direct* method, first described by Oakley Coles in 1872, gum arabic and flour were mixed and painted on the tongue. After the selected functional exercises had been performed, the contacts on the palate and teeth were transferred onto the cast of the upper jaw with red ink.

The *indirect* palatographic technique was first used by Kingsley. He prepared an upper plate of black India rubber and covered the tongue with a mixture of chalk and alcohol. The contacts seen on the palatal rubber plate were then transferred on the cast, as in the direct method just described.

The current direct method entails covering the superior surface of the tongue with a precise impression material (e.g., Imprex). A thin even layer is applied to the tongue with a spatula. After functional exercises a Polaroid print is made of the palatal region with the help of a surface mirror. The evaluation of the palatogram is possible by direct measurements on the picture (Fig. 5-41).

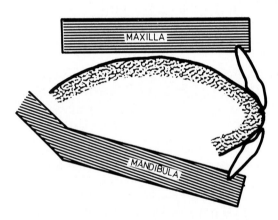

Fig. 5-39. In horizontal growth patterns a tongue thrust habit can cause procumbency of both upper and lower incisors.

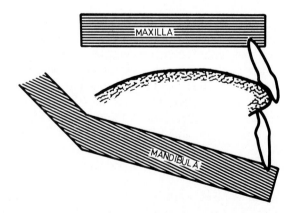

Fig. 5-40. In vertical growth patterns a tongue thrust habit is more likely to cause labial tipping of the upper and lingual tipping of the lower incisors.

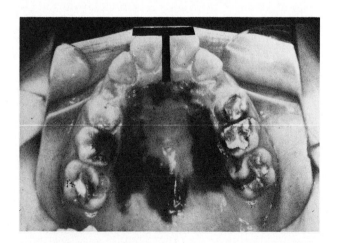

Fig. 5-41. Palatogram with measurement of the distance between the tongue tip and incisal edges.

Speech assessment is also desirable from an orthodontic point of view. The tongue, together with the pharynx, velum, palate, and teeth, plays a central role in phonation. The movements of the tongue during speech are sophisticated and dependent on local conditions. In malocclusions with malposed teeth there may also be a malposition of the tongue, which can impair normal speech. Usually the tongue, with its inherent flexibility, is able to compensate for atypical morphologic relationships; and this compensatory potential is an important diagnostic clue as the clinician establishes a treatment plan and prognosis for functional appliance therapy. The ability to compensate or adapt can be assessed from the palatographic record (Fig. 5-42).

Therapeutic requirements for various tongue dysfunctions. The variety of aberrations of tongue function requires a functional therapeutic approach that is tailored to the problem. The skeletal pattern is a conditioning factor. If the abnormal tongue function is the primary

etiologic basis of the malocclusion, causal therapy can be instituted to eliminate it and restore the integrity of the teeth and investing tissues by means of functional appliances. This approach is likely to succeed in both anterior and lateral open bite problems, provided the growth direction is horizontal or at least average. Other malocclusions have additional factors as causative elements, and still others with just as excessive overjet and sagittal discrepancies require control of not only these problems but the tongue abnormality as well. In other words, more than one muscle or muscle group may be involved in the enhancement of a morphologic aberration and treatment planning should take this into account.

Thumb- and finger-sucking effects. One specific kind of malocclusion, which is also a consequence of abnormal function, requires a combined treatment—active mechanical appliance as well as functional appliance in the mixed dentition (Fig. 5-43). Finger-sucking

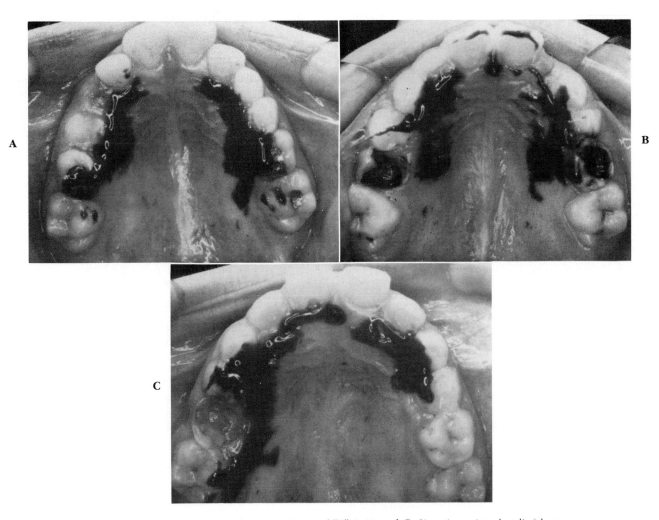

Fig. 5-42. Palatogram during the pronunciation of "S." **A,** Normal. **B,** Sigmatismus interdentalis (abnormal). **C,** Sigmatismus lateroflexus (abnormal).

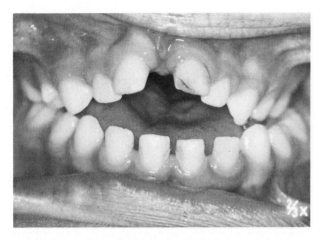

Fig. 5-43. Open bite malocclusion with cross-bite, a consequence of abnormal tongue posture and function. Frequently a prolonged fingersucking habit is the instigating factor.

can cause an open bite, with simultaneous narrowing of the maxillary arch. The adaptive tongue function aggravates and prolongs the malocclusion. With bilateral narrowing the patient often compensates with a lateral shift to one side or the other to gain maximum chewing surface contact. This functional type of cross-bite, or convenience cross-bite, is not skeletal in the initial stages but adaptive. Before beginning functional appliance therapy, it is advisable to expand the maxillary arch with a split palate jackscrew type of active plate. Sometimes a small wire crib can be incorporated to block the tongue in the cross-bite area or at least set up an exteroceptive engram that initiates tongue retraction. In some severe dysfunction cases treatment may begin with the oral screen and the active plate will be used later. This is often done in the deciduous dentition.

In a skeletal open bite that gets progressively worse because of a severe vertical growth pattern, successful causal therapy is not possible. Since the tongue dysfunction in these cases is secondary to the primary morphogenetic basis, therapeutic demands are more rigorous. Fixed appliances, often with tooth sacrifice, offer a more effective approach. In extreme cases orthognathic surgery is the only viable alternative, after completion of growth. In the early mixed dentition, however, a partial improvement may be achieved by eliminating some of the dysfunction; but this does not materially alter the growth pattern, which will require other therapeutic methods later on (Figs. 5-44 and 5-45). Nevertheless, a vertical growth pattern can be influenced by strong orthopedic forces or a specially designed activator. Heavy vertical pull fixed orthopedics can alter the direction of mandibular growth, while restricting buccal segment eruption, whereas the activator has the potential of af-

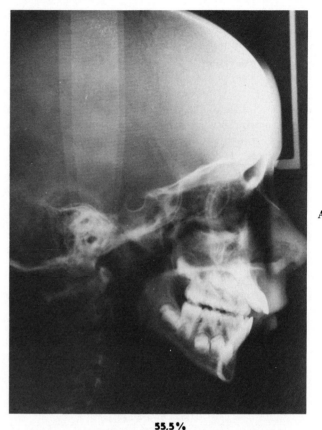

A

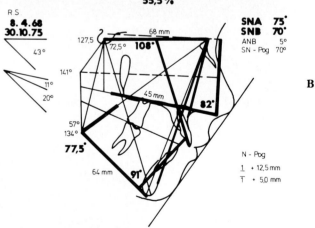

B

Fig. 5-44. Open bite malocclusion and vertical growth pattern in a 7½-year-old girl. **A,** Lateral cephalogram. **B,** Cephalometric tracing showing a not unfavorable posterior-to-anterior face height ratio. In most cases of this type, there is supraeruption of posterior segments and a minimal or nonexistent freeway space.

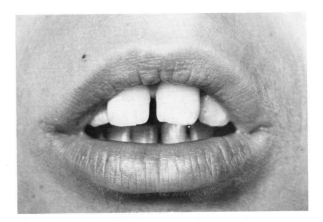

Fig. 5-46. Incompetent lip posture associated with mouth breathing, excessive epipharyngeal lymphoid tissue, etc.

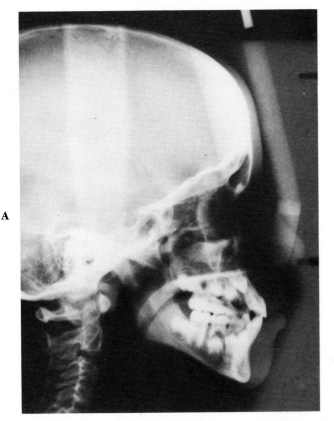

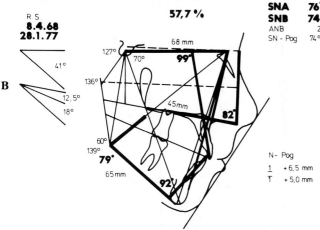

R S			SNA	**76°**
8.4.68			SNB	**74°**
28.1.77			ANB	2°
			SN - Pog	74°

Fig. 5-45. Improvement of the open bite malocclusion in the same patient as in Fig. 5-44 after elimination of the dysfunction. This result is in spite of persistence of the vertical growth pattern. **A,** Lateral cephalogram. **B,** Cephalometric tracing. Significant dental compensation has been achieved.

fecting the inclination of the maxillary base. It is stressed again that an analysis of the growth pattern is also needed, in addition to the functional study, to determine the therapeutic approach most likely to be successful.

Examination of the lips. As part of the functional continuum, the lips must be carefully examined. The external balancing muscle factors are as important as the internal factors. The configuration of the lips should be studied in the relaxed position. If the lips are trained, any patient can achieve a lip seal, at least under conscious effort, but we want to know what the lip relationship is most of the time.

1. If there is only a slight contact or a very small gap between the upper and lower lips, they are said to be competent.
2. If there is a wide gap or if the lips, primarily the upper lip, are too short, they can be considered incompetent. Improvement with orthodontic treatment and exercises is possible only in the early stages (Fig. 5-46).
3. If the lips seem normally developed but the upper incisors are labially tipped, making closure difficult, Ballard and Tulley call this potential lip incompetency. The incisal margins interpose between the lips, resting on the lower lip, and prevent the normal lip seal. The lower lip trap then enhances the already excessive overjet, tipping the incisors further forward into a more dangerous zone where any trauma may result in breakage. Even hypermobility is possible in the incisor area, with the lower lip pushing the upper incisors labially while often retroclining and crowding the lower incisors at the same time. Treatment of these problems early is an important preventive measure (Fig. 5-47).

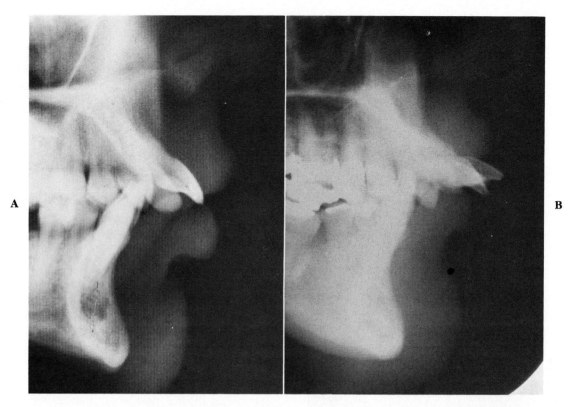

Fig. 5-47. A, Potential lip incompetency associated with excessive overjet. The lower lip cushions to the lingual of the maxillary incisors whereas the upper lip is short and hypofunctional. In trying to effect a lip seal during the deglutitional cycle, the mentalis muscle is hyperactive. **B,** Severe lip incompetency leading to actual mobility of the upper incisors. The strong hyperactive mentalis muscle is quite capable of forcing the upper incisors labially against the hypotonic upper lip. Constant jiggling of these teeth can cause periodontal involvement and ultimate bone loss.

4. If the lower lip is hypertrophic, everted, and re-dundant (i.e., with an excess of tissue), little can be done to improve the situation by orthodontic ther-apy.

There are various methods for evaluating the lip pro-file. Photographs and lateral cephalograms can be used effectively.

Schwarz analysis (lateral cephalogram). A. Martin Schwarz devised an analysis that is quite useful. Three reference lines are constructed for this method (Fig. 5-48).

H line—corresponding to the Frankfort horizontal
Pn line—perpendicular to the H line at soft tissue nasion
Po line—perpendicular from orbitale to the H line

Between the two constructed perpendicular lines is what Schwarz terms the GPF or gnathic profile field. In normal proportions the upper lip touches the Po line whereas the lower lip lies one third the width of the GPF posterior to it. The oblique tangential line (T) is constructed by joining subnasale, at the junction of the

upper lip and nose, to soft tissue pogonion, the most anterior point on the profile curvature of the symphysis. In the ideal case the T line bisects the vermilion border of the upper lip and touches the anterior vermilion cur-vature of the lower lip.

Ricketts lip analysis. The reference line used by Rick-etts is similar to the Schwarz T line but is drawn from the tip of the nose to soft tissue pogonion. In a normal relationship the upper lip is 2 to 3 mm and the lower lip 1 to 2 mm behind this line (Fig. 5-49).

Steiner lip analysis. The upper reference point for the Steiner analysis is at the center of the **S**-shaped curve between the tip of the nose and subnasale. Soft tissue pogonion is the lower terminus. If the lips lie behind the reference line, they are too flat; if in front, too prom-inent (Fig. 5-50).

Holdaway lip analysis. This is a quantitative assess-ment of lip configuration. Holdaway measures the angle between the tangent to the upper lip from soft tissue pogonion and the N-B line, which he calls the H angle (Fig. 5-51). With an A-N-B of 1 to 3 degrees, the H angle

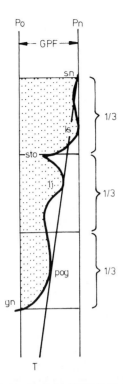

Fig. 5-48. The gnathic profile field *(GPF)* (A.M. Schwarz) permits assessment of the profile from the lateral cephalogram. *Po,* Perpendicular to the Frankfort plane at orbitale; *Pn,* perpendicular to the Frankfort plane at nasion; *Sn,* subnasale; *ls,* labium superius oris; *li,* labium inferius oris; *sto,* stomion; *pog,* pogonion; *gn,* gnathion.

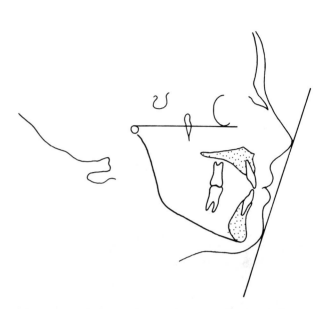

Fig. 5-49. Reference line used by Ricketts for assessing the soft tissue profile.

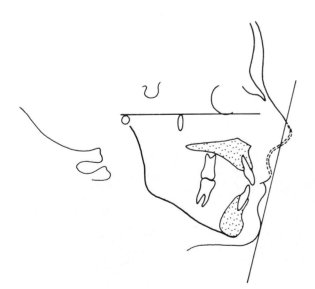

Fig. 5-50. The Steiner lip analysis.

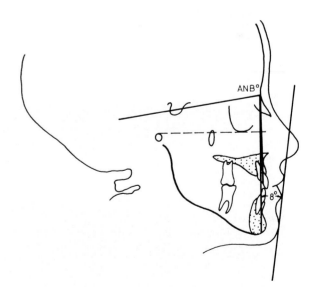

Fig. 5-51. The Holdaway lip analysis.

should be 7 to 8 degrees. Changes in the A-N-B mean changes in the ideal H angle. Holdaway defines the ideal profile as follows:

A-N-B angle of 2°, H angle of 7° to 8°
Lower lip touching the soft tissue line that connects pogonion and the upper lip extended to S-N
Relative proportions of nose and upper lip balanced (soft tissue line bisecting subnasal **S** curve)
Tip of nose 9 mm anterior to the soft tissue line (normal at age 13 years)
No lip tension on closure

The upper lip is tense if the difference between the thickness of the soft tissue (A to S-N) and the thickness of the vermilion border of the upper lip is greater than ±1 mm (Holdaway). After the elimination of lip tension, each 3 mm retraction of the incisors will result in 1.0 mm retraction of the upper lip.

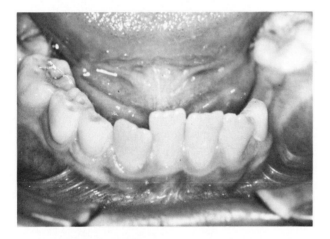

Fig. 5-52. Crowding of the lower incisors caused by lip sucking or by a confirmed hyperactive mentalis muscle.

The length and thickness of the lips are not only age dependent but also correlated with the various malocclusions. The following chart is based on examination of 12-year-old children, giving the averages derived:

	Class I	Class II	Class III
Length of upper lip (mm)	23.0	22.0	20.9
Length of lower lip (mm)	37.0	36.5	36.0
Thickness of upper lip (mm)	11.5	10.8	12.4
Thickness of lower lip (mm)	12.5	14.0	11.8

These differences between the various types of malocclusions disappear during orthodontic treatment.

Dysfunction of the lips. A number of lip muscle abnormalities have been identified and characterized. The most common is sucking or biting of the lower lip, known as a mentalis habit because of the crinkling "golf ball" appearance of the symphyseal tissue with excessive mentalis activity. In this type of dysfunction there is usually contact between the tongue and the lower lip that can be observed during swallowing. The consequences of the combined muscle abnormality can be not only the opening of the bite anteriorly but also the lingual tipping of the lower incisors with crowding and labial malpositioning of the upper incisors. The pernicious "lip trap" thus works against the integrity of both the upper and the lower dentitions (Fig. 5-52). There can actually be a retraction or dehiscence of the labial gingival tissue overlying the lower incisors (Fig. 5-53).

Similar to nail biting or pencil biting, upper lip biting is a habit frequently seen in schoolchildren. It is a stress-strain relief syndrome. The tongue function can be normal, with the hyperkinetic behavioral activity and abnormal lip habit as the main factors. Of course, an inherent morphogenetic pattern type of Class II malocclusion can

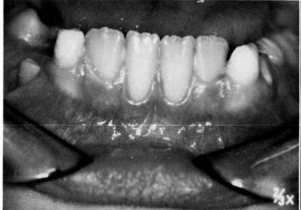
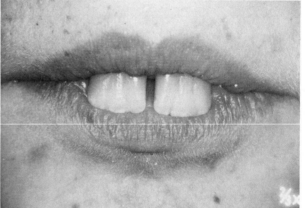

A   B

Fig. 5-53. A, Retraction of the gingival margin. A dehiscence of this type is frequently seen with abnormal perioral muscle function (e.g., perverted lip habit) as illustrated in **B.**

provide the overjet that requires lip compensations, which in turn exacerbate the original overjet.

As with tongue habits, lip sucking can be either a primary or a secondary factor. In cases in which it is the primary causative factor, there is overjet with labial tipping of the upper and lingual tipping of the lower incisors and only a slight skeletal sagittal discrepancy. The lip habit enhances the original slight to moderate overjet. In cases in which it plays only a secondary role the original overjet is due to a significant sagittal discrepancy, usually with mandibular underdevelopment. The inclination of the incisors can be normal. The lower lip cushions in the gap between the upper and lower incisors primarily as an adaptation to the morphologic malrelations. Lip activity may not be so intensive, but more adaptive. As with tongue problems, functional therapy is successful only in cases of primary dysfunction. In the cases of secondary role of the lip, functional therapy is subservient to other orthopedic and orthodontic (or surgical) methods.

Respiration. The mode of respiration is of interest for several reasons:

1. Mouth breathing or disturbed nasal breathing can be considered an etiologic factor or at least a predisposing cause for some malocclusion symptoms. In 1968 Ricketts described the "respiratory obstruction syndrome," with the following symptoms: visceral-type swallowing, predisposition to open bite, unilateral or bilateral cross-bite, and slight deflection of the head. In examinations by the author a significantly high frequency of the following symptoms is observed in patients with disturbed nasal respiration: Class II, Division 1, malocclusion; narrowness of the upper arch; crowding of the upper and lower arches; vertical growth pattern (Fig. 5-54).

2. It is not possible to treat with some functional appliances if the patient has disturbed nasal breathing. If the tonsils and adenoids are enlarged, with a compensatory anterior tongue posture, the patient cannot tolerate a bulky acrylic appliance in the oral cavity. There are other appliances that can be used in cases of habitual mouth breathing (Fig. 5-55).

3. In mouth breathing patients the lip seal is usually inadequate. The tongue has a low posture and disturbed function. If this condition persists after treatment is finished, the result is not likely to be stable, with relapse as a consequence. If at all possible, it is advantageous to establish normal nasal respiration prior to orthodontic therapy. Unfortunately, in some patients with allergies or a deviated nasal septum, it is not possible to do this during the growth period.

• • •

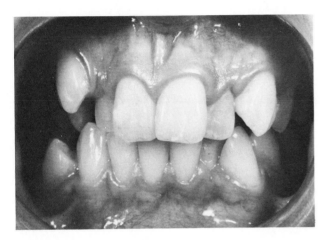

Fig. 5-54. Crowding associated with habitual mouth breathing. This may not be a primary etiologic factor, however. Other concerns such as morphogenetic patterns or premature loss may be more important.

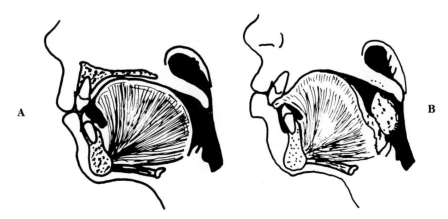

Fig. 5-55. Normal sagittal section, **A,** and anterior positioning of the tongue, **B,** in a patient with enlarged tonsils. (After Moyers.)

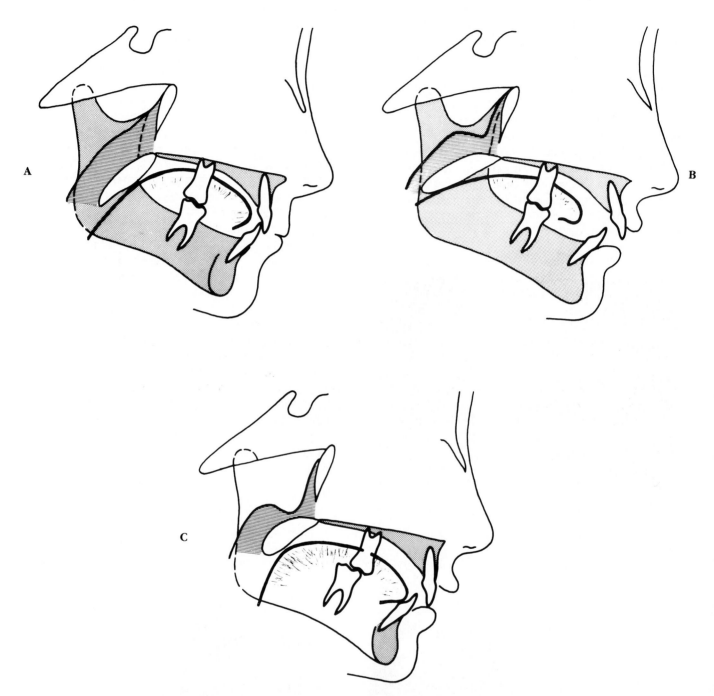

Fig. 5-56. Assessing the size of the adenoids on headplate tracings. This should be a routine diagnostic exercise. It is particularly important in patients with allergic histories and mouth breathing or abnormal lip posture. **A,** No adenoids. **B,** Small and, **C,** large adenoids.

The assessment of disturbed nasal function is not always easy. The case history data can give some idea of the frequency of ENT diseases and mode of sleeping, habits, allergies, etc. The clinical examination should determine whether the lips are competent or not. Lip incompetency does not necessarily mean mouth breathing but suggests that this might be the case. Further clinical examination with a mirror or cotton swab is possible but not really reliable. It can be helpful to have the patient hold a sheet of cardboard between his lips, or some water in his mouth, to see whether he can breath through the nose without difficulty.

The presence and size of the adenoids and tonsils can also be estimated on the lateral head film. This indicates whether the nasopharyngeal passage is free or partially or totally obstructed. The work of Moyers and Linder-Aronson in this field shows the potential effect of epipharyngeal lymphoid tissue blockage, with resultant tongue posture compensation and mouth breathing, so this part of the examination is important. There are various ways of assessing the size of adenoids and tonsils. An arbitrary scale of small, medium, or large can be used, from both the clinical examination and the lateral cephalogram (Fig. 5-56). It should be remembered that there is spontaneous regression of epipharyngeal lymphoid tissue with development. At 10 years of age, 180% of the lymphoid tissue is present that will still be there at 18 years of age. So obstructive adenoids usually regress without surgical intervention.

The nasal respiratory resistance can also be measured by an indirect plethysmographic approach. In habitual mouth breathing the respiration resistance is low whereas in structurally conditioned mouth breathing it is high. The use of a small piece of paper held under the nose while the patient is breathing will also determine whether respiratory air is escaping from the nostrils. If the paper does not flutter at all, at least some obstruction is likely. Visualization of the nasal turbinates by looking through the nostrils is also of some help. The diagnosis of "mouth breathing" is probably best made by the otolaryngologist, however, and a consultation is to be recommended if there is a problem.

The scope of functional therapy with respiratory problems can be summarized as follows:

1. In habitual mouth breathing with small respiratory resistance, functional therapy is indicated. Exercises can be prescribed. Holding a sheet of cardboard between the lips is one very satisfactory means of enhancing lip seal.
2. When there are structure problems, with excessive adenoid tissue, allergies, etc., it is advisable to seek an otolaryngologic consultation and possible treatment. If successful, orthodontics can then begin.
3. If the structural conditions are unalterable, functional appliance therapy cannot be instituted. In such cases

only active fixed appliance mechanotherapy is likely to produce the changes desired. Even then, the stability of the results is open to question unless autonomous improvement occurs.

Significance of functional analysis in treatment planning with removable appliances

The importance of functional analysis in the examination of various types of malocclusions is universally recognized.

Class II malocclusions. The postural rest position of the mandible can be anterior or posterior to the habitual occlusal position. More frequently, however, it is anterior. Together with a large freeway space and mandibular overclosure and deep bite, the prognosis for treatment with functional appliances is usually good.

Early TMJ symptoms can frequently be seen in Class II malocclusions, especially in cases of deep overbite, horizontal growth pattern, and abnormal perioral muscle function. The dysfunction of the tongue should be evaluated as well as the lips, mentalis muscle, facial, and supra- and infrahyoid musculature, with an eye toward localized effects on dentoalveolar growth. Respiratory disturbances have a potential interfering role with regard to the accomplishment of a normal growth and developmental pattern and should be eliminated, if possible, before orthodontic treatment.

Class III malocclusions. As with Class II malocclusions, the postural rest position of the mandible can be anterior or posterior to the habitual occlusal position. If it is anterior, then there is a true Class III malocclusion. If it is posterior, then it is a tooth guidance problem, or forced bite (pseudo–Class III), since the lower incisors move past their maxillary counterparts in the closing maneuver, with the lingual surfaces of the lower incisors engaging the maxillary incisal margins as the posterior teeth are brought into contact. The path of closure and condylar position in the fossa should be checked carefully. The skeletal pattern must also be evaluated so a differentiation can be made between true and pseudo–Class III malocclusions.

Tongue posture and function should be checked both clinically and cephalometrically. Functional appliance therapy is particularly indicated in pseudo–Class III malocclusions with normal tongue posture. A true skeletal Class III malocclusion does not offer a favorable prognosis for functional appliances. Respiratory conditions must also be studied in this malocclusion category. Breathing disturbances and enlarged tonsils and adenoids seem to cause a compensatory forward positioning of the tongue, with a flattening of the dorsum, as the unconscious reflex action keeps the airway open. The maxillary arch is thus unopposed by normal tongue support and can collapse both transversely and sagittally because of the effective low tongue posture.

Open bite malocclusions. These problems can be primary or secondary and, depending on the localization of the dysfunction, anterior or posterior. In primary dysfunctions with abnormal muscle action as a major etiologic factor, the growth pattern is usually average or horizontal. When the growth pattern is mostly vertical, the dysfunction may be more secondary or adaptive. Functional appliances are increasingly likely to be successful in cases with primary dysfunction and at least an average growth pattern.

Gnathologic considerations

A gnathologic instrumental registration may be incorporated as part of the functional analysis in the permanent dentition, after active treatment, or in TMJ disturbances.

In the mixed dentition transitional period with autonomous changes in sagittal and occlusal plane inclination, gnathologic assessment is not appropriate. Functional abnormalities may be determined by looking for the path of closure, initial or premature contacts, and any deflections that occur in the postural rest–to–habitual occlusal position stroke. The amount of interocclusal clearance is also a diagnostic criterion.

A differentiation between tooth-guided slides and skeletal problems creating the same habitual occlusion is necessary both before and after treatment. In dentoalveolar slides the cause is premature contact or abnormal intercuspation. Then orthodontic tooth movement or equilibration can correct the problem. In skeletal slides a compensation may exist by virtue of the mandible's sliding into a forced position; often an excessive overjet is compensated by an anterior sliding or posturing of the mandible, creating the so-called dual bite. This kind of problem requires a major assault on the multisystem involvement—with orthopedic therapy, possible selective extraction, growth guidance over a fairly long time, and possibly a surgical correction later, if the problem is really severe.

The goal is the same for both functional and fixed multiattachment orthodontic appliances (i.e., a functional and stable occlusion). To evaluate the result, the same criteria are used. The objectives for a normal Class I occlusion as far as position, inclination, and angulation of teeth are concerned are well expressed by Andrews in his "six keys of occlusion" concept. Since these objectives are not always possible with removable appliances alone, a combination approach may be necessary to achieve as many of the objectives as possible. Bodily movement, changing axial inclination, torque, correcting rotations, closing spaces in a parallel fashion, and controlling extraction sites usually require the precise control that only multiattachment fixed mechanotherapy can provide.

APPLYING THE PRINCIPLES OF OCCLUSION

In treatment with removable appliances, the principles of optimum static and functional occlusion should be considered as much as is possible.

1. Eruption and axial inclination, particularly of the canine teeth, can be controlled. The erupting teeth can be guided into a correct position by grinding and reshaping the acrylic guiding planes of the appliance. It is possible to control the axial inclination of the canines to a large degree by loops on the labial bow of the activator concurrently with the recontouring of the acrylic (Fig. 5-57). By means of active plates, especially expansion plates, the axial inclination is subjected to certain methods to prevent buccal tipping of the crowns (Fig. 5-58).

2. To control the lingual crown torque of teeth in the buccal segments, it is necessary to consider the transverse curve of Wilson during therapy. In the course of expansion therapy a buccal crown torque or tipping can be created, with elongation of the lingual canines and

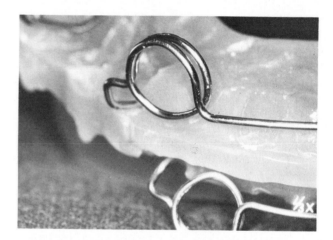

Fig. 5-57. Loops on the labial bow of an activator to control the axial inclination of the canines.

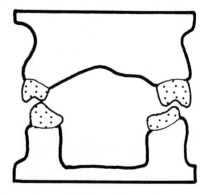

Fig. 5-58. Overexpanded upper dental arch with a disturbed occlusion.

resultant traumatic occlusal interference and instability. This undesirable phenomenon can occur both with rapid palatal expansion and with increases achieved by the jackscrew type of active expansion plate. Slow expansion during the mixed dentition is less likely to produce this iatrogenic reaction. However, the limitation of expansion therapy should be recognized at the proper time and other means employed if necessary to attain the treatment goal; or therapy should be terminated when optimum bodily expansion and maintenance of normal buccolingual cusp contact with opposing teeth have been attained.

3. The curve of Spee can be concave, flat, or convex (Fig. 5-59). Leveling it when it is abnormal is possible during the mixed dentition since eruption of the posterior teeth is stimulated or guided by the functional appliance. After the eruption of the permanent teeth, control of the curve of Spee is more difficult with removable appliances. To level the occlusal plane and control the vertical dimension require using fixed multiattachment appliances.

4. Force application is interrupted with the use of removable appliances. The teeth can be moved into traumatic positions and can then migrate back during the static intervals. The clinican must be careful not to cause this "jiggling" during the use of removable appliances, or must keep it to a minimum, while correcting crossbite conditions.

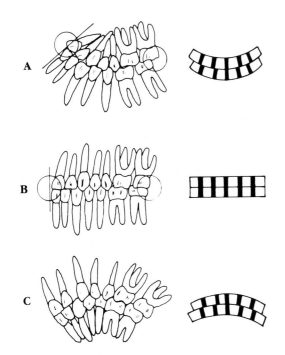

Fig. 5-59. Variations in the curve of Spee (after Andrews). **A,** Concave. **B,** Flat. **C,** Convex.

5. After the completion of active treatment some occlusal interferences may still exist. It may be necessary to resort to selective grinding or equilibrative procedures. In such cases a gnathologic articulator may be beneficial in mounting the casts first to check the possible areas of interference. To project the possible need for future equilibration, it is necessary to consider the growth direction during active treatment.

a. In a horizontal growth pattern, selective grinding procedures should be employed in the molar but not the incisal region. This is because the bite can deepen and incisal guidance can worsen during the terminal stages of mandibular growth, leading to incisor crowding. The final equilibration in this area should be postponed until growth has ceased.

b. In a vertical growth pattern, equilibration can be done in the incisor region but should be postponed in the buccal segments until later. The molar guidance can become worse in the last stages of jaw growth, leading to a relapse into open bite. Correction by equilibration can be done only to a moderate extent, and even then in the post-growth period.

6. Examination of the condylar guidance in the mixed dentition is of interest from an informational point of view, but it should be recognized that condylar guidance is not stabilized during the transitional dentition period.

a. The activator directly influences condylar structures during the growing period. The condylar guidance can become flatter or steeper during orthopedic treatment. Asymmetry that exists in the steepness of condylar guidance before treatment may be amenable to correction during activator therapy. In other cases the opposite condition is observed, with the creation of an asymmetry. This is especially true if a midline correction has been undertaken using an incorrect construction bite for the activator.

b. Prior to expansion treatment with active plates, particularly during treatment of cross-bite, there is asymmetric condylar guidance. The results of such treatment can and should correct this condition in the temporomandibular joint as well as in the dentoalveolar area. Otherwise, the probability of TMJ problems exists later on.

c. A simple method of assessing condylar guidance in the mixed dentition has been developed. The sagittal measurement of the condylar guidance is performed using a condylar facebow (Fig. 5-60). The registration tray for the upper arch is modified. It can be adapted to dental arches of various sizes. The palate is left open (Fig. 5-61). Fixation is achieved by impression material, and the tray is

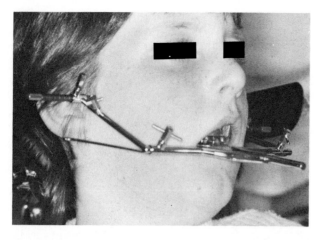

Fig. 5-60. Facebow for simplified extraoral registration in the mixed dentition.

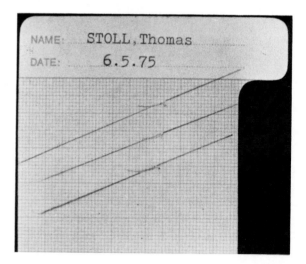

A

B

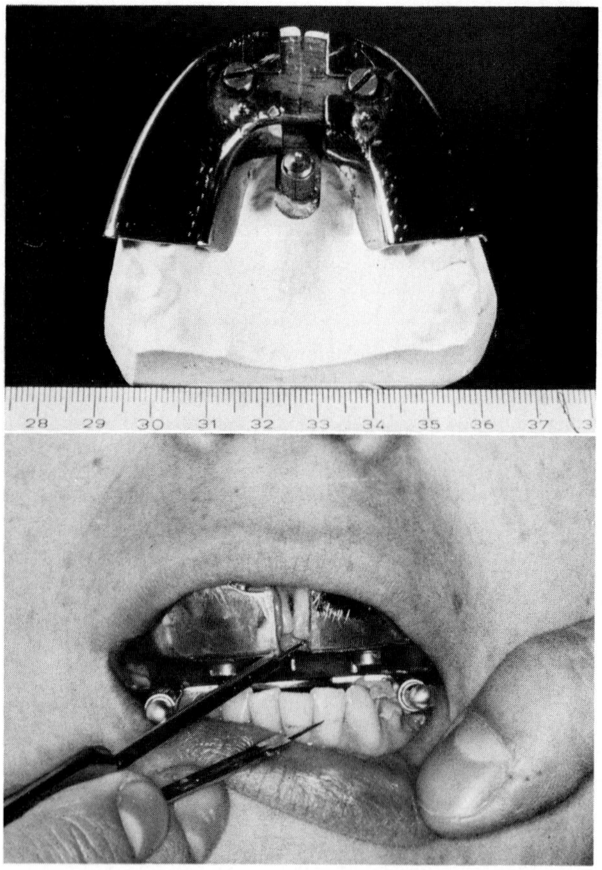

Fig. 5-61. A, Adjustable tray for registration. **B,** Fixed in the mouth with impression material.

anchored only dentally. It has triple support to eliminate any rolling or unwanted movement. The condylar guidance is registered three times on the Gerber registration chart on both left and right sides. The average is then used for the evaluation (Fig. 5-62).

We can conclude from the foregoing that some gnathologic principles should be considered, even in the mixed dentition period, and with removable appliance treatment. Specifically, these are as follows:

1. The eruption and axial inclination of the teeth, particularly the canines, can be controlled.
2. The curve of Wilson can be controlled, particularly during expansion treatment.
3. The curve of Spee can be leveled out during the eruption of the posterior teeth.
4. Occlusal trauma should be eliminated during orthodontic tooth movement.
5. The indications for and timing of equilibrative procedures should be anticipated and applied at the proper time.

CONCLUSIONS

Functional analysis transcends all diagnostic records, although it utilizes each one in a special way. As much as anything, it is a philosophy of diagnostic interpretation. The orthodontist is so used to employing the static set of plaster casts (related in habitual occlusion), the lateral cephalogram (again with the teeth in occlusion),

Fig. 5-62. Triple registration of the condylar guidance.

the panoral radiograph with the teeth in a manipulated incisal relationship to keep them all within the focal trough, and the facial photographs (which usually record the teeth in occlusion and the facial muscles in repose) or intraoral photographs (which duplicate the interdental relationships on the study models) that a dynamic assessment of these records alone requires a new orientation.

Even the clinical examination is usually an appraisal of morphologic and interarch relationships for many clinicians—with some lip service paid to the way the draping musculature appears. How many orthodontists put their patients through deglutitional, masticatory, and speech exercises? How many check the temporomandibular joint in various functional exercises and positions? How many really delve into the patient's anamnestic history for information on these areas? There may be questions on finger-sucking or tongue thrusting, but they are only part of the functional diagnostic mosaic.

A total approach is indicated for any form of orthodontic treatment, but especially for functional appliances. An appreciation of what the muscles have done can be converted into therapeutic utilization of these same dynamic intrinsic forces. American orthodontists have been quite skilled in using extrinsic forces to achieve a predetermined "norm" of tooth-to-tooth relationship. Now, however, they must also enlist the intrinsic forces, which may have caused or exacerbated the original malocclusion, in the corrective process. Only then will optimal accomplishment and stability of results be achieved.

CHAPTER 6

THE ACTIVATOR

DEVELOPMENT, CONSTRUCTION, AND MODE OF ACTION

Conventional orthodontics has as its arena of operation the dentoalveolar area. Moffett terms this the second order of craniofacial articulation, since he considered the tooth socket an articulation, with the periodontal ligament providing the cellular elements to create the change (Fig. 6-1).

Extending the effects of orthodontic guidance to the third order of articulation, as classified by Moffett (i.e., the sutures and the condylar joints), however, is not new. Historically there is evidence that facial sutures were influenced as early as 1803 by Fox, with extraoral force. Therapeutic intervention in the condylar area, the TMJ, of course, involves the mandible rather than the maxilla. Since the mandible is the only freely functional osseous structure on the body and is tied to its contiguous structures by 13 muscle attachments, its position in space, sagittally, transversely, and vertically, is of concern to the orthodontist. The possibility of influencing the mandibular position by altering the TMJ arrangement of parts and morphology has intrigued orthodontists for many years.

In 1879 Kingsley introduced the term and concept of "jumping the bite" for mandibular retrusion patients. He did this with a vulcanite palatal plate consisting of an anterior incline that guided the mandible to a forward position when the patient closed on it. This maneuver was done to correct the sagittal relationship but not to tip the lower incisors forward. Clinical experience by Kingsley and others demonstrated the difficulty of holding the forward position of the lower jaw, so the technique is seldom used any more—except as indicated by Hotz, whose *Vorbissplatte* was a modified Kingsley plate. Hotz used the appliance in cases of deep bite retrognathism, in which there was the likelihood of a functional retrusion caused by the overbite, and when the lower incisors were lingually inclined by hyperactivity of the mentalis muscle and lower lip.

The ideas of Kingsley did have an influence on the development of functional jaw orthopedics, however. The activator was originally used by Viggo Andresen (1908) with vertical extensions to contact the contiguous lingual surfaces of the mandibular teeth. Yet, almost 75 years later, the possibility of achieving a permanent forward positioning of the mandible is still controversial in some circles despite treatment of many thousands of patients by this method. Too many cases exist in which a forward "jumping of the bite" has been done, with the result that after appliance removal a dual bite exists (Fig. 6-2). In these cases the patient habitually positions the mandible forward from a more retruded centric relation into a habitual occlusion that appears to be correct when looking at the buccal occlusion but actually is a postural maneuver initiated by the protracting musculature to achieve a full occlusion. This type of relationship

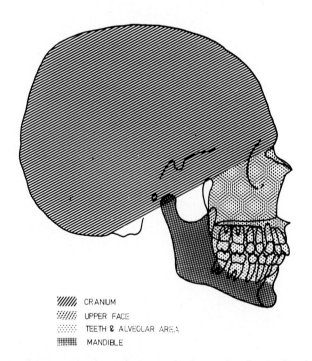

Fig. 6-1. Craniofacial articulation—occlusal, periodontal, sutural, and condylar joints. With functional appliances it is possible to perform therapeutic measures in all these areas.

CRANIUM
UPPER FACE
TEETH & ALVEOLAR AREA
MANDIBLE

150

is potentially damaging to the temporomandibular joint. It causes jiggling of the teeth as the mandible drops back during actual excursive function associated with mastication. Yet, in other cases a "jumping of the bite" can be successfully achieved. These, however, are functional retrusion problems with a forced retropositioning of the condyle in the fossa as a result of dominant retrusive activity of the posterior temporalis, deep masseter, and hyoid musculature associated with vertical overclosure or deep bite. Similar mandibular repositioning can also be observed sometimes after elimination of traumatic occlusion, cross-bite conditions, etc.; but this is not functional jaw orthopedics in the strictest sense, for functional jaw orthopedics is concerned with permanently altering the position of the mandible by influencing and redirecting the growth processes. One of the pitfalls of activator therapy, accounting for dual bite, has been improper diagnosis and case selection, attempting to "jump" the bite in the wrong type of malocclusion.

A second postulate of Kingsley, associated with his original concepts, has often been overlooked in recent functional orthopedic therapy. The jumping of the bite should be performed without proclination of the lower incisors. This requisite of Kingsley highlights a dichotomy that too often exists. The axiom requires no labial tipping of lower incisors, although the literature is replete with admonitions that activators can indeed protrude these teeth. This clinical fact too often means a failure of activator therapy since the overjet is reduced by proclination of teeth instead of bodily anterior positioning of the mandible itself.

Impressed by the Kingsley concepts and appliances, Andresen developed a loose-fitting appliance modification. Being mobile, it transferred functioning muscle stimuli to the jaws, teeth, and supporting tissues. Actually the progenitor of the appliance was a modified Kingsley plate, which Andresen used as a retainer over summer vacation for his daughter when he removed fixed appliances that had been used to correct a distoclusion. Seeing the continued improvement with this "retainer," he called it a biomechanical working retainer. He used it following the removal of fixed appliances, not only to stabilize the result achieved but also as a biomechanically functioning appliance, particularly over the summer holidays, when patients were gone for long periods.

Some years before Andresen started experimenting with his working retainer, Pierre Robin had created an appliance that was quite similar in objectives. The "monobloc," as he called it (since it was a single block of vulcanite), was used to position the mandible forward in patients with glossoptosis and severe mandibular retrognathism. These patients were in danger of occluding their airway with the tongue mass. Forward mandibular posture reduced this hazard, and he noted significant improvement in the jaw relationship also. Actually the problem, usually associated with cleft palate, became known as the Pierre Robin syndrome. Despite the similarity of the two appliances, Andresen's inspiration came from Kingsley and he did not even know of the Robin appliance. These developments were independent of each other.

When Andresen moved from Denmark to Norway, he became associated with Karl Häupl at the University of Oslo. Häupl, a periodontist and histologist, was impressed with results obtained by Andresen's functioning retainer. His special concern was its effect on the underlying tissues. He became convinced that the appliance induced growth changes in a physiologic manner and stimulated or transformed the natural forces with an intermittent functional action transmitted to the jaw, teeth, and investing tissues. Familiar with the work of Roux, who subscribed to the shaking-the-bonding-substance-of-bone hypothesis, Häupl felt that this was indeed a clinical validation of the concept. By the time Andresen

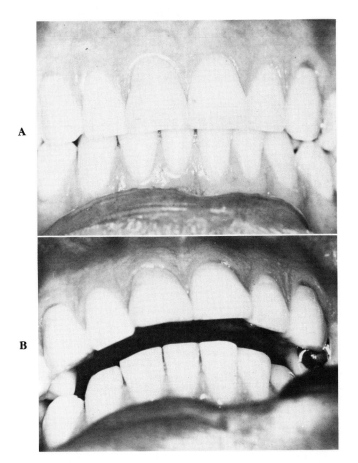

Fig. 6-2. Dual bite—can be a late consequence of activator treatment with a false indication. **A,** Habitual occlusion. **B,** Centric relation.

and Häupl teamed up to write about their appliance and interpretations of its action, the name *activator* was used, because of its ability to activate the muscle forces.

Some ideas of Häupl have already been discussed in the previous chapter. One point not mentioned is the importance of understanding the influence of the activator on the growth process and its limitations. As to whether the activator promotes mandibular growth, the answer is qualified by the term "individual optimum." It is not possible to create a large mandible from a small one with an activator, but the optimum size consistent with morphogenetic pattern can be achieved for that individual patient. Häupl considered this the goal of activator treatment. Even today, to calculate this individual optimum for each case is undeniably a difficult task. Yet the philosophy of treatment was to stimulate condylar changes by relocating the mandible anteriorly and thus reach the desired occlusion. Growth prediction, growth direction, and growth timing were all vague concepts as far as clinical orthodontics was concerned at the time. It is a tribute to these pioneers that so many patients did actually benefit from the activator. Nevertheless, it should be remembered that the task of the appliance was to influence the sagittal posture of the mandible and the reciprocal effect of the appliance on the maxillary growth was essentially ignored.

The original appliance was really an upper and a lower plate joined together at the occlusal plane. Only one wire element was used—a labial arch for the upper anterior teeth (Fig. 6-3). To achieve expansion, the appliance was split in the center and a flexible Coffin spring was incorporated (Fig. 6-4) For more sophisticated use of the appliance, various springs were added later on. Even jackscrews, an ancient and venerable appliance adjunct, were used, not primarily for expansion but for adjustment.

Andresen and Häupl, in cooperation with Petrik, pro-

duced the fifth edition of their book on functional jaw orthopedics in 1953. Many additional wire elements were described (Fig. 6-5). Eschler (1952) had developed some modifications of the labial bow, with intermaxillary effectiveness. One part was active, moving the teeth; the other was passive, holding the soft tissue of the lower lip away and thus enhancing the tooth movement desired. The principle of the bow action was a progenitor for later developments, serving to eliminate undesirable soft tissue pressure on the one hand while delivering force to precise tooth targets on the other (Fig. 6-6).

All the original appliances had a basic vulcanite or acrylic fabrication consisting of joined maxillary and mandibular components. Since the appliances were

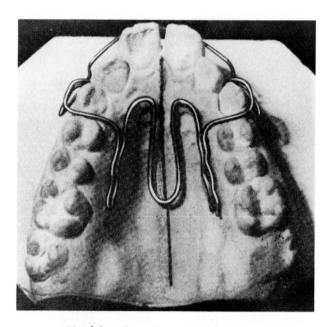

Fig. 6-4. Coffin springs used for expansion.

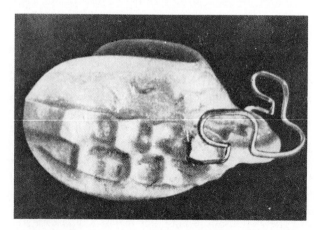

Fig. 6-3. Original activator according to Andresen and Häupl.

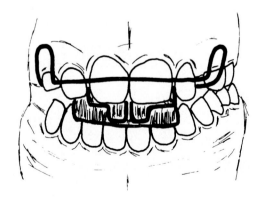

Fig. 6-5. Additional elements for moving the incisors used by Petrik.

worn only at night, their bulkiness was not so critical. However, subsequent modifications have been made to reduce the unwieldiness and bulk, allowing an increase in wearing time. Two types of modification can be differentiated:

1. Appliances consisting of one rigid acrylic mass for maxillary and mandibular arches but with reduced volume or bulk

   a. Some of these appliances are reduced in the anterior palatal region and are called open activators. The idea is also to restore exteroceptive contact between the tongue and palate, which is prevented by the classical activator (Fig. 6-7). Patients prefer these appliances since they are reduced in the linguoincisal area and do not obstruct the oral cavity. However, the open activator also has some disadvantages. The construction bite cannot be opened too much vertically, because tongue function is not under control. If too high a vertical registration is made, the tongue may thrust into the anterior interincisal gap, creating a postural and functional abnormality (Fig. 6-8). A further disadvantage of the elastic open activator, introduced by Klammt in 1955, is the lack of support in the cutaway area of the appliance, especially where guidance of erupting teeth or expansion is necessary.

   b. These are appliances with reduction in the alveolar region and with a cross-palatal wire instead of a full acrylic plate. They are supported (or anchored) dentally. Because of the tooth-borne anchorage, the indication for them (as introduced by Balters) is limited and the management difficult. Again, the labial bow serves to eliminate abnormal muscle pressure by extending into the buccal vestibular area, opposite the canine and premolar regions (Fig. 6-9).

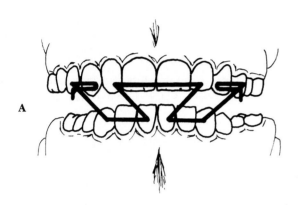
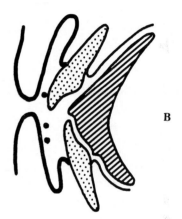

Fig. 6-6. Combined labial bow according to Eschler. **A,** The upper part touches the teeth. **B,** The lower part holds the lower lip away from the lower incisors.

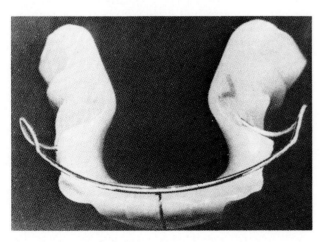

Fig. 6-7. Open activator. The palatat acrylic is cut away.

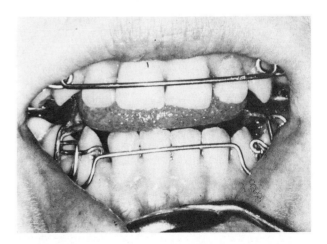

Fig. 6-8. Tongue thrust habit that arose during the wearing of an open activator with a high construction bite.

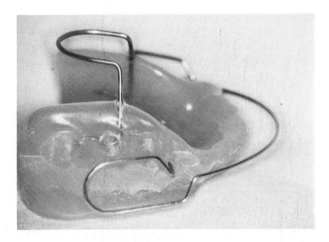

Fig. 6-9. Balters' appliance—the Bionator.

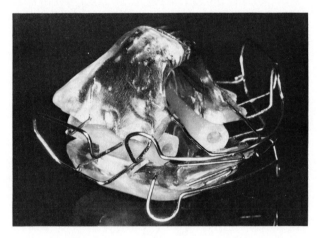

Fig. 6-10. Elastic activator—the Kinetor according to Stockfish.

2. Appliances consisting of two parts (upper and lower) joined with wire bows
   a. The muscle impulses are reinforced by wire elements incorporated in the design. The flexibility or elasticity of the appliance permits mandibular movements in all directions (Fig. 6-10). The Schwarz double plate is one of the earlier modifications of this type.

There is a significant difference in mode of action between the rigid one-piece appliance and the flexible two-piece joined by intermaxillary wiring. The rigid activator does not permit muscle shortening, and therefore contractions that arise are isometric in nature. Isometric contractions develop higher tension than do isotonic ones. A longlasting tonic stretch reflex contraction can be observed when elicited by the proper appliance construction. The elastic construction does permit muscle shortening, and there is thus less force magnitude. The momentary stretch in these flexible construc-

tions gives rise to a transient phase reflex contraction.

The elastic activators are not bulky, and the movements of the mandible are not impeded. As noted earlier, the wearing time can be increased with relative patient comfort. However, the effectiveness of the appliance is decreased because of the lesser-magnitude isotonic contractions elicited. The increase in efficiency is gained by the longer wearing time. This means that the rigid activator is at least as effective as the elastic counterpart but it takes a shorter time. A further limitation of the flexible activator is that it is possible to take the construction bite only in an edge-to-edge relationship.

Further recent modifications have been designed in consideration of the morphogenetic pattern and growth direction prediction. Variations in the horizontal and vertical components of the construction bite can be made, depending on the goal of treatment, with different kinds of force activation.

EFFICACY OF THE ACTIVATOR

According to the concepts of Andresen and Häupl, the activator is effective in exploiting the interrelationship between function and changes in internal bone structure. During the growth period there is also an interrelationship between function and external bone form. The activator induces musculoskeletal adaptation by introducing a new pattern of mandibular closure. The neuromuscular adapatation to the increased distance and the change in direction is the basic requirement for reeducating the orofacial musculature.

The adaptational process in the functional pattern caused by the activator also includes and affects the condyles. The condylar adaptation to the anterior positioning of the mandible consists of growth in an upward and backward direction to maintain the integrity of the temporomandibular joint structures. This adaptational process is induced by a loose appliance. The mandible is not opened beyond postural rest position by the construction bite (i.e., generally no more than 4 mm). Myotatic reflex activity is stimulated, causing isometric muscle contractions. It is this muscle force being transmitted by the appliance that moves the teeth. Thus the appliance works by using kinetic energy.

Although the original concept and working hypothesis by Andresen and Häupl have been discussed and utilized for 45 years, it is still open to debate—being partially or totally accepted by some authorities while rejected by others.

One explanation for the continuing controversy is given by Rolf Grude (1952). He suggested that the mode of action of the activators, according to the Andresen-Häupl concepts, can be observed only if the mandible is not displaced beyond postural rest position. If the mandible is prevented by the construction of the appliance from assuming this required position, the resultant mode of action is completely different. If the mandible is opened beyond the 4 mm limit, the appliance does not work in the manner suggested by Andresen and Häupl but by stretching the soft tissues or by the visco-elastic properties of the muscles.

This statement by Grude can be accepted only with reservation:

1. An opening of 4 mm from the occlusal position does not induce the same muscle activation in every patient. There is a wide range of dimensions for the interocclusal clearance. The distance varies not only from individual to individual but within the same individual from time to time.

2. The postural rest position is assessed when the patient is in an upright standing or sitting position. The suspension of the mandible by the motivating musculature is dependent on head and body posture, the degree of wakefulness or sleep, the intraoral vacuum, etc. Alteration of the head posture causes a different gravity vector, resulting in a new relationship of parts and a new postural rest vertical dimension. Examination of patients wearing the activator while asleep has shown that these alterations are not decisive but a clearance of some millimeters must be considered. There is a different reaction and a different force system is maintained by opening the mandible slightly or extensively. Between these two extremes are various transitional positions.

Classification of views. In studying the literature, we can classify the writings of various authors into three groups, according to their different views:

1. Some authors (Petrovic, McNamara) substantiate the Andresen-Häupl concept that the myotatic reflex activity which arises and the isometric contractions induce the musculoskeletal adaptation by introducing a new mandibular closing pattern. Grude had suggested that such adaptation was possible only with a small bite opening. In his experiments on skeletal adaptation, McNamara observed a progressive disappearance of the modified neuromuscular pattern. The stimuli from the activator and muscle receptors, as well as the periodontal mechanoreceptors, promote displacement of the mandible. The superior heads of the lateral pterygoid muscles have the most important role in this adaptation, because they assist in the skeletal adaptations. Petrovic came to similar conclusions based on his very important and extensive study of the condylar cartilage. The fundamental requirement for condylar growth stimulation is the ability to activate the lateral pterygoids. An appliance holding the mandible rigidly in an anteriorly displaced position does not activate these muscles and so does not stimulate condylar growth. (See Petrovic research, Chapter 2.)

Based on their research, Petrovic and McNamara support the view that variations in the mode and direction of dislocation of the mandible are decisive factors in activator therapy.

2. A second group of authors (Selmer-Olsen, Herren, Harvold and Woodside) does not accept the theory of myotatic reflex activity with isometric muscle contractions as being the inducing basis of skeletal adaptation. According to their views, the viscoelastic properties of muscle and the stretching of the soft tissues are decisive for activator action. During each force application, secondary forces arise in the tissues, introducing a bioelastic process. Thus not only the muscle contractions but also the viscoelastic properties of the soft tissues are important in stimulating the skeletal adaptation. Depending on the magnitude and duration of the applied force, the viscoelastic reaction can be divided into the following stages:

Emptying of vessels
Pressing out of interstitial fluid
Stretching of fibers
Elastic deformation of bone
Bioplastic adaptation

The proponents of this explanation of activator action recognize only a modest skeletal adaptation in the vertical plane and no alteration in the sagittal.

Selmer-Olsen (1937) was the first author to disagree with the Andresen-Häupl explanation. He suggested that the mandible normally assumes a position of equilibrium, determined by the forces acting from intraoral and perioral tissues. An opening beyond this equilibrium position requires active work from the opening muscles to overcome the resistance of the stretched fibers of the soft tissues. Thus the forces responsible for moving the teeth in activator therapy are not due to muscle function, per se, but to the stretching of the soft tissues.

Recent support for Selmer-Olsen comes from other authors like Herren and Harvold and Woodside. For them the primary requirement for eliciting a stretch of the soft tissues is the dislocation of the mandible anteriorly or opening beyond the postural rest vertical dimension. Herren overextends in the sagittal plane, moving the mandible anteriorly into an incisal cross-bite relationship. Harvold and Woodside open the mandible with the construction bite as much as 10 to 15 mm beyond the postural rest vertical dimension. The muscle tension, rising as a consequence of the stretching of the tissues, varies with the degree of mandibular displacement. The overextended activator, stretching the soft tissues like a splint, induces no myotatic reflex activity but instead applies a rigid stretch and buildup of potential energy.

The rationale behind the Harvold-Woodside theory is that the mandible normally drops open when the patient is asleep. If it is opened only 3 or 4 mm by the appliance, one of two things may happen: either the appliance may fall out or it may be ineffective because the wider open sleep position does not permit it to advance the mandible and thus does not call on the dental and possible skeletal adaptation. Harvold and Woodside question how much actual muscle contraction there can be when the patient is asleep. They can be relatively sure that the appliance will stay in, with the wide open construction bite, and can thus assess the actual force likely to be directed at the teeth and jaws.

3. Between the two extremes, exemplified by Andresen and Häupl versus Selmer-Olsen, there are a number of authors who take a higher construction bite without the extreme extension advocated by Harvold. Using an opening of 4 to 6 mm, these authors feel that the ultimate decision as to whether the force delivered is kinetic energy (isometric muscle contractions) or potential energy (viscoelastic properties), or a combination of both, depends on the nature of the malocclusion, the interocclusal clearance, the head posture, the state of mind, the level of wakefulness or sleep, etc.

Schmuth, Witt, and Witt and Komposch write of their experiences using activator construction bites that displace the mandible 4 to 6 mm below the intercuspal position. They have observed long periods of continuous pressure from the mandibular teeth against the activator. Thus the teeth are subjected to forces that act almost continuously. For this reason a vertical opening of more than 4 mm beyond the habitual occlusion is not considered to be functional jaw orthopedics in the traditional sense.

Eschler defined the techniques that open the vertical dimension beyond 4 mm in the construction bite as the "muscle-stretching method," working alternately with isotonic and isometric muscle contractions. He described the cycle: At insertion of the appliance the mandible is elevated by isotonic muscle contractions. When the mandible assumes a static position in contact with the appliance, isometric contractions arise. Since the mandible cannot reach the postural rest position, the elevators remain stretched. When fatigue occurs, the contracting muscles relax and the mandible drops. As soon as the muscles have recovered, the cycle begins again.

Ahlgren's electromyographic research shows that the activator functions as an interference, producing new contraction patterns in the jaw muscles. The innervation pattern can be adjusted after a while and the mandible repositioned forward.

Synopsis. The various concepts can be summarized as follows: depending on the construction of the appliance, the activator can initiate the myotatic reflex activity, induce isometric muscle contractions (sometimes also inducing isotonic contractions), or have its effectiveness based on the viscoelastic properties of the stretched soft tissues. According to the mode of action, there are two main principles. A third approach combines the two rationales.

1. According to the original Andresen-Häupl concept the forces generated in activator therapy are due to muscle contractions and myotatic reflex activity. There is stimulation of the muscles by a loose appliance, and the moving appliance moves the teeth. The muscles function with kinetic energy, and intermittent forces are of clinical significance. A successful treatment depends on muscle stimulation, the frequency of movements of the mandible, and the duration of the effective forces. Activators with a low vertical dimension construction bite function this way.

2. According to the second working hypothesis the appliance is squeezed between the jaws in a splinting action. The appliance exerts forces that move the teeth in this rigid position. The stretch reflex is activated, inherent tissue elasticity is operative, and there is strain without functional movement. The appliance works using potential energy. For this mode of action an overcompensation of the construction bite in the sagittal or vertical plane is necessary. An efficient stretch action is achieved by the overcompensation and the viscoelastic properties of the contiguous soft tissues.

3. The third approach enlists the modes of action of the preceding two. It can be called a transitional type of activator action, which alternately uses muscle contraction and viscoelastic properties of soft tissues. The appliances in this group have a greater bite opening than recommended by Andresen and Häupl, but they do not overcompensate as do Harvold and Woodside. The stretch reflex resulting from activators in this group is seen as a longlasting contraction. The intermittent forces induced by the contractions are not as pronounced as in the original construction. Eschler observed the occurrence of both isometric and isotonic contractions when this appliance construction was used.

All the modes of action are dependent on the direction and degree of opening of the construction bite. By taking into account the individual characteristics of the facial skeleton, the individualized growth processes, and the goal of treatment, the clinician can fabricate the appliance to work according to the desired mode of action.

SKELETAL AND DENTOALVEOLAR EFFECT OF THE ACTIVATOR

During craniofacial growth the activator is capable of influencing the third level of articulation, as outlined by Moffett (i.e., the sutures and the temporomandibular joint). The efficiency of its action is determined by the construction bite. It is also effective in the dentoalveolar region, particularly during tooth eruption. The dentoalveolar effect is achieved primarily by the correct trimming of the acrylic contiguous to selected teeth.

1. As might be expected, any *skeletal effect* from the activator is dependent on the growth potential. Two divergent growth vectors propel the jaw bases in an anterior direction.

a. The sphenoccipital synchondrosis moves the cranial base and nasomaxillary complex upward and forward.

b. The condyle translates the mandible in a downward and forward direction (Fig. 6-11). The activator is most effective in controlling the lower vector, or the downward and forward growth of the mandible. This effect can also be designated as an articular one, because of the promotion or redirection of condylar growth. When the mandible is being positioned anteriorly, growth direction is more important than growth increments. Only the upward and backward growth of the condyle is capable of moving the mandible anteriorly.

The possibility of influencing condylar growth with functional orthodontic appliances is conditioned by phylogenetic and ontogenetic peculiarities of the condylar cartilage. In contrast to primary cartilages (epiphyses, sphenoccipital synchondroses) growth is regulated to a high degree by local exogenous factors. According to Moss, Petrovic, and others, condylar growth is an expression of a locally based homeostasis for the establishment and maintenance of a functionally coordinated stomatognathic system. As the research by Petrovic has

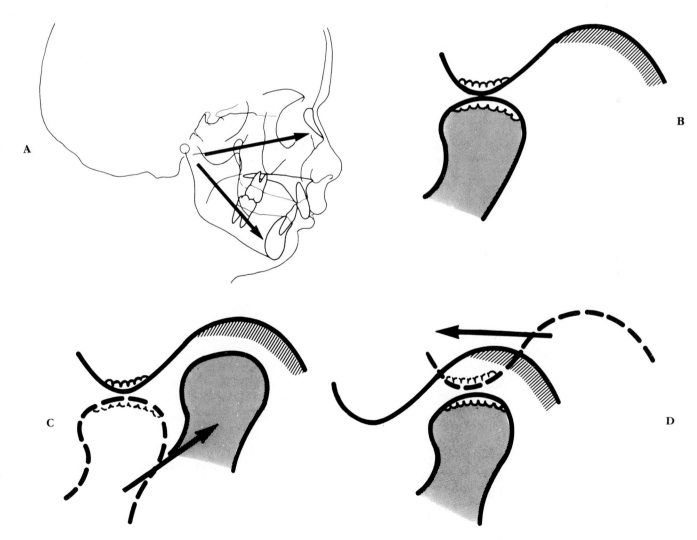

Fig. 6-11. A, Divergent growth vectors that move the jaw bases in a forward direction. **B,** The articular effectiveness of the activator moves the condyles into a forward-downward position. **C,** Adaptation to the new position through condylar growth. **D,** Adaptation to the new position by remodeling in the fossa.

shown, the lateral pterygoid muscle has a decisive role in this growth. Forward posturing of the condyle activates the superior head of the lateral pterygoid. In young individuals this induces a cell proliferation in the condyle and a growth response.

A favorable growth direction is necessary in addition to incremental stimulation, for treatment success. The activator can, to a limited degree, control the upper growth vector, supplied by the sphenoccipital synchondrosis, which moves the maxillary base in a forward direction. If the mandible cannot be positioned anteriorly, then maxillary growth can be inhibited and redirected. The growth and translation of the nasomaxillary complex can be influenced, particularly by activators of a special construction. (See "Construction Bite," facing page.) Of course, maxillary growth can also be affected by extraoral force (Chapter 2).

In addition to sagittal considerations, the vertical skeletal relationship must be assessed and altered, if need be, by the activator. Rotations of mandibular growth vectors can be compensated by changing the maxillary base inclination. A downward displacement of the maxillary base allows an adaptation of the maxilla to a vertical rotation of the mandible. When the rotation of the jaw bases during growth is unfavorable, activator therapy cannot be completed successfully. (See "Cephalometric analysis," p. 160.) If the activator is constructed with a vertical opening of the bite only (or with minimal sagittal change), the effect is primarily on the midface development in the subnasal area. Both vertical maxillary growth and eruption of the teeth are restricted. Woodside believes that a small vertical opening restricts only the horizontal midface development whereas a wide vertical opening achieves the restriction by downward displacement of the midface area. A decrease in the S-N-A angle can be observed unless the bite opening is extreme. In such cases the maxillary plane is then tipped upward and point A moves forward some.

2. The *dentoalveolar efficiency* of the activator is a primary treatment objective. The space between the two divergent growth vectors is filled in with teeth and bone. The dentoalveolar effect of the activator is to control tooth eruption and alveolar bone apposition. For this reason the activator is most effective when used in the early mixed dentition.

Various tooth movements have been observed during activator therapy, especially in the lower incisor area. Some authors have observed a forward displacement of the lower anterior segment (Björk, Parkhouse) or a bodily displacement of the incisors (Jacobsson). A labial tipping (Richardson) or a lingual tipping (Moss) of the lower incisors has also been observed. These movements are dependent on the design of the appliance and the extension of the acrylic in the lower incisor area. By

proper trimming of the appliance, different movements can be performed and the eruption of the teeth can be guided.

FORCE ANALYSIS IN ACTIVATOR THERAPY

When the muscles are activated by the functional appliance, various types of forces are created—static, dynamic, rhythmic.

1. Static forces are of a permanent type and can vary in magnitude and direction. They do not appear simultaneously with movements of the mandible. In this category are the forces of gravity, posture, and elasticity of soft tissues and muscles.

2. Dynamic forces are of an interrupted nature. They appear simultaneously with movements of the head and body and have a higher magnitude than do static forces. The frequency of these forces also depends on the design and construction of the appliance and the reaction of the patient. Swallowing gives rise to a dynamic force. Some clinicians are prone to see only the active or dynamic force mechanisms of the activator. However, in addition, the static forces must be considered because of their constancy and long duration.

3. The rhythmic forces are associated with respiration and circulation. They are synchronous with breathing, and their amplitude varies with the pulse. These trophic stimuli are considered quite important in activating cellular activity. The rhythmic vibrations of the mandible are transmitted to the maxilla. The applied forces are intermittent and interrupted. Force application to the teeth and mandible is intermittent. The removal of the activator from the mouth constitutes the interruption of these forces.

Activator effectiveness during sleep depends on the frequency of movements, the kind of construction bite, alterations in the interocclusal space and on muscle tone.

According to the original concept of Andresen and Häupl, the only forces operative in activator therapy are the natural ones transformed and transferred by the activator to the jaws and teeth. However, recent modifications with different designs and the incorporation of additional elements (springs, jackscrews, pads) have made it possible for the active forces created to be used along with the endogenous forces of the stomatognathic system. The appliance can also perform its function by interfering with endogenous forces. Hence there are two principles employed in the modern activator.

Force application—the source is usually muscular

Force elimination—the dentition is shielded from normal and abnormal functional and tissue pressures by pads, shields, wire configurations, etc.

The types of force employed in activator therapy may be categorized as follows:

1. The growth potential, including the eruption and migration of teeth, gives rise to natural forces. These can be guided, promoted, or inhibited by the activator.
2. Muscle contractions and stretching of the soft tissues initiate forces when the mandible is relocated from its postural resting position by the appliance. The contractions are stimulated and transformed by the activator. Whereas the forces may be functional (muscular) in origin, their activation is artificial. These artificial functioning forces can be effective in all three planes of space.
   a. In the sagittal plane the mandible is propelled forward, with the result that muscle force is delivered to the condyle and a strain is produced in the condylar region. A slight reciprocal force can be transmitted to the maxilla during this maneuver.
   b. In the vertical plane the teeth and alveolar processes are either loaded with or relieved of normal forces. If the construction bite is high, a greater strain is produced in the contiguous tissues. If transmitted to the maxilla, these forces can have an inhibitory effect on growth increments and direction and can influence the inclination of the maxillary base.
   c. In the transverse plane it is possible also to create forces with midline corrections.
3. Various active elements (e.g., springs and screws) can be built into the activator and confer an active biomechanical type of force application.

The mode of force application, magnitude, and direction are dependent on the three-dimensional dislocation of the mandible, which is determined by the construction bite.

CONSTRUCTION BITE

One important aspect of proper activator fabrication is the determination and reproduction of the correct "construction" or "working" bite. The purpose of this mandibular manipulation is to relocate the jaw in the direction of the treatment objectives. This creates artificial functional forces, and thus the mode of action of the appliance can be assessed. Before the construction bite is taken, a careful preparation must be made with a detailed study of the plaster casts, cephalometric and panoral head films, and the patient's functional pattern.

Diagnostic preparation

Patient compliance is essential. Hence it is important not only to assess clinically the somatic and psychologic aspects of the patient but also to determine the patient's motivation potential. This may be enhanced in Class II malocclusions by creating an "instant correction"—mov-

ing the mandible forward into an anterior, more normal sagittal, relationship. The patient sees the potential and objectives of the correction to be brought about by the functional appliance and is more likely to work toward this goal than to just realize the dental health and functional improvement (Fig. 6-12). As Fränkel points out, this clinical maneuver at the beginning of treatment also tells the clinician whether the therapeutic goal is really an improvement. In some problems of maxillary protrusion and excessive vertical dimension and reduced symphyseal prominence, a forward positioning will not make the profile look better. Then other therapeutic measures may be required.

Study model analysis. Preparatory to constructing the activator, the most important information to be derived from the cast analysis is gleaned from the following:

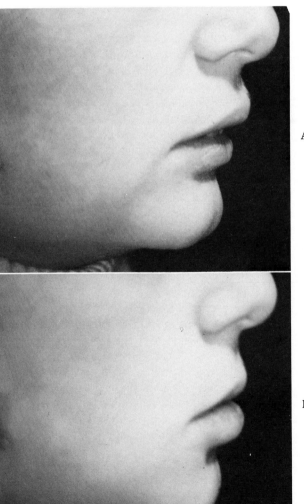

Fig. 6-12. A, Occlusal position. **B,** Construction bite position.

1. First permanent molar relationship in habitual occlusion
2. Nature of the midline discrepancy, if any; if the midlines are not coincident, a functional analysis should be made to determine the path of closure from postural rest to occlusion; if the midlines change, there is a likely functional problem (amenable to correction in the appliance); dentoalveolar noncoincident midlines cannot be corrected by functional appliances
3. Symmetry of the dental arches; any asymmetries should be evaluated, since some of them (e.g., segmental open bite) may be corrected by the activator.
4. Curve of Spee; this should be checked to see whether it can or should be leveled by the activator; if severe and with the premolars already erupted, the leveling needed is beyond the capabilities of the activator.
5. Crowding and any dental discrepancies; these are measured because, in conjunction with the cephalometric analysis, they help determine the requirements and possibilities of lower incisor movement.

Functional analysis. Before the construction bite is taken, a functional analysis is performed to obtain the following information:

1. Precise registration of the postural rest position (since the vertical opening of the construction bite depends on this)
2. Path of closure from postural rest to habitual occlusion (any sagittal or transverse deviations are recorded)
3. Prematurities, point of initial contact, occlusal interferences, and resultant mandibular displacement, if any (some of these can be eliminated with the activator, but some will require other therapeutic measures)
4. Clicking, crepitus, etc. in the TMJ (might be indicative of a functional abnormality or the need for some modification of appliance design)
5. Interocclusal clearance or freeway space (checked several times and the mean amount recorded)
6. Respiration; with allergies or disturbed nasal respiration, the patient cannot wear a bulky appliance; in such cases an open activator may be used or the respiratory abnormalities may be eliminated first.

Particular attention must be paid to epipharyngeal lymphoid tissue. The size of tonsils or adenoids should be recorded, even if nasal breathing does not seem to be affected. If the tonsils are enlarged and the tongue has assumed a compensatory anterior position to maintain an open airway, the patient will not be able to tolerate the appliance. A consultation with an otolaryngologist may be needed first, and possible removal of

diseased or excessive epipharyngeal tissue should be considered in such cases.

Cephalometric analysis. This essential diagnostic requisite enables us to establish the nature of the craniofacial morphogenetic pattern to be treated. The most important information required for planning the construction bite is the following:

1. Direction of growth—average, horizontal, or vertical (implication is that growth rotation follows a logarithmic spiral)
2. Differentiation between position and size of the jaw bases (relation to cranium, sagittal apical base relationship, etc.)
3. Morphologic peculiarities, particularly of the mandible (may assist in determining the timetable for development; in many patients in the mixed dentition, characteristics and symptoms aid in forecasting whether the growth pattern will be more horizontal or vertical in subsequent years)
4. Axial inclination and position of the maxillary and mandibular incisors (provides important diagnostic and prognostic clues for determining the anterior positioning of the mandible required and the details of the appliance design for the incisor area)

Treatment planning

The next step after accumulating and analyzing the diagnostic information is to plan for the construction bite. The extent of anterior positioning for Class II malocclusions and posterior positioning for Class III malocclusions should be determined.

Anterior positioning of the mandible. The usual intermaxillary relationship for the average Class II problem is end-to-end incisal. However, it should not exceed 7 to 8 mm or three quarters of the mesiodistal dimension of the first permanent molar (Fig. 6-13). Anterior

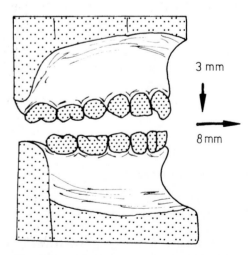

Fig. 6-13. Construction bite in edge-to-edge relationship with slight opening.

positioning of this magnitude is contraindicated when any of the following pertain:

1. The overjet is too large. In extreme cases it can approach 18 mm. Then the anterior positioning becomes a stepwise progression, accomplished in two or three phases (Fig. 6-14).
2. Labial tipping of the maxillary incisors is severe. These should probably be uprighted first, if possible, by a prefunctional appliance.
3. An incisor (usually a lateral) has erupted markedly to the lingual. Then the mandible must be postured anteriorly to an edge-to-edge relationship with the lingually malposed tooth; otherwise it will not be possible to move this tooth labially. Eschler termed the condition a "pathologic" construction bite. As with severely proclined upper incisors, it is usually advisable now to institute a short prefunctional appliance alignment of lingually malposed teeth before starting activator treatment, thereby eliminating the need for the "pathologic" construction bite.

Opening the bite. The vertical considerations are as important as the sagittal determination and are intimately linked to it. There are some guiding principles in maintaining a proper horizontal-vertical relationship and determining the height of the bite.

1. The mandible must be dislocated from the postural resting position in at least one direction—sagittally or vertically. This is essential to activate the associated musculature and induce a strain in the tissues.

2. If the magnitude of the forward position is great (7 or 8 mm), then the vertical opening should be minimal so as not to overstretch the muscles (Fig. 6-15). This type of construction bite means an increased force component in the sagittal plane, enabling a forward positioning of the mandible to be achieved. According to Witt, the approximate sagittal force that develops is in the 315 to 395 g range whereas the magnitude of the

vertical force approximates 70 to 175 g. The primary neuromuscular activation is in the elevator muscles of the mandible.

3. If extensive vertical opening is needed, the mandible must not be anteriorly positioned. If the bite opening is more than 6 mm, mandibular protraction must be very slight (Fig. 6-16). Myotatic reflex activity of the muscles of mastication can then be observed, as can a stretching of the soft tissues. A more extensive bite opening is possible in functionally true deep-bite cases. If the bite registration is high, both the muscles and the viscoelastic properties of the soft tissues are enlisted. The vertical force is increased, while the sagittal force is decreased. This type of construction bite is obviously not effective in achieving anterior positioning of the mandible, but the inclination of the maxillary base can be influenced. One possible indication for such a construction bite is the case with a vertical growth pattern. Then the vertical relationship, either deep bite or open bite, can be therapeutically affected by the activator. The disadvantages of a wide-open construction bite are the

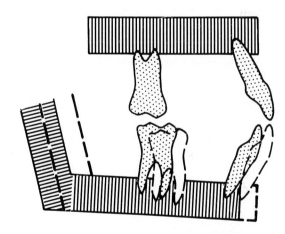

Fig. 6-15. Anterior positioning of the mandible from the rest position.

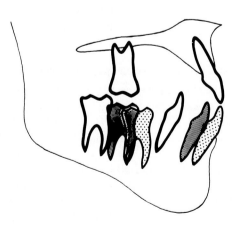

Fig. 6-14. Anterior positioning of the mandible in two phases—first phase, *dark;* second phase, *dotted.*

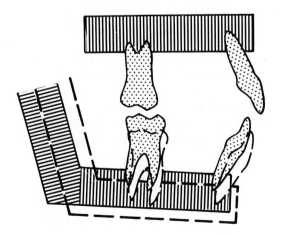

Fig. 6-16. Opening the mandible below the rest position.

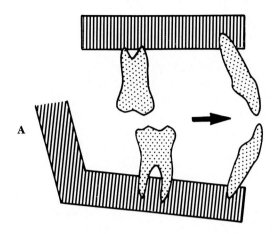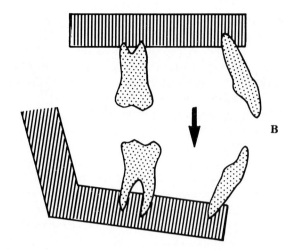

Fig. 6-17. A, Sagittal force component, which arises during anterior positioning of the mandible. **B,** Vertical force component, which arises during opening the mandible.

difficulty in wearing the appliance, with an increased difficulty of adaptation to the new relationship and to the appliance itself. Muscle spasms often occur, and the appliance tends to fall out of the mouth. The high construction bite also makes lip seal difficult if not impossible. Yet the reestablishment of normal lip seal is an important and essential requisite of functional appliance therapy.

General rules for the construction bite. The assessment of the construction bite determines the kind of muscle stimulation, the frequency of mandibular movements, and the duration of effective forces (Fig. 6-17).

1. In a forward positioning of the mandible of 7 to 8 mm, the vertical opening must be slight to moderate (2 to 4 mm).
2. If the forward positioning is no more than 3 to 5 mm, then the vertical opening should be 4 to 6 mm.
3. Lower midline shifts or deviations can be corrected by the activator only if there is actual lateral translation of the mandible itself. If the midline abnormality is due to tooth migration, there is no asymmetric relationship between the mandible and the maxilla. An attempt to correct this type of dental problem could lead to iatrogenic asymmetry. Functional cross-bites in the funtional analysis can be corrected by taking the proper construction bite (Fig. 6-18).

It should be stressed that all preconditions for successful treatment with the activator, even small variations in mandibular position, have a significant alteration potential in activator force application as a consequence.

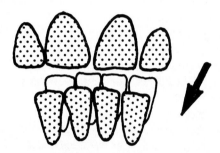

Fig. 6-18. Correction of midline shift with the construction bite.

Both experimental research and clinical experience have shown that an increase in muscle activation with overextended appliances does not increase the efficiency of the activator. According to Sander, the frequency of maximal biting into a 6 mm high construction bite is 12.5% of the sleeping time whereas in an 11 mm high construction bite it is only 1.1%, and if this is increased to 13 mm, as prescribed by Harvold, it is only 0.8%.

Execution of the construction bite technique

1. A horseshoe-shaped wax bite rim is prepared for insertion between the maxillary and mandibular teeth. It should have proper arch form and size, be wide enough, and be 2 to 3 mm thicker than the planned construction bite. It can be made for either the upper or the lower arch occlusal surfaces. If the rim is first placed on the lower arch, however, the mandible can be guided into the desired anterior position required for treatment of the specific Class II malocclusion (Fig. 6-19).

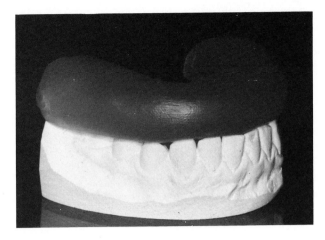

Fig. 6-19. Wax rim on the cast.

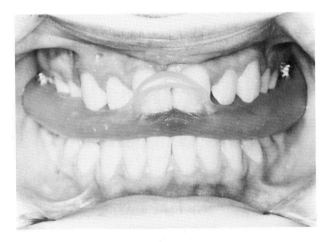

Fig. 6-20. Wax rim in the mouth. When the bite is being taken, midline shift should be controlled.

placed in the mouth as described for Step 1. The wax should not be too soft. During the closing movement the operator controls the edge-to-edge incisal relationship and the midline registration (Fig. 6-20). The wax should be cut away from the labial of the central incisors so the midlines can be visualized and a correct reproduction of the incisal relationship established.

4. In the final step the wax is carefully removed from the mouth without distorting and is checked on the upper and lower models. After it has been fitted on the casts, the margins are trimmed with a scissors so the operator can be sure that the wax is close to all the cusps of the teeth. Then the hardened wax bite is chilled and checked once again in the mouth.

It is to be emphasized that the construction bite should be taken only after careful planning and must always be taken on the patient, not on the articulated models. A construction bite prepared on casts has the following disadvantages:

- It does not fit.
- There is asymmetric biting on it.
- The patient is not really comfortable, and there are more frequent disturbances during sleep.
- The likelihood of unwanted lower incisor procumbency is greater, since the appliance exerts undue stress on these teeth.

Technique for a low construction bite with markedly forward mandibular positioning

The mandible is positioned anteriorly to achieve an edge-to-edge relationship, parallel to the functional occlusal plane. In Class II functional retrusion cases, which show posterior displacement from postural rest to habitual occlusion, the mandible can be positioned anteriorly to a greater degree than in true Class II malocclusions, with a normal path of closure. A rule-of-thumb limitation is that the construction bite should always be at least 3 mm posterior to the most protrusive positioning possible. The mandible should remain within the limits of the interocclusal clearance and should not exceed its postural resting position for the vertical registration.

When the mandible moves mesially to engage the appliance, the elevator muscles of mastication are activated. When the teeth engage the appliance, the myotatic reflex is activated. In addition to the muscle force arising during biting and swallowing, the reflex stimulation of the muscle spindles also elicits reflex muscle activity.

The activator that is constructed with a low vertical opening registration and a forward bite is appropriately designated as the horizontal H activator (Figs. 6-21 and 6-22). With this type of appliance the mandible can be postured forward without tipping the lower incisors la-

If the operator chooses to place the softened wax bite rim on the upper arch, the mandible can be moved easily into a more retruded position required for the construction of a Class III activator.

2. Before taking the wax bite registration, the operator has the patient sit upright. This should be a relaxed posture, not a strained one. Then the mandible is gently guided into the predetermined position. The operator guides but does not force the jaw to the desired sagittal relationship. This exercise is repeated three to four times, with the patient's chin being manipulated between thumb and forefinger. The patient is asked to repeat the exercise on his own and then to hold the forward position for a short-time to set up an exteroceptive engram that can be replicated when the wax is placed between the teeth.

3. When the operator is relatively sure that the patient can replicate the exercise, the softened wax bite rim is

bially. The maxillary incisors can be uprighted, and the anterior growth vector of the maxilla is slightly inhibited. There is no effect on the inclination of the maxillary base, however. As might be expected, this type of appliance is most effective when an anterior sagittal relationship of the mandible is the primary treatment objective. It is indicated in Class II, Division 1, malocclusions with sufficient overjet.

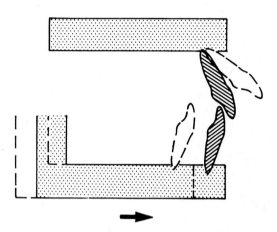

Fig. 6-21. Effectiveness of the H activator—anterior positioning of the mandible, lingual tipping of the upper incisors. Only a modest influence on the maxillary base in the sagittal plane can be achieved.

Class II caused by mandibular overclosure that results in a functional retrusion. In such cases the activator can, in effect, "jump the bite." An example is shown in Fig. 6-23. The patient, a 10-year-old girl, was treated with a horizontal activator. The mandible was anteriorly positioned in postural rest but slid into a posteriorly guided functional retrusion position in habitual occlusion. With a large anterior positioning for the construction bite, the retrognathism was reduced and the upper incisors were tipped lingually into a more normal position. The lip trap was eliminated. A second activator was then constructed to elicit the maximum dentoalveolar effectiveness of the appliance. By judicious grinding, the occlusion was guided into a more favorable relationship. The active phase of orthodontic therapy was completed in 2 years (Fig. 6-24).

Additional indication for the horizontal H activator. Class II, Division 1, malocclusions with posterior positioning of the mandible caused by a growth deficiency but with the likelihood of a future horizontal growth pattern are suitable candidates for treatment with the H activator. In these cases it is advantageous to plan for lingual tipping of the maxillary incisors and pretreatment labial tipping of the lower incisors. Treatment is more difficult in patients with labially inclined lower incisors, but it is possible to posture the mandible

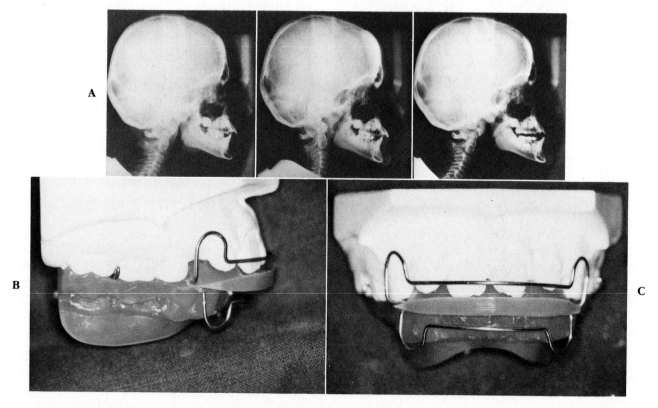

Fig. 6-22. A, Anterior positioning of the mandible in construction of the H activator. *Left,* occlusion; *middle,* rest; *right,* construction bite. **B** and **C,** H activator, lateral and frontal views.

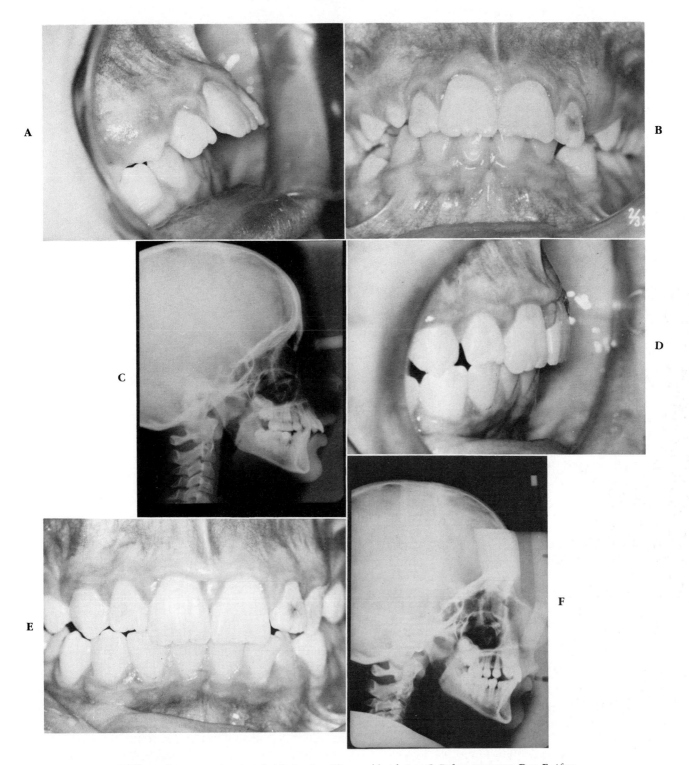

Fig. 6-23. Class II, Division 1, malocclusion in a 10-year-old girl. **A** to **C,** Before treatment. **D** to **F,** After "jumping the bite." Note the lingual tipping of the upper incisors.

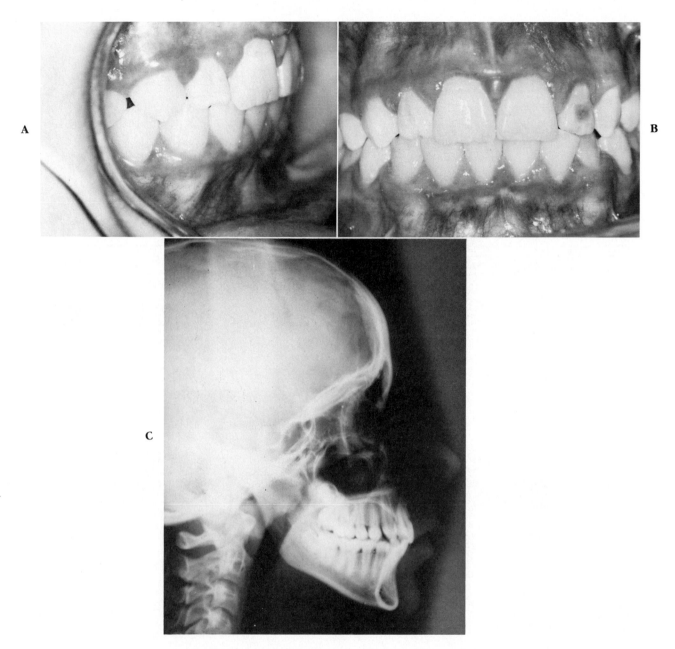

Fig. 6-24. Same patient as in Fig. 6-23 after seating of the occlusion.

forward and simultaneously upright the labially tipped lower incisors. (See also Chapter 7.)

An example of this type of **H** activator use, a 10-year-old girl with an average growth trend and retrognathic skeletal pattern, is shown in Fig. 6-25. There was only a slight skeletal discrepancy, with an A-N-B difference of 3 degrees. The maxillary and mandibular bases were of average length; the ramus was short. The upper and lower incisors were inclined labially, with spacing between the uppers. The overjet was caused by the labial inclination and position (+ 8.5 mm anterior to the nasion-pogonion plane) of the upper incisors. The lower lip was trapped between the upper and lower incisors in the excessive overjet. The lips were potentially incompetent, the swallowing was somatic, and the respiration was nasal. The mandible and symphysis were well developed. An important consideration was the likelihood of a horizontal growth direction shift in subsequent years.

A horizontal type of activator was prescribed. With an

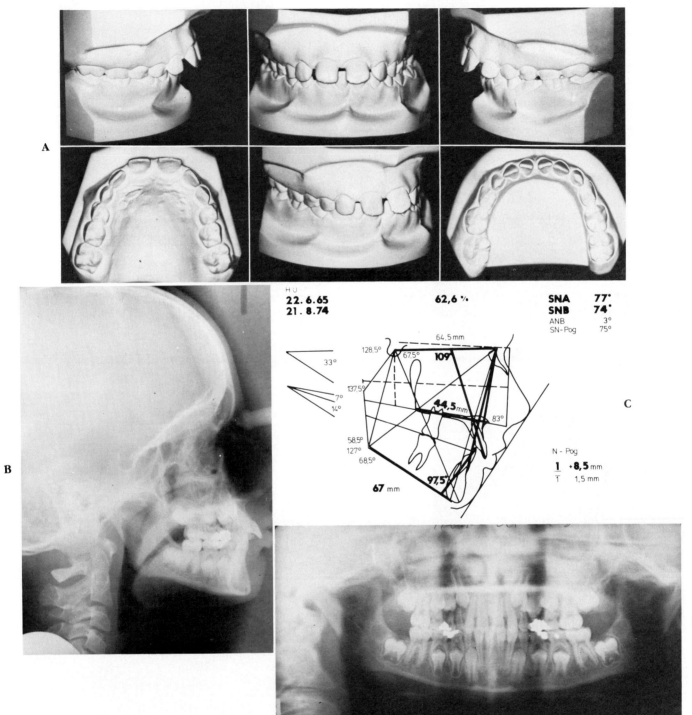

Fig. 6-25. Before treatment, 9-year-old patient. **A,** Casts. **B,** Headplate. **C,** Cephalometric tracing. **D,** Orthopanthomogram.

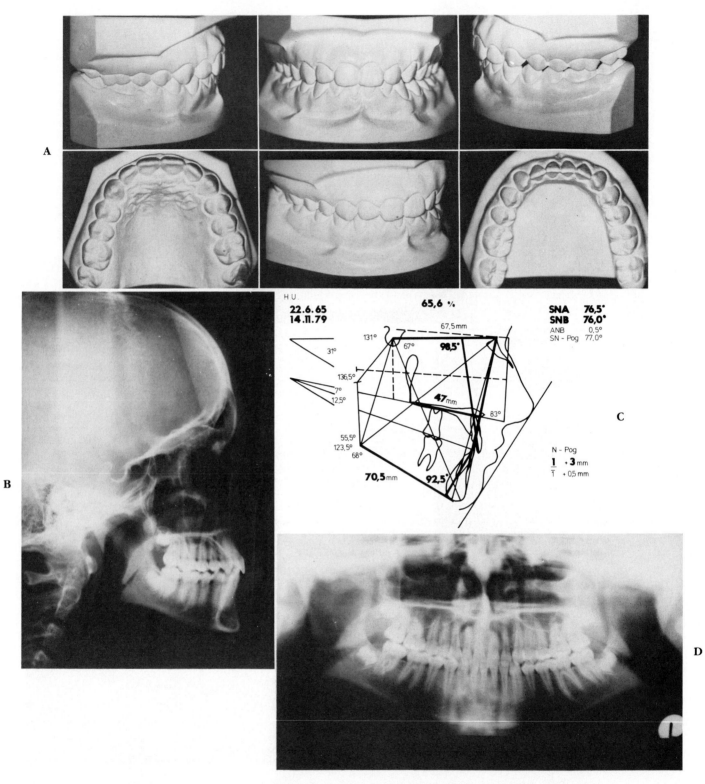

Fig. 6-26. After treatment, same patient as in Fig. 6-25. **A,** Casts. **B,** Headplate. **C,** Tracing. **D,** Orthopanthomogram.

overjet of 6 mm and an overbite of 4.5 mm, the therapeutic objective was a slight anterior positioning of the mandible and uprighting of the upper and lower incisors. The mandible was positioned only 5 mm anteriorly and opened 6 mm vertically with the construction bite, to enable the muscles to exert an uprighting effect and still have enough space for the lower incisal covering by the labial acrylic cap.

Active treatment was 3 years for this patient. The mandible assumed an anterior position with a growth increment of 3.5 mm (0.4 mm less than average). The ramus height growth was 6.0 mm, which was significantly large (3.4 mm above average). The basal relationship of Ar-A and Ar-Pog improved from 12 to 19 mm. Both the upper and the lower incisors were uprighted. Significantly, with a forward rotating growth direction, the growth pattern became more horizontal (Fig. 6-26).

It is important to note that the indication for an anterior posturing of the mandible is not only an originally posterior position but also the likelihood of a favorable growth pattern—direction as well as incremental change. The goal of the functional appliance therapy is to influence the growth of the mandible favorably, achieving optimum growth direction and amounts, and to eliminate any dysfunction or posteriorly retruded habitual occlusion. This type of therapy cannot be done in a vertical growth pattern. Another type of appliance must be constructed.

Technique for a high construction bite with slightly anterior mandibular positioning

In this type of construction bite the mandible is positioned less anteriorly, only 3 to 5 mm ahead of the habitual occlusion position. Depending on the magnitude of the interocclusal space, the vertical dimension is opened 4 to 6 mm, a maximum of 4 mm beyond the postural resting vertical dimension registration. The appliance induces the myotatic reflexes in the muscles of mastication. It is also possible that an additional force is elicited with the stretching of the muscles and soft tissues, causing a response of the viscoelastic properties of the soft tissues involved. This greater opening of the vertical dimension in the construction bite allows the myotatic reflex to remain operative even when the musculature is more relaxed (i.e., while the patient is sleeping). The frequency of maximal biting into the appliance is less than with the **H** type of activator, however. The stretch reflex activation with the increased vertical dimension may well influence the inclination of the maxillary base.

This appliance is indicated in cases with vertical growth patterns and can be properly designated as the vertical **V** activator (Figs. 6-27 and 6-28).

The Class II, Division 1, malocclusion with a vertical growth direction cannot be significantly improved sagittally by anterior positioning of the mandible. The mandible may be postured forward but the danger of a dual bite is great, as the original experiences of Kingsley indicate.

The goal of activator treatment in this case is not just a minimal forward positioning of the mandible because of the vertical growth pattern but an actual adaptation of the maxilla to the lower dental arch. This can be only partially achieved by a retroclination of the maxillary base. This skeletal adaptation must be supported by dentoalveolar compensation, which requires differential guidance of eruption of lower buccal segments, withholding of maxillary buccal segment eruption (as described by Harvold), lingual tipping of the maxillary incisors, and labial tipping of the mandibular incisors. To achieve this, it is necessary to hold the upper incisors with a labially extended acrylic groove. The lower incisors can be supported on the lingual surfaces by acrylic and tipped labially until contact with the upper incisors is attained.

An example of this type of case is shown in Fig. 6-29. The patient is an 8-year-old girl with a Class II, Division 1, malocclusion and a vertical growth pattern. Her posterior/anterior height ratio was 56.4% and the cranial base–mandibular plane angle was 42 degrees. The face was retrognathic, with an A-N-B angle of 8 degrees. The jaws were normally developed but the ramus was extremely short. The upper and lower incisors were tipped labially. Because of the vertical growth pattern and the labial tipping of the lower incisors, the facial pattern was considered unfavorable for conventional activator therapy. On the other hand, some of the functional relationships could benefit from functional orthopedic guid-

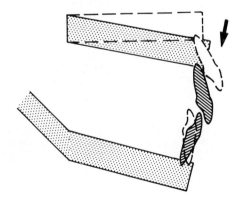

Fig. 6-27. Effectiveness of the vertical activator—changed inclination of the maxillary base, slight anterior positioning of the mandible, dental compensation.

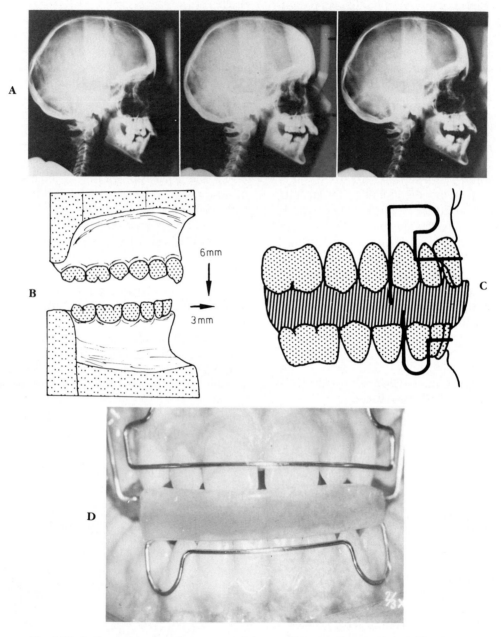

Fig. 6-28. A, Forward-downward positioning of the mandible in construction of the V activator. *Left,* occlusion; *middle,* rest; *right,* construction bite. **B,** Opening and slight anterior positioning of the mandible. **C,** Schematic of the V activator. **D,** In the mouth.

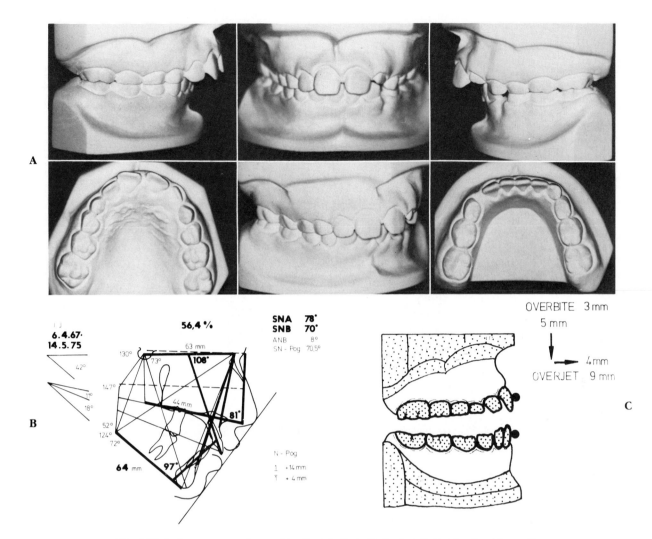

Fig. 6-29. Before treatment, 8-year-old patient. **A,** Casts. **B,** Tracing. **C,** Construction bite position.

ance. The posterior position of the mandible could be slightly improved, if the abnormal retruding force of the musculature were eliminated. The vertical growth pattern could be compensated somewhat by retroclining the maxillary base. The upper incisors could be tipped lingually, to compensate dentally for the Class II characteristics, although a further labial tipping of the lower incisors would be needed to complete this compensation.

The treatment was performed with a vertical activator. The bite was opened for the construction bite 5 mm, but the anterior positioning of the mandible was only 4 mm. The upper incisors were tipped lingually with the labial bow and then supported with the acrylic cap (which extended over the labial). The acrylic was trimmed away on the incisal edges, and on the lingual, to permit maximum upper incisor lingual compensation. The lower incisors were held with the labial bow

and supported lingually with the acrylic. The selective trimming of the activator in the maxillary arch was to stimulate intrusion in the buccal segments while permitting extrusion of the anterior teeth. The successful clinical result after 2 years of therapy is shown in Fig. 6-30.

The posttreatment analysis showed an average growth increment. There was a slight anterior posturing of the mandible and a decrease in the S-N-A angle, with further retroclination of the maxilla—a skeletal compensation for the sagittal malrelationship. There was also a dentoalveolar compensation, achieved by lingual tipping of the upper and slight labial tipping of the lower incisors. Mandibular posterior segment eruption exceeded maxillary counterpart eruption. It is clear from a study of the posttreatment cephalogram that the ideal incisor axial inclination could not have been achieved in vertically growing Class II malocclusions of this type. To do so

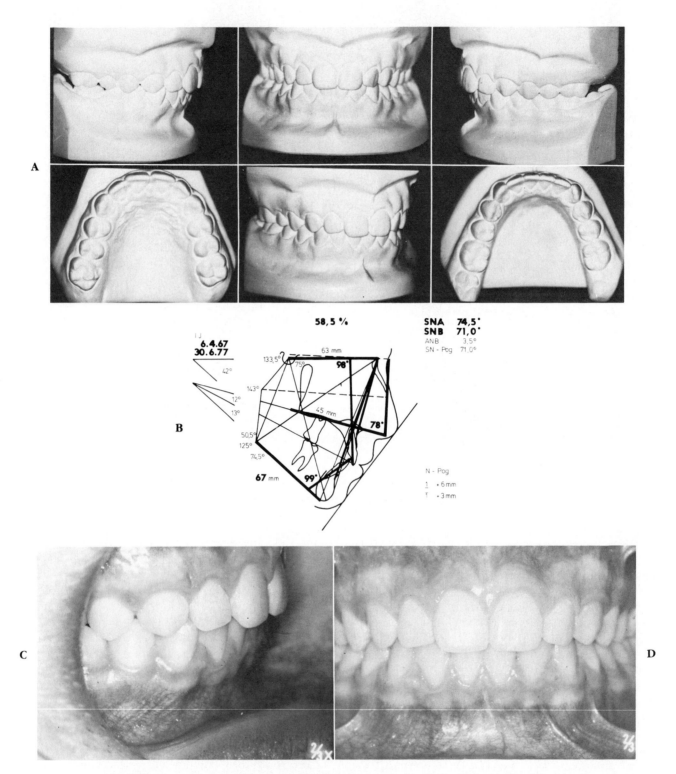

Fig. 6-30. After treatment, same patient as in Fig. 6-29. **A,** Casts. **B,** Tracing. **C** and **D,** Lateral and frontal views.

would have left an excessive overjet and potential lip trap; and with the incisors unsupported by normal function, they would have been relatively more unstable.

Technique for a construction bite without forward mandibular positioning

A forward positioning of the mandible is not indicated in activator construction when there is no need for a sagittal correction. Such appliances are used primarily in vertical dimension problems (deep overbite and open bite) and in selected cases of crowding (Fig. 6-31).

Vertical problems

Deep overbite malocclusions. These can be of either dentoalveolar origin or a skeletal nature.

In *dentoalveolar overbite* problems the deep overbite can be due to infraclusion of the buccal segments or to supraclusion of the anterior segment. Deep overbite cases with infraclusion of molars can be treated by activators designed and trimmed to permit extrusion of these teeth. Problems in this category are usually functionally true overbite cases, with a large clearance. Yet there can be a retrusive sagittal relationship associated with the mandibular overclosure. The construction bite may be either moderate or high depending on the size of the freeway space.

In deep overbite cases caused by supraclusion of the incisors, the interocclusal space is usually small. The activator should not be constructed with a high construction bite in these cases. Intrusion of the incisors is possible to only a limited extent when an activator is being used. Any correction is attained by loading the incisal edges with acrylic cover. Depression is relative, rather than absolute, since the other teeth are free to erupt and to accomplish the predetermined growth pattern. In such cases a successful result requires a significant increment of growth in the vertical direction.

The *skeletal deep overbite* malocclusion usually has a horizontal growth pattern, which can be compensated

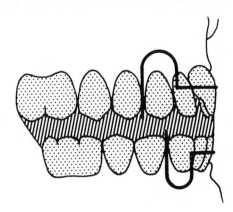

Fig. 6-31. Activator with vertical opening only and no anterior positioning of the mandible.

by forward inclination of the maxillary base. A slight forward inclination is achieved by loading the incisors, as with supraclusion of the incisors. The acrylic cap engages these teeth while freeing the molars to erupt. With this therapeutic approach the construction bite should be high enough to exceed the postural rest vertical dimension of the patient. This enlists stretch reflex response and the viscoelastic properties of the muscles and soft tissues as they are stretched. The opening is beyond the 5 to 6 mm freeway space, in a construction similar to that prescribed by Harvold and Woodside. A dentoalveolar compensation is simultaneously possible by extrusion of the lower molars and distal driving of the upper molars with stabilizing wires.

Open bite malocclusions. An anterior positioning of the mandible is not necessary or desirable if the skeletal relationship is orthognathic. The dentoalveolar open bite can be treated by proper trimming of the acrylic of the appliance. These procedures will be described in the next chapter. The bite is opened 4 to 5 mm to develop a sufficient elastic depressing force and load the molars that are in premature contact. The vertical growth pattern in these cases can be influenced by properly constructed activators that follow this principle. A precondition for successful therapy, however, is a retroclination of the maxillary base with a restriction of the patient's vertical growth pattern. This literally means to "close the V" between upper and lower maxillary bases, depressing the posterior maxillary segments with the activator in a manner analogous to that done by orthognathic surgery. In surgical open bite cases the posterior segments are impacted, allowing autorotation of the mandible. If there is divergent rotation of the bases, the treatment of open bite malocclusions with the activator is not possible.

Arch length deficiency problems. Malocclusions with crowding can sometimes be treated with activators. In the mixed dentition period there can be problems of anchorage with regular expansion plates. In such cases the activator can be used to accomplish the desired expansion since it is anchored intermaxillarily.

The appliance works like two active plates with jackscrews in the upper and lower parts. There is a low construction bite since jaw positioning and growth guidance by selective eruption of teeth are not desired. The treatment objective is expansion, using an appliance stabilized by intermaxillary relationships (Fig. 6-32).

The force application from this type of appliance is reciprocal, an advantage in situations in which the demands are usually bilateral (Fig. 6-33). With the same appliance a reciprocal force can also be developed in the sagittal plane. If the incisors are lingually inclined and the molars must be moved distally to increase arch length, the protrusive force loading the incisors can be directed onto the stabilizing wires that fit in the contact embrasures, producing a molar distalization response.

An example is shown in Fig. 6-34, of an 8-year-old girl with a retrognathic face but a balanced skeletal pattern and an A-N-B angle of only 2 degrees. The length of the mandibular base was slightly deficient, about 3 mm below the average when related to the cranial base. (A de-

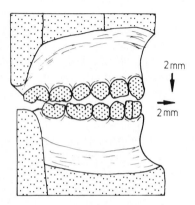

Fig. 6-32. Construction bite with slight forward-downward positioning of the mandible.

ficiency of 3 mm at this age does not yet indicate a significant growth deficiency.) The maxillary base was 41 mm, which was judged quite short, but greater growth increments can be expected in this area. The growth direction was assessed as horizontal. The overbite was not extremely deep, and there was a slight compensation in the vertical relationship stemming from the small forward inclination of the maxillary base. The upper and lower incisors were tipped lingually. A crowding condition existed in both dental arches, with an overall pattern of Class II, Division 2–type, problems, as indicated by the position of the upper inciors and the Class II molar relationship.

A study of the diagnostic records indicated that expansion of the dental arches both transversely and sagittally was therapeutically desirable. Since exfoliation of deciduous teeth in the buccal segments would be a problem in the future, perhaps accelerated by the use of a conventional expansion plate, an activator was recommended. Another reason was the sagittal malrelationship. Since the vertical dimension was essentially normal, only a slight opening of the construction bite was made for the activator.

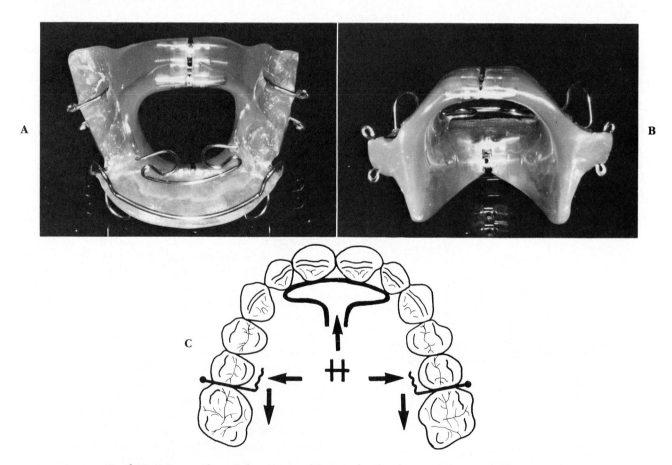

Fig. 6-33. Activator with two jackscrews. **A** and **B,** Frontal and oral views. **C,** Reciprocal effectiveness in the sagittal and transverse planes.

The objective of treatment in this case was not to activate the muscles and contiguous soft tissues, as is the case for most activators, but to provide sufficient long-term anchorage to accomplish the arch width and arch length expansion. Hence the force enlisted was not from the muscles but was provided by two expansion screws in the transverse direction with maxillary lingual protrusion springs and stabilizing wires in the anteroposterior dimension. The labial tipping of the lower incisors was accomplished by allowing the acrylic to contact the lower incisors on the lingual. The upper and lower labial bows did not contact the teeth but did help eliminate labial tissue strain and assisted in labial movement of the anterior teeth by force elimination, in a manner similar to the lip pads used on the Fränkel appliance.

The treatment, which was active until the eruption of the permanent teeth, improved the retrognathic profile. The growth rate for the maxillary base was high. Post-treatment measurements showed normal proportional relations between the maxillary and mandibular bases and the cranial base. There was no alteration in the hor-izontal growth pattern and the inclination of the maxillary base. The axial inclinations of the upper and lower incisors were improved, and the Class II relationship was corrected. The primary objective of correcting the crowding with transverse and sagittal expansion was accomplished (Fig. 6-35).

Construction bite with opening and posterior positioning of the mandible for Class III malocclusions

The construction bite sagittal change depends on the category of malocclusion and the objectives of treatment. In Class III malocclusions the goal is a posterior positioning of the mandible. The construction bite is taken by retruding the lower jaw (Fig. 6-36). The extent of the vertical opening depends on the amount of retrusion possible.

Tooth guidance or functional protrusion Class III malocclusions. The assessment of a possible forced bite is relatively easy. The mandibular incisors hit prematurely in and end-to-end contact and the mandible

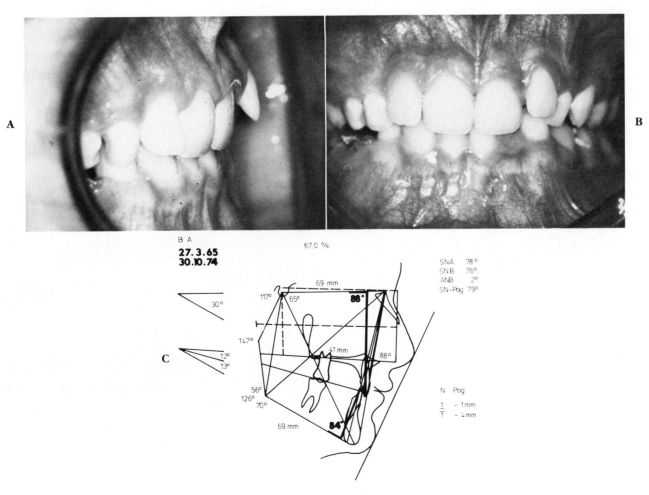

Fig. 6-34. Before treatment, 9-year-old patient. **A** and **B,** Lateral and frontal views. **C,** Tracing.

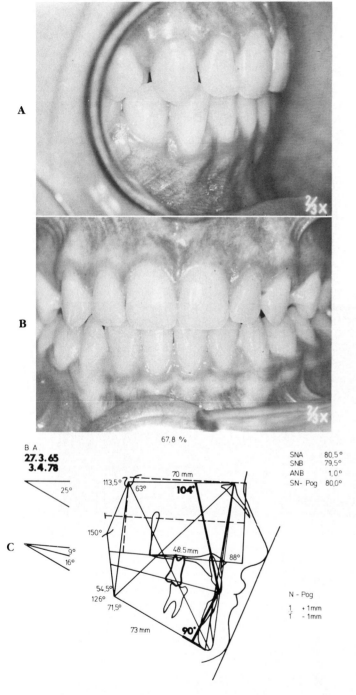

Fig. 6-35. After treatment, same patient as in Fig. 6-34. **A** and **B,** Lateral and frontal views. **C,** Tracing.

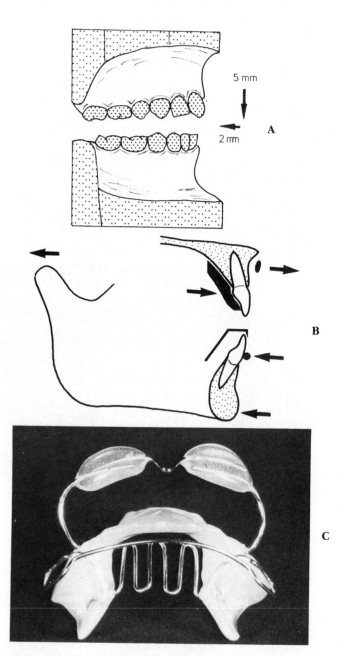

Fig. 6-36. A, Construction bite in the retruded position. **B,** Effectiveness of the reversed (Class III) activator. **C,** Class III activator with upper pads and lower tongue crib.

then slides anteriorly to complete the full occlusal relationship. In these cases the vertical dimension is opened far enough to clear the incisal guidance for the construction bite. This eliminates the protrusive relationship with the mandible in centric relation. In these cases it is possible to achieve an edge-to-edge bite relationship with the posterior teeth still out of contact.

The prognosis for pseudo–Class III malocclusions is good, especially if therapy is started in the early mixed dentition. At this stage the skeletal manifestations of this type of malocclusion are not usually severe since the malocclusion develops progressively. If it is possible to hold the mandible in a posterior position and guide the maxillary incisors into their correct labial relationship, a good incisal guidance can be established. If this is done in the early mixed dentition, there is an adaptation of

the maxilla to the prognathic mandible, resulting in a balanced relationship.

An example of this type of problem is shown in Fig. 6-37, a 7½-year-old boy with the maxillary incisors already erupted and in a lingual cross-bite relationship. The profile was retrognathic and the jaw bases short. The A-N-B angle was −1 degree. As might be expected, the growth pattern was horizontal and the gonial angle extremely small. The maxillary incisors were tipped lingually, which is a favorable characteristic in Class III therapy.

Therapy consisted of a rocking open of the mandible by the activator to a more posterior position, allowing the condyle to drop back in the fossa. At the same time the maxillary incisors were tipped labially to provide the proper incisal guidance. Concurrently, force was elimi-

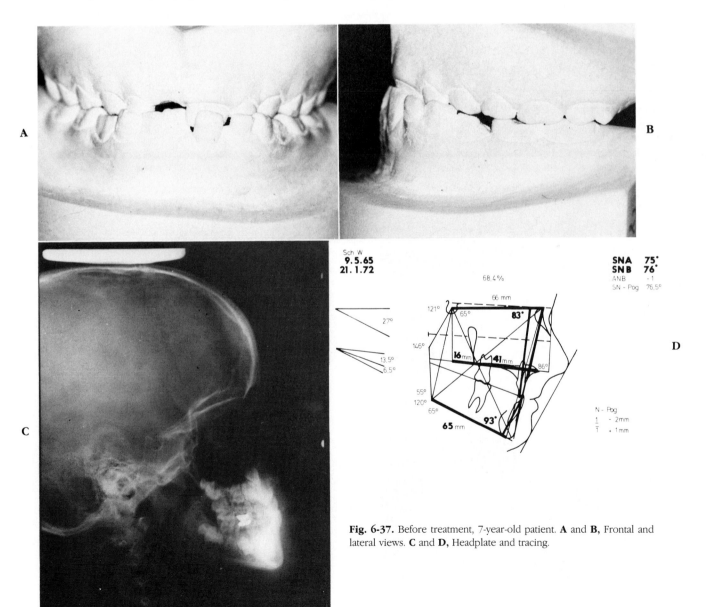

Fig. 6-37. Before treatment, 7-year-old patient. **A** and **B,** Frontal and lateral views. **C** and **D,** Headplate and tracing.

nated in the upper arch with maxillary lip pads to allow the fullest extent of the growth potential in this seemingly deficient area, during the eruption of the incisors. The construction bite was opened only 3 mm to permit retruding the mandible to an edge-to-edge incisal contact. The mandible was held in this posterior position with the labial bow and an acrylic cap on the lower anterior segment. The acrylic was relieved on the lingual of the lower incisors, and the maxillary incisors were supported with close contact.

During treatment, posterior positioning of the mandible could be observed. The S-N-A angle increased, and the A-N-B angle changed to +2 degrees. The articular angle increased because of the posterior positioning of the mandible. The mandibular plane opened slightly,

and the maxillary incisors were tipped labially (Fig. 6-38).

Skeletal Class III malocclusion, with a normal path of closure from postural rest to habitual occlusion. Treatment with functional appliances is not always possible. The opening of the vertical dimension for the construction bite depends on the possibility of achieving an end-to-end incisal relationship. If the overjet is large, the construction bite requires a larger opening. Indications for functional treatment of true Class III problems are limited. Usually only combined therapy with fixed and removable appliances, maxillary orthopedic protraction, etc. is likely to be successful. Even then, orthognathic surgery is always a possibility to achieve proper sagittal and transverse relationships.

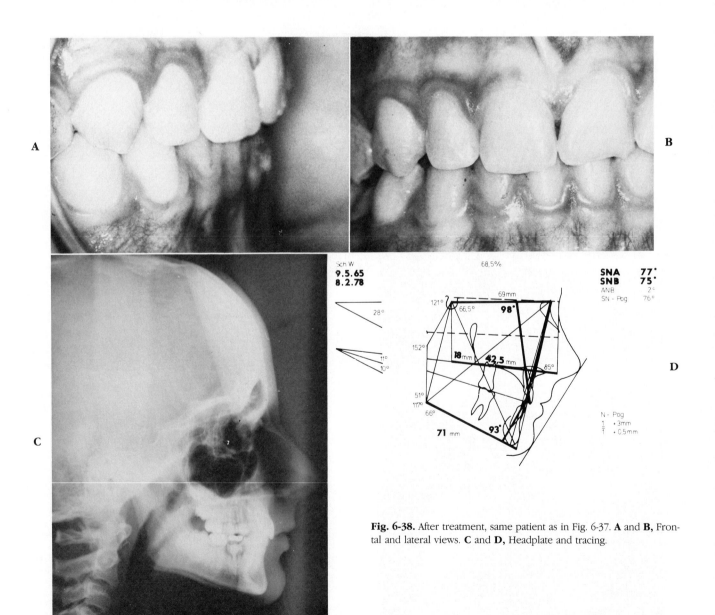

Fig. 6-38. After treatment, same patient as in Fig. 6-37. **A** and **B**, Frontal and lateral views. **C** and **D**, Headplate and tracing.

However, if treatment is initiated in the early mixed dentition, an improvement can be achieved. If the bite can be opened and incisal guidance established, adaptation of the maxillary base to the prognathic mandible can be expected to a certain degree. Correct incisal guidance prevents anterior displacement of the mandible.

An illustration of the type of case that responds to activator guidance is shown in Fig. 6-39. The patient was a 7-year-3-month-old boy. The profile was retrognathic, with a midface concavity. The maxilla was small and retrognathic; the mandible, of normal size. The A-N-B angle was a −3 degrees in habitual occlusion. The path of closure was normal, with no anterior tooth guidance. Cephalometric analysis indicated an average growth pat-tern. Both maxillary and mandibular incisors were lingually tipped. The assessment was that this was a true Class III, with a deficient maxilla the major problem.

Therapy was started with an activator. The bite was opened, and it was possible to establish an end-to-end bite relationship. This required a 5 mm open construction bite. The acrylic portion of the appliance contacted the maxillary incisors to move them labially. As noted in the cephalometric analysis, the original axial inclination was favorable for labial tipping. Lip pads were placed in the vestibular region to stimulate all possible apical base improvement in the maxilla. The lower incisors were held with a labial bow and acrylic cap. Lingual tipping of these incisors was not considered necessary, even though the inclination was less than ideal at this time.

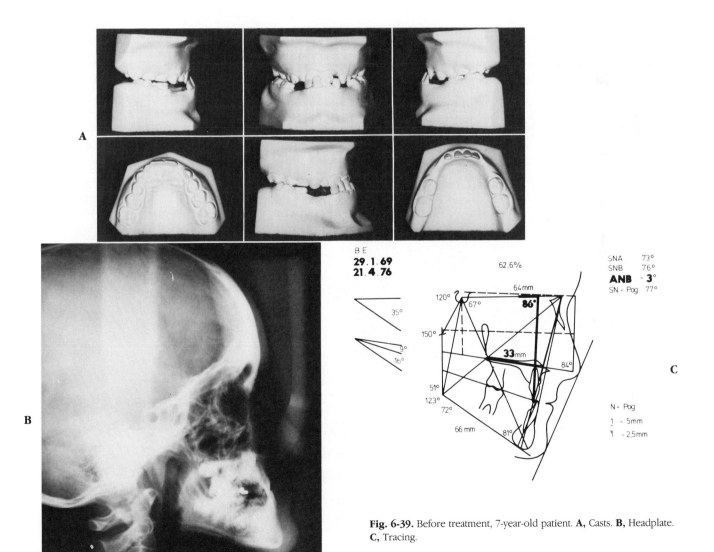

Fig. 6-39. Before treatment, 7-year-old patient. **A,** Casts. **B,** Headplate. **C,** Tracing.

To assist in the compensation with a potential dentoalveolar adaptation, the buds of the lower first premolars were removed.

After 1½ years of treatment, there was definite posterior positioning of the mandible as well as evidence of stimulation of the maxillary apical base. Before treatment the maxillary base had been 11 mm too short in relation to the mandibular base. After this first phase activator guidance, the discrepancy was reduced to 5 mm. The A-N-B angle was improved by 2 degrees. The upper incisors were tipped labially, and the lower inci-

sors were markedly lingual (probably as a result of the enucleation of the lower first premolars). When permanent tooth eruption occurred, the treatment objective would be to close spaces in the lower arch with fixed appliances, lingual root torque on the lower incisors, etc. (Fig. 6-40).

As important as the proper construction bite registration is, the full effectiveness of the activator can be achieved only with proper trimming of the acrylic at the proper time. The details will be covered in the next chapter.

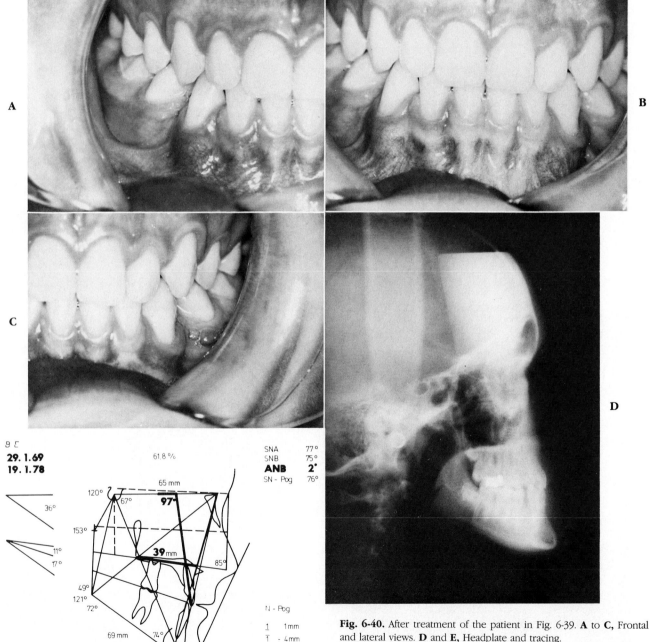

Fig. 6-40. After treatment of the patient in Fig. 6-39. **A** to **C,** Frontal and lateral views. **D** and **E,** Headplate and tracing.

CHAPTER 7

FABRICATION AND MANAGEMENT OF THE ACTIVATOR

PREPARATION

Certain preliminary steps are required before the actual construction of the activator appliance. After the construction bite is taken and checked on the patient, and rechecked on the stone working models, the working models are mounted on a fixator. Some clinicians prefer to send the models and wax bite separately to the laboratory and let the technician mount the models. However, if they are shipped in the construction bite on the fixator, there is less likelihood of damage to or deformation of the bite in transit. Since this is a critical step in the fabrication process, all care must be taken to safeguard the construction bite.

The actual design of the appliance is dictated by a series of diagnostic measurements and decisions. The different categories of Class II malocclusion, as determined by the cephalometric and functional analyses, demand structural modifications. This has been covered in Chapters 3 and 6, but proper fabrication of the appliance can save much chair time and ensure greater patient compliance.

The fabrication demands proper communication with a technical laboratory. The extension of the acrylic body and flanges is drawn on the upper and lower working models with an indelible pencil. It also helps to draw the wire elements on the models. Then a prescription form is filled out in detail for the laboratory technician. (These forms are supplied by most laboratories, which are as anxious as the clinician that the appliance be made properly and work correctly.) A detailed drawing of the construction can be made separately or on the diagram provided by the laboratory. This is important, especially if the appliance is complicated (Fig. 7-1). Wrapping the working models, bite, and fixator in foam rubber for shipping is strongly recommended.

LABORATORY PROCEDURES

As already mentioned, the activator consists of a combination of acrylic and wire components. An important part of the fabrication process is to transfer the construction bite accurately onto the activator. With all the advances in *materia technica* (i.e., rapid-set self-curing acrylics, soft acrylics, good separating media, exotic wire formulas), the success or failure of an appliance can well depend on the appliance replication of the clinically determined correct sagittal and vertical posturing of the mandible. More appliance failures are due to an improper construction bite or improper fabrication than to any other cause. If the clinician has not already mounted the stone working models in the construction bite and placed them on the fixator, this is the first step for the technician. If there is any doubt that the relationship is incorrect, this is the time to call the referring doctor and discuss the problem or to make arrangments for a new construction bite. The fixator (Fig. 7-2) allows the upper and lower parts of the activator to be made separately, and then both parts can be united in the correct construction bite on the fixator.

Preparation of the wire elements

After the casts have been mounted, the detailed instructions on the prescription form read, and the penciled markings on the casts checked, the wire elements are bent. The usual design requires an upper and a lower labial bow for the classic activator.

Labial bow. The major wire elements of the activator are the upper and lower labial bows. They consist of a horizontal middle section, two vertical loops, and wire extensions through the canine–deciduous first molar embrasure into the acrylic body. The horizontal portion contacts the labial surfaces of the four incisors. Depending on the vertical dimension (deep overbite or anterior open bite), the wire crosses the incisors above or below the area of their greatest convexity (Fig. 7-3). The bow can be either negative or positive (passive or active) depending on the prescription. The negative labial bow influences the soft tissues without touching the teeth, almost as a screening appliance.

For the upper labial bow the vertical U-shaped loops that start with a 90° bend at the lateral incisor–canine embrasure form gentle continuous curves above the gingival margin and return to pass freely through the

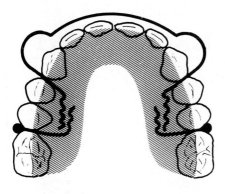

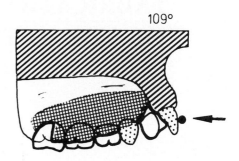

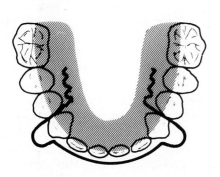

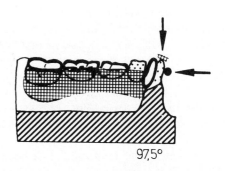

Fig. 7-1. Construction diagram of the appliance.

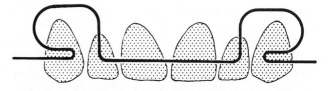

Fig. 7-3. Labial bow with loops for the canines and contact with the incisors in the incisal third.

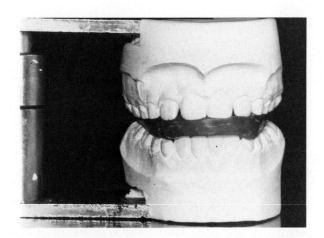

Fig. 7-2. The casts are trimmed in the construction bite relationship on the fixator and mounted sideways..

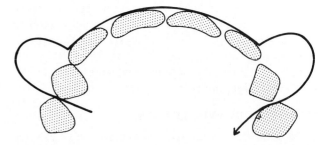

Fig. 7-4. Labial bow activated for distal driving of the premolars *(right).*

canine–first deciduous molar (or first premolar) embrasures to anchor in the lingual acrylic. The wire, however, approximates the mesial marginal ridge of the first deciduous molars in case it is needed to exert a distalization force vector on these teeth (Fig. 7-4).

For the lower labial bow, which is of similar configuration to the upper, the middle horizontal portion is longer since the bend for the vertical loops starts more distally, in the mesial third of the canines. It returns in the canine–deciduous first molar (or first premolar) embrasure. This makes the U-shaped vertical loop somewhat narrower.

The gauge of the labial bow wire is different for active and passive labial bows. For the active bow, the spring-hardened type of stainless steel wire is 0.9 mm thick; for the passive bow, only 0.8 mm.

Additional elements. Depending on the prescription, additional spurs or elements may be needed. If so, they are formed at this time. The needs and designs of these wire appurtenances have been described in Chapter 6.

Fixation of the jackscrews and wire elements

The proper-sized jackscrews are first attached to the cast. The size and magnitude of the opening needed are determined, partly by palatal configuration and partly by the type of malocclusion. For appliances with two screws (one in the upper and one in the lower cast), it is necessary to saw a groove in the midline. The screw is then affixed in this groove with sticky wax (Fig. 7-5). The next step is to fix the wire elements on the labial surfaces of the teeth. The areas that should be free of acrylic are isolated with a layer of wax.

Fabrication of the acrylic portion

The appliance consists of upper, lower, and interocclusal parts (Fig. 7-6). In the upper and lower parts the dental and gingival portions can be differentiated. Especially in the lower cast, the gingival part can be extended posteriorly. If the construction bite is high, as for a vertical activator, the extension of the flanges is greater than for a horizontal type of activator, which positions the mandible more anteriorly. This extension is important to enhance the retention of the appliance, particularly for the vertical activator, because the patients habitually have an open mouth posture (Fig. 7-7).

The flanges for the upper part are 8 to 12 mm high in the gingival area, covering the alveolar crest. The palate is free (Fig. 7-8). If the acrylic plate is thin, it does not encroach on the tongue space; but this may cause too much appliance flexibility. To increase the rigidity, a palatal bar can be used. The bar is similar to that used in the standard Bionator appliance and is made up from 1.2 mm thickness stainless steel. The only purpose of the bar is appliance stabilization. The lower acrylic plate is 5 to 10 mm wide on the average although in the molar area it is sometimes greater, with flanges of 10 to 15 mm (Fig. 7-9).

Despite the fact that appliance fabrication is common knowledge and the services are almost always per-

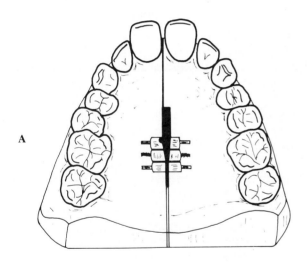

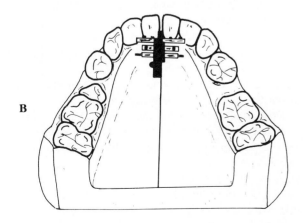

Fig. 7-5. Jackscrews fixed on the casts. **A,** In the upper arch. **B,** In the lower arch.

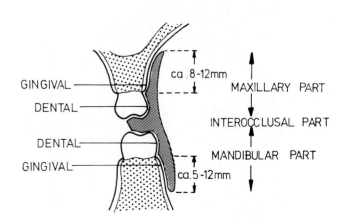

Fig. 7-6. Individual acrylic parts of the activator.

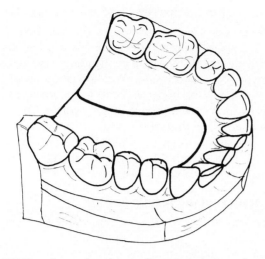

Fig. 7-7. Lingual extension of the appliance in the lower molar region.

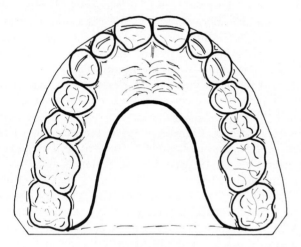

Fig. 7-8. Limits of the appliance base acrylic in the upper jaw.

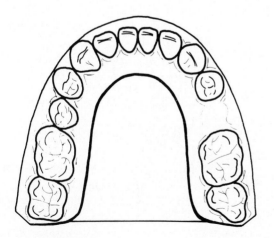

Fig. 7-9. Limits of the appliance in the lower jaw.

formed by technicians, a brief outline will be given here of the acrylic technique:

1. Before the acrylic portion is made up, the casts are put in a water bath for 20 minutes, dried, and isolated.
2. After fixation of the wire elements and covering of the acrylic-free areas with baseplate wax, the upper and lower portions are molded from self-curing acrylic.
3. The casts are placed on the fixator, and the upper and lower portions are joined with endothermic acrylic at the interdental area (Fig. 7-10).
4. The Dentaurum fixator allows simultaneous acrylic application of the interocclusal part from both lingual and buccal sides.
5. After polymerization the appliance is ground and polished. However, it is not trimmed in the laboratory for specific tooth guidance. This is done later by the clinician, with the patient in the chair.
6. The appliance is shipped back to the operator, along with a copy of the original prescription.

MANAGEMENT OF THE APPLIANCE

After the appliance has been returned and checked to ensure that the instructions were followed, a "trimming plan" is developed, with diagnostic records to record each grinding procedure needed and the expected movement. This is done with the patient in the chair, allowing frequent spot checks to see whether the acrylic guiding planes are indeed functioning as desired. Some operators prefer that the appliance be worn for a week with no grinding so the patient can get used to it. Then the trimming plan is carried out per the written outline that has been developed.

It is impossible to overemphasize the importance of communication with the patient and parents. Time spent in the beginning, establishing a high level of patient compliance, is well spent. Videotapes, demonstrations, and patient information booklets are all beneficial. Most important, however, is the doctor-patient relationship and the sincere interest and enthusiasm of all the staff in maintaining a high level of patient motivation during the entire treatment time.

Before leaving the office, the patient must know how to place the appliance in the mouth himself. The usual instructions call for wearing the appliance 2 or 3 hours during the day for the first week. During the second week the patient must sleep with the appliance as well as wear it 1 to 3 hours each day. The appliance is checked by the operator in 3 weeks to see whether the trimming has been accurate and is working as desired. Guide plane contact areas are usually shiny if functioning properly, but these can be reshaped and corrected as needed. If the patient has difficulty wearing the appli-

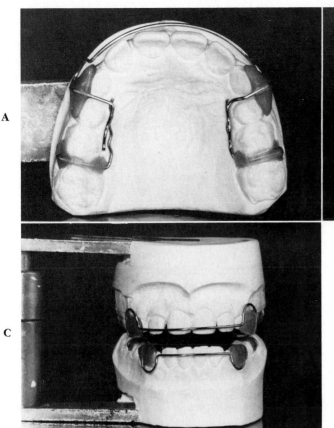

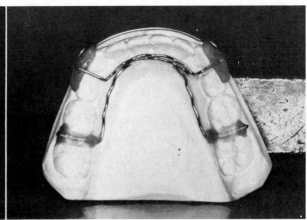

Fig. 7-10. A, Upper cast prepared with wire elements. **B,** Lower cast prepared with wire elements. **C,** Casts with wire elements in the fixator prepared for molding the acrylics.

ance for the whole night, then more daytime wear is needed to compensate for this until-full nighttime wear is routine. Sometimes, in addition to postponing the trimming for the first adjustment appointment, the sealing or addition of self-cure soft acrylic to the lower flanges will improve retention during the early accommodative stages.

If the patient can wear the activator without difficulty and is following instructions, it is sufficient to make checkup appointments every 6 weeks. During these office visits, in addition to maintaining a rapport with the patient and reinforcing the motivational potential, the following steps should be performed.

1. All guiding planes that have been ground and all areas in contact with the teeth should be checked for shiny surfaces to see whether the appliance is being correctly worn and is working properly.
2. Reshaping of acrylic guide areas may be needed after the initial trimming to improve the action; but it is also needed during the course of treatment to ensure continued tooth movement, particularly in the upper arch, where retrusion or distalization is desired. If teeth are erupting, reshaping is also necessary.

3. Guiding acrylic contact planes often must be resealed or recontoured by adding self-curing soft acrylic in a very thin layer to maintain the proper functional activation on the desired teeth. Clinical examination as well as examining the acrylic inclined planes for shiny spots will help determine when and how much sealing should be done.
4. The labial bow or bows and any additional wire elements must be checked for action and possible deformation. Constantly moving the appliance up and down in the mouth may change wire configurations and will occasionally fatigue a wire sufficiently to cause it to fracture. The active bow should touch the teeth. The passive bow is away from the teeth, in contact with the soft tissues. The guiding and stabilizing wires are activated by the patient's biting into the appliance.
5. The lip pads, if used, should be checked for possible irritation in the sulcus area. They may need reshaping. They should not contact the alveolar process or the teeth.
6. In expansion treatment the jackscrews are normally activated not by the operator but by the patient at 2-

week intervals. However, the operator should check this activation for too frequent or infrequent activation for the particular problem. Too much activation prevents the appliance from fitting properly. It may be necessary to change the activation interval.

7. The construction bite position may need to be altered occasionally. This can be performed by various methods.

   a. (direct method) An acrylic layer can be ground away on the dental surface of the lower plate and new self-curing acrylic added, positioning the mandible as desired. This is definitely required when the operator has decided to advance the mandible in steps instead of all at one time.

   b. (indirect method) New impressions can be taken, a new construction bite made as originally done, and the casts mounted in the laboratory. Acrylic modification is done on the newly mounted casts on the fixator.

   c. The upper and lower portions of the activator can be separated interocclusally and then rejoined in the new construction bite position by endothermic acrylic.

CHAPTER 8

TRIMMING OF THE ACTIVATOR

PRINCIPLE OF THERAPEUTIC TRIMMING FOR TOOTH GUIDANCE

To stimulate the functional activity of the perioral musculature with a loose appliance so the movement and eruption of selected teeth can be guided, certain areas of the acrylic that contact the teeth should be ground away.

After the activator has been fabricated in the laboratory, it is placed in the mouth for a check of the fit and correctness of the construction bite. Normally the acrylic is interposed between the upper and lower occlusal surfaces of the buccal segments and is a negative reproduction of tooth surface anatomy. If only forward posturing is desired, then this tightly fitting appliance will serve as a handle on the dentition to hold the mandible in the planned protraction. However, merely holding the mandible in a forward position is not enough to achieve the proper relationship of teeth in the three planes of space. Selective guidance of the eruption of teeth and the development of arch form are necessary, in addition to the elimination of all possible functional retrusive muscle activity and attempts to get the best possible condylar growth adaptation to the more correct sagittal relationship. Carefully planned grinding or trimming of the appliance in the tooth contact area makes it effective in the dentoalveolar region. The aim of trimming is to achieve a loosely fitting appliance that the patient can manipulate yet one that maintains the correct sagittal relationship while stimulating or restricting selective eruption and movement of anterior and posterior teeth.

The principles of force application in the trimming process are determined by the kind, direction, and magnitude of force created by the loosely fitting activator:

1. The force is intermittent. This kind of application allows dynamic and rhythmic muscle forces to act in such a manner that the appliance works by kinetic energy.
2. The direction of the desired force is determined by selective grinding of the acrylic surfaces that contact the upper and lower teeth. After proper grinding the desired force will contact predetermined areas of the teeth and create force in the direction of needed tooth movement. Any surfaces that might impede this movement are relieved or cut away.
3. The magnitude of the force delivered can be roughly estimated by determining the amount of actual acrylic contact with the tooth surfaces. If the force is delivered to a small portion of the tooth surface, it will be greater than if there is a broad contact between the acrylic and a larger tooth surface. The acrylic surfaces that transmit the desired intermittent force and contact the teeth are called *guiding planes*.
4. Pretrimming rules must be followed. After the appliance has been carefully checked for proper fit in the mouth, an exact plan of needed tooth movement is developed. Approximate trimming can be done on the plaster casts. However, the final grinding must be done in the mouth. Any undercut acrylic surfaces that might interfere with the planned tooth guidance must be removed. This potential problem can be checked with an explorer (Fig. 8-1) or visualized by checking the shadows created on the acrylic by undercut surfaces (Fig. 8-2). Since there is always a bit of adjustment and "give" to be expected while the appliance is worn during the first couple of weeks, the final trimming is not done until the second visit in most cases to achieve the best possible efficiency. The acrylic areas that contact the teeth are likely to become polished, and thus the area of force delivery can be well identified. Then careful grinding can be done to direct the force more accurately where it is required.

Because of the variability of behavioral activity and difference in maturity levels, the grinding procedure is sometimes varied. Since a tightly fitting appliance adapted to the teeth is somewhat more easily accommodated to in the early stages, the first stage of trimming does not fully establish the loose functional fit desired. A few contacts are left that stabilize the appliance until the patient adjusts. Then the remainder of planned trimming is done, on the second or third visit. Meanwhile the patient has adjusted to the forward posturing of the

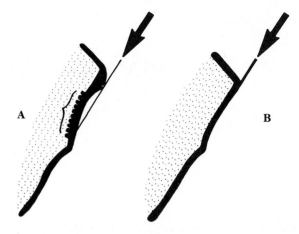

Fig. 8-2. Shadow test. **A,** Before and, **B,** after trimming.

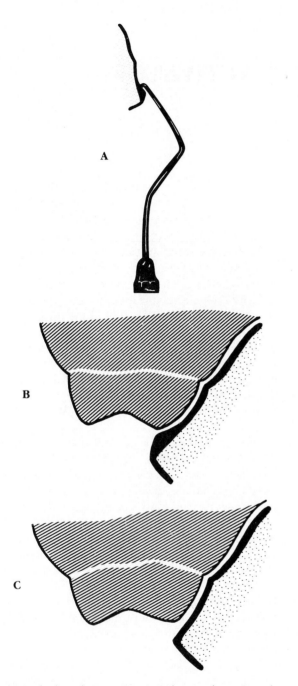

Fig. 8-1. Checking the trimming. **A,** With an explorer. **B,** Undercut surface in the acrylic. **C,** Acrylic surface after trimming.

mandible and can better accept the loose appliance while still protracting the mandible. When expansion is needed for a very narrow maxillary arch, the appliance may actually be squeezed between the buccal segments, exerting light force for the whole treatment period as decrowding occurs.

Trimming should be done in stepwise progression. Single tooth movements are analyzed as to where each tooth should ultimately be with respect to contiguous teeth. Then the total planned grinding procedure is

written up and checked off as each trimming procedure is performed. Done in this systematic and careful manner, tooth movement in the vertical, sagittal, and transverse directions is possible.

TRIMMING THE ACTIVATOR FOR VERTICAL CONTROL

Two movements occur, intrusion and extrusion. Only limited intrusion is possible with the loosely fitting activator, however, despite the fact that relative intrusion is a viable treatment objective, since some teeth are selectively prevented from erupting while others are free to do so or are actually stimulated by acrylic guiding planes. Selective extrusion in the mixed dentition is a major and valid treatment objective, affecting both vertical and horizontal tooth relationships, if done properly.

Intrusion of teeth

Intrusion of incisors can be achieved by loading the incisal edges of these teeth (Fig. 8-3). Ground properly, they become the only loaded or contacting surfaces, with no other contact between the incisor teeth and the acrylic, even in the alveolar area. When the simultaneous use of an active labial bow is indicated (active because it touches the labial surfaces of the incisor teeth), the contact between the bow wire and the incisors is below the area of greatest convexity, or on the incisal third (Fig. 8-4). This location does not interfere with intrusive movement of the incisors and may actually stimulate it somewhat. Such intrusive loading is indicated in deep overbite cases.

Intrusion of molars is performed by loading only the cusps of these teeth (Fig. 8-5). The acrylic detail is ground away from the fossae and fissures, to eliminate any possible inclined-plane (oblique) stimulus to molar movement, when only a vertical depressing action is desired. Ground this way, the activator can thus deliver higher forces. If larger occlusal surfaces are loaded, a

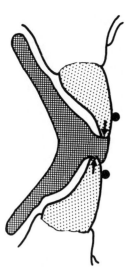

Fig. 8-3. Intrusion of the incisors via acrylic capping.

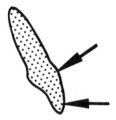

Fig. 8-4. Labial bow position for intrusion (incisal third) or extrusion (gingival third) of the incisors.

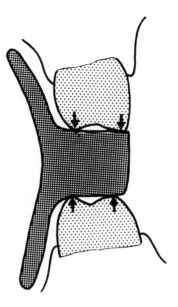

Fig. 8-5. Acrylic contact for intrusion of the molars.

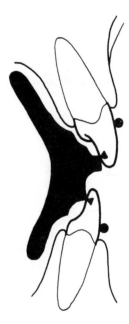

Fig. 8-6. Extrusion of the incisors by placement of the labial bow below the area of greatest convexity.

reflex mouth opening occurs more frequently, resulting in less effective depressing action by the appliance. Molar depression and loading are indicated in open bite problems, when there is minimal or nonexistent interocclusal clearance.

Extrusion of teeth

Extrusion of incisors requires loading their lingual surfaces in the maxilla above and in the mandible below the areas of greatest concavity. Although generally this is not too effective because of the anatomy of the teeth, the extrusion can be enhanced nonetheless by placing the labial bow above the area of greatest convexity (Fig. 8-6). Such extrusion modifications are indicated for open bite problems, particularly chronic finger-sucking cases in which the incisors are relatively intruded.

Extrusion of molars can be facilitated by loading the lingual surfaces of these teeth above the area of greatest convexity in the maxilla or below the greatest convexity in the mandible (Fig. 8-7). Molar and premolar extrusion is indicated in deep bite problems. The trimming of the activator for molar extrusion can be done at one time for all molars. It is not necessary to anchor the

appliance dentally since it is sufficiently stabilized in the alveolar regions by the acrylic extensions. If the buccal segment teeth in the upper and lower jaws are extruded simultaneously, there is inadequate control. The teeth can overerupt or move mesially. This reduction of a deep bite may be more rapid but less desirable from a sagittal point of view. As Balters has recommended in trimming his Bionator, it is imperative that controlled differential eruption guidance be employed for the best interdental and occlusal plane relationships. Particularly

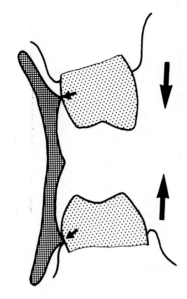

Fig. 8-7. Acrylic contour for extrusion of the molars.

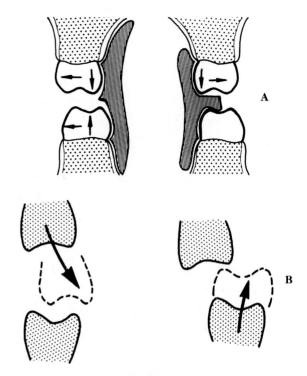

Fig. 8-9. Selective trimming. **A** *(left)* Both molars are extruded simultaneously; *(right)* only the upper molar is extruded. **B** *(left)* selective eruption of the upper molars for correction of a Class III relationship; *(right)* selective eruption of the lower molars for correction of a Class II relationship.

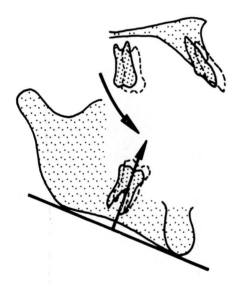

Fig. 8-8. The eruption pathway of the molars should be considered in selective trimming.

where there is a flush terminal plane relationship, proper selective grinding can convert an impending Class II or Class III malocclusion into a Class I interdigitation.

Selective trimming of the activator

During selective trimming procedures only the upper or lower molars are extruded. After these teeth have erupted sufficiently, the eruption of the antagonists can be controlled. Thus the sagittal and vertical relationships can be influenced.

When a selective grinding is being planned, the path of eruption of the molars must be taken into consider-

ation. The lower molars erupt in an upward and slightly forward direction; the upper molars downward and forward, with a greater mesial migration component if left unattended (Fig. 8-8). In Class II malocclusions, if the eruption of the maxillary molars is inhibited while that of the mandibular molars is stimulated, the upper molars will remain in their mesiodistal position with respect to the basal structures but the lower molars will improve their sagittal relationship (Fig. 8-9). This is particularly important in flush terminal plane relationships, wherein an end-to-end bite exists until the deciduous molars are shed and the differential migration to take up the leeway space is completed. The resultant improvement of sagittal relationships by differential eruption and holding the upper molars in a distal relationship can cause a mandibular vertical rotation, which has the initial effect of accentuating the mandibular retrognathism. This reactions can be favorable, however, in cases with a horizontal mandibular growth direction and deep overbite. In cases with a vertical growth pattern and tendency to open bite, the distal position of the molars can be altered before their final eruption. After the lower molars have erupted, the distal surfaces of the upper second deciduous molars may be sliced. This will then permit the upper molars to migrate slightly to the mesial, closing down the bite and reducing the mandibular retrognathism, but care must be taken not to create a Class II malocclusion again in the process.

If eruption of the upper molars is stimulated while lower molar eruption is inhibited, the upper molars will move mesially. This reaction can be used to help correct a Class III malocclusion that is not too severe. The mesial positioning of the upper molars results in a closing down of the bite and a more horizontal growth vector, which is not favorable in Class III malocclusions. For vertical growth patterns or open bite cases, however, the reaction is a favorable one, with the alveolodental compensation reducing the apparent dysplasia. Distal driving of the upper molars, as is often done with a Kloehn headgear, will open the bite more although it is possible to get more vertical eruption of upper molars if desired. In such cases the mesial movement is impeded by spurs from the acrylic body of the appliance.

The method of trimming can be more sophisticated if its objective is to control not only eruption of the molars but also the dental anchorage of the appliance. The dental anchorage assumes greater importance in modifications of the activator, when the acrylic bulk is reduced in the alveolar and palatal regions. The method of trimming for these skeletonized activators will be described in Chapter 9.

TRIMMING THE ACTIVATOR FOR SAGITTAL CONTROL

When there are specific goals of protruding or retruding the incisors or mesially or distally changing the molar sagittal relationship, they can be achieved by judicious appliance control.

Protrusion and retrusion of incisors can be accomplished only by combined grinding of the acrylic and guide planes plus adjustment of the labial bow wire. When the labial bow touches the teeth, it can either tip them lingually or retain them in position. In such cases it is called an active bow. When it is away from the teeth and preventing soft tissue contact (e.g., in the Bionator), it is termed a passive bow (Fig. 8-10).

The *active* bow may contact the incisors on the gingival third of their labial surfaces to promote extrusion in open bite cases or on the incisal third to inhibit extrusion in deep overbite cases. To retrude incisors, bow placement may be either gingival (to reduce the tipping vector while lingualizing these teeth) or incisal (to accentuate tipping of severely protruded incisor crowns when there is space present). Thus the axial inclination of incisors is subject to some control. The labial bow does not work as a spring force, however. It is fabricated from a relatively thick (0.9 mm) wire and is activated only when the mandible closes in the construction bite position. All wire appurtenances in the activator are thick nonspring types and work according to the same principle.

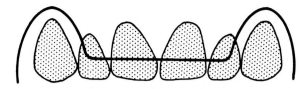

Fig. 8-10. Upper labial bow.

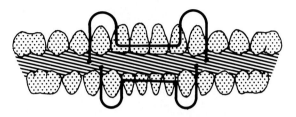

Fig. 8-11. Upper and lower labial bows.

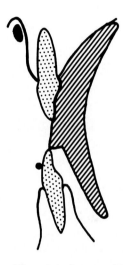

Fig. 8-12. Placement of lip pads in the upper labial fold for a Class III malocclusion.

By relieving pressures and muscle strain of the lips and checks on the dentition, the *passive* bow permits labial or buccal movement of selected teeth. In the pure activator, when the bow does not extend distally to the canine its effect is primarily to permit labial tipping or holding of the maxillary and mandibular incisors. For this reason some of the appliances are constructed with an upper and a lower labial bow (Fig. 8-11). The only exception is the Class III activator, which has lip pads similar to the Fränkel appliance instead of a labial bow (Fig. 8-12).

Protrusion of incisors

The incisors can be protruded by loading their lingual surfaces with acrylic contact and screening away the lip strain with the passive labial bow (or lip pads). Loading can be achieved by either of two methods:

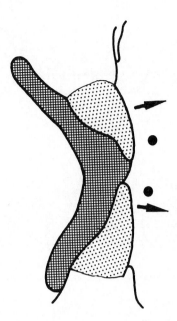

Fig. 8-13. Protrusion of the incisors by loading the whole lingual surface.

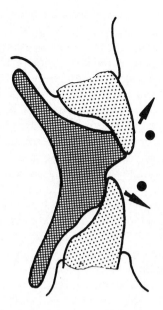

Fig. 8-14. Labial tipping of the incisors by loading the incisal third of the lingual surfaces.

1. The *entire* lingual surface is loaded (Fig. 8-13). To avoid opening spaces between the teeth, only the interdental acrylic projections are trimmed. By this mode of labial tipping the incisors can be moved labially with a low magnitude of force since the applied force is spread over a large surface. Some tipping can be expected, despite total acrylic contact in the beginning.

2. Only the *incisal* third of the lingual surfaces is loaded (Fig. 8-14). This variation results in labial tipping of the incisors using a higher degree of force, since the contact surface is small. When the incisal third is loaded, the axis or rotation is closer to the apex of the incisors.

Incisor protrusion can also be accomplished by means of auxiliary elements.

1. *Protrusion springs.* These are continuous or closed springs of fairly heavy wire (0.8 mm) that are activated only when the teeth are closed into the appliance (Fig. 8-15).

2. *Wooden pegs.* Instead of springs embedded in the lingual acrylic, small wooden pegs are inserted with minimal projection. The wood swells when wet, and the pegs thus project more and exert a small degree of increased force when the teeth are fully seated in the activator (Fig. 8-16). The protrusion springs or wooden sticks usually contact the incisors in the middle or gingival third of the lingual surfaces (Fig. 8-17). The labially tipped incisors can then be partially uprighted by an active labial bow that contacts the incisors at their incisal third. However, extensive torque or bodily movement is not possible with an activator.

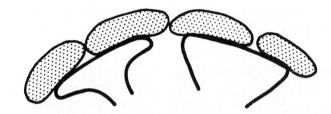

Fig. 8-15. Protrusion springs for labial tipping of the incisors.

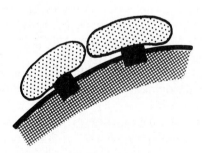

Fig. 8-16. Protrusion of the incisors performed with wooden sticks.

3. *Gutta percha.* Gutta percha may be added to the lingual acrylic; however, this time honored approach has been superseded by the use of a thin layer of soft acrylic added where desired. The self-curing acrylics (e.g., Coe-Soft) are ideal not only behind the teeth but also in the alveolar crest portion. A special indication is in moving the maxillary centrals and supporting alveolar bone labially as they erupt in Class III malocclusions.

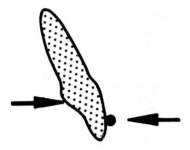

Fig. 8-17. If the protrusion springs are placed gingivally, the labially tipped incisor can be uprighted with an incisally placed labial bow.

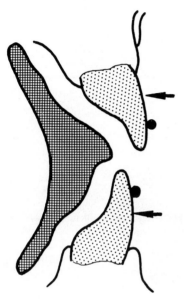

Fig. 8-18. Retrusion of the incisors by grinding the acrylic away completely.

Retrusion of incisors

The acrylic is trimmed away from behind the incisors to be retruded. The active labial bow, which contacts the teeth during functional movements, is the source of force for moving these teeth.

The acrylic can be completely ground away from behind the incisors and the alveolar process (Fig. 8-18). If the labial bow touches the teeth in the incisal margin region, the center of rotation approaches the apex. If the labial bow contacts the gingival third of the incisors, the centrum is moved coronally toward the junction of the apical and middle thirds. The gingival position can elongate the incisors at the same time, depending on the degree of labial convexity. This type of effect is desirable only in open bite cases, when both retrusion and elongation are desired. In labially inclined incisor problems, when there is a deep bite, every attempt should be made to minimize any extrusion of the incisors as they are being axially uprighted.

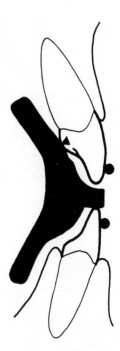

Fig. 8-19. Retrusion of the incisors with a fulcrum in the cervical region.

If it is desired to have the axis of rotation in the middle third of the incisors, the acrylic is trimmed away only in the coronal region leaving a cervical contact point or fulcrum. The labial bow contacts the incisal third of the labial surfaces, providing some motivation force and also preventing incisor extrusion during retraction (Fig. 8-19). It is important to recognize this need for vertical control during incisor retraction. A very important task of the activator is to try to control the axial inclination of the lower incisors. This cannot be solved with simple single movements such as retrusion or intrusion. The status of the malocclusion and the whole appliance design must be considered.

Design of the lower incisor area. As has been stressed before, the design of the appliance in the lower incisor area is of particular importance. The conventionally made appliance that loads the lingual surfaces of the lower incisors tips these teeth labially because of the reciprocal intermaxillary reaction built into the construction bite and design of the nighttime wear appliance. This movement is desirable if there is lingual inclination of the lower incisors because of hyperactive mentalis function and a lip trap.

As an example, Fig. 8-20 shows a 9-year-4-month-old boy with a Class II, Division 1, malocclusion and a retrognathic profile but no severe skeletal malrelationship. The growth pattern was horizontal, with the jaw bases short and the symphysis wide. The large overjet was due to a confirmed lip trap and perioral malfunction, with

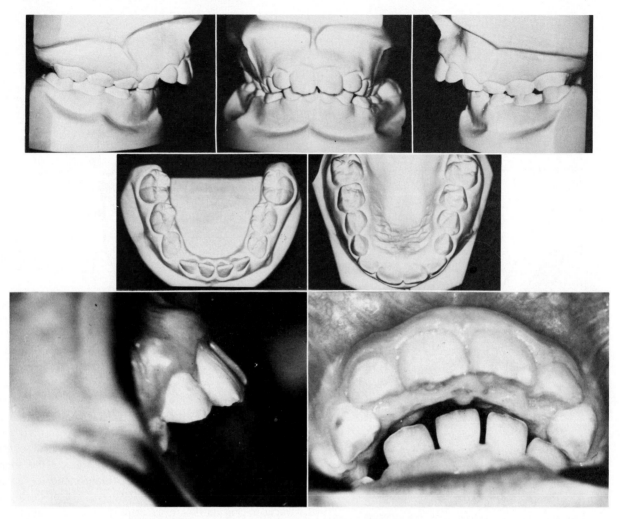

Fig. 8-20. Patient H.A. before treatment. Excessive overjet and lingually inclined lower incisors are due to a lip trap habit. Note the narrow maxillary arch and the unilateral cross-bite.

the maxillary incisors tipped labially some 9 mm in front of the N-Pog line. The upper dental arch was narrow because of excessive buccinator mechanism pressures, leading to a convenience bite swing and crossbite of the first molars on the right side.

Treatment was begun for this patient with an expansion plate to align the upper dental arch and correct the cross-bite. Then an activator was employed. Since the overjet was 12 mm, the construction bite was positioned in steps, with the first bite 8 mm anterior to habitual occlusion (Fig. 8-21). The overbite was 9 mm but was opened only 4 mm. Because of the very deep bite, the lower incisors were loaded lingually and capped with acrylic to prevent eruption. The lower labial bow was passive. The acrylic was ground away from the lingual of the upper incisors, including the alveolar area, with only the incisal edges supported to prevent elongation during retrusion. The upper active labial bow contacted

the teeth on the incisal third. The acrylic was trimmed for extrusion in the molar area. A stabilizing spur was added mesially to the upper molars to exert a distalizing component as these teeth erupted. After 2½ years of treatment and 1½ years of retention, the results of treatment are shown in Fig. 8-22.

The patient had a high growth increment, especially in the mandibular area (2.3 mm above average), and the facial profile became orthognathic with a pronounced horizontal growth vector. Despite this, the overbite improved because of molar extrusion and retarded incisor eruption, leveling the curve of Spee. The lower incisors were tipped labially, which reduced the overbite somewhat. This was in spite of the incisal acrylic cap over these teeth, since the addition of self-curing soft acrylic on the contiguous lingual surfaces exerted both a labial and an intruding component. With extrusion of the upper incisors controlled, the usual extrusive tendency

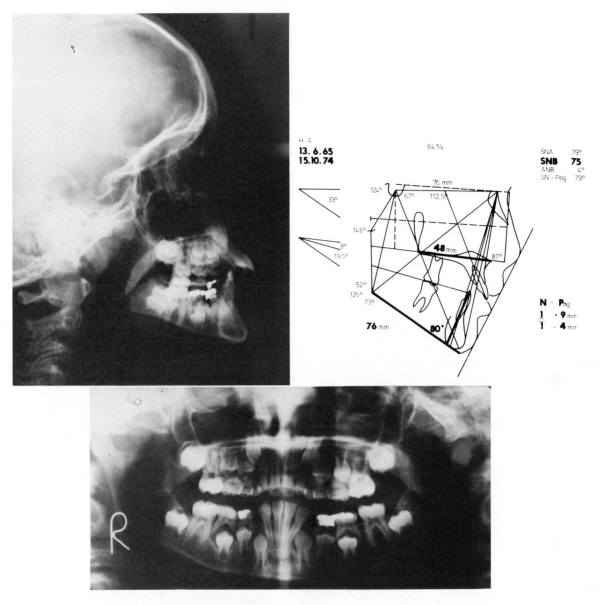

Fig. 8-20, cont'd. For legend see opposite page.

was prevented during incisor retraction. The appliance design was important in this case, impeding the usual extrusion expected with lingual tipping of incisor teeth. The uprighting of the upper and lower incisors helped improve the overjet, as did the labial movement of the lower incisors, which also opened space for the canines.

On the final cephalogram the lower incisors were 3 mm behind, and the upper incisors 3 mm ahead of the N-Pog line. The satisfactory result was due not only to movement of the incisors but also to the growth-conditioned forward positioning of the mandible and resultant displacement of the N-Pog line.

If the lower incisors are tipped labially before treat-

ment is started for a Class II, Division I, malocclusion, then classical activator therapy is probably contraindicated. Further protrusion of the incisors not only makes the axial inclination worse, as well as the lip line profile, but also prevents the successful correction of the sagittal Class II malrelationship. Such a result is also unstable, and the following consequences are possible:

Given the fact that the lower incisors are excessively procumbent, they then contact the lingual of the maxillary incisors, eliminating the overjet before the buccal segment sagittal malrelationship is completely corrected.

If the mandible cannot be postured anteriorly

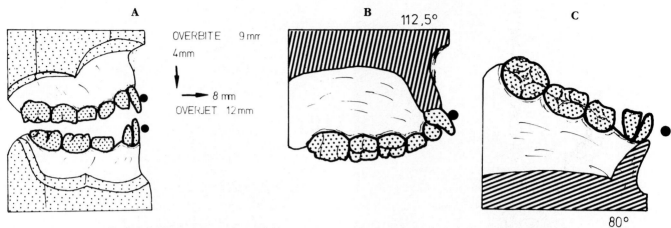

A

OVERBITE 9 mm
4 mm
↓
→ 8 mm
OVERJET 12 mm

B 112,5°

C 80°

Fig. 8-21. A, Casts in the construction bite. **B,** Active upper and, **C,** passive lower labial bows. (Same patient as in Fig. 8-20.)

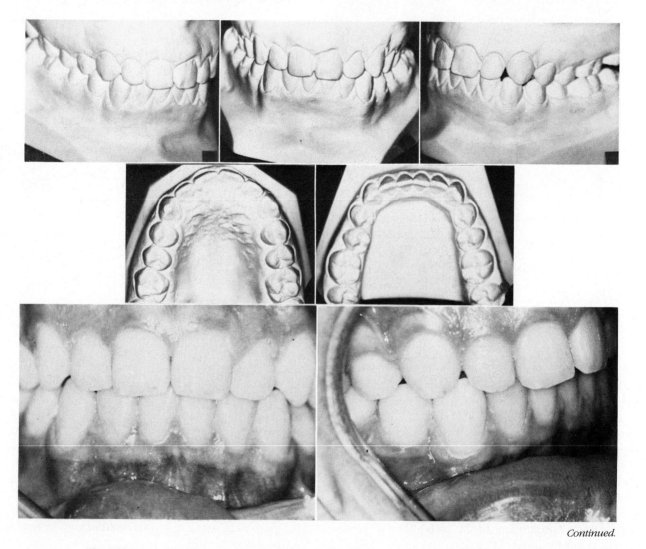

Continued.

Fig. 8-22. Patient H.A. after treatment. Superimposition of cephalometric tracings before and after treatment.

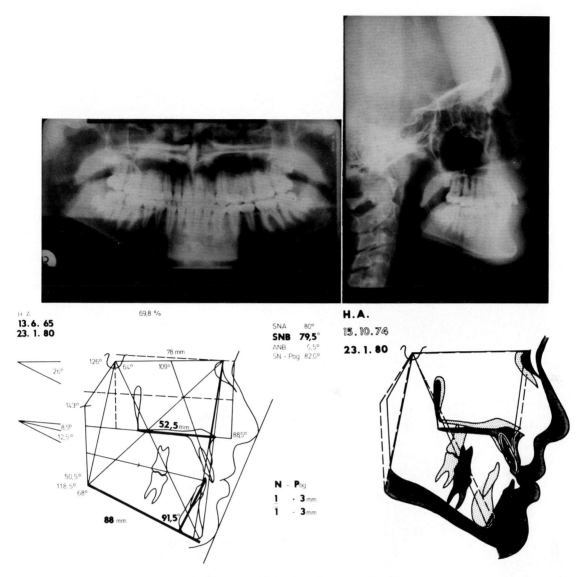

Fig. 8-22, cont'd. For legend see opposite page.

enough, then there is dental compensation of an original skeletal discrepancy. This is acceptable only in cases of a vertical growth pattern. In average or horizontal growth vectors it is a poor treatment regimen for the mixed dentition period.

If the mandible continues to grow anteriorly after appliance therapy, as it is likely to do, outgrowing the maxilla, then there is crowding of the lower incisors, particularly in horizontal growth patterns. What may look good clinically right after termination of activator wear deteriorates rapidly, making the whole procedure suspect.

The following is a case in point:

Fig. 8-23 shows the before-treatment records of an 8-year-9-month-old girl, with a retrognathic face and an average growth pattern. The mandible was in a posterior position but of average length. The ramus height was very small (43 mm). The maxilla was judged slightly retrognathic but with a long base. Despite the good axial inclination of the upper incisors, they were 10.5 mm ahead of the N-Pog line. The lower incisors were labially inclined at almost 100 degrees.

Conventional activator treatment was started. Because of the full Class II molar relationship, activated springs were used to assist in distalizing these teeth. The upper incisors were held with an acrylic cap to prevent their being tipped lingually while activating the labial bow. (See design of the upper incisor area). The lower incisors were loaded lingually and the lower labial bow was passive.

A good clinical result was achieved after 3 years of treatment (Fig. 8-24). The cephalometric analysis

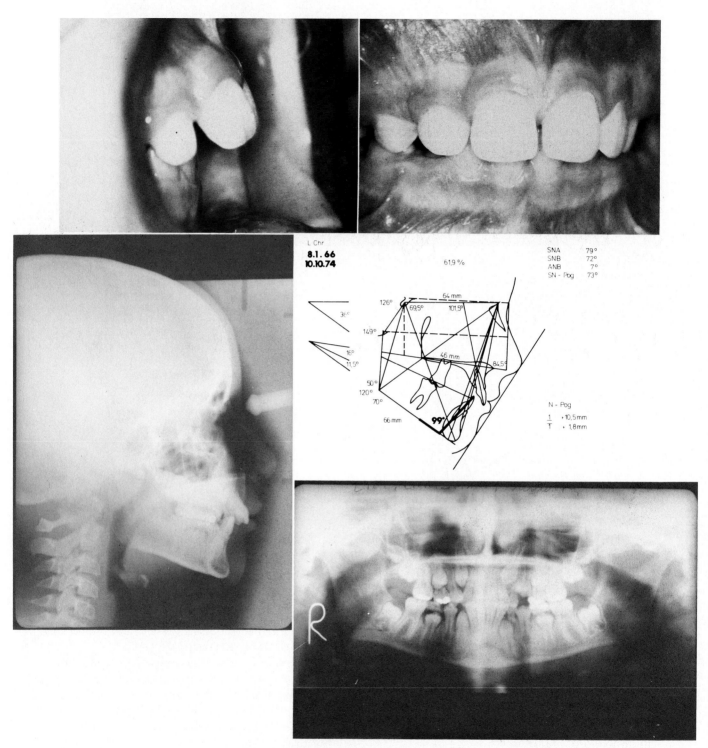

Fig. 8-23. Patient L.C. before activator treatment.

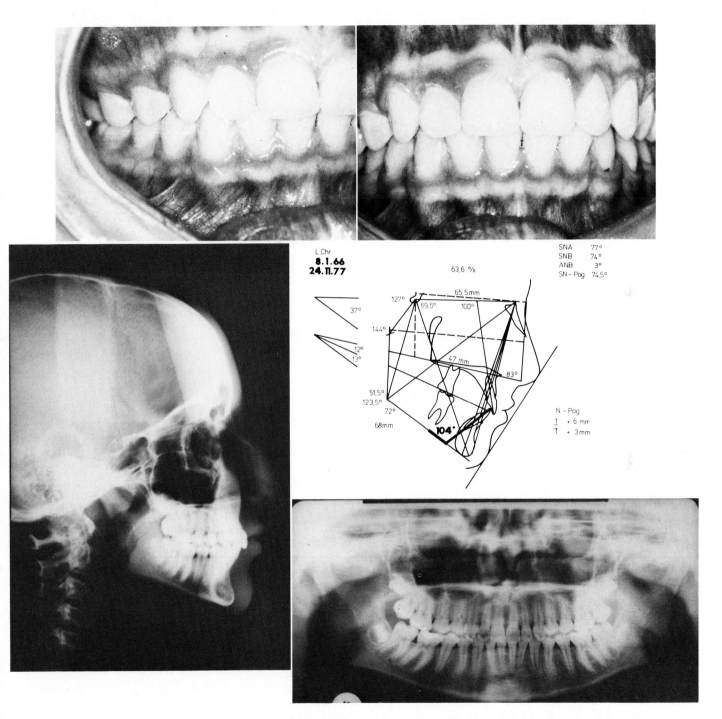

Fig. 8-24. Patient L.C. after 3 years of treatment.

showed an improvement of the sagittal skeletal relationships, with a 4-degree reduction of the A-N-B angle to 3 degrees. The growth increment of the mandibular base (−1.9 mm below average) and of maxillary base (−2.5 mm below average) was low whereas that of the ramus was average. The basal relationship Ar-Pog to Ar-A improved from 13 to 20 mm. The axial inclination of the lower incisors worsened, tipping forward to 104 degrees. The result was not considered stable since a greater growth increment of the mandibular base was likely to occur in the next several years, with consequent lower incisor uprighting and crowding.

Based on the previous case and the observations made, what design factor changes should be made for these problems? Depending on the axial inclination and position of the incisors, there are three possibilities:

1. Labial tipping of the lower incisors
2. Holding the incisors in their initial position
3. Uprighting the lower incisors while the mandible is being anteriorly positioned

If it is necessary to procline the lower incisors, this can be done (as already described) by loading the entire lingual surface or only the incisal third. The labial bow is passive. In open bite cases no incisal groove is provided whereas in deep bite cases a flat acrylic rim only lightly touching the incisal edges discourages extrusion.

If it is necessary to hold the incisors in their position, the acrylic should be trimmed only interdentally and left contracting the teeth lingually, with an acrylic cap extending over onto the labial of the incisors (Fig. 8-25).

If a retrusion or uprighting of the incisors is required while positioning the mandible anteriorly, the design of the lower incisor area should be managed in a more sophisticated manner (Fig. 8-26). There must be no contact between the teeth and the acrylic on the lingual, not even during the functional movements of the mandible. An acrylic labial cap contacting on the labial incisal holds the incisors. In deep overbite cases the incisal edges are loaded, but only from the labial side, creating a lingual movement component through the inclined-plane action while preventing extrusion. The incisal edges are not loaded in open bite cases. The labial bow is active, moving the incisors lingually and extruding if possible.

Another case report is pertinent here:

G.C., a 9-year-6-month-old girl with very proclined incisors (104 degrees) when she presented for treatment, had a skeletal Class II relationship with a retrognathic mandible. The mandibular base was extremely short, the maxillary base of average length. The growth pattern was average. In addition to proclination of the lower incisors, there was labial tipping of the uppers (Fig. 8-27).

A horizontal type of activator was constructed with an

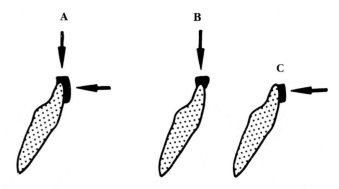

Fig. 8-25. Acrylic groove or cap holding the incisors, **A,** incisally and labially, **B,** incisally, and, **C,** labially.

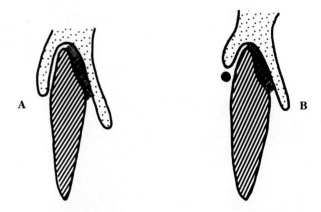

Fig. 8-26. Acrylic groove, **A,** holding the incisors and, **B,** uprighting them with a labial bow.

opening of 4 mm in the construction bite to enable the upper and lower incisors to be retruded. This could be performed easily because of the spacing between the teeth. The incisors were capped on the labial with acrylic, and the acrylic was ground away on the lingual in the alveolar and dental areas. The molars were extruded with guided eruption. The lower incisors were uprighted more than the uppers. The upper molars were guided distally with stabilizing wires at the mesial embrasures.

After 4½ years of treatment and retention the Class II relationship had improved, with the mandible positioned more anteriorly. The growth increment of the mandibular base was average whereas that of the maxillary basal growth was +2.5 mm above average. For this reason, not only the S-N-B but also the S-N-A angle increased. The basal relationship of Ar-Pog to Ar-A improved only from 10 to 15 mm. The growth pattern became horizontal. In spite of the not too favorable reaction of the maxillary base to therapy, the lower incisors were uprighted during the anterior positioning of the mandible from 104.0 to 95 degrees (Fig. 8-28).

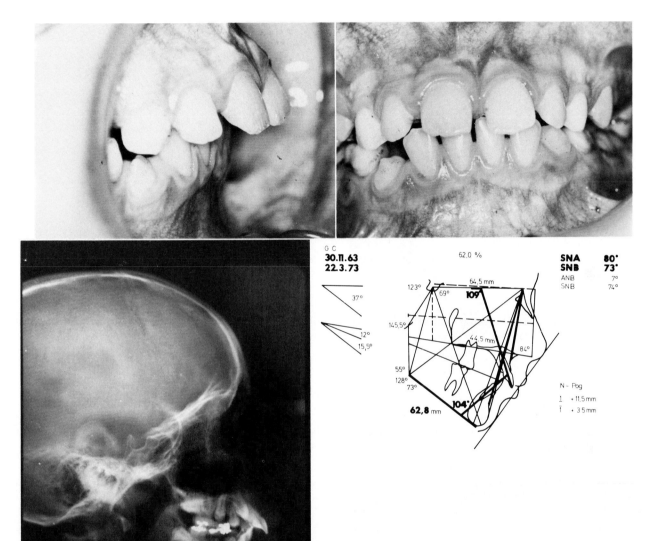

Fig. 8-27. Patient G.C. before treatment. Note the labially tipped upper and lower incisors.

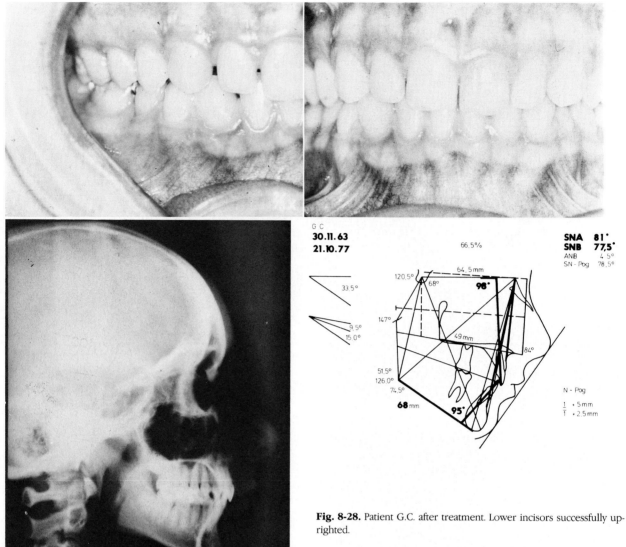

Fig. 8-28. Patient G.C. after treatment. Lower incisors successfully uprighted.

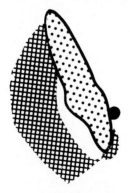

Fig. 8-29. Extension of the acrylic labially on the upper incisors and grinding in the dental area lingually. The labioincisal cap guides the incisors lingually. The labial bow is active.

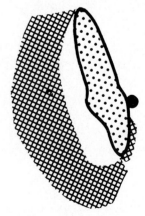

Fig. 8-30. Design for an upper V activator. The acrylic is extended labially up to the middle third of the labial surface and lingually over the whole dentoalveolar and palatal area.

Design of the upper incisor area. Some variations in activator design in the upper incisor area have already been described. In deep overbite cases the incisal edges are loaded with the acrylic rim. In open bite cases the acrylic is ground away to enable the teeth to be extruded. For protrusion the lingual surfaces are loaded.

A special design for the upper incisor area is required for retrusive movements and in the construction of the vertical activator. For retrusion of the upper incisors it requires that the acrylic be ground away and the labial bow be active. During retrusion the incisors are extruded. In deep overbite cases, however, extrusion is undesirable so the construction demands a labial acrylic capping with incisal contact. This creates an oblique guide plane at the labioincisal, effectively guiding the incisors lingually while not allowing them to erupt (Fig. 8-29). The acrylic is ground away on the lingual up to the labioincisal margin and inclined plane just described. The labial bow is active. The incisors are thus moved lingually along the path dictated by the acrylic guide plane on the incisal margin, with extrusion.

In constructing the vertical activator, the design for the upper incisor area is similar to that required for retrusion and deep overbite cases. However, some differences in design do exist:

1. The labial acrylic cap is extended up to the area of greatest convexity, at about the junction of the incisal and middle thirds of the labial surface (Fig. 8-30).
2. The acrylic is completely ground away on the lingual of the incisors and away from the palatogingival tissue contiguous with the incisor alveolar support area.
3. The labial bow contacts the teeth on the gingival third.

This design has a twofold objective: it should influence the axial inclination of the teeth, but also it is hoped that it will affect the inclination of the maxillary base in vertically growing patterns. (This inclination change is possible because of the vertical force created by the high construction bite.)

Movements of the posterior teeth in the sagittal plane. The buccal segment teeth can be moved mesially or distally by the activator. Although large mesiodistal bodily movements are not possible with the activator, modest movements of these teeth can be achieved in Class II or Class III malocclusions. When activator therapy begins in the early mixed dentition, the permanent first molars should be sagittally controlled by the appliance. During eruption the premolars can also be guided toward their desired position by grinding the activator properly. As indicated earlier, the molars can be moved mesially or distally by the way the guiding acrylic planes are made to contact the teeth.

For distalizing movements the guide planes load the molars on the mesiolingual surfaces (Fig. 8-31). The guide plane extends only up to the greatest convexity in the mesiodistal plane. A distalizing movement is indicated for the maxillary arch in Class II nonextraction problems. The extent of this movement is limited with activator use. Guiding the eruption of the teeth is an important part of treatment. For increasing the distalizing effect, additional elements can be incorporated in the activator (as outlined previously).

Stabilizing wires or spurs are rigid (0.9 mm) projections from the lingual acrylic that contact the mesial surface of the first permanent molars interproximally (Fig. 8-32). It is possible to prevent mesial movement with these wires. When treatment is begun with a headgear or lip bumper and continued with an activator, stabilizing wires should be used to prevent mesial migration of the first molar teeth. The stabilizing wires also serve to implement distalizing eruption guidance for the first molars. This can be accomplished with a slight activation of the wires, bending them distally or using the reciprocal force created by a protruding adjustment on the maxillary incisor teeth where needed.

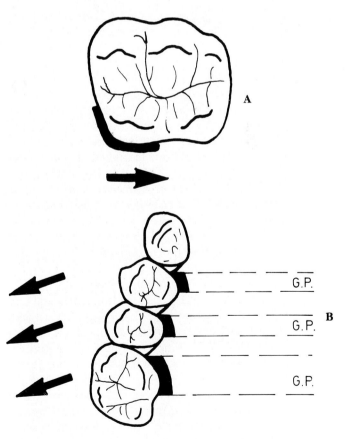

Fig. 8-31. Distal movements of the molars. **A,** Loaded area and, **B,** guide planes.

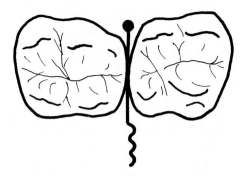

Fig. 8-32. Stabilizing wire. Used also for distalizing the molars or preventing their mesial movement.

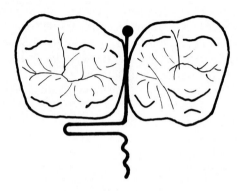

Fig. 8-33. Active open spring. To effect sagittal tooth movement.

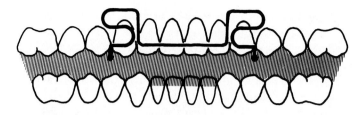

Fig. 8-34. Labial bow with loops for the canines. To effect distalization.

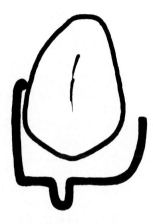

Fig. 8-35. Guiding wires. Developed by Petrik, these move the canines distally.

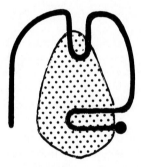

Fig. 8-36. Retraction spring for the canines. These are 0.6 mm in diameter and are active springs.

Distalizing guidance of maxillary molars is also possible with active open springs (Fig. 8-33).

Occasionally, particularly in first premolar extraction cases, a distalizing of the canine teeth is needed. This can be done with various additional appurtenances.

1. Originally the labial bow was modified to move the canines distally (Fig. 8-34). The lateral U-shaped bends of the bow were connected with the horizontal middle portion by loops. This design had one major disadvantage: it was difficult to activate the loops for distalizing the canines and the middle portion of the bow for retruding the incisors at the same time.

2. Petrik suggested the use of guiding wires for this purpose (Fig. 8-35). These work independently of the labial bow. They are rigid (0.8 to 0.9 mm) and contact the mesial surfaces of the canines. They have a U-shaped outline to permit their adaptation.

3. Another variation in canine retraction is the use of retraction springs (Fig. 8-36). These contact the canine mesiolabially over a large surface. They can be pulled back or activated by a parallel movement, enabling the canines to be moved back with only a slight tipping. The springs are active wires of 0.6 mm diameter.

Mesial movement of buccal segment teeth is accomplished by having the acrylic guide planes of the activator contact the teeth on the distolingual surfaces. The guiding planes extend up only to the greatest lingual circumference in the mesiodistal plane (Fig. 8-37). A mesial movement of the posterior teeth is indicated only in the upper dental arch in Class III malocclusions without crowding.

In Class II malocclusions the guiding planes for the lower posterior teeth are ground not for mesial movement but for either expansion or extrusion. There is already a mesial force component present because of the reciprocal intermaxillary anchorage created by the con-

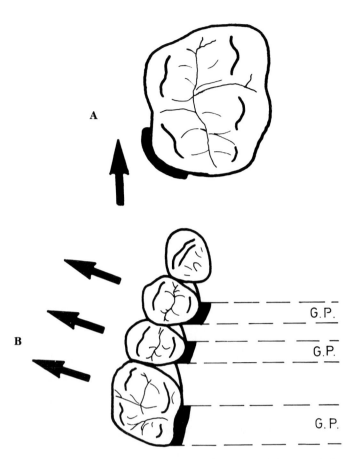

Fig. 8-37. Mesial movements of the molars. **A,** Loaded area and, **B,** guide planes.

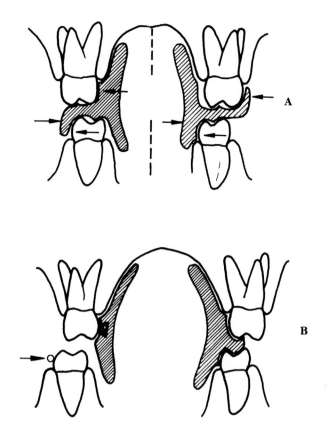

Fig. 8-38. Transverse effectiveness of the activator. **A,** In cross-bite cases. **B,** By anchoring the appliance on one side and moving the teeth on the opposite side with pegs or springs or the addition of soft acrylic.

struction bite and the influence of the stretched retractor muscles on the anteriorly positioned mandible. A mesial driving of the lower teeth could aggravate the labial inclination of the lower incisors (Björk). This is seldom needed, as has been pointed out previously.

Movements of the teeth in the transverse plane. It should be pointed out that if the construction bite is shifted to one side or the other an asymmetric action is created in the transverse plane (Fig. 8-38). This is a contralateral reciprocal force and could be needed for the alignment of an asymmetric narrow maxillary arch on one side and a narrowness of the mandibular arch on the other. Such treatment cannot be controlled very well, however, and alignment of asymmetric dental arches is done better with other appliances.

It is possible to trim the activator to stimulate expansion of the buccal segment teeth, although the opportunities are limited compared to those available with active plates, jackscrews, etc. To achieve transvere movement, the lingual acrylic surfaces opposite the posterior teeth must be in contact with the teeth (Fig. 8-39). If a higher level of force is required in one dental arch or tooth area, this can be obtained by adding a thin layer

of self-curing soft acrylic. More effective expansion is obtained by using expansion-type jackscrews while trimming the appliance to enhance the expansion. To achieve a symmetric force application, the expansion screw is placed in the anterior intermaxillary portion of the appliance (Fig. 8-40). This construction is quite bulky, however, and pushes the tongue posteriorly. The appliance can also be made with two eccentrically placed jackscrews in the upper and lower portions. (See also Chapter 6.) The anterior acrylic portion can then be partially cut out.

Single teeth can also be moved laterally. If there is a cross-bite condition for one or more teeth, the malocclusion can be corrected with two springs and corresponding grinding of the appliance (Fig. 8-41). The upper molar is moved buccally with a closed loop spring, the lower molar in buccal cross-bite is moved lingually with a frame loop. The acrylic is ground away on the lingual of the lower molar.

Transverse mesiodistal movements in the incisor region for single teeth can be achieved using guiding or rigid wire elements and are often needed to close existing spaces.

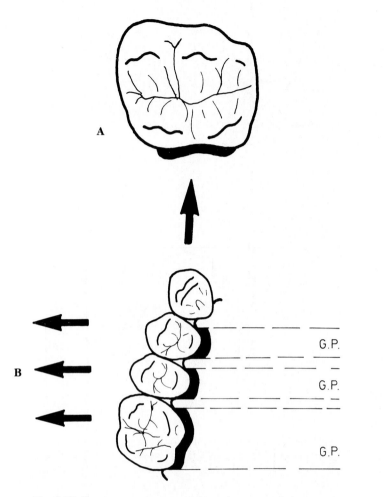

Fig. 8-39. Transverse movement of the molars. **A,** Loaded area and, **B,** guide planes.

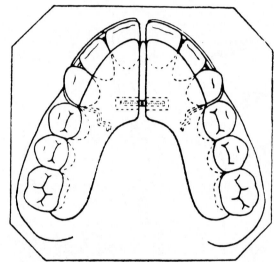

Fig. 8-40. Expansion jackscrew built into the activator.

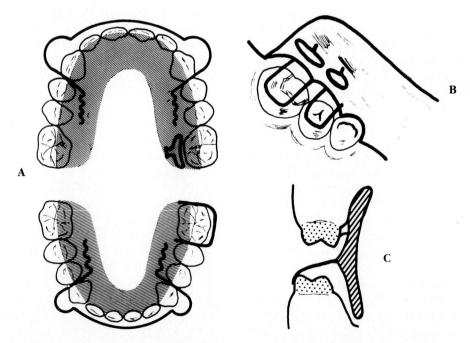

Fig. 8-41. Modification for the cross-bite correction of single molars. **A,** Protrusive spring in the upper and closed loop in the lower molar areas. **B,** Both springs from above. **C,** Springs in cross section.

Guidelines

Although single tooth movements have already been discussed, in activator therapy only combined movements are done simultaneously on anterior and posterior teeth in various directions. Before selective grinding of the activator begins, some sort of treatment plan should be made, listing the areas to be trimmed and the reason for each grinding procedure. For the general categories of malocclusions, general trimming procedures can be described, not losing sight of the fact that individual variation may be necessary for specific individual problems.

Activator trimming in Class II malocclusions (Fig. 8-42)

For incisors. The upper incisors are to be retruded, and the labial bow is active. In some cases an acrylic capping is necessary to prevent extrusion along with the retrusion. The lower incisors are to be protruded, and the labial bow is passive. There are a number of modifications in the acrylic design depending on the requirements of holding or retruding the lower incisors or of preventing eruption, as in a deep bite case, using acrylic capping when possible to prevent excessive labial inclination of these teeth.

For posterior teeth. The upper posterior teeth are to be moved posteriorly or are withheld from mesial movement by guide planes and stabilizing wires. To guide eruption and level the curve of Spee, the acrylic is trimmed away next to the lower posterior teeth. The lower teeth tend to move mesially as they erupt, however, so this is expected to make a small contribution to correction of the sagittal malrelationship. The eruption of the upper teeth should be prevented as much as possible, to reduce the rocking open of the mandible (which increases the retrognathism). Selective grinding of the acrylic, so the guiding planes will contact the mesiolingual cusp surfaces of the buccal segment teeth, enhances the Class II correction. Stabilizing wires or spurs may also assist in the distalizing process as the first molar teeth erupt to some degree.

Activator trimming in Class III malocclusions (Fig. 8-43)

For incisors. The upper incisors are loaded for protrusion, and the labial bow is passive. If the upper incisors are in the process of eruption, they can be guided labially along acrylic guide planes or by adding a thin layer of self-cure cold acrylic lingual to the teeth. Lip pads may be used instead of a labial bow to stimulate all possible basal maxillary development. The lower incisors should be retruded. The acrylic to the lingual of the lower incisors is ground away, and there is a labial acrylic cap. The lower labial bow is active. The acrylic does not touch either the lingual of the lower incisors or the alveolar crest. The lower anterior portion of the activator can be completely trimmed away or left open, because no force application is required in this area. The activator cannot influence the flat position of the tongue, so often seen in Class III malocclusions. Al-

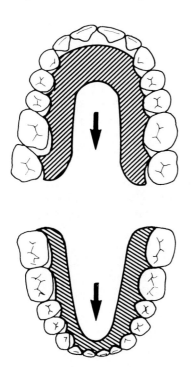

Fig. 8-42. Plan of trimming the acrylic interdental projections for distal driving of the upper teeth and mesial movement of the lower in Class II malocclusions.

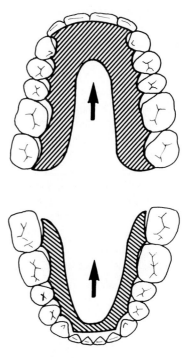

Fig. 8-43. Plan of trimming for mesial movement of the upper teeth and distal driving of the lower in Class II malocclusions.

though leaving the anterior portion of the acrylic out and the space open makes the appliance less bulky, the incorporation of a wire crib for tongue control is recommended in some cases.

For posterior teeth. The guide planes for the upper posterior teeth are trimmed for mesial movement. Eruption is encouraged in a downward and forward direction. The lower posterior teeth have guide planes trimmed to contact the mesiolingual cuspal surfaces for all possible posterior vector stimulus as these teeth erupt. The eruption is kept to a minimum, however.

Activator trimming in vertical dysplasia–type malocclusions

Deep overbite malocclusions. The incisor area is trimmed for intrusion, the molar area for extrusion. The labial bow is active and contacts the teeth at their incisal third.

Open bite malocclusions. The incisor area is ground away for extrusion, the molar area for intrusion. The labial bow is active and contacts the incisor teeth at their gingival third.

SUMMARY

Both skeletal and dentoalveolar changes can be achieved in activator functional appliance therapy. However, the functional method has its limitations. The best time to approach most malocclusions is in the mixed dentition. The activator can solve many of the problems that become more severe if left unattended. The restoration of normal function is a major contribution to the morphofunctional interrelationship. If treatment objectives require more orthodontic guidance, therapy can continue with or may replace the functional appliance method using fixed or removable appliances in the permanent dentition. Sometimes combination therapy is indicated, even in the mixed dentition, as the activator is combined with expansion plates or extraoral force.

The construction bite varies for different types and degrees of abnormality. Depending on the timing, technique, and trimming, significant facial and occlusal changes can be achieved. Next to the elimination of abnormal perioral muscle function, growth guidance is the major contribution of functional therapy. The correction of functional retrusions (Class II), protrusions (Class III), or lateral functional shifts is simple with the activator. The trimming technique permits guidance of eruption and individual tooth movements. Occlusal changes

can be seen in all three planes of space. In the sagittal plane it is possible to reposition the mandible, protrude and retrude incisors, and move buccal segment teeth mesiodistally. In the vertical plane routine objectives include guiding the inclination of the maxillary base (and its growth direction) and extruding teeth. In the transverse plane one can correct a functional crossbite, expand the dental arches, and correct single tooth crossbites.

The limitations of functional appliance therapy should be recognized. First, it should not be considered a "stand-alone" regimen, a method for full correction of all malocclusions. The elimination of abnormal perioral muscle function and the guidance of growth and eruption of teeth are important treatment objectives, but there are other facets of malocclusions that respond better to other biomechanics and that can be used separately or in conjunction with the activator or its modifications. The degree of success in skeletal problems depends on growth timing, direction, and magnitude. Dentoalveolar changes are best accomplished during the eruption of teeth.

The functional appliance is quite effective in the treatment of mandibular retrognathism in patients with a horizontal growth pattern. It is less effective in its influence on maxillary prognathism or a vertical growth pattern, being contraindicated in some instances and requiring special modification in others. And it is inappropriate for certain situations—extensive bodily movement, torque, rotation, and intrusion of teeth.

The clinician must consider the special characteristics of each malocclusion before fabricating the activator, since the appliance can and should be designed for the individual. The construction bite, the grinding technique, the function and placement of the labial bow, and the possible need for other appurtenances are all subject to discretionary diagnosis and treatment planning ahead of time. For example, the degree of protrusion or opening for the construction bite, the anchorage of the appliance, and the relationship of teeth to the appliance are prime considerations.

A popular and effective modification of the classic activator is the so-called Bionator, introduced by Balters, and modified subsequently by other clinicians. Because of its special design and anchorage considerations, as well as the trimming technique, it is discussed in the next chapter.

CHAPTER 9

THE BIONATOR—
A MODIFIED ACTIVATOR

PRINCIPLES OF BIONATOR THERAPY

The bulkiness of the activator and its limitation to nighttime wear only put significant constraints on its use and success for clinicians interested in attaining the greatest potential of functional growth guidance. During sleep, function is obviously minimal or nonexistent; hence the term "functional appliance" for an activator is not completely correct in the strictest sense. To meet this criticism, a number of modifications have been made to produce a less bulky appliance, a more elastic appliance, one that can be worn during both the day and the night, and one that has the highest possible degree of efficiency.

The Bionator is the prototype of a less bulky appliance. Its lower portion is narrow and its upper has only lateral extensions, with a cross-palatal stabilizing bar. The palate is free for proprioceptive contact with the tongue; the buccinator wire loops hold away potentially deforming muscular action; the appliance may be worn all the time except during meals. Balters developed this appliance during the early 1950s, at the same time that Bimler was working (in the same direction) with a skeletonized activator. Although the theoretical principles of the Balters appliance are based on the works of Robin, Andresen, and Häupl, there are basic differences from the activator.

According to Balters the equilibrium between the tongue and circumoral muscles is responsible for the shape of the dental arches and intercuspation (Fig. 9-1). The functional space for the tongue is essential to the normal development of the orofacial system. This hypothesis supports the early function and form concepts of van der Klaauw and the later functional matrix theory of Moss. To Balters the tongue, as the center of reflex activity in the oral cavity, was the most important factor. A discoordination of its manifold functions could lead to abnormal growth accomplishment and to actual deformation. The purpose of the Bionator was to establish good functional coordination and eliminate these deforming growth-restricting aberrations.

Balters was of the opinion that the position of the tongue must be considered carefully in planning therapy since it was responsible for certain types of malocclusions. For example, posterior displacement of the tongue could lead to a Class II malocclusion; low anterior displacement could cause a Class III malocclusion; narrowing of the arches, with resultant crowding, particularly of the maxillary arch, was the result of diminished outward pressure during both postural rest and function, as opposed to the forces from the buccinator mechanism on the outside; and open bite was the consequence of hyperactivity and forward posturing of the tongue.

Nevertheless, despite the initial ostensible similarity of this concept to the functional matrix theories of Moss, which came later, there was a significant difference. Balters felt that only the role of the tongue was decisive. With his lateral wire configurations to relieve the forces of the surrounding neuromuscular structures, he took only secondary consideration of the neuromuscular envelope. According to the research of Winders in 1956, however, the tongue exerts three to four times as much force on the dentition as the buccal and labial musculature does; so this would seem to support the Balters

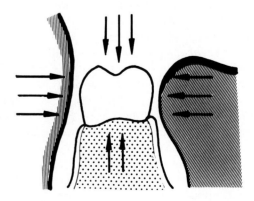

Fig. 9-1. In the transverse plane, muscle forces influence the position of the teeth; in the vertical plane, occlusal forces do this.

thesis, if resting force and other factors (tissue rigidity, the elastic index, atmospheric pressures, and intercuspation) are not considered.

Because of his conviction about the dominant role of the tongue, Balters designed his appliance to take advantage of tongue posture. He constructed it to position the mandible anteriorly with the incisors in an edge-to-edge relationship, which he considered important for natural bodily orientation; and since the forward posturing of the mandible was what enlarged the oral space, bringing the dorsum of the tongue into contact with the soft palate to help accomplish lip closure, this was used to help patients learn the normal functional patterns.

The principle of treatment with the Bionator is not to activate the muscles but to modulate muscle activity, thereby enhancing normal development of the inherent growth pattern and eliminating abnormal and potentially deforming environmental factors. In light of this, the Bionator falls between the simpler screening appliances and the activator.

Unlike the construction bite of the activator, however, that of the Bionator cannot accommodate to facial pattern and growth direction by variations in vertical opening as the mandible is postured forward. The bite cannot be opened and must be positioned in an edge-to-edge relationship. If the overjet is too large, however, the forward posturing can be done step-by-step, but still not opening the bite. Balters reasoned that there could not be adequate control of tongue function with a high construction bite and that the patient could actually acquire a tongue thrust habit as the mandible dropped open and the tongue instinctively moved forward to maintain an open airway.

Since there is no allowance for the vertical component except in guiding eruption of the posterior teeth, the indications are reduced for this appliance. Myotatic reflex activity with isotonic muscle contraction is stimulated, and the loose appliance works with kinetic energy. The viscoelastic properties of muscles and soft tissues and the stretch reflex response are not utilized in the vertical dimension as with the Harvold-Woodside type of activator. The behavior of the lips and tongue is directly influenced by the labial bow and palatal bar. It is possible, however to create sagittal and vertical dentoalveolar changes with the appliance in certain sucking habits. Nevertheless, the main consideration still is to influence the function of the tongue, in contradistinction to that with the Fränkel appliance, whose main aim is to influence the outer neuromuscular envelope. With the creation of normal function, desired changes will then occur. It is common knowledge now that abnormal tongue function can be secondary, adaptive, or compensatory because of skeletal maldevelopment; but this was not taken into consideration by Balters in the original version of his appliance.

The main advantage of the Bionator lies in its reduced size, which means that it can be worn day and night. The appliance exerts a constant influence on the tongue and perioral muscles, because of the screening effect of the labial bow and its lateral extensions (which hold off muscle contact with the dentoalveolar area, particularly in the usually narrowed maxillary arch of Class II, Division 1, malocclusions). Since unfavorable external and internal muscle forces are prevented from exerting undesirable and restrictive effects on the dentition and supporting structures for a longer time, the action is faster with the Bionator than with the classic activator. Constant wear results in more rapid sagittal adjustment of the musculature to the forward mandibular posture since the mandible retracts only during eating (or a small percentage of the time).

The main disadvantage of the Bionator lies in the difficulty of correctly managing it. This is because of the simultaneous requirements of stabilization of the appliance plus selective grinding for eruption guidance. The normalization of function can occur only if the inherent growth pattern is normal in the first place, with no environmental influences to prevent accomplishment of that pattern. In the case of skeletal disturbances, however, the effectiveness of the Balters Bionator is very limited, even as it is for any functional appliance. The various activators can be modified for different growth directions (the **H** or **V** activator constructions). A correct differential diagnosis is essential for successful Bionator treatment; and problems must be functional-type retrusions, with relatively normal skeletal potential and sufficient growth increments to permit a favorable change. A further potential disadvantage, shared with other skeletonized activators (the Bimler appliance particularly), is the vulnerability to distortion, since there is far less acrylic support in the alveolar and incisal region.

Of course, the Bionator can be modified, as other functional appliances have been, to satisfy some of these criticisms.

BIONATOR TYPES

There are three basic constructions of the Bionator: the standard, the open bite, and the reversed or Class III.

Standard appliance (Fig. 9-2)

The standard appliance consists of a lower horseshoe-shaped acrylic lingual plate extending from the distal of the last erupted molar around to the corresponding point on the other side. For the upper arch the appliance has only posterior lingual extensions that cover the molar and premolar regions. The anterior portion is open from canine to canine. The upper and lower parts, which are joined interocclusally in the correct construction bite relationship, extend 2 mm above the upper and below the lower gingival margin. The upper anterior portion is kept free so as not to interfere with tongue function. However, tongue function is kept under control by the edge-to-edge incisal contact relationship, leaving no space for thrusting activity. When it is possible to establish this relationship, no acrylic capping of the lower incisors is done. If there is some space between the upper and lower incisors in the construction bite, then acrylic can be extended to cap the lower incisors. This does not really hinder the potential procumbency of these teeth, however, since the labial wire does not contact them and the capping is only partially successful in preventing labial tipping—a limitation of the Bionator, particularly when lower incisors are already labially inclined.

The function and posture of the lips and cheeks are guided by two wire constructions, the palatal bar and the labial bow with buccal extensions. The palatal bar is formed of 1.2 mm hard stainless steel wire extending from the top edges of the lingual acrylic flanges in the middle area of the deciduous first molars (Fig. 9-3). The palatal bar lies approximately 1 mm away from the palatal mucosa and runs distally as far as a transpalatal line between the distal portions of the maxillary permanent first molars to form an oval posteriorly directed loop that reinserts on the opposite side in mirror fashion.

The cross-palatal bar stabilizes the appliance and si-multaneously orients the tongue and mandible anteriorly to achieve a Class I relationship. The forward orientation of the tongue, according to Balters, is accomplished by stimulating its dorsal surface with the palatal bar. This is the reason for the posterior curve of the palatal bar.

The labial bow, made of 0.9 mm hard stainless steel wire (Fig. 9-4), begins above the contact point between the canine and deciduous upper first molar (or premolar). It then runs vertically upward, making a rounded 90-degree bend to the distal along the middle of the crowns of the posterior teeth, and extends as far as the embrasure between the deciduous second molar and the permanent first molar. Scribing a gentle downward and forward curve, it runs anteriorly at about the same position with respect to the buccal surfaces of the lower posterior teeth as far as the lower canine. From there, at a sharp angle obliquely upward, it extends toward the upper canine, bends to a level line at approximately the incisal third of the incisors, and runs to the canine on the opposite side. It ends in mirror-image form on the opposite side and inserts again into the acrylic. The labial portion of the bow should be approximately the thickness of a sheet of ordinary typewriter paper from the incisors.

This position of the wire gives rise to a negative pressure, with the wire supporting lip closure. In the course

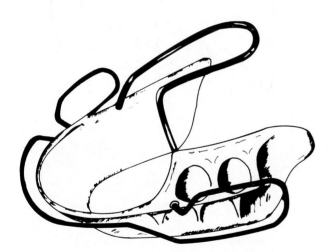

Fig. 9-2. The Balters Bionator basic appliance.

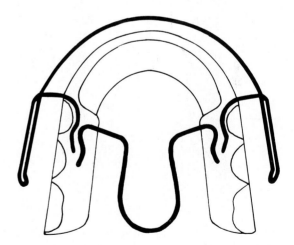

Fig. 9-3. Palatal bar of 12 mm hard stainless steel for the basic appliance.

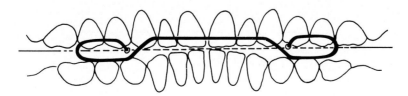

Fig. 9-4. Labial bow of 0.9 mm hard stainless steel for the basic appliance.

of treatment, however, the wire should upright the incisors and provide space when the dental arch is widened. The posterior portions of the labial bow are designed as buccinator loops, screening muscle forces in the vestibule (Fig. 9-5). The loops are sufficiently away from the teeth to allow for expansion but not so far as to cause discomfort to the cheeks. The buccinator loops screen the buccinator muscles, and the lingual acrylic parts prevent both the cheeks and the tongue from interposing in the interocclusal space. Thus, with proper trimming, it is possible to stimulate selective eruption.

Open bite appliance (Fig. 9-6)

The open bite appliance is used to inhibit abnormal posture and function of the tongue. The construction bite is as low as possible, but a slight opening allows the interposition of posterior acrylic bite blocks for the posterior teeth to prevent their extrusion. To inhibit tongue movements, the acrylic portion of the lower lingual part extends into the upper incisor region as a lingual shield, closing off the anterior space without touching the upper teeth.

The palatal bar has the same configuration as in the standard Bionator, with the function of moving the tongue into a more posterior or caudal position.

The labial bow is of similar form to that in the standard appliance, differing only as the wire runs approximately between the incisal edges of the upper and lower incisors (Fig. 9-7). The labial part of the bow is placed at the height of correct lip closure, thus stimulating the lips to achieve a competent seal and relationship. The vertical strain on the lips tends to encourage the extrusive movement of the incisors, after elimination of the adverse tongue pressures.

Class III or reversed Bionator (Fig. 9-8)

The Class III or reversed Bionator type of appliance is used to encourage the development of the maxilla. The construction bite is taken in the most retruded position possible, as with the Function Regulator of Fränkel, to allow labial movement of the maxillary incisors and at the same time exert a slight restrictive effect on the lower arch. The bite is slightly opened, about 2 mm of interincisal space, for this purpose. The lower acrylic portion is extended incisally from canine to canine. This extension is positioned behind the upper incisors, which are stimulated to glide anteriorly along the resultant inclined plane. The acrylic is trimmed away behind

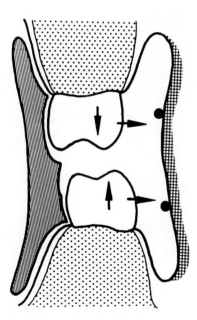

Fig. 9-5. Buccinator loop in the deciduous molar region. It screens excessive force of the muscle.

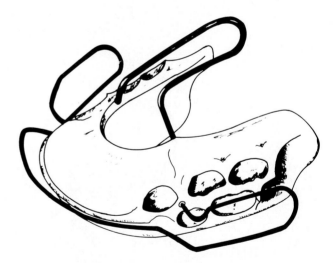

Fig. 9-6. The open bite Bionator appliance.

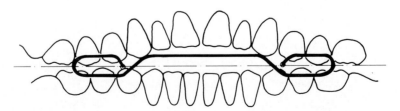

Fig. 9-7. Labial bow for the open bite appliance. It crosses the interincisal area.

the lower incisors about 1 mm so as not to tip the lower incisors labially.

The palatal bar configuration runs forward instead of posteriorly, with the loop extending as far as the deciduous first molars or premolars (Fig. 9-9). From this point the wire runs back to the upper margin of the acrylic, posterior to the distal surface of the permanent first molar, where it enters the acrylic with a right-angle bend. The tongue is supposedly stimulated to remain in a retracted position and in its proper functional space. It should contact the anterior portion of the palate, encouraging the forward growth of this area.

The labial bow runs in front of the lower incisors rather than in front of the upper incisors as in the standard appliance (Fig. 9-10). It emerges from the acrylic in the same manner as in the standard appliance, but the labial part runs straight along the lower incisors without a bend in the canine region. The wire either touches the labial surfaces lightly or stands away the thickness of a sheet of paper.

TERMINOLOGY USED IN TRIMMING THE BIONATOR APPLIANCE

Since the volume of the appliance is reduced, its anchorage is more difficult than that of the activator. The trimming of the appliance must be selective because of the simultaneous requirements of anchorage. To understand these problems, Balters introduced some new terms:

1. *Articular plane.* This is the plane that extends from the tips of the cusps of the upper first molars, premolars, and canines to the mesial margin of the upper central incisors. Running parallel to the alar-tragal line, it is considered important for the assessment of the mode of trimming (Fig. 9-11).

2. *Loading area.* The palatal or lingual cusps of the deciduous molars (or premolars) and permanent first molars are relieved in the acrylic part of the appliance. The grinding away of acrylic here enhances the achorage of the appliance (Fig. 9-12).

3. *Tooth bed.* Some parts of the loading areas are trimmed away to the articular plane. Acrylic surfaces prepared in this manner are termed the tooth bed (Fig. 9-13).

4. *Nose.* Between the tooth beds, interdentally, there are acrylic fingerlike projections called "noses" (Fig. 9-14). These extensions act both as guiding surfaces and as sources of anchorage for the appliance in the sagittal and vertical planes.

5. *Ledge.* Depending on the tooth movements desired, the appliance acrylic is trimmed and the "nose" reduced. A reduced plastic extension placed only on the occlusal third of the interdental area is called a "ledge" (Fig. 9-15). The nose is mostly on the mesial margin of the first permanent molars whereas the ledge is between the premolars or deciduous molars.

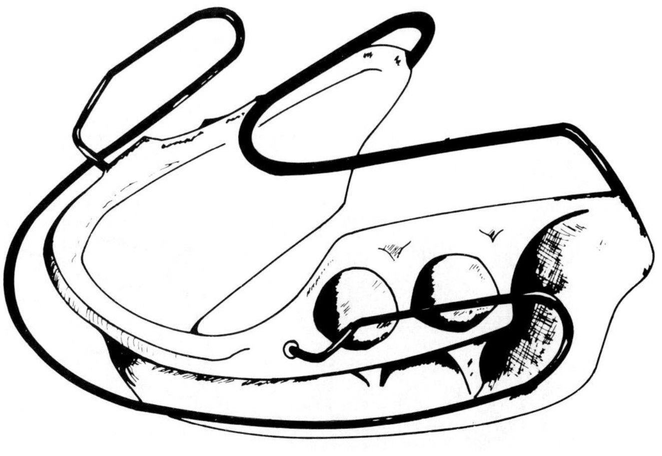

Fig. 9-8. The reversed Bionator appliance for Class III malocclusions.

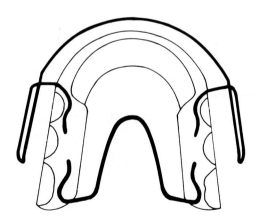

Fig. 9-9. Palatal bar for the reversed appliance. The loop extends anteriorly to the canine–deciduous first molar embrasure.

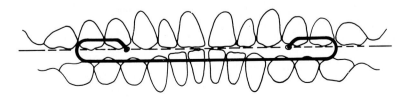

Fig. 9-10. Labial bow for the Class III reversed appliance.

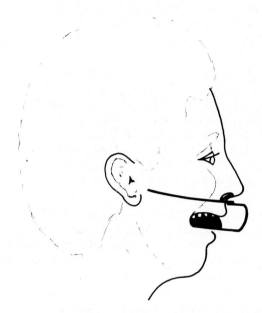

Fig. 9-11. Assessment of the articular plane before impression taking. It should parallel the alar-tragal line.

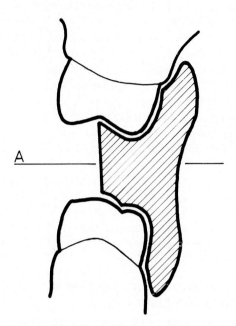

Fig. 9-12. Loading area. *A,* Articular plane.

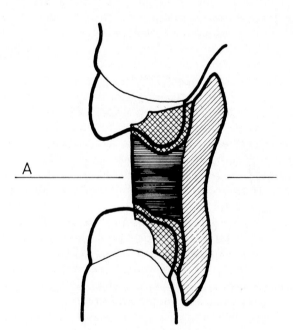

Fig. 9-13. Tooth bed. Acrylic is trimmed to a thin cap over the opposing teeth. *A,* Articular plane.

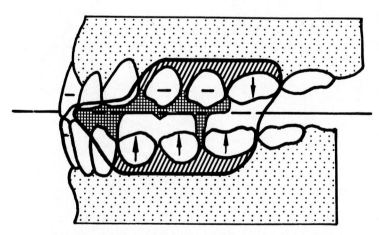

Fig. 9-14. "Nose" in the lower first molar region (acrylic interdental projection).

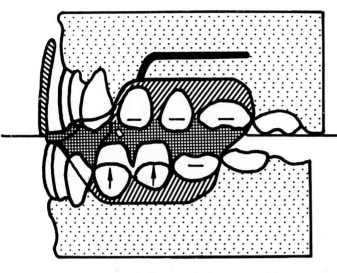

Fig. 9-15. Ledge between the lower premolars.

ANCHORAGE OF THE APPLIANCE

Since the bulk, volume, and extension of the appliance are reduced, there are special requirements for anchorage. When treatment is begun with the Bionator, it is not possible to trim all the guiding acrylic planes simultaneously for all the areas. Some acrylic surfaces are used for stabilization of the appliance; others can be ground as needed to effect the desired tooth movement stimulus. In the second stage of treatment it is necessary to alternate the loaded or stabilizing areas with the areas being trimmed for tooth guidance. Stabilization or anchorage of the appliance is obtained from the following:

1. Incisal margins of the lower incisors, by extending the acrylic over the incisal margin as a cap
2. Loading areas, since the cusps of the teeth fit into the respective grooves in the acrylic
3. Deciduous molars, which can always be used as anchor teeth
4. Edentulous areas, after premature loss of the deciduous molars
5. "Noses" in the upper and lower interdental spaces
6. Labial bow, which, if correctly placed, will prevent posterior displacement of the appliance

TRIMMING THE BIONATOR

The anchorage of the Bionator permits an anterior posturing of the mandible, which is determined by the construction bite. As on the activator, trimming of the occlusal surfaces on the Bionator is essential to allow certain teeth to erupt further while fully erupted teeth are prevented from further eruption by contact with the acrylic. Balters' terminology refers to stimulation of eruption as "unloading" or "promotion of growth" and prevention of eruption as "loading" or "inhibition of

growth." By trimming of the acrylic "tooth beds" and elimination of the influence of tongue and cheeks, the teeth are free to erupt until they reach the articular plane. Once there, they should be allowed to erupt no further so the loading can be accomplished by the addition of self-curing acrylic as needed. The appliance can be trimmed or ground periodically until the teeth reach the desired relationship with the articular plane. Because of the need to anchor the appliance (as pointed out already), this procedure cannot be performed in all areas at the same time. Thus it is necessary to load and unload the same area periodically. This means that the same tooth can function as an anchor and then later be allowed to erupt.

The difficulty in managing the classic Bionator is the alternate loading and unloading of certain areas. On one visit acrylic will be added to load a specific tooth. On the next visit it may be ground away in the same area. Especially in cases of deep overbite, there must be enough space to allow for the full eruptive potential of the teeth. Deciduous teeth, if present, are used as anchors. The types of anchorage, according to Ascher, are as follows:

Dentition	Anchorage
1, 2, III-V, 6	IV, V—upper and lower
1, 2, III-V, 6	V and space after IV
1, 2, II-6	alveolar process—IV, V
1, 2, III, 4-6	6 and alveolar process

If there are deciduous molars present, the anchorage is not difficult. If the premolars are already erupting, however, a change in the loading and unloading areas is necessary.

Since the method of trimming or selective grinding on the Bionator is similar to that on the activator, only the main differences will be described here.

1. To allow extrusion of the posterior teeth, some acrylic is always left interdentally at the level of the occlusal (articular) plane, forming the so-called tooth bed (Fig. 9-16). The upper and lower molar regions should be trimmed first. Then the lower premolars are trimmed while the molars are loaded. Finally, the upper premolars are stimulated while the lower premolars and molars are loaded. Care must be taken to ensure that the lingual acrylic surfaces do not interfere with eruption (Fig. 9-17).
2. The acrylic projections between the teeth (the "noses") are left untouched, or they can be replaced with self-curing acrylic. Their role is similar to that of the stabilizing spurs of the conventional activator—a distalizing influence on the permanent first molars. Instead of the noses, guiding wires of 0.8 to 0.9 mm can be used. These are fabricated of

stainless steel, as with the activator. This is especially true if space opening is required or if treatment has been begun with extraoral force. The noses in the areas of the lower molars must be well defined to prevent the mandible from dropping back.

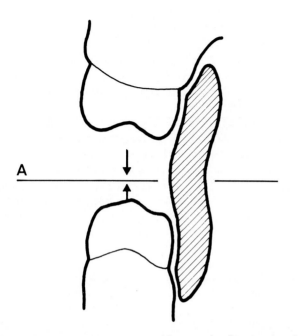

Fig. 9-16. Unloading of the upper and lower molars for extrusion. *A,* Articular plane.

3. To facilitate transverse movement, the occlusal surfaces of the Bionator are trimmed. However, on closure, the cusp tips should remain in contact with the so-called tooth bed. In cases of open bite the posterior teeth are fully loaded for intrusion (Fig. 9-18).

CLINICAL MANAGEMENT OF THE BIONATOR TREATMENT

For maximum beneficial effect, the Bionator must be worn both day and night. The time interval between visits are 3 to 5 weeks depending on the state of eruption of the individual teeth.

The labial bow should be checked to ensure that it touches the teeth only lightly if at all. The buccinator loops should be away from the deciduous first and second molar areas but should not irritate the cheek mucosa. If expansion is required, the loops can be activated. In the final stages minor spaces can be closed by active retraction of the bow.

In accordance with the plan of anchorage and growth promotion, the loading and unloading of acrylic areas or planes must be done according to whether tooth movement is to be stimulated or retarded. Again, it should be emphasized that this is true of the first molars initially, the lower premolars (if present) secondly, and the upper premolars thirdly—alternating the unloading and loading for anchorage purposes to stabilize the appliance.

During the first phase of treatment it is quite usual for rapid horizontal and vertical changes to occur in the

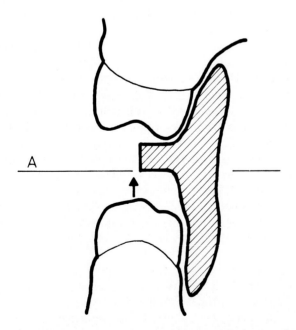

Fig. 9-17. Loading of the upper and unloading of the lower molars. *A,* Articular plane.

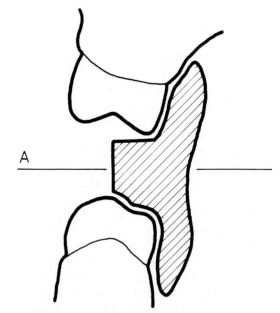

Fig. 9-18. Loading of the upper and lower molars, with expansion effect for the uppers. *A,* Articular plane.

mandibular position. This first change is a muscular adaptation to the new position, with a foreshortening of the lateral pterygoid muscle (as shown by Petrovic and associates). The rapid changes lead to an open bite in the posterior segments. It is in the second stage that articular and dentoalveolar adaptation occurs, following neuromuscular adaptation. The dentoalveolar changes in the deciduous molar area are often insufficient; thus the posterior open bite in this area persists until the premolars can be guided into full occlusion, under the corrective stimulus of the appliance.

INDICATIONS FOR BIONATOR THERAPY

There is a broad gamut of opinions about the clinical usefulness of the Bionator as Balters envisioned and used it. Some clinicians believe that the appliance is less effective than the activator; others that it can be used in every type of malocclusion. No doubt exists, however, that those who use it without the proper diagnostic study and indications, or the proper clinical acumen, have many failures.

The main objective of the appliance, according to Balters, is to establish a muscular equilibrium between the forces of the tongue and the outer neuromuscular envelope. The form and shape of the dental arches depend on this functional equilibrium. Changes in the equilibrium can lead to deformities that will be manifested in the growth period. The consequences of these dysfunctions may be localized primarily in the dentoalveolar area, which is the reason why the Bionator is so effective in this region (as recent research by Ingrid Janson has shown). Although there are many cases in which treatment with the Bionator alone is possible, in most instances a combination of various therapeutic measures is needed to produce the best result.

Special tooth movements (e.g., rotations, torquings, bodily movements for space closure, or distalizations for opening space) cannot be performed with the Bionator, any more than they can be with the conventional activator, even though the wearing time is doubled. Other mechanisms are available to satisfy these treatment objectives. The treatment of Class II, Division 1, malocclusions in the mixed dentition by using the standard Bionator is indicated under the following conditions:

1. The dental arches are well aligned originally.
2. The mandible is in a posterior position (i.e., functional retrusion).
3. The skeletal discrepancy is not to severe.
4. There is a labial tipping of the upper incisors.

The Bionator is not indicated if the following can be said to be true:

1. The Class II relationship is caused by maxillary prognathism.

2. There is a vertical growth pattern.
3. There is labial tipping of the lower incisors. (An anterior posturing of the mandible with simultaneous uprighting of the lower incisors cannot be performed with the Bionator.)

Cases of deep overbite can also be successfully managed with the standard type of Bionator, after grinding away of the acrylic in a manner that permits uninhibited eruption of the buccal segment teeth. This means a step-by-step trimming in the area of the molars and premolars. The best treatment time is during the eruption of the premolars. However, treatment will be successful only if the deep bite is caused by infraocclusion of the molars and premolars, which is due primarily to lateral tongue posture or thrust. It will not work if the overbite is due to supraclusion of the incisors. In buccal segment infraclusion the freeway space is usually large, which is a good precondition for both the Bionator and the activator. In cases with a strong horizontal growth pattern the Bionator is not indicated for treatment of a deep overbite.

Malocclusions with crowding should be treated with the Bionator, despite some buccal segment expansion that might be achieved because of the buccinator loops. Cases with crowding can be better managed with a specially modified activator or, after eruption of the premolars, with active plates. Of course, fixed appliances provide the best individual tooth control in such cases.

Open bite cases can be handled with the open bite Bionator, in which the buccal segment teeth are loaded for all possible intrusive stimulus. The Bionator is particularly successful in open bite cases that are the consequence of abnormal habits such as finger-sucking, retained infantile deglutitional patterns, or aberrant tongue function. Other methods, however, are indicated in open bite problems with skeletal etiology.

Although Balters recommended his reverse type Bionator for Class III–type malocclusions, other clinicians have had only limited success. The explanation for this failure is as follows:

The design of the appliance loads the mandibular teeth and unloads the upper anterior alveolar portion, where growth stimulation is desired, especially during eruption of the incisors. The objective envisioned by Balters was a functional loading of this maxillary lingual area by increased tongue function. He thought that this could be stimulated by guiding the tongue forward with the palatal bar. This in turn would move the incisors and supporting alveolar process labially. Studies by Rakosi and associates, however, have shown that the palatal bar usually only flattens the dorsum of the tongue and does not move it anteriorly. Whether the loop is opened anteriorly or posteriorly is of no consequence, according to the cinefluorographic records made on patients. The reversed appliance does seem to tip the maxillary incisors labially but does not stimulate basal bone forward movement. Thus the only indication for this type of appliance is in pseudo–Class III problems in which the upper incisors are tipped lingually, causing an anterior mandibular displacement on closure from postural rest to habitual occlusion.

BIONATOR AND TMJ CASES

A special use for the Bionator, with which considerable success has been achieved, is in temporomandibular joint problems. This is especially true in adult patients. A majority of TMJ problems have coincidental bruxism and clenching during the REM period of sleep. Wearing a Bionator at night tends to relax the muscle spasms that occur, particularly of the lateral pterygoid. The design of the appliance for this purpose is similar to that of the standard appliance, the difference being that the construction bite need not move the mandible as far forward. The main purpose is to prevent the riding of the condyle over the posterior edge of the disk, which causes the clicking. By checking clinically, first in habitual occlusion and then in a forward-postured mandible, the operator can determine how far forward the mandible must be brought to eliminate the clicking on the opening maneuver. It can be observed that the clicking usually disappears in these cases when the mandible is opened in the forward posture. This means that the condyle no longer rides over the posterior disk margin, onto the retrodiskal pad. Such action is ultimately damaging to both the disk and the pad, causing objective pain and dysfunction symptoms, headaches, etc. The Bionator maintains the forward position, preventing the deleterious parafunctional effects at night. The construction bite is also opened slightly, and the lower incisors can then be capped. No grinding is done; thus when the acrylic is worn, it grasps or loads both upper and lower buccal segments, guiding the mandible forward during the clenching or bruxing activity. Bionator therapy, together with local heat applications and muscle relaxants, can provide almost immediate and dramatic relief for patients. In many instances adult Class II patients learn an accommodative forward position as the muscles adapt. The apparent reason is the foreshortening of the protracting muscles of the mandible, not a stimulus of growth or morphologic changes in the condyle. However, appliance wear must be indefinite as a splint at night for this to happen.

SUMMARY

The Bionator is an effective appliance for treating functional or mild skeletal Class II malocclusions in the mixed and transitional dentitions, provided that they are chosen after a careful diagnostic study, that the appliance is made properly and managed properly by loading and unloading different areas as indicated during the eruption of the premolars, and that patient compliance is excellent for both daytime and nighttime wear. A special indication is in the treatment of TMJ patients who have bruxism and clenching, clicking, and/or crepitus. Such problems are amenable to Bionator therapy, and relief of the objective symptoms is dramatic.

CHAPTER 10

THE FRÄNKEL FUNCTION REGULATOR

The philosophy of functional appliances and their indications, use, and success have already been covered in previous chapters. Essential diagnostic procedures have been discussed in detail to help the clinician assess the original malocclusion and determine whether it is, indeed, a "functional appliance case." The biologic basis of the workings of these appliances has been extensively studied and is validated in the first two chapters. No longer does the American clinician doubt that a potent tool is there, ready and waiting to be used for the right case at the right time. However, major questions remain: What functional appliance should be used? Are they all the same? What are the criteria for appliance selection and use? Which is preferable—nighttime or full-time wear? Does it make a difference whether a classical Andresen activator, Bimler appliance, Stockfisch Kinetor, Balters Bionator, or Herren, Harvold, or Hamilton wide open bite activator is used? What about the Fränkel appliance?

To answer some of these questions, a full appreciation of the concepts of Rolf Fränkel and the appliances he uses is imperative. Fränkel has had a greater impact on American orthodontics than has any proponent of functional appliances. His four visits to the United States in the past dozen years have been outstandingly successful, as judged by the great numbers of orthodontists who have attended his courses under the aegis of the Kenilworth Research Foundation, the G.V. Black Institute for Continuing Education, the University of Chicago, the Ann Arbor Orthodontic Study Club, and the University of Detroit. His appearances on the annual programs of the American Association of Orthodontists have been before packed houses. For American orthodontists, trained with fixed multiattachment appliances and taught that European methods were inferior or socioeconomic compromises, this is quite a tribute. Their curiosity has not been without good reason. Fränkel, the meticulous scientist, the consumate clinician, has passed the major test—he has "put the plaster on the table."

Credit is gratefully given to Rolf Fränkel for most of the illustrations in this chapter.

And very good plaster it is, too. And the serial radiographic cephalometric records substantiate that plaster, as do the facial and intraoral radiographs. Nord of the Netherlands referred to the Fränkel technique as a "revolution in orthodontics." For American orthodontists it took a revolution of at least 180 degrees to accept and try the Fränkel appliances.

As is so often the case, the disciple is not immediately able to duplicate the results attained by the master. Teaching a whole new way of approaching orthodontic problems and correcting them cannot be done in a series of 2-day courses or in 45-minute lectures to national meetings. Most of Fränkel's writings are in German, and the chapter in the Graber-Neumann textbook and in periodical articles in English can hardly replicate the German volumes. Self-teaching is effective when there is feedback from a computer or a learned teacher, but most American clinicians have not had the benefit of firsthand guidance. Using a Fränkel appliance for the first time has been likened to learning to use a sailboard. Anybody who has climbed on one of these fascinating and challenging crafts knows what it feels like to be dunked in the drink a number of times before mastering the art of sailing. So there has been some disappointment for many of its users. Articles have appeared in the literature purporting to show that "it ain't necessarily so!" Still, using the sailboard analogy, these experiences are like those of the neophyte, with no firsthand lessons, who has been half-drowned trying to stay on the board and have smooth sailing and then deciding to write about his experiences after the first 50 unceremonious dunkings. It is even worse than this. You can assume that the sailboards are made properly and are balanced and work well in the right hands; but for the Fränkel appliance user, untrained in taking a construction bite, who then sends his impressions off to a laboratory that does not know how to fabricate the appliance properly, the chances are not very good that success will be the reward. Add to this the very real continuing challenge of maintaining patient compliance with an appliance that requires considerable effort to wear in the beginning weeks, an appliance that makes normal speech very difficult at first, and you can be sure the treatment goals will not be achieved. Like any misused orthodontic appliance, even iatrogenic response is possible, with labial tipping of lower incisors or actual labiogingival dehiscence from improperly made lip pads.

Because of the problems encountered by many beginning Fränkel appliance users, this chapter will address itself primarily to those aspects of FR management that are most critical to success—the different philosophy, the construction of the Fränkel appliances (FR I, II, III, IV), the construction bite, laboratory proceedings, the mode of action of the various FR modifications, the clinical handling of the appliance, and successful treatment considerations.

FRÄNKEL PHILOSOPHY

The basic philosophy of functional appliances has been elucidated in other sections of this book and will not be repeated here. Rather, the differences recommended by Rolf Fränkel will be described.

Unlike conventional activators, the major part of the Fränkel appliance is confined to the oral vestibule (Fig. 10-1). The buccal shields and lip pads effectively hold the buccal and labial musculature away from the teeth and investing tissues, eliminating any restrictive influence that this "functional matrix" might have (Fig. 10-2). Fränkel believes that this active muscle and tissue mass (the buccinator mechanism and the orbicularis oris complex) has a potential restraining influence on the outward development of the dental arches, particularly during the transitional period of development. Abnormal perioral muscle function has the ability to exert a deforming action that prevents full accomplishment of the optimal growth and developmental pattern. This approach is in contrast to the conventional "push out from within" action of other removable appliances, which ex-

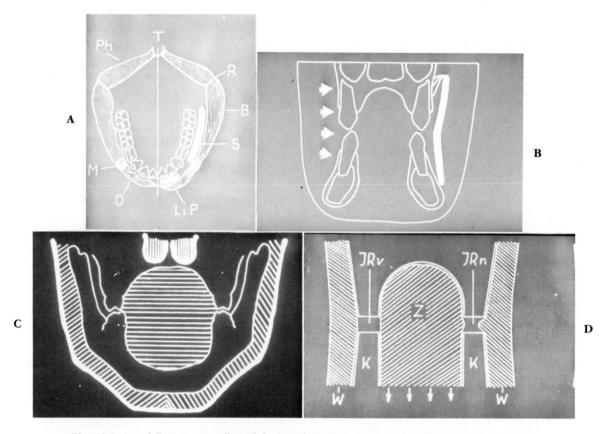

Fig. 10-1. A and **B,** Screening effect of the buccal shields and lip pads, holding off the buccinator mechanism and orbicularis oris pressures. The continuous band of muscles, anchored at the pharyngeal tubercle *(T),* passes around the pharynx through the constrictor muscles to the pterygomandibular raphe *(R)* and continues anteriorly through the buccinator *(B)* and orbicularis oris *(O)* to form a continuous restrictive band. *Ph,* Pharyngeal musculature; *S,* shield; *M,* corner of mouth; *LiP,* lip pad. **C,** Counterbalancing effect of the tongue if the dorsum is in contact with the palate. On swallowing, a negative atmospheric pressure is created that sucks the cheeks into the interocclusal space, **D,** to help maintain the interocclusal space at postural resting position before the mandible drops at the end of the deglutitional cycle. *W,* Cheeks; *K,* dentoalveolar area; *JRv,* interocclusal space; *JRn,* interocclusal space with cheek invagination. (Courtesy Rolf Fränkel.)

pand without relieving external muscle forces and literally coerce the new dentoalveolar morphology to adapt. Fränkel visualizes his vestibular constructions as an artificial "ought-to-be" matrix that allows the muscles to exercise and adapt. Implicit in this protection from constant neuromuscular constriction of the dentition, particularly mesial to the deciduous second molars, is the fact that when the buccinator mechanism pressures are

screened from the dentition significant *expansion* may be attained in the critical intercanine dimension. This relieves the crowding so often seen in the lower anterior segment, and so often the basis for removal of four first premolars in fixed multiattachment mechanotherapy. Fränkel shows extensive long-term data to support this working hypothesis in the form of plaster casts before and well beyond treatment and in anteroposterior

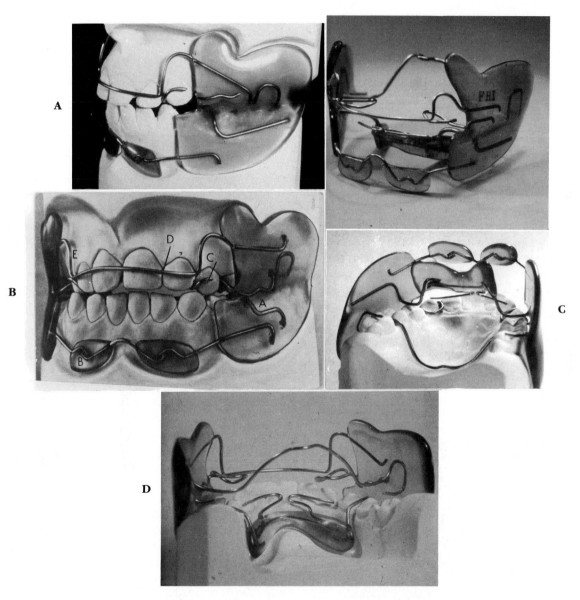

Fig. 10-2. Fränkel Function Regulator (FR Ib). **A,** Buccal shields, lip pads, labial wire, and lingual appliance components on and off the plaster casts. **B,** Shields *(A),* lip pads *(B),* canine clasp *(C),* labial arch *(D),* and labial arch loop *(E)* identify the major vestibular components. **C,** Appliance in place on the maxillary cast. The palatal bow, molar occlusal rests, and canine clasps are visible on the left. Note that the appliance is "locked" on the maxilla as the palatal bow and canine clasps pass through the embrasures mesial to the permanent first molar and first premolar. **D,** Lingual acrylic pad, lingual wires, and crossover hanger wire, in addition to the wire configurations mentioned, on the mandibular cast.

cephalograms showing significant apical base expansion when compared to controls. The autonomous improvement and stability of this treatment accomplishment are little short of amazing for an appliance that does not even touch these teeth.

A prime consideration is the concept that the Fränkel appliance is truly an exercise device, stimulating normal function while eliminating the lip trap, hyperactive mentalis, and aberrant buccinator and orbicularis oris action. To achieve the stated objectives means full-time wear, not just nighttime wear when asleep. It is the daily functional exercise that is so important for Fränkel appliance success. To Fränkel (and other users of daytime wear functional appliances) "functional" means continuously repetitive and frequent activity, not possible during sleep time only.

Frantisek Kraus, a pioneer in "screening" therapy from Czechoslovakia, espoused the same philosophy in his book in 1956, so the concept is not new. Simple oral screens have been used for years, and the Mühlemann-Hotz propulsor has some of the same features, albeit to a very limited degree. The routine expansion achieved by proper buccal shield and lip pad construction has been amply demonstrated, and long-term assessment of posttreatment results shows an amazing stability not seen with conventional fixed appliance expansion procedures. There is no question that expansion can be achieved from within and without; but the adaptation of the contiguous musculature to the vestibular artificial functional matrix constriction, along with appropriate exercises, clearly indicates that the musculature plays a significant role in the ultimate status of the arch form and size (Fig. 10-3).

The analysis of the effects of buccal shields and lip pads in the previous paragraphs does not mention the role of the tongue. It is not that Fränkel ignores it. He believes that the tongue plays a significant role in the ultimate outward progression of the teeth and investing tissues. He also thinks, however, that its effect has been overstressed, to the exclusion of the equally important buccal musculature. Much of tongue function may be compensatory or adaptive to dentoalveolar morphology and not necessarily the primary causative factor in the existing malocclusion.

As might be expected in an analysis of functional appliances, Fränkel emphasizes the form-function relationship. He calls for an understanding of the physiology of deglutition. This was stressed again in his May, 1983, course at the University of Chicago. Normally, with anterior lip seal and a posterior oral seal provided by the tongue and soft palate during the deglutitional process, a negative atmospheric pressure is set up within the oral cavity. The cheeks are actually sucked into the interocclusal space as the mandible returns to postural rest position in the terminal phase of the swallowing process (*JRn,* Fig. 10-1). The effect is both a constricting effect on the dentoalveolar process and a prevention of eruption of the buccal segments by virtue of the interposed cheek tissue. The partial vacuum created inside the arch has the momentary effect of greater external pressure, offsetting the intrinsic force potential of the tongue. The FR buccal shields prevent the pressure of the buccinator mechanism from being exerted on the dentoalveolar area both during deglutition and at rest. The net effect is outward expansion to the "ought-to-be" acrylic shield functional matrix. Worn at a critical time in dental development, with maximum eruption in the direction of least resistance, it can induce optimal downward and outward movement of both teeth and investing tissues—as has, indeed, been validated by numerous studies.

Another difference between the Fränkel Function Regulator and conventional activator therapy is the manner in which the anteroposterior correction is achieved. Fränkel is not the only one to criticize the tendency for the conventional tooth-borne acrylic mass of the classic Andresen appliance (as well as the Herren, Harvold-Woodside, Hamilton, L.S.U., and Williamson modifications) to procline the lower incisors excessively. Björk pointed this out long ago. The loose-fitting appliance cannot help contacting the teeth in the anterior and posterior segments as the patient moves it up and down. At the very least, there is a tendency for the activator to rest on the lower incisors at night, when the mouth is partly open. To prevent this undesirable action, Fränkel has designed his appliance so there is no actual tooth contact at all in the lower arch. The forward posturing for the construction bite is achieved by lingual wire loops of the FR Ia or by a relatively thin acrylic pad that contacts the infradental mucosa only behind the lower

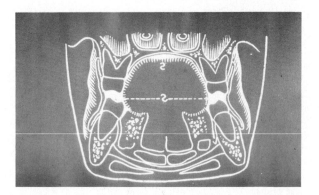

Fig. 10-3. Contiguity of buccal musculature and tongue to the teeth and supporting structures. Note the lingual inclination of the mandibular buccal segments. Abnormal perioral muscle function allows the tongue to drop and tips the maxillary buccal segments lingually. There is normally little effect on mandibular width, however. (Courtesy Rolf Fränkel.)

anterior segment in the FR Ib or FR II (Fig. 10-4). It serves more as a proprioceptive signal and pressure-bearing area for maintenance of mandibular propulsion than as a physical barrier to the return to the original sagittal relationship. The design and construction of the vestibular acrylic and wire configuration augment this proprioceptive trigger to maintain forward posturing.

An important part of the Fränkel philosophy is the fact that the FR is anchored to the maxillary dental arch in a very positive manner. The no. 1 priority for appliance use is that this objective be achieved in the mixed dentition via wires between the contacts at the mesial of the permanent maxillary first molars and the distal of the

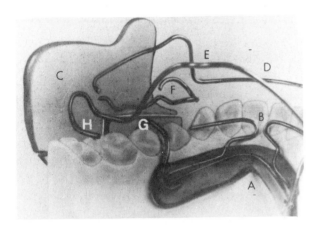

Fig. 10-4. FR Ia mounted on the lower cast. Lingual pad *(A)*, passive lingual springs *(B)*, shield *(C)*, labial wire *(D)*, palatal bow *(E)*, canine clasp *(F)*, crossover hanger wire *(G)*, and molar rest *(H)*.

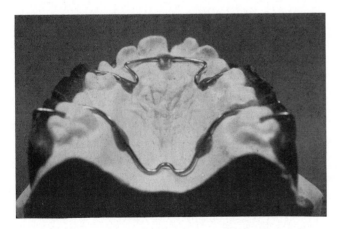

Fig. 10-5. FR II under construction (occlusal view). Palatal and lingual incisor wires are anchored in the embrasures mesial to the permanent first molars and first premolars or deciduous first molars if present. This is essential to ensure proper Function Regulator action. To allow proper seating below the marginal ridge, it is usually necessary to disk (or notch) the deciduous teeth at the embrasure.

deciduous maxillary canines (Fig. 10-5). The teeth *must* be separated to allow the wires to pass through the contacts, below the occlusal surfaces. This may mean actual disking of the distal surfaces of the deciduous canines and second molars. Simply allowing the wires to rest on these embrasures from the occlusal is totally inadequate and allows the same undesirable effect of lower incisor labial tipping as is seen so often with the conventional activator. Added to this is the potential for damage to the labial gingival tissue by the lip pads as the appliance bobs up and down during the day. Recent articles in the periodical literature demonstrate that this can be the cause for appliance failure to achieve treatment objectives. Indeed, it is blatant misuse of the appliance and is a direct criticism of the clinician who has ignored this axiom and then writes up his "objective assessments" of the FR therapy results.

As Harvold, Woodside, Rakosi, and others have shown, freeing the lower posterior teeth from acrylic or wire restraints while holding the bite open allows the unrestricted upward and forward movement of these teeth, contributing to both vertical and horizontal correction of the malocclusion. Maxillary molars are prevented from downward and forward movement by the FR appliance, anchored as it is on the maxillary arch. Some expansion is possible, of course. The differential eruption can be counted on for 1 or 2 mm toward the usually needed 6 to 7 mm for establishment of a correct sagittal interdigitation.

The labial wire of the Fränkel appliance rests on the maxillary incisors; but it is not activated or "pinched up," as is often done with a Hawley appliance, to close spaces. This action tends to tip the incisors excessively to the lingual and their apices labially if the teeth rock on the lingual alveolar plate. It may even restrict full mandibular horizontal growth as the bite is deepened and the upper anterior segment exerts a retruding effect on the lower incisors and mandible at full closure when the appliance is not worn. There is some restraining effect on the maxillary teeth and arch, however, although McNamara's research indicates that this is minimal; but Lee Graber has shown that in selected cases the FR actually has a headgear effect, holding back the maxillary downward and forward progression. Incisors can be tipped lingually, and spaces closed if needed, by pre-functional appliance treatment with fixed or removable appliances, and this is preferred to activation of the FR labial wire.

Fränkel has stressed another theoretical action of the buccal shields and lip pads. In addition to holding off deforming muscle action and permitting the teeth to erupt downward and outward, he believes that by extension of the shields and pads into the actual depth of the vestibule he can put the tissue under tension without

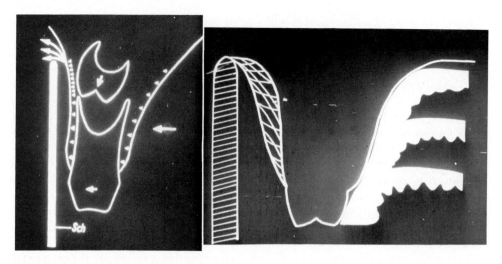

Fig. 10-6. Relief of the buccinator mechanism forces on the dentoalveolar area. The shield extends to the depths of the vestibule, exerting pressure on tissue attachments to the alveolar bone. In addition to relieving the external pressure, particularly when it is strongest (during deglutition), the shields exert an indirect tension on the periosteum overlying the bone. This has been shown experimentally to enhance osseous proliferation, according to our research, and results in more bodily tooth movement of both erupted and unerupted teeth, with changes in the buccal and lingual bony surfaces.

A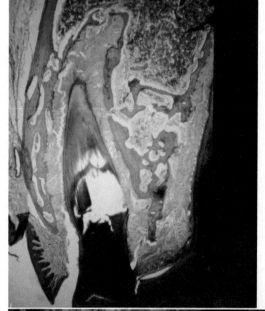

Fig. 10-7. Experimental results of studies on squirrel monkeys by Graber et al. Buccal shields extended into the maxillary vestibular depths from Fränkel-type appliances pinned to the palate substantiate the clinical claims made by Fränkel. The histologic section, **A,** shows the erupting tooth, with resorption on the contiguous buccal plate and deposition on the lingual alveolar process as well as the external surface of the buccal plate. This response is illustrated better in **B** and its diagram, **C.** The section of the buccal alveolar crest clearly shows the resorptive processes contiguous to the buccal surface of the tooth, with lamellar deposition at the crest and on the buccal surface, in animals wearing buccal shields. It also shows bodily eruption of the premolar tooth.

B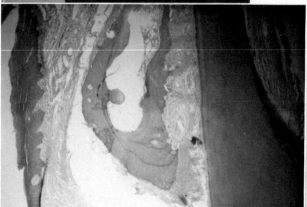

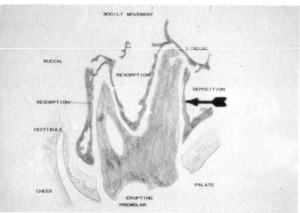 **C**

creating irritation. This tension conceivably exerts a pull on the contiguous periosteal tissue of the maxillary bone (Fig. 10-6). Experiments by Enlow, Hoyt, and Moffett have shown that periosteal pull can elicit increased bone activity in contiguous osseous structures. If it works, the maxillary basal bone would be widened as the thin alveolar shell over the erupting teeth proliferated laterally. AP cephalograms of many of Fränkel's cases do, indeed, show apical base widening. The working hypothesis is valid, but experimental work thus far has had a difficult time pinpointing this effect. In an NIH-sponsored research project on primates at the ADA Research Institute by Graber, Graber, Verrusio, Muller, Helmi, and Voss, it has been clearly shown that the buccal shields do stimulate *bodily* buccal movement of posterior teeth and buccal plate activity far beyond what is observed in controls (Fig. 10-7). As far as periosteal pull is concerned, however, the effect seems to be temporary, confined to the first 2 weeks of appliance wear. How much of the significant expansion is achieved by periosteal pull versus relief of the restraining effect of the musculature is conjectural at this point. Again, implicit in this design is the fact that the vestibular constructions serve as a base for oral gymnastics—prescribed exercises by the patient each day—to accomplish as much as can be done. Lip seal exercises are a most important part of patient management (as will be stressed later). Primates are not capable of being trained to do this, and herein may lie the reason for inability to see the total effect possible on the periosteal tissue. One phase of the ADA study is on 50 Class II, Division 1, malocclusion patients in the mixed dentition. The results obtained with Fränkel appliance wear corroborate the claims by Fränkel and McNamara and others who use the FR *properly*.

Visual treatment objective diagnostic test (FR-VTO)

At the initial clinical examination a very simple yet important maneuver can give the operator an excellent clue as to whether the Fränkel appliance, or any functional appliance that postures the mandible forward, will improve the facial appearance and profile. First, the patient is asked to swallow and then lick the lips and relax. Sometimes a few syllables are repeated to achieve the relaxed mandibular position and an approximation of postural rest. Then the patient is instructed to close the teeth in habitual occlusion, again licking the lips first, and to keep the teeth lightly together with the lips relaxed. These two profile relationships are carefully studied and may be photographed to obtain an instant print. The patient is then asked to *posture the mandible forward* into a correct sagittal relationship, reducing the overjet. A photograph of this profile may be taken and compared to the original Polaroid view with the teeth in occlusion (Fig. 10-8). If this clinical exercise makes the

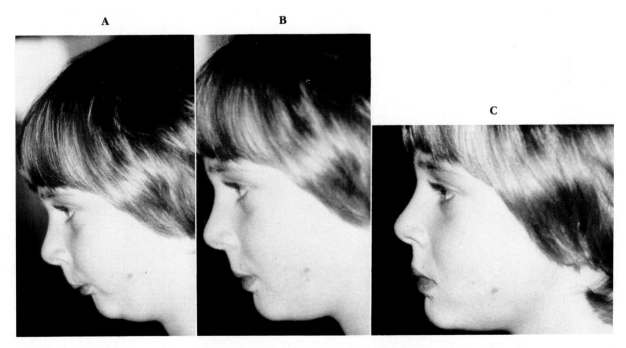

Fig. 10-8. A marked Class II, Division 1, malocclusion with full occlusion, **A,** 3 mm of mandibular protraction, **B,** and 6 mm of cuspal advancement into a Class I buccal segment relationship, **C.** The dramatic change produced provides a VTO (visual treatment objective) for potential Fränkel appliance users. If the profile is not improved by this maneuver, some other appliance may be needed.

facial balance look better, then the Fränkel appliance will probably be beneficial. It is good patient management to give the photographs to the patient and parent to show the significant improvement in the facial profile and to motivate the patient toward an achievable treatment goal. If the profile is not improved by forward mandibular posturing or is actually made worse, then other forms of treatment are probably needed. This is possible in patients with excessive anterior face height, procumbency of the lower incisors, deficient symphyseal development, and a very steep mandibular plane. Obviously a cursory visualization is no substitute for a comprehensive cephalometric analysis to determine whether the FR is to be the best possible appliance. Patients with an anteriorly rotating growth pattern, functional retrusion, deep overbite, and excessive interocclusal clearance but a normally positioned maxilla are good candidates. The previous chapters on principles of functional appliances, on cephalometric and functional diagnosis, on Class II treatment, and on deep overbite discuss the indications and contraindications for functional appliance treatment. Essentially the same criteria are applicable to Fränkel appliance treatment and will not be repeated.

CONSTRUCTION BITE AND FABRICATION OF THE FRÄNKEL APPLIANCE

The primary use of functional appliances in the United States has been as a deficiency appliance and a deterrent of abnormal perioral muscle function. This means that most cases are Class II, Division 1, malocclusions. To a lesser degree the activator has been used in Class II, Division 2, and open bite problems. The same case selection constraints apply to the Fränkel appliance. Rolf and Christine Fränkel have presented dramatic evidence of the efficacy of the FR IV in properly chosen cases of skeletal open bite, and this is also reported in the *American Journal of Orthodontics*.

Four basic variations of the FR appliance have been designed by Fränkel. The FR I is for correction of Class I and Class II, Division 1, malocclusions. The FR II is for Class II, Division 1 and 2, cases. The FR III is for Class III problems. The FR IV is used for open bites and bimaxillary protrusions. This section of the chapter, devoted to appliance construction, is detailed primarily for the FR I and FR III. There is minimal variation for the FR II and IV. Classic nonextraction treatment is described, which does not mean that the FR cannot be used in extraction cases, with some appliance changes (Fränkel has illustrated a number of successful extraction cases). However, the more sophisticated uses of the FR are beyond the scope of this book.

The first impression of the Fränkel appliance to both operator and patient is that it is a complicated and possibly fragile appliance. The insistent demands by Fränkel

for precise fabrication and the minimal tolerances during construction are not likely to attract the nondescript clinician. However, such precision and care pay off, with few subsequent adjustments needed during active therapy other than advancing the lip and lingual pads or correcting appliance distortions. Well-trained and competent laboratories are now available to make appliances properly to prescription—a situation that did not exist in the early days of FR usage in the United States. Many of the early failures (too many) were due to improper fabrication.

FR I

There are actually three FR I appliance modifications. However, the original FR Ia, with a lingual wire loop instead of an acrylic lingual mandibular pad, is now seldom used (Fig. 10-9). Perhaps the best use of the FR I has been in Class I cases, with minor crowding or with delayed development of the basal bony and dental structures. Fränkel recommends the FR Ia for Class I deep bite cases with protruded maxillary and retruded mandibular incisors. Although the appliance is occasionally used for Class II, Division 1, malocclusions in which the overjet does not exceed 5 mm, the lingual acrylic construction of the FR Ib is generally preferred now (Figs. 10-2 and 10-4).

The vestibular shields are a unique component of the Fränkel appliances (Figs. 10-1, 10-2, 10-4, 10-6, 10-9, and 10-10). The labial lip pads, or pelots (as Fränkel calls them), are analogous to some of the lip bumpers that have been used with various fixed appliances in the United States to eliminate the lip trap and hyperactive mentalis muscle function, but their placement and fabrication must be very precise. As Fig. 10-2 shows, in addition to connecting wires between the shields and pads, there is also a maxillary labial bow with canine loops.

Instead of the bulky acrylic of most activators that covers the palate, the FR has a palatal bow shaped like a Coffin spring with the open end facing mesially. The buccal extensions of the loop pass through the embrasures between the permanent first molars and deciduous second molars and are anchored on each side in the buccal shields (Fig. 10-10). It is imperative that these lateral extensions insert below the occlusal surfaces of the embrasures to lock the appliance on the maxillary arch and prevent a free float. As pointed out earlier, the locking of the FR appliance on the maxillary arch is accomplished largely by this firm insertion in the embrasure. Special elastic separators are available to create sufficient space; but if they are difficult to place, it may be necessary to disk or notch the distal convexity of the deciduous upper second molar. It is a good idea actually to separate the molar and canine embrasures, even before taking the impressions, and then to replace the

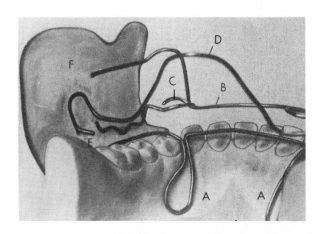

Fig. 10-9. FR Ia on the mandibular cast. Wire loops *(A)* instead of the acrylic lingual pad, are used to posture the mandible forward. Other parts identified are the maxillary labial wire *(B)*, maxillary canine clasp *(C)*, palatal wire *(D)*, maxillary molar occlusal rest *(E)*, and buccal shield *(F)*. The hanger wire (passing between the upper and lower occlusal surfaces) is an extension of the lingual loops *(A)*. It is passive and does not contact the upper or lower posterior teeth.

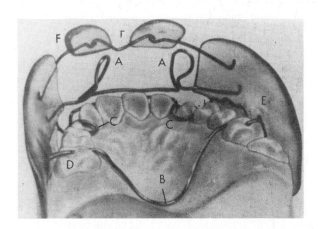

Fig. 10-10. FR Ia mounted on the maxillary cast. Identified are the mandibular lingual posturing loops *(A)*, transpalatal wire *(B)*, canine clasps *(C)*, occlusal rest *(D)*, buccal shield *(E)*, and lip pads *(F)*. Note that the palatal and canine wires pass through the notched proximal embrasures, in direct contact with the maxillary first molar and first premolar–canine area. This locks the appliance on the maxillary dentition and is essential for proper use.

heavy separators. The ends of the palatal bow can be bent back to terminate on the maxillary first molars as occlusal rests (Fig. 10-10). The maxillary canine loops also project from the lingual part of the shield into the canine–deciduous first molar embrasure, wrapping around the lingual of the canines and terminating on their labial surface. They assist in anchoring the appliance on the maxilla as well as guiding the erupting canines into place. They also exert a mild distal pressure on the deciduous first molars to prevent these teeth from coming forward (Figs. 10-2, 10-4, and 10-10).

On the mandible there is either a lingual bow with U loops extending downward to the floor of the mouth to fit against the lingual tissue below the incisors, as in the FR Ia (Fig. 10-9), or an acrylic pad replacing these wires, as will be discussed under the FR Ib (Figs. 10-2 and 10-4). The objective in each case is to provide a signal to the mandible to remain in the forward position when the appliance is worn to correct a Class II condition, being held forward by the protracting muscles and not by the appliance itself (although the ends of the lower loops do contact the apical base lingual tissue). This bilateral foreshortening of the lateral pterygoid muscles is quite important and may lead to actual permanent changes in the muscle itself. The lingual wire that joins the loops, crossing the lower incisors at their cingula does not exert any pressure on the incisors. In rare instances when it is desirable to procline incisors, the wire can be activated for this purpose.

To hold this new position, the mandible is stabilized against the maxillary teeth by cross-occlusal wires at the first molar–canine-premolar embrasures, as previously described. The interproximal wires are aided by a passive labial bow on the maxillary incisors. The cross-palatal Coffin-spring type of stabilizing wire is needed to provide rigidity for the appliance since there is no palatal acrylic (Fig. 10-10). The occlusal supports between the mesiobuccal and distobuccal cusps of the first molars keep the FR I from being dislodged superiorly, which would force the periphery of the shields into the sulcus tissue and allow the cross-palatal wire to impinge on the tissue. These supports also prevent upper molar eruption; the lower molars, however, are free to erupt mesially in Class II corrections.

The buccal shields (Figs. 10-1, 10-2, 10-4, 10-9, and 10-10) are contiguous to the buccal surfaces of the molars and premolars, extending as deeply into the vestibular limits as the tissue and patient comfort will allow while still maintaining a slight tension. To relieve pressures from the buccinator mechanism, the buccal shields stand away from the maxillary dentition and basal alveolar bone. As pointed out earlier, the aim is to allow all possible alveolodental development and needed bodily expansion of the teeth in the buccal segments (Fig. 10-1). The extension of the peripheral portions of the shields into the vestibular depths creates a slight tension on the connective tissue fibers in the sulci (Fig. 10-6). The objective is to stimulate periosteal pull with an intermittently outward force aided by lip seal exercises. The working hypothesis, as noted already, is that this unidirectional pull will enhance basal bone development and allow the teeth to erupt bodily into a more buccal position.

The lip pads (Fig. 10-2) act in a manner similar to that of the buccal shields, by eliminating the abnormal perioral muscle activity, particularly of the hyperactive and

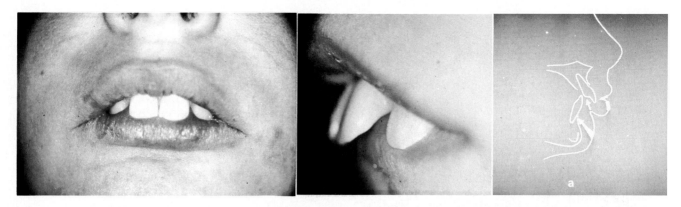

Fig. 10-11. Deforming activity of the lip trap, with the lower lip cushioning to the lingual of the maxillary incisors during function. Under these conditions normal lip seal is not possible. Not only are the maxillary incisors moved forward against a hypotonic upper lip, but the hypertonic lower lip and hyperactive mentalis muscle exert a lingualizing and crowding effect on the lower anterior segment *(arrows).*

potentially deforming mentalis muscle. By intercepting the lip trap, with the lower lip cushioning to the lingual of the maxillary incisors, the deforming muscular activity is controlled in both arches (Fig. 10-11). Fränkel has suggested that there is also a periosteal pull labially from the lip pad pressure in the anterior vestibular depth which exerts a bone-growth stimulus, reducing the pronounced mentolabial sulcus. The lip pads also serve another function. They form the labial boundary of the mandibular posturing trough. Together with the lingual loops (or acrylic pad in the FR Ib), they maintain the mandible in its forward construction bite for Class II correction.

FR Ib. The FR Ib has largely replaced the FR Ia. With the exception of substituting a lingual acrylic pad for the lower anterior wire loops to maintain forward mandibular posture, it is essentially the same (Figs. 10-2 and 10-4).

In the FR Ib, instead of a single wire crossing the lingual surfaces of the lower incisors, two passive recurved springs rest gently above the cingula. The skeletal wires that help form the lingual acrylic pad insert into the buccal shields, passing between the upper and lower occlusal surfaces in the deciduous molar region. Care must be taken that the cross-occlusal wires do not contact any teeth when the appliance is fully seated. Fränkel suggests the use of this appliance in Class II, Division 1, malocclusions with a deep bite and an overjet that does not exceed 7 mm. As is true of most functional appliances, the prognosis with the FR Ib is better if the molars do not exceed an end-to-end sagittal cuspal relationship. The construction is simpler than for the FR Ia, and it is easier for the patient to become accustomed to the lingual acrylic pad than to the U-loops.

The preliminary clinical procedures and laboratory fabrication of the FR Ib are described next.

Separation. It is recommended that separation be placed in the maxillary canine–deciduous first molar and deciduous second molar–permanent first molar contact areas before the impression-taking procedure. If this is done 5 to 7 days before taking the impressions, the need for disking or notching is reduced. Special heavy elastic separators are available for this purpose. As already emphasized, it is imperative that the appliance be anchored on the maxillary arch when placed or as soon as possible thereafter (Figs. 10-5 and 10-10). The separators usually provide sufficient room in the embrasures for seating of the palatal loop extension and canine loop crossover wires without cutting away tooth structure. However, in mixed dentition treatment it is often necessary to slice the distal contact of the deciduous upper second molars as well as the mesial marginal ridges of the deciduous upper first molars to assure proper locking of the appliance on the maxilla in the critical period of initial adjustment (Fig. 10-12). An occlusal rest is then placed on the deciduous upper second molars.

Impression taking. As with other functional appliances, impression taking, with the FR Ib is critical. Indeed, the technique is more demanding since the impressions should reproduce the whole alveolar process up to the depths of the sulci, including the maxillary tuberosities.

In his various trips to the United States, Fränkel has stressed the importance of impression taking and the construction bite procedures more than any other phase of management; and he has found mistakes in these areas more frequently, too. With all the need for total extension of the coverage, care must be exercised not to distort the soft tissues and muscle attachments. The metal flanges of the impression trays should not reach too far into the sulci (Fig. 10-13). Rimming the trays with

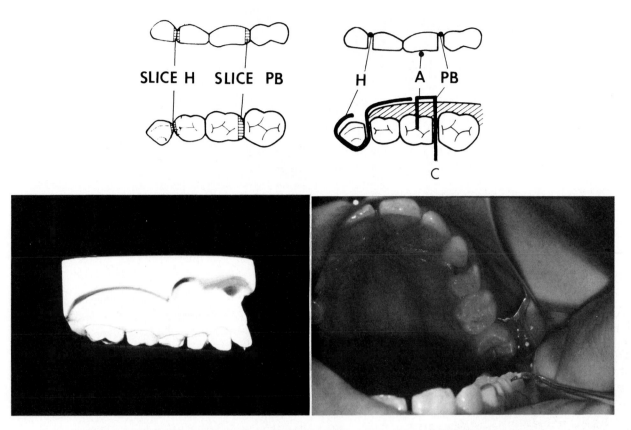

Fig. 10-12. Space between the maxillary first molar and deciduous second molar, and at the canine–deciduous first molar embrasure, is essential before placing the FR appliance. If separators do not create sufficient room to anchor the appliance on the maxillary arch, the proximal areas can be "sliced" or disked (as shown on the drawing). Care must be taken, however, not to injure any permanent teeth. Slice *H* is for the canine clasp; *PB* for the palatal bow. On deciduous dentitions the maxillary molar rest *(A)* is bent mesially to overlie the deciduous second molar.

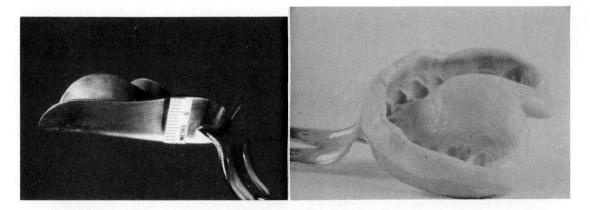

Fig. 10-13. The proper tray should not be overextended, since this will distort the musculature and muscle attachments. A distance of 15 mm from the bottom of the tray to the top is about as far as the tray should extend. A relatively thin peripheral roll is needed on the impression so as not to distort the contiguous tissue.

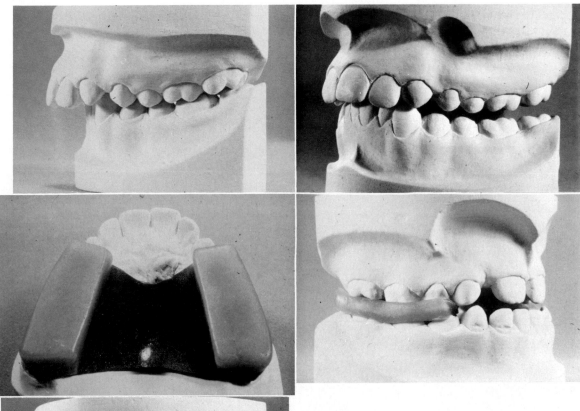

Fig. 10-14. In the Fränkel technique the construction bite is not opened any more than needed to allow the crossover wires to pass through the interdental space. This is necessary for effective lip seal exercises. The amount of forward positioning is usually about 3 mm, or half the width of a cusp. In mild Class II malocclusions this can correct the sagittal discrepancy in one step. Fränkel uses an adapted baseplate to which wax is added and softened for the construction bite. By leaving the anterior region open, he visualizes the midlines for proper registration in all three dimensions.

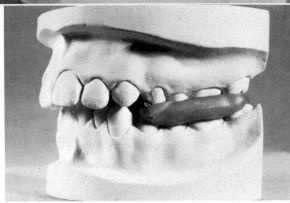

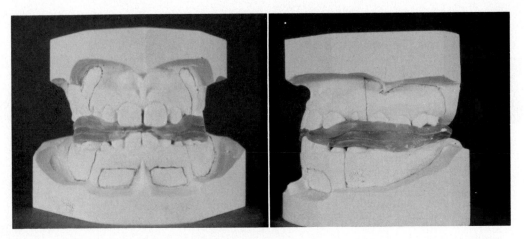

Fig. 10-15. The horseshoe-shaped wafer is made up of three layers of softened beeswax. It is cut away on the incisal to permit determination of the correct vertical, sagittal, and midline registration. Lip pads and buccal shields are already outlined on the stone models.

a soft utility wax (or similar compound) permits individualizing the trays for a more faithful reproduction. The consistency of the impression material should be enough to give a good but *thin* peripheral roll, displacing the tissue gently and reproducing the muscle attachments (Fig. 10-13). The idea is to reproduce the resting vestibular sulcus and not to overextend or distort the tissues. Preformed disposable styrofoam trays are usually inadequate. One of the more successful techniques makes use of a thermal-sensitive acrylic tray that can be softened in hot water (175°), fitted to the model, and then inserted and adapted to the individual morphology. A custom tray can also be fabricated based on the study models if desired. The proper tray choice, beading, and impressions will improve the detail needed while cutting down on the amount of cast trimming.

Construction bite (Figs. 10-14 and 10-15). There are differences of opinion currently on just where the mandible should be postured for functional appliances. Procedures vary in both the degree of opening vertically and the amount of forward posturing of the mandible. As with all physiologic phenomena, adaptation is likely for a range of vertical and horizontal positionings. Fig. 10-14 shows one way, suggested by Fränkel, that allows complete visualization of the incisor relationship for correct midline and vertical opening. The following procedure is based on our own experiences with the Fränkel appliances:

For minor sagittal problems (2 to 4 mm) the construction bite is taken in an end-to-end incisal relationship, as with the Bionator, *care being exercised that no obvious strain of facial muscles is induced.* The balance must not be disturbed between protractor and retractor muscles. It is good clinical practice to have the patient hold the mandible in the desired forward position, with midlines correct, for 3 to 5 minutes and to repeat the maneuver of moving the mandible forward several times (Fig. 10-16). A practice construction bite, placing the softened **U**-shaped roll of bite wax on the lower teeth and having the patient close into the desired for-

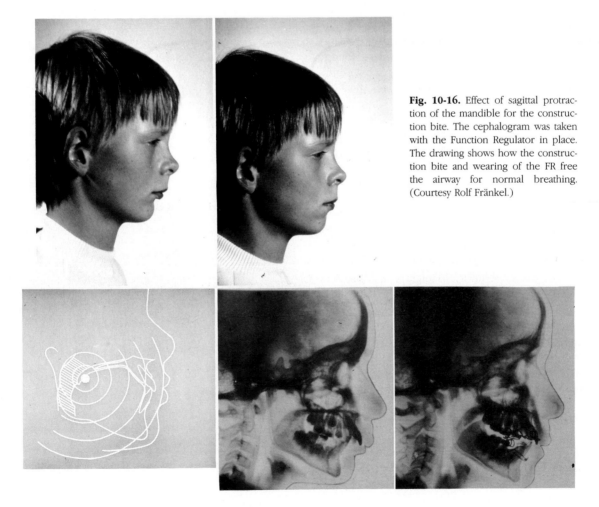

Fig. 10-16. Effect of sagittal protraction of the mandible for the construction bite. The cephalogram was taken with the Function Regulator in place. The drawing shows how the construction bite and wearing of the FR free the airway for normal breathing. (Courtesy Rolf Fränkel.)

ward position, is a valuable exercise. Fränkel now recommends that the construction bite not move the mandible further forward than 2.5 to 3.0 mm. The vertical opening should be only large enough to allow the crossover wires through the interocclusal space without contacting the teeth. For most activators, however, the construction bite requires a larger horizontal and more vertical posturing. Schmuth notes that 4 to 6 mm of advancement and opening is easily tolerated by most patients and will allow an end-to-end incisal relationship to be established for most Class II malocclusions. Fränkel originally subscribed to this amount of posturing, but clinical and experimental research showed that step-by-step activation produced a better and more continuous tissue reaction, particularly in the condyle, than did the "great leap forward." Patient acceptance was better, also. It still frees the airway for enhancement of normal nasal breathing (Fig. 10-16).

If an end-to-end relationship, or no more than 6 mm forward posturing, is used, then the incisal contact will determine the vertical opening. There must be at least 2.5 to 3.5 mm clearance in the buccal segments to allow the crossover wires to pass through in the Fränkel appliance, so the incisal vertical relationship usually results in discluding these teeth. A tongue blade is sometimes placed between the teeth during taking of the construction bite to establish sufficient vertical clearance for the crossover wires. For many functional appliance clinicians a good rule of thumb is that the greater the horizontal movement the less the vertical opening should be. For both the Bionator and the Fränkel appliances, however, vertical opening is kept to a minimum.[14]

Recent histlogic research by Petrovic and associates confirms the clinical impression that correcting the sagittal discrepancy in two or three stages may be more effective from a tissue response point of view as well as for patient adjustment to the forward posturing. Optimal prechondroblastic activity in the condyle is observed by staged construction bites. The construction bite technique and the important research at the tissue, cell, and molecular level are covered in Chapters 2 and 5 to 7 of this book.

For the Fränkel appliance, if 6 mm of sagittal movement is needed to correct the anteroposterior relationship, a construction bite of 3 mm forward posturing permits easy adaptation by the patient, less likelihood of dislodgment during both day and night, and reduced possibility of muscle strain or fatigue. The design and construction of the FR permit staged advancement of the mandible after a favorable response to treatment from the original construction bite has been noted. This is usually after 6 months of appliance wear. The patient readily adjusts to the new advancement of the lip pads and lingual acrylic flange, since the appliance is already comfortable in other aspects.

Even though the step-by-step forward posturing procedure is used for the FR, the vertical opening still cannot be increased much beyond an end-to-end bite, or only enough to allow the wires to pass through the posterior interocclusal space without endangering lip closure and lip seal exercises or losing control of tongue activity and increasing the danger that the appliance will bob up and down. Some clinicians consider this a limitation of the Fränkel appliance—in contrast to the other functional appliances, in which the height of the bite can be modified to take advantage of the different directions of growth (the **H** versus the **V** or Harvold-Woodside type–activators). This topic is well covered in previous chapters by Rakosi.

The construction bite can either be made into a softened roll of beeswax or used as a semisoft horseshoe wafer made up of three thicknesses of yellow wax. (See Chapter 7 for details and ilustrations.) For both the trial or practice bite and the final construction bite, the wax is only semisoftened in warm water. If it is too hot, the outside portion will become mushy while the inside remains too hard to obtain the correct occlusal relationship. To permit checking of midline relationships, the wax should be cut away at the midline. An improper midline registration may mean inability of the patient to adapt, with treatment failure the ultimate outcome. If the dental midlines do not coincide in habitual occlusion, the skeletal midlines must be determined and then used for taking the construction bite. Midline discrepancies are usually due to tooth drift and should not be corrected in the bite by manipulation during forward posturing. Such discrepancies, if correctable, may be han-

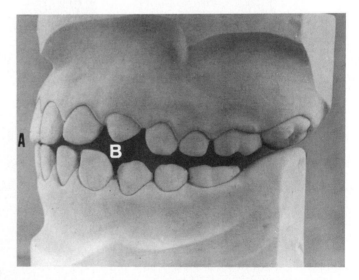

Fig. 10-17. In a mild Class II malocclusion an end-to-end incisal relationship *(A)* should be registered in the construction bite *(B)*. If there is not enough room for the crossover wires, however, then the bite must be opened slightly. The less the vertical opening, the easier it is for the patient to perform effective lip seal exercises.

dled later with fixed appliances. After the practice bite has been obtained (with commendation of the patient for cooperation), the final bite is taken. It should be removed carefully, chilled in cold water, and placed on the models to double-check the fit. The chilled wax is then pressed on the upper arch (Figs. 10-15 and 10-17). The patient is instructed to posture the lower jaw gently forward until it fits into the bite. The teeth and bite are checked for midline registration and full seating, and both the vertical and the horizontal openings are reevaluated to ascertain that the proper registration has been achieved. (See Chapter 7.)

After it has been determined that the construction bite is correct, the heavy elastic separators are replaced in the maxillary canine and first molar embrasures. The patient is instructed that if they are lost he should come to the office immediately so they can be replaced. Adequate space *must* be present when the appliance is delivered 2 or 3 weeks later. This is essential if the appliance is to fit properly and lock on the maxillary arch.

Working model pour-up and trimming. The newly taken impressions are poured immediately in yellow stone, with an adequate base to permit proper carving of the models and mounting on the articulator. It is important that the model extend outward, away from the alveolar process at least 5 mm, to allow subsequent application of wax relief. Care must be taken that the tuberosity areas are not cut away too closely when trim-

ming the stone to the level of the vestibular sulcus (Fig. 10-18).

After the working models have been separated from the impressions, they are carefully trimmed for the lip pads and buccal shields. Fränkel believes this is necessary since, even with the best trays and impressions, the depths of the sulci are not adequately reproduced to permit full extension of the acrylic for periosteal pull and maximum benefit from the lip seal exercises. The carving can be done by either the orthodontist or the technician. However, it is preferable that the operator do it before sending the models to the laboratory. Furthermore, if this can done with the patient present, the anatomic conditions of the particular areas can be inspected while carving for the buccal and anterior sulci. The carving should be done with meticulous care to produce the tissue tension necessary to stimulate appositional bone development in the basal areas and yet not ulcerate the mucosa by overextension. If the buccal shields do not extend enough into the sulci, the cheek will invaginate into the space and either dislodge the shield or fold inside it, negating its activity. It is better to have to polish the peripheral portions somewhat because of overextension after the first visit than to undershoot the mark on the buccal shield and lip pad extension.

LIP PADS. Since the impression-taking procedure may distort the tissue and actually diminish sulcular depth, the stone of the mandibular model is carefully carved back about 5 mm from the greatest curvature of the alveolar base with a pear-shaped carbide bur and office knife. Again, this is to ensure optimum extension, to put the sulcus connective tissue under slight tension, and to

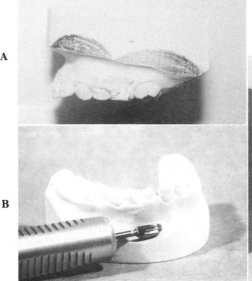

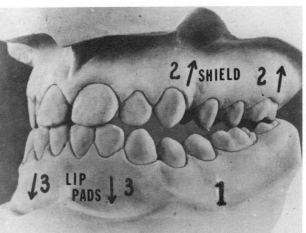

Fig. 10-18. Correct model trimming prior to appliance fabrication is required. The desired amount of stone to be cut away can be outlined in pencil, **A,** and then cut away with a round or oblong acrylic bur, **B.** Final detailing is done with a plaster knife, **C.** No trimming is needed for the buccal shields on the mandible *(1),* but extension is required for the maxillary buccal shield periphery *(2)* and the mandibular lip pads *(3).* Care must be taken not to disturb muscle attachments. (Courtesy Max Hall and Dick Allessee.)

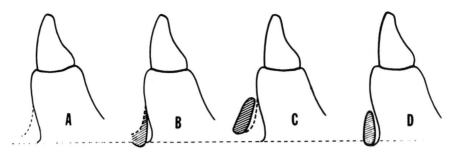

Fig. 10-19. Correct and incorrect trimming and lip pad position are shown in this drawing. **A** and **C,** Inadequate carving and wrong positioning of the lip pad. **B** and **D,** Proper carving and parallel pad orientation. Actual tissue damage may result from improper model carving and pad fabrication. (Courtesy Rolf Fränkel.)

prevent the lip mucosa from working in between the pads and the labial mucosal tissue of the alveolar process. In Fig. 10-19, *A* and *C,* the solid line marks the real depth of the sulcus whereas the dotted line delineates the corrected peripheral limits, allowing for possible distortion by the impression-taking technique. The correct trimming is shown in Fig. 10-19, *B* and *D.* A profile view of the working model should show the alveolar surface to be nearly vertical after the carving. The lower relief should be at least 12 mm below the gingival margin, according to Fränkel, to permit the wire framework for the lip pads to lie 7 mm below the incisor gingival margin. This allows properly formed rhomboid acrylic lip pads to be made over the wire skeleton. The technician may do some further fine carving, but this should be minimal since no record of the original extent of the sulci exists after the impression. It is better that either the operator or the laboratory technician, not both, have the trimming responsibility. Any overextension of acrylic can be polished from the pads at appliance placement.

BUCCAL SHIELDS. The maxillary stone model must also be trimmed, after first removing the excess from the base. In the trimming for the buccal shields, the sulcular depth must be 10 to 12 mm above the gingival margin of the posterior teeth. Attention must be paid particularly to the muscle attachments and the tuberosity area. The region next to the muscle attachment over the deciduous first molar and the superior limit of the lateral incisor depression, just mesial to the canine, must be well defined. This allows optimum extension of the buccal shields for all possible appositional bone growth (Fig. 10-18).

Trimming of the lower buccal vestibular sulcus is not required for the shields.

SEATING GROOVES. If adequate space has not been created by the special heavy elastic separators, then seating grooves must be cut in the permanent first molar–deciduous second molar and deciduous canine–first molar embrasures. To permit lateral expansion, these must be

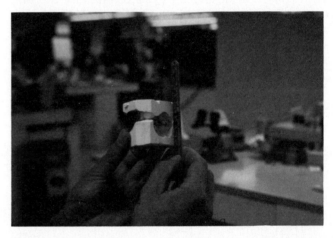

Fig. 10-20. The backs of the working models must be properly trimmed with the casts mounted in the construction bite, either before sending to the technician or by the technician before he mounts the models on the fixator. Backs should be parallel and in the same plane. (Courtesy Max Hall and Dick Allessee.)

parallel. Prior separation usually makes seating grooves unnecessary, but a 1.5 mm wide groove can be made with a sharp blade or saw on the cast. It is better to have the grooves too deep than too shallow, so the seating wires are deep enough to anchor the inserted FR firmly on the maxillary dentition (Figs. 10-5, 10-9, and 10-12). The seating grooves that are cut on the model must be duplicated in the patient's mouth at the time the appliance is placed. This means that if the heavy separators have not created enough room the mesial marginal ridges of the deciduous first molars must be notched as well as the distal marginal ridges of the deciduous second molars. Care must be exercised not to injure the permanent first molars.

FINAL TRIMMING. Before the working models are sent to the technician, the wax construction bite should be replaced and the backs of the models trimmed so they are flush, much like the original study casts (Fig. 10-20). This allows the technician to check the bite when the

Doctor _____

Address _____

_____ Zip _____

Patient's Name _____

Original Malocclusion—Class_____ Division _____

Date shipped by Doctor _____

Appliance Placement Date_____

WAX RELIEF FOR EXPANSION

The standard relief on the FR1, FR2, and FR4 is 3mm on the upper and ½mm on the lower. The standard relief on the FR3 is 3mm on the upper and 0 on the lower.

☐ Standard Relief   ☐ Alternate Relief — use diagram →

MODEL PREPARATION

Please trim the backs of the models parallel, with the wax construction bite in place. This will help insure accuracy in mounting the casts.

☐ Do not alter models in any way.
☐ Trim vestibules to best height and symmetry.
☐ Flatten lower sulcus to ____ mm depth.

DISCING TEETH

Deciduous — Notching of the model interproximal to the c's and d's and the distal of the e's on the upper.
☐ Yes ☐ No

Permanent — Notching of the model interproximal to the upper 3 and 4, 5 and 6, with equal amounts removed on each (this should duplicate the space created by the separators placed by doctor).
☐ Yes ☐ No

SPECIAL INSTRUCTIONS

_____

_____

_____

_____

PLEASE CONSTRUCT THE FOLLOWING TYPE OF FRANKEL APPLIANCE ON THE ENCLOSED MODELS:

☐ FR I   ☐ FR III
☐ FR II   ☐ FR IV

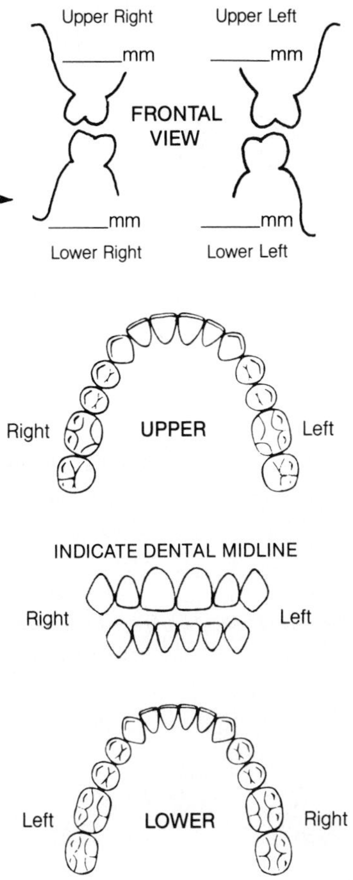

Upper Right   Upper Left
____ mm   ____ mm

FRONTAL VIEW

____ mm   ____ mm
Lower Right   Lower Left

Right   UPPER   Left

INDICATE DENTAL MIDLINE

Right   Left

Left   LOWER   Right

Fig. 10-21. Typical prescription pad used by orthodontic laboratories for instructions for FR fabrication. Proper attention to detail at this point can prevent problems later on. (Courtesy Max Hall and Dick Allessee.)

casts are received and the operator to double check it when the finished appliance is returned.

Laboratory prescription and procedures. Since few clinicians fabricate their own Fränkel appliances and because precise and specific instructions are required by the laboratory for proper appliance fabrication, prescription pads (Fig. 10-21) have been developed.

Different laboratories will require different information, but the prescription blank shown provides the important information needed by the technician to make the appliance as desired. If the notching described has not already been done by the operator, then the laboratory should be given precise instructions on the prescription blank.

It is important that the laboratory know (on the pre-

scription blank) of any midline deviation or other abnormalities. The appointment time for appliance placement must be clearly marked. Furthermore, the operator should not hesitate to call and discuss fabrication personally, if there is any question, or to leave instructions for the technician to call, because the precision demanded for FR construction requires complete clarity of the clinician's needs and desires.

Working model mounting. After carefully unpacking and checking the casts and construction bite, the laboratory personnel will assemble the parts to be sure that nothing has gone wrong in the shipping. The first step then is to mount the models on a straight line fixator or articulator, with both fully inserted in the wax bite. After the casts have been mounted with plaster, the

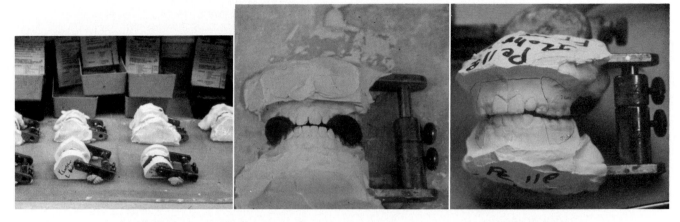

Fig. 10-22. When the models reach the laboratory, they are assembled on fixators, after it has been determined that the backs of the casts are trimmed correctly with the construction bite in place. After mounting, the Dentaurum 072-000 fixator permits easy separation and replacement of casts in the correct relationship without the wax bite in place. (Courtesy Max Hall and Dick Allessee.)

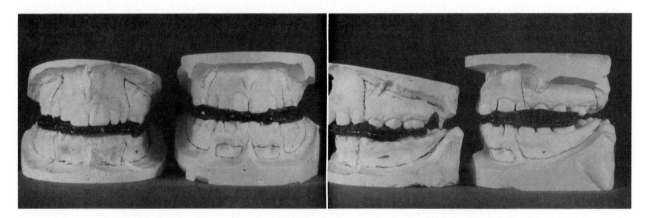

Fig. 10-23. After the models are properly trimmed (Fig. 10-18), buccal shields and lip pads are outlined on the casts in pencil preparatory to applying the wax relief and acrylic. (Courtesy Max Hall and Dick Allessee.)

wax bite is removed. A minimum of 2.5 mm interocclusal space must be present for the crossover wires. A number of different kinds of fixators are available, but the one most commonly recomended is made by Dentaurum (072-000) (Fig. 10-22).

Wax relief. Since the buccal shields must stand away from the teeth and tissues if the desired expansion is to be achieved, the prescription should incorporate information for thickness of wax relief in the various areas. It is a good procedure to outline the lip pads and buccal shields with pencil on the mounted work models before waxing them up (Fig. 10-23). Then the buccal surfaces are covered with layers of wax (Figs. 10-24 and 10-25). The thickness is determined individually by the amount of desired expansion needed, but it should not exceed 4 or 5 mm in the tooth area or 2.5 to 3 mm in the maxillary alveolar region. Only 0.5 mm thickness is needed at the mandibular shield periphery. To obtain the correct thickness of wax, pink baseplate wax of a known thickness can be applied in layers; or 3 mm thick red boxing wax can be used in the thickest portions, and baseplate wax then added to fill in the rest of the penciled outlines in the prescribed thicknesses. Fränkel uses a pointed explorer-like instrument with millimetric markings on the tip to ensure the correct depth of the wax (Fig. 10-25). Sometimes the maxillary buccal contours are curved, or convex, and the wax relief must exceed 3.0 mm to allow the appliance to be inserted and withdrawn properly over an undercut (particularly in the maxillary canine area). The wax covering is especially important in the region of the deciduous maxillary first molars, because this is the region of greatest

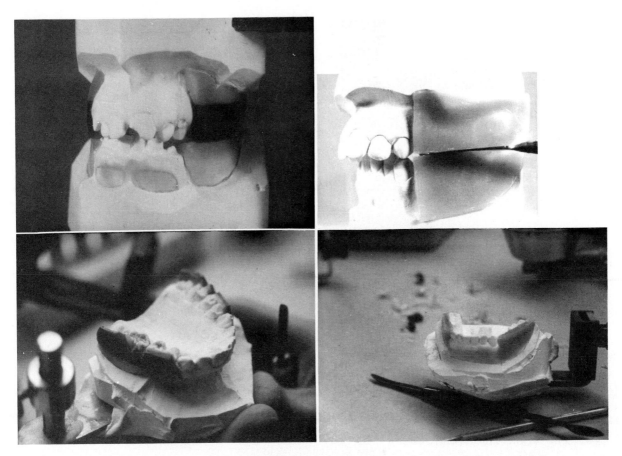

Fig. 10-24. Wax relief is applied to the maxillary and mandibular casts in the correct thickness. Only 0.5 mm is needed on the mandibular cast, but 2.5 to 3.0 mm is required in the maxillary alveolar region. Not more than 4 mm relief should be used in the tooth area. Red boxing wax (3.0 mm) can be used for the thicker portions. Only a thin layer of wax is needed under the lip pads. Each cast may be waxed separately and then the wax is joined when the models are placed together on the fixator. (Courtesy Max Hall and Dick Allessee.)

arch narrowing in most Class II, Division 1, malocclusions. It must be remembered, however, that if the space between the shields and tissue over the alveolar bone at the depth of the vestibule is too great it is almost impossible to prevent invagination of the cheek into this area, which will negate the desired periosteal pull effect.

Lower arch waxing requires only a very thin layer over the apical base (0.5 mm), thinning out to a rounded knife edge in the lower sulcus, where transverse changes are usually not desired. If the wax layer is too thick, it will make the appliance too bulky and the patient wil have a harder time adapting to it. The relief wax thickness is much greater in the dentition area, however, where as much as 4 or 5 mm is possible depending on the need for arch expansion. The usual amount needed is 3.0 mm. Upper and lower casts are waxed separately and then joined at the occlusal plane

so the outer surface has a gentle flowing concave curve. Usually a thin layer of pink baseplate wax is placed under the lip pads to reduce the danger of abrasion of gingival tissue by the lip pads and the possible dehiscence of the canine or incisor gingival margins if the patient bobs the appliance up and down in the mouth during daytime wear. This iatrogenic effect is of particular concern for appliances not properly locked on the maxillary arch by notching.

Wire forming. The wires are formed and placed as shown in Figs. 10-26 to 10-30 after the waxing has been completed. The palatal bow and occlusal rests are heavier (0.040 and 0.51 inch respectively), since they are stabilizing and connecting wires. The tooth-moving wires, which are seldom indicated with the FR appliance, are a smaller gauge (0.028 inch). To prevent abrasion and irritation, the stabilizing and connecting wires should not contact the tissue. Wires situated in the vestibule that are

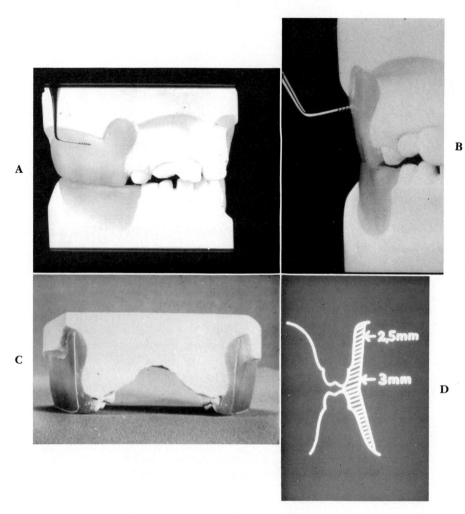

Fig. 10-25. A and **B,** One technique used by Fränkel to ensure the correct thickness of wax is to make millimetric markings on an explorer and use this to measure the thicknesses applied. **C,** Wax application thickness from the posterior before being finished down to a smooth surface. **D,** Minimal thickness recommended.

not covered by acrylic should be 1.5 to 2.0 mm from the alveolar mucosa. On the lingual aspect the wires should be 1.0 to 2.0 mm from the mucosa and palate. To avoid impingement and irritation of the soft tissues, wire bending should follow the natural tissue contours.

Lower lingual support wire. This heavy 0.051-inch stainless steel wire can be either three components soldered together or one continuous wire (Fig. 10-26). It is easier to bend the crossover wires and horizontal reinforcing wires separately and then solder them together or to pick up the free ends in the cold-cure acrylic pad when it is fabricated. The horizontal reinforcing wire element follows the contours of the lingual apical base at approximately 1 or 2 mm from the muscosa and 3 to 4 mm below the lingual gingival margin of the incisors, to permit adding acrylic for the pad. The crossover wires pass between the occlusal surfaces, at the embrasure between the deciduous first and second molars (or first and second premolars), care being taken not to con-

tact the upper and lower teeth. The ends are then bent at about 90 degrees to insert into the buccal shields. It is important that the ends be parallel to each other as well as to the occlusal plane to allow for advancement of the anterior section later if needed. This is discussed in the latter part of this chapter. The wire must slide through the shield in the advancement procedure; it must be perfectly straight. To prevent breakage, all wire bends in the Fränkel appliance (or any functional appliance) must be gradual. A right-angle bend can fatigue the wire and result in fracture during wear.

Wire parts that are embedded in the acrylic should not contact the wax (Fig. 10-27), nor should they stand away more than 1.0 mm from the wax surface (Fig. 10-30). This will prevent the buccal shields from becoming too thick and bulky.

Lower lingual springs. The 0.8 mm (0.028 inch) recurved spring wires are contoured to the lingual surfaces of the lower incisors right above the cingula, with the free ends about 3 mm below the incisal margins.

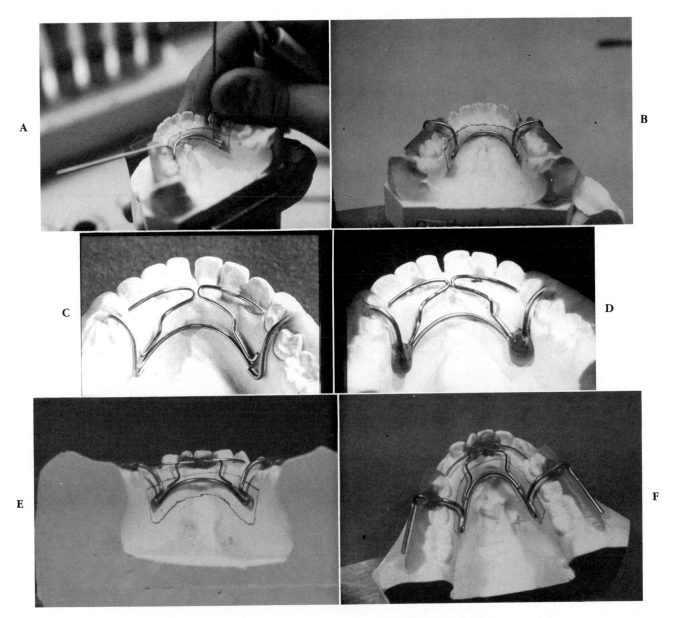

Fig. 10-26. Lower lingual wires are formed after the lower model on the fixator has been separated. **A** and **B,** In forming the lingual pad skeleton wire that crosses over between the upper and lower deciduous molars or premolars, care must be taken that the hanger wire does not touch upper or lower occlusal surfaces. **C** and **D,** The passive lingual springs are then formed and affixed to the cast with sticky wax, along with the hanger wire skeleton. **E** and **F,** The buccal ends are bent parallel to the buccal surface and stand away 1.0 mm from the relief wax so they can be encased in the acrylic shield. (Courtesy Max Hall and Dick Allessee.)

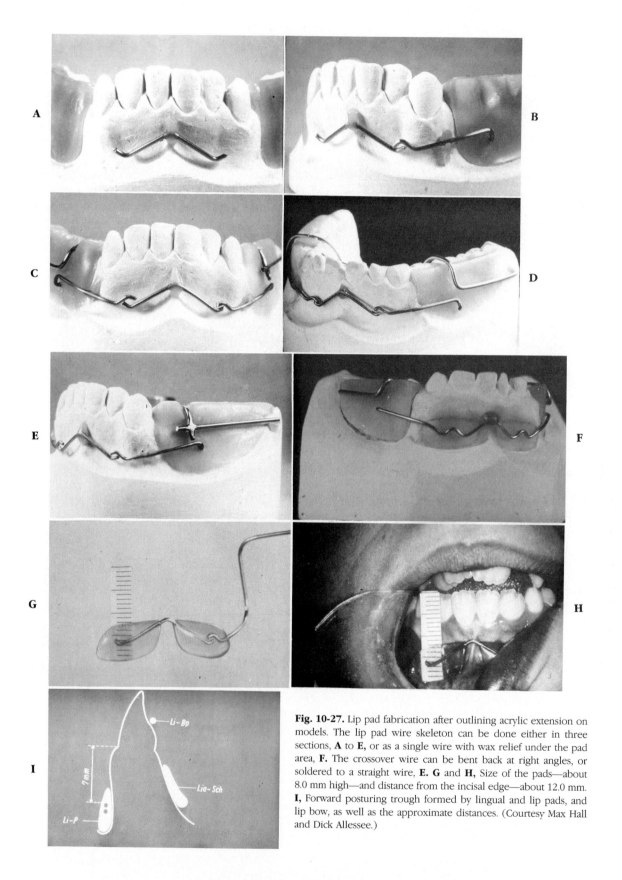

Fig. 10-27. Lip pad fabrication after outlining acrylic extension on models. The lip pad wire skeleton can be done either in three sections, **A** to **E,** or as a single wire with wax relief under the pad area, **F.** The crossover wire can be bent back at right angles, or soldered to a straight wire, **E. G** and **H,** Size of the pads—about 8.0 mm high—and distance from the incisal edge—about 12.0 mm. **I,** Forward posturing trough formed by lingual and lip pads, and lip bow, as well as the approximate distances. (Courtesy Max Hall and Dick Allessee.)

(Fig. 10-26) The primary objective for these elements is to prevent extrusion of the lower incisors, but care must be taken not to activate them. This will tip the lower incisors labially, an all too common problem with functional appliances. Fränkel stresses that these wires should usually be passive. If they are to be used for some special tooth-moving task, which is rare, then a smaller-gauge wire (0.5 or 0.6 mm) would probably be better suited to apply spring pressure. Tooth movements should really be done, pre-Fränkel or post-Fränkel therapy, with fixed or different removable appliances.

Lower labial wires. These 0.9 mm (0.036 inch) wires serve as the skeleton for the lower lip pads. (Fig. 10-27). Fränkel prefers three wires for this unit instead of one, which is more prone to breakage. The lateral wires emerge from the buccal shields in a slightly inferior direction and follow the contour of the muscosa around to the lateral incisor embrasure at a distance of about 1.0 mm from the tissue so they may be covered lingually and labially with the acrylic of the lip pads. The wire framework should be at least 7 mm below the gingival margin. The middle wire, or third component, is bent in the shape of an inverted **V** to prevent impingement on the labial muscle attachment.

Palatal bow. The 1.0 mm (0.040 inch, 18 gauge) thick palatal bow has a slightly posterior curve as shown in Figs. 10-3 and 10-4. The curve provides an extra length of wire to facilitate slight lateral expansion adjustment. This is necessary sometimes when the alveolodental area develops transversely and begins to contact the buccal shields. The wire should cross the maxillary occlusal surfaces in the grooves that have been cut just mesial to the maxillary first molars to enhance the seating on the maxillary arch (Fig. 10-28). The wire makes a loop in the buccal shield and emerges to lie between the maxillary first molar buccal cusps, ending in the fossa as an occlusal rest. The molar rests remain passive, unless the wire in the interproximal space moves up too high and impinges on the gingival tissue between the first molar and deciduous second molar. In this case the rests are bent slightly occlusally to reduce tissue contact (Figs. 10-5, 10-9, and 10-28). The rests should be parallel to the occlusal plane so the molars will be free to expand laterally. If the FR Ib is used in the deciduous or mixed dentition and the permanent first molars have not erupted sufficiently, the occlusal rests can be bent mesially instead of distally, with the ends lying in the central fossae of the deciduous second molars (Figs. 10-15 to 10-19).

Maxillary labial bow. The 0.9 mm (0.036 inch, 19 gauge) maxillary labial bow shape and position are illustrated in Figs. 10-2 and 10-29. The bow originates in the buccal shields and lies in the middle of the labial surfaces of the incisors. The wire leaves the acrylic with a slight bend toward the sulcus and then curves downward in the natural depression between the canine and lateral incisors to form the canine loops. The canine loops form larger and more gentle curves, with the apex of each loop crossing the middle third of the canine root, about 2 mm away from the mucosal surface. This configuration is important to permit canine eruption and expansion without danger of contacting the labial wire. The loops should be wide enough to allow constriction later, if needed, to close maxillary incisor spaces. However, the labial bow is normally not used for tooth movement, which can be done before or after Fränkel appliance orthopedic growth guidance with active plates or fixed appliances. The wire is straight and is not adapted to the individual tooth malpositions in the anterior segment. It should be emphasized that tipping of the maxillary incisors lingually with pinching up of the labial bow loops, as is done so often with a Hawley retainer, is not a treatment objective with the Fränkel appliance. Research by the author has shown that lingually tipped maxillary incisors can actually prevent full accomplishment of the mandibular growth pattern and thus reduce the benefit of forward posturing of the lower jaw. In addition, lingual tipping can cause the FR to become unseated from the maxillary interproximal grooves, letting the appliance drop and lose its maximal effectiveness. In the FR II there is a lingual wire behind the upper incisors to prevent lingualizing of the maxillary anterior segment. This wire may be used to tip the central incisors labially in a Class II, Division 2, malocclusion.

Canine loops. The canine loops (0.9 mm, 0.036 inch, 19 gauge) are embedded in the buccal shield at the occlusal plane level. They turn sharply toward the gingival margin of the deciduous maxillary first molars and fit in the embrasures between the deciduous first molars and canines, helping the palatal bow extensions at the first molar embrasures to anchor the FR on the maxillary arch. If the wires are formed properly, they can be bent occlusally to prevent interference with the erupting first premolars and canines. The loops wrap around the lingual surfaces of the canines and emerge labially at the canine–lateral incisor embrasures, curving distally over the canine cusps (Fig. 10-28). The free ends can be bent occlusally if required.

Fabrication of acrylic portions of the FR. After the wires are bent and properly adapted to the models as just outlined, they are secured with sticky wax (Fig. 10-30). The articulator should be closed again to ensure that the hangers or crossover wires do not touch either the upper or the lower tooth surfaces. Because of stress

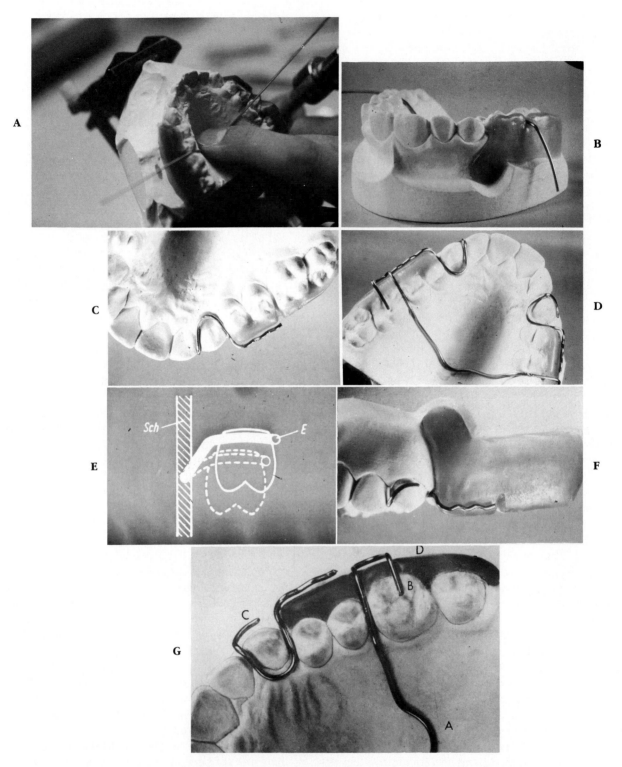

Fig. 10-28. Maxillary lingual wires. **A** and **B,** The heavy palatal wire is formed partly by thumb and finger pressure and partly with a no. 139 pliers for the center loop. The bird-beak pliers also works well for the canine clasps (Fig. 10-29). **C** and **D,** Note that the palatal bow crosses over in the embrasure between the permanent first molar and deciduous second molar or second premolar in the groove provided and then is bent around to form an occlusal rest. In the permanent dentition the maxillary rest is on the permanent first molar. If the deciduous second molar is present, the occlusal rest is bent forward to lie on this tooth. **E** and **F,** The canine clasp also passes through the embrasure provided by separation or slicing at the canine–first premolar region. As it passes through, it is bent occlusally; thus it may be adjusted downward so as not to interfere with eruption of these teeth. In **G** the palatal aspect includes *(A)* palatal bow, *(B)* occlusal rest, *(C)* canine clasp, and *(D)* wax relief.

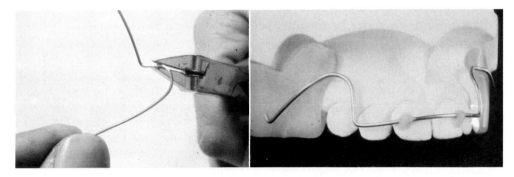

Fig. 10-29. Fabrication of the passive maxillary bow is relatively simple with a bird-beak no. 139 pliers. The bow is affixed to the model with sticky wax and must stand away enough for acrylic to incorporate the wire ends in the shield completely.

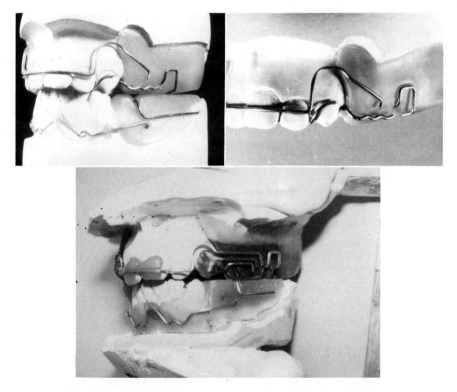

Fig. 10-30. Wire ends to be incorporated in the buccal shields. Each wire is held by sticky wax so it is not disturbed by the application of acrylic.

at this point, Eirew recommends double hangers through the interdental space on each side to reduce breakage.

The lip pads, buccal shields, and lingual pads are usually fabricated in cold-cure acrylic. Different laboratories vary the technique, but one (McNamara & Huge) completes the acrylic fabrication for the lower lingual pad and the labial lip pads first and then forms the maxillary wires and does the acrylic construction. Other laboratories bend the wires for the whole appliance and then do the acrylic work at the same time. It is easier to form the lingual pressure pad in the two step process, but the buccal and lip pads can be done easily either way. (See Figs. 10-33 to 10-36.)

Before the acrylic work for the buccal shields is done, the upper and lower wax portions are joined and the interdental space sealed to make a smooth lingual surface and to prevent the acrylic from seeping through. The shields and pads are formed with alternate applications of monomer and polymer (the "salt and pepper" technique). Some laboratories prefer to mix the entire mass and mold the acrylic, claiming that the surface is more dense and the consistency better. With either technique the name and phone number of the patient can be typed on a small piece of onionskin paper and incorporated in the buccal shields during the buildup phase. As the acrylic polymerizes, it can be molded to form the approximate desired shape. The total thickness of the shields and pads should not be greater than 2.5 mm. If the polymerized appliance is then placed in a pressure cooker for 15 to 20 minutes at 25 to 30 pounds of pressure, the consistency and density will be improved (Fig. 10-37). To facilitate separation of the appliance from the models after they are removed from the pressure cooker, the articulator should be placed in icewater to harden the wax. To prevent distortion, wires are gently freed from the models before separating the appliance from the work models. Rough polishing and shaping can be done with a sandpaper arbor chuck or cherrystone-type bur (Fig. 10-38). Because of the inherent complexity of the FR appliance and difficulty in polishing some of the lingual surfaces, extreme care must be exercised not to nick the wires or catch the appliance on a rag wheel in the polishing process. Distortion is likely in such cases, or the wires will break soon after the patient starts wearing the appliance. For some reason, Fränkel appliance repairs are needed more frequently than other functional appliance repairs—with even the heaviest wires breaking at the exit point from the shields. Important wearing time and patient compliance can be lost if the appliance must be sent back to the laboratory. It is important to round off and polish all margins, particularly where they put sulcus tissue under tension.

The lip pads look somewhat like a parallelogram (Fig. 10-2); but the individual anatomy permits variation to prevent unnecessary impingement and irritation, especially at the frenum borders. The superior periphery of the lip pads should be at least 5 mm from the gingival margin. Figs. 10-19 and 10-27 illustrate the proper position and inclination of the pads. This attention to detail is quite important in eliminating the mentalis muscle hyperactivity and abnormal functional lip trap that enhance the overjet.

Before the FR is inserted in the patient's mouth, it should be replaced on the models and checked carefully for tolerances, adaptation, and wire conformity. The anterosuperior margin of the vestibular shield should extend past the canine–deciduous first molar embrasure to the middle of the canine. Some clinicians actually carry this into the depression over the lateral incisors (Fig. 10-35) as suggested by Diers. The posterior periphery of the shield should extend distally beyond the last erupted tooth.

FR Ic. The FR Ic is recommended by Fränkel for the more severe Class II, Division 1, malocclusions in patients with an overjet of more than 7 mm and a sagittal dysplasia that exceeds an end-to-end cuspal relationship. As has been pointed out, it is neither feasible nor desirable to posture the mandible forward into a Class I relationship and eliminate the excessive overjet in one step. Tissue response is less favorable and patient compliance is much poorer. Thus the mandibular protraction is done in two, or occasionally, three steps.

To accomplish the advancement procedures and dispense with the need for a new appliance, a simple maneuver is possible. The buccal shields (Fig. 10-31) are split horizontally and vertically into two parts. The anteroinferior portion contains the wires for the lingual acrylic pressure pad and for the lower lip pads. To allow for this maneuver, the heavy through-the-bite hanger wire that connects the lingual pad and buccal shields has been formed to permit advancement of the mandibular trough (formed by the lip pads on the labial and the lingual pad on the inside). The ends of the hanger wires are incorporated in the buccal shield and are horizontal. This allows the movement of the free portion in an anterior direction—after the acrylic cut has been made—by pulling the anterior section forward, with the wire slipping forward within the posterior part of the shield to accommodate the forward movement of the lingual pressure pad and labial lip pads. As Fig. 10-31 shows, the vertical split is pried open with an office knife to the desired position by a 2 to 3 mm advancement and is then filled in with cold-cure acrylic and polished. A new tactile engram is thus constructed for mandibular position, with both lip and lower lingual pads giving new exteroceptive and proprioceptive signals.

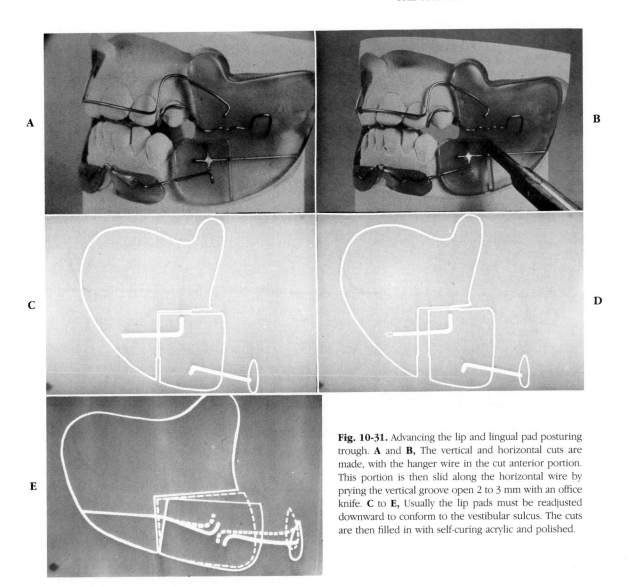

Fig. 10-31. Advancing the lip and lingual pad posturing trough. **A** and **B,** The vertical and horizontal cuts are made, with the hanger wire in the cut anterior portion. This portion is then slid along the horizontal wire by prying the vertical groove open 2 to 3 mm with an office knife. **C** to **E,** Usually the lip pads must be readjusted downward to conform to the vestibular sulcus. The cuts are then filled in with self-curing acrylic and polished.

Occasionally adjustments must then be made in the lip pads, bending the wires downward slightly. Parallelism with the contiguous tissue must be checked so there is no abrasion on placement and removal or during function. Also, because of the further mandibular advancement, the posteroinferior buccal shield periphery may irritate the sulcus and require trimming.

In actual practice the FR Ic is seldom used any more, since the FR Ib and FR II can be modified the same way, making the horizontal and vertical cuts for the advancement when needed rather than ahead of time. The same connecting wire is pulled forward in the posterior part of the shield, opening the vertical slots to the desired 2 or 3 mm advancement of the lingual and labial pads. The slots are then filled in with cold-cure acrylic. An early variation of the FR Ic was to incorporate jackscrews in the slots of the buccal shields, permitting bilateral

advancement as desired. This modification has been resurrected by some laboratories and is available on prescription. The thickening of the buccal shield to accommodate the jackscrews has been considered a disadvantage by Fränkel (Fig. 10-32).

Pre–Fränkel appliance fixed or removable mechanotherapy. Before a description of the FR II is undertaken, a few words on pre–Fränkel appliance mechanotherapy are in order. The Fränkel appliance is a deficiency appliance and an exercise device. It has been designed primarily to eliminate abnormal perioral muscle function and the deleterious effects on the dentition and optimal growth increments. It is *not* a tooth-moving appliance. Appurtenances can be added, as with any other functional appliance, but such modifications are usually not very efficient. More important, they jeopardize the effectiveness of the Fränkel appliance and increase the

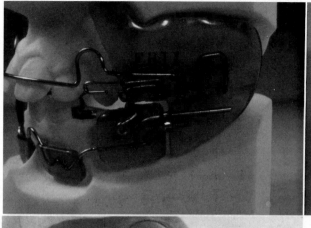
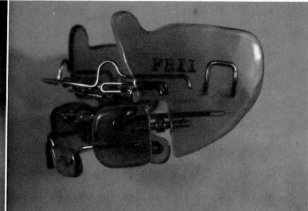
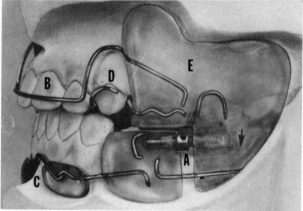

Fig. 10-32. Advancing the shields with a jackscrew. This can be done gradually in two or three steps, as desired, or at one time (after 3 or 4 months) as shown in Fig. 10-31. Jackscrew *(A),* labial wire *(B),* lip pads *(C),* canine clasp *(D),* buccal shield *(E).* Arrow on the shield shows the direction to turn the jackscrew to open it.

likelihood of its being unseated from the maxillary arch. This then produces undesirable lower incisor procumbency and possible labiogingival stripping in the lower arch.

However, it is frequently desirable to do minor expansion of the upper arch, to correct rotations, change axial inclinations, or close spaces before placing the FR. Such movements would actually enhance the Fränkel appliance success. So careful diagnosis is called for. The clinician should not hesitate to use a simple active plate or direct-bonded attachments to achieve one or more of the aforementioned objectives ahead of time. (See Chapter 11.) Such limited corrective procedures also may be done afterward. However, it is stressed that the Fränkel appliance does not exclude use of other forms of therapy but often demands it for optimal efficiency. This type of therapy is beyond the scope of the present chapter. Nevertheless, it can be stated with assurance that 3 to 6 months of pre-Fränkel tooth movement can pay off in a better final result for the patient.

FR II

Although the FR II has been used by Fränkel mostly for Class II, Division 2, malocclusions, more and more of his disciples are using it for Class II, Division 1, patients (Fig. 10-33). It is estimated that 80% to 90% of all Fränkel appliances now being made in the United States are the FR II type. The complaint encountered from some clinicians is that the FR I canine loop can interfere with eruption of the permanent canines and that the FR II canine loop is less likely to do this. Fränkel also has used active plates to align the maxillary anterior teeth before placing the FR II. However, our experience with fixed appliances prior to FR II placement for such cases has been more rewarding, as already noted. FInal detailing may also be necessary after the eruption of canines and premolars. This is particularly true of the maxillary canines, which often do not seat completely with Fränkel appliance therapy alone. Thus a post-Fränkel appliance period of fixed mechanotherapy is frequently needed, too, to provide the optimum result that American orthodontics has come to strive for and expect.

In any event, routine alignment of maxillary anterior teeth in Class II, Division 2, malocclusions is suggested prior to FR II placement. Such pre–functional appliance fixed mechanotherapy for the maxillary anterior segment is needed in one third to one half of all Class II patients.

FR II construction. The FR II is modified by adding a

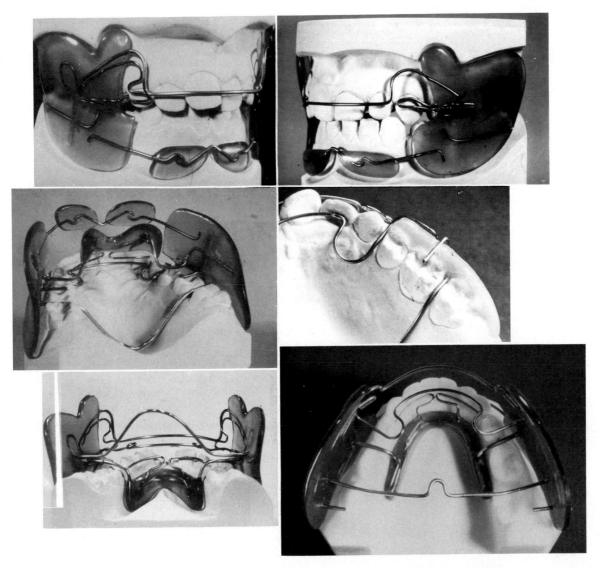

Fig. 10-33. The FR II appliance has canine clasps that do not wrap around the canine and thus are less likely to interfere with eruption. The clasps continue through the distal canine embrasure and form a stabilizing lingual palatal bow. Formerly called a protrusion bow, because of its use in Class II, Division 2, malocclusions, it now is made of heavier wire and is passive, helping to anchor the appliance on the maxilla. The shields, lip pads, palatal bow, and lower lingual pad and wires are the same as for the FR I. Note the maxillary molar rest bent mesially to lie in the occlusal fossa of the deciduous second molar.

stainless steel lingual bow (0.8 mm, 0.032 inch, 20 gauge) behind the maxillary incisors. This serves to maintain the pre–functional appliance alignment achieved and stabilizes the appliance by helping to lock it on the maxillary arch, a prime requisite of FR therapy (Figs. 10-5 and 10-33). An added factor, relative "depression" of the maxillary anterior teeth, has also been suggested. Fränkel originally called this a protrusion bow; but it no longer functions in this manner, with fixed or removable appliance pre-Fränkel mechanotherapy.

Since pre-FR therapy has achieved individual tooth alignment, there is no need for a resilient lingual bow. A heavier stabilizing wire is thus recommended for improved structural support (0.030 to 0.036 inch). This assists the crossover wires in the embrasures between the permanent maxillary first molars and deciduous second molars and between the maxillary canines and deciduous first molars, as described previously. On his visits to the United States, Fränkel keeps emphasizing, after seeing cases by various clinicians or reading articles showing improper use of his appliance in the literature, that one of the major reasons for failure of FR therapy is the lack of a positive maxillary stabilization of the appliance. The deleterious consequences of an unseated and free-floating appliance are seen in the proclining of lower incisors, mucosal irritation, and actual dehiscences in the lower canine and incisor areas, with wearing away of gingival mucosa.

The maxillary lingual bow of the FR II originates in the vestibular shield and passes to the lingual through the canine–deciduous first molar embrasure, which has been previously notched. The wire forms loops that approximate the palatal mucosa and recurve vertically to contact the incisors at the canine–lateral incisor embrasure (Fig. 10-33). A 90-degree bend allows the wire to follow the lingual contours of the four incisors, right above the cingula. The main objective of the FR II is to improve the mandibular sagittal relationship. Since evidence exists that little reciprocal retrusive maxillary response occurs in most cases, the additional lingual stabilizing wire has the desirable objective of preventing lingual tipping of the maxillary incisors (Fig. 10-34). As

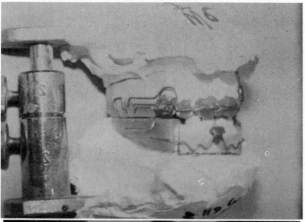

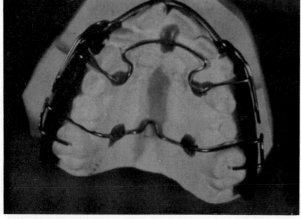

Fig. 10-34. Waxing for the FR II is similar to that for the FR I; the lingual and labial wires are affixed with sticky wax prior to the application of acrylic. The lower lip pad wire is a single piece in this particular appliance but can be made in three pieces if preferred.

pointed out earlier, lingually tipped maxillary incisors could prevent optimal mandibular forward posturing. It is a known fact that so-called lingual tipping with the round wire labial bow of removable appliances is in reality a partial labial root tipping as the incisors rotate about a centrum somewhere between the root apex and the gingival margin. It is seldom desirable to produce labial root tipping on most Class II malocclusions. Pre- and postorthodontic therapy with fixed appliances can prevent such undesirable sequelae, but the lingual bow also reduces this tendency. The lingual bow of the FR II passes through the notch created in the deciduous first molar–canine embrasure to insert into the buccal shields. It performs the same function as the canine loops of the FR I do in helping to seat the appliance on the maxilla.

The FR II canine loops are modified. They continue to originate in the buccal shields, but they contact the canines on the buccal only as a recurved loop (Fig. 10-33). These 0.8 mm (0.032 inch 20 gauge) loops actually serve as an extension of the buccal shields in the canine area, which is narrowed most by the abnormal perioral muscle function associated with the malocclusion. Placing these wires 2 to 3 mm away from the deciduous canines eliminates the restrictive muscle function, permitting the needed width development. Diers actually extends the buccal shields forward into the canine fossa for the same reason (Fig. 10-35).

As with the FR I, the therapeutic effect of the FR II is three-dimensional. Selective eruption is encouraged to provide vertical dentoalveolar adjustment. The need for bite opening is greater in Class II, Division 2, malocclusions; therefore the FR II can and must be used to enhance selective eruption of the lower buccal segments. Maxillary expansion is often not needed in Class II, Division 2, patients, who have broad dental arches. In such cases there is minimal carving of the work model in the vestibular area. The buccal shields need not stand away from the alveolar mucosa in the vestibule.

Since there is usually a strong mentalis muscle activity in Class II, Division 2, malocclusions, lip pads are well rounded and polished to prevent mucosal irritation. In some cases of deep bite Class I or Class II, Division 2, malocclusions, with deep overbite and infraclusion of lower posterior segments, in which lip length and contact are ample, the vertical dimension can be opened to a greater degree without endangering lip seal. Particularly in an anteriorly rotating growth pattern, this tends to open the bite and direct mandibular growth in a more vertical direction, reducing the tendency to grow into a deeper bite during and after active treatment (Fig. 10-36). This variation of vertical dimension of the construction bite to affect growth direction is discussed in Chapter 7.

The processing of the FR II is the same as for the FR

I. After waxing and wire forming, the wire elements are affixed to the model with sticky wax (Fig. 10-37). The acrylic may be added either with the "salt and pepper" technique or by mixing first to a moldable consistency and then applying by kneading and molding with the fingers. The claim is made that the acrylic is denser with the latter method, but most laboratories prefer the direct alternate monomer-powder method illustrated. In any event, the appliance is then placed in a pressure cooker as with acrylic retainer fabrication to provide a more dense finished product. Polishing of the appliance requires great care so as not to distort the wire elements (Fig. 10-38).

Modifications are to be discouraged for the neophyte, but some experienced clinicians have tried to incorporate extraoral force at night. Buccal tubes can be placed in the buccal shields at about the deciduous second molar area (Fig. 10-39). A facebow with light force placed by the patient on retiring enhances the maxillary retraction potential, where needed. McNamara has shown minimal "headgear effect" or retrusion of the maxillary complex with his conventional FR-treated cases. Case selection and patient cooperation are critical, however. Monitoring also is vital to prevent any possible unfavorable sequelae (e.g., dehiscence of the lower incisors).

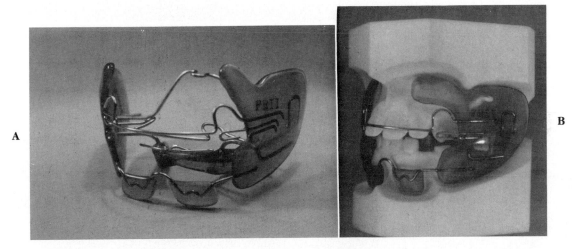

Fig. 10-35. A, The appliance is polished after trimming and is ready for insertion. **B,** The FR II has been modified according to Diers, with the buccal shields projecting into the maxillary canine and lateral incisor fossae to screen off any deleterious or restricting effects on basal bone growth.

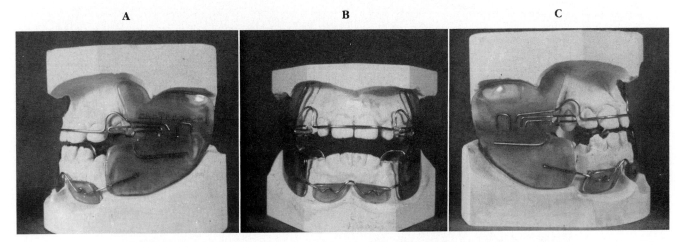

Fig. 10-36. The FR II, with a wider open vertical construction bite, is used when greater posterior eruption is needed and when lip length is adequate and will not be affected (as far as lip seal exercises are concerned) by the vertical increase. The wider opening is increasingly likely to produce a more vertical growth direction for anterosuperiorly rotating patterns, which tend to grow into deep overbites (e.g., in Class II, Division 2, malocclusions). Note the interocclusal position of the hanger wires and space between the shields and the maxillary alveolar process, **B.**

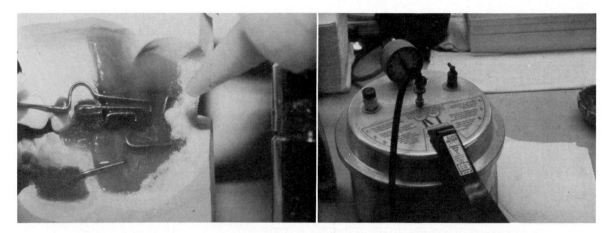

Fig. 10-37. The "salt and pepper" technique of adding acrylic powder and monomer is most frequently used; but these materials can be mixed ahead of time, kneaded and rolled into a pliable mass, and applied by finger pressure with a light coat of petrolatum on the fingers to prevent sticking. In either case the curing appliance is then put into a pressure cooker under 20 pounds of air.

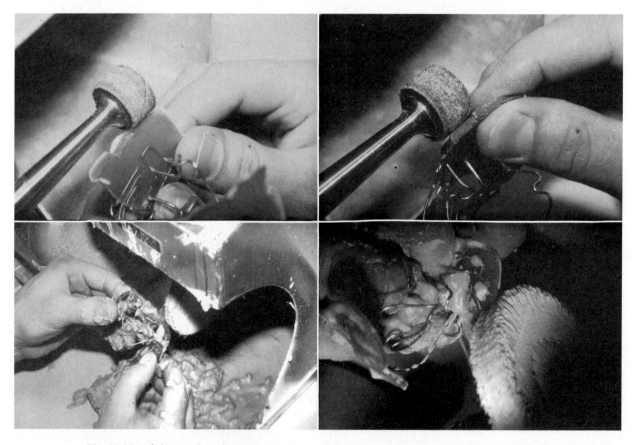

Fig. 10-38. Polishing is done in a manner similar to that used for Hawley retainers. However, the skeleton framework makes it easier to catch and distort the appliance. Greater care is required with both the sandpaper arbor and the rag wheel and pumice.

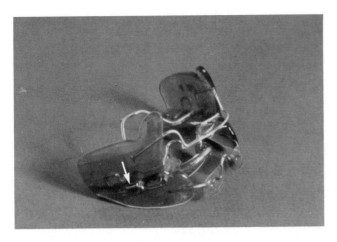

Fig. 10-39. Recently some modifications have been introduced by Fränkel appliance disciples. Since there is little function during sleep, it is possible to incorporate extraoral force for Class II malocclusions with maxillary protractions. The appliance is anchored on the maxilla, and light oblique or vertical pull force can be tolerated without dislodgment. Note the horizontal buccal tube embedded in the buccal shield *(arrow)*.

Normally this is not likely to occur during sleeping since the mandible tends to drop open. Nevertheless, the FR must be firmly anchored on the maxillary arch by the palatal bow at the molar, and the lingual palatal incisor wire at the canine, area or the results will be disastrous; but if the extraoral force does not dislodge the appliance (by virtue of a vertical pull paralleling the Y-axis), greater maxillary retraction is possible with the combined appliances. (Combinations of functional and extraoral force appliances are discussed in more detail in Chapter 11.)

Examples of successful FR I and FR II treatment are illustrated in Figs. 10-40 to 10-45.

FR III

The concepts described for the FR I and FR II also apply to the FR III, which is still a deficiency appliance. However, there is usually a deficiency in the maxillary arch instead of the mandible. (Fig. 10-46).

The *lip pads* are situated in the labial vestibular sulcus

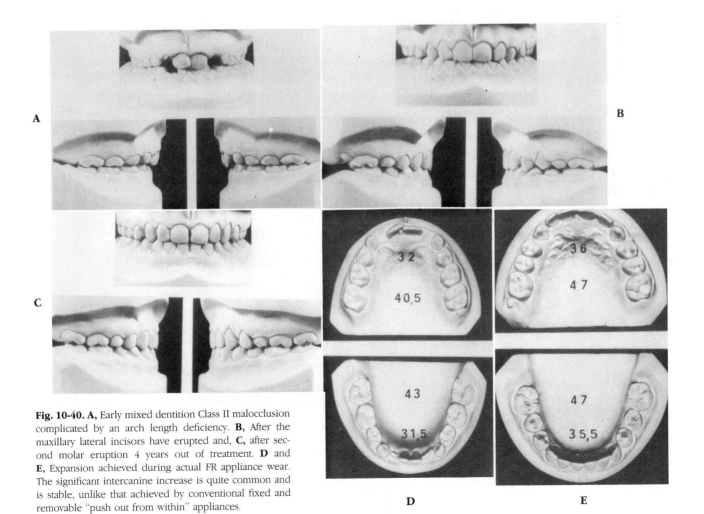

Fig. 10-40. A, Early mixed dentition Class II malocclusion complicated by an arch length deficiency. **B,** After the maxillary lateral incisors have erupted and, **C,** after second molar eruption 4 years out of treatment. **D** and **E,** Expansion achieved during actual FR appliance wear. The significant intercanine increase is quite common and is stable, unlike that achieved by conventional fixed and removable "push out from within" appliances.

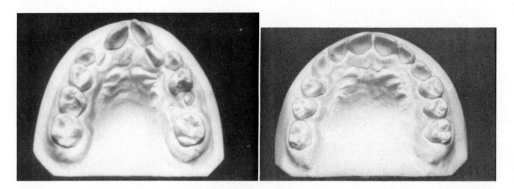

Fig. 10-41. Another example of significant maxillary arch widening under the influence of screening buccal shields and lip seal exercises. As in the case in Fig. 10-40, the results proved stable. The autonomous arch length increase in the maxillary arch was almost 5 mm.

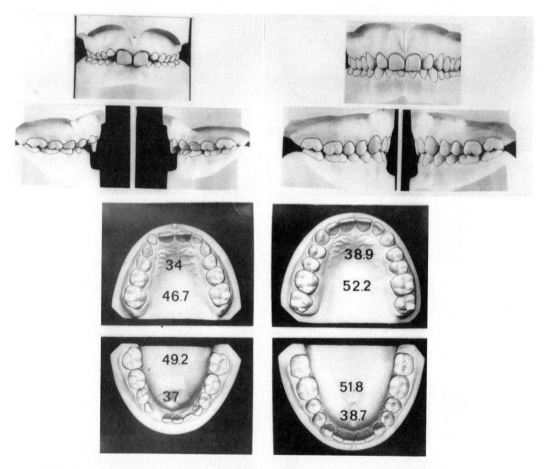

Fig. 10-42. Class II, Division 1, malocclusion treated during the mixed dentition. The excessive overbite and overjet have been eliminated, and the expansion achieved has corrected the arch length deficiency. Again there is a large and stable maxillary intercanine increase of almost 5 mm.

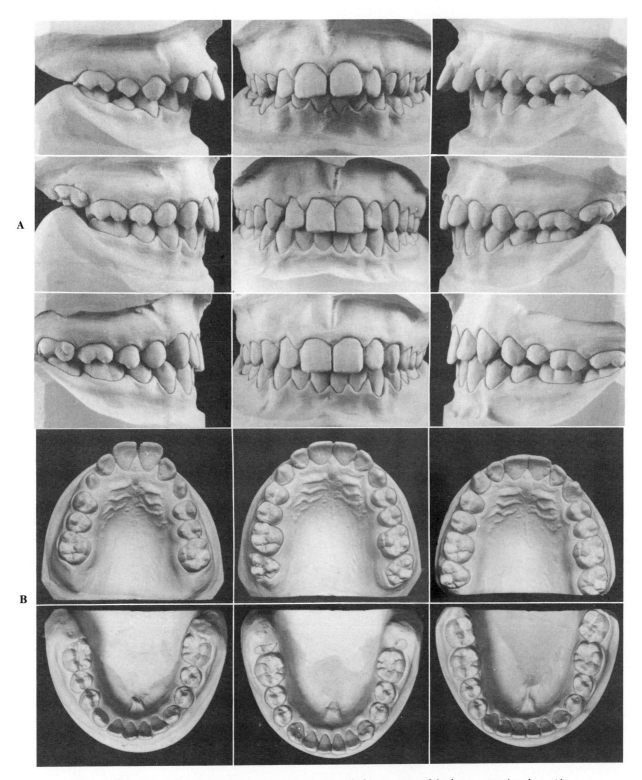

Fig. 10-43. A, Class II, Division 1, malocclusion treated after eruption of the lower second molars with a Fränkel Function Regulator. The middle row of casts shows improvement during therapy, and the lower row the final stable result achieved at 16 years of age. **B,** Expansion achieved and retraction of maxillary incisors. Lower incisor irregularity has been corrected, but there is no proclination of these teeth.

Continued.

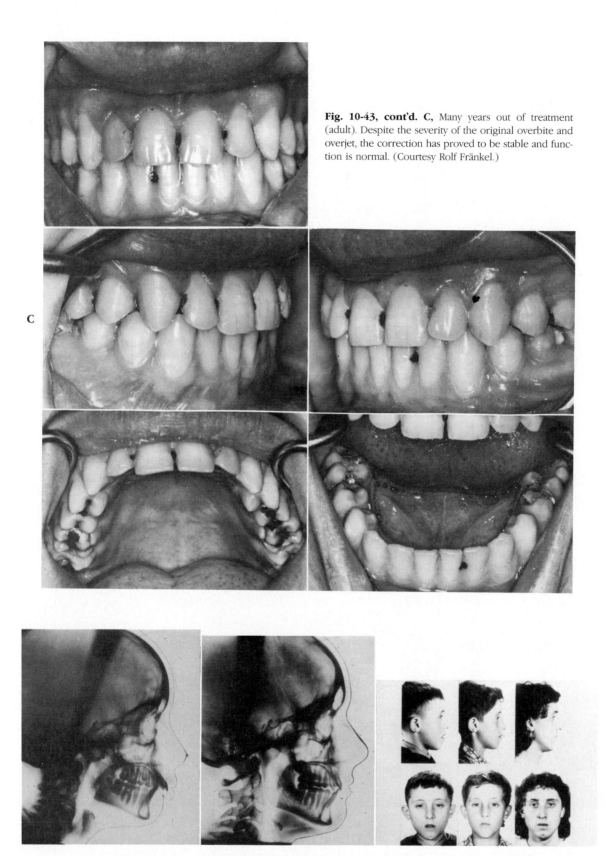

C

Fig. 10-43, cont'd. C, Many years out of treatment (adult). Despite the severity of the original overbite and overjet, the correction has proved to be stable and function is normal. (Courtesy Rolf Fränkel.)

Fig. 10-44. Before and after FR treatment of a Class II, Division 1, malocclusion. The elimination of perverted perioral muscle function and the lip seal exercises have together reduced the anterior face height and provided better facial balance.

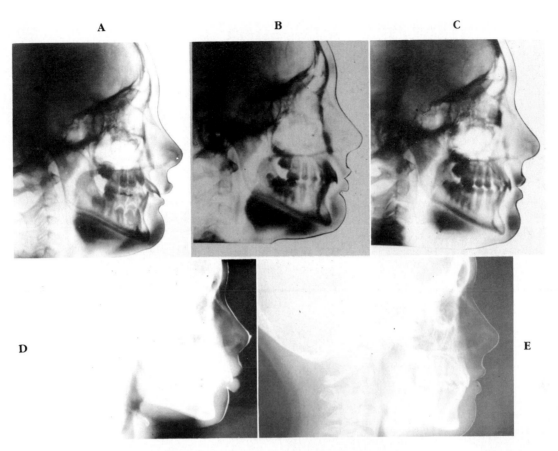

A   B   C

D   E

Fig. 10-45. Major sagittal change accomplished in the FR treatment of a Class II, Division 1, mixed dentition problem. **A,** Pretreatment, **B,** at the end of treatment, and, **C,** 4 years later. The apical base relationship is normal. **D** and **E,** Both soft and hard tissue changes, achieved by Function Regulator therapy and lip seal exercises. (Courtesy Rolf Fränkel.)

of the upper incisor segment, instead of the lower (Figs. 10-46 and 10-47). The pads stand away from the mucosa and underlying alveolar bone in the same manner as with the FR II. The supporting metal framework is made up of 0.040-inch stainless wire. The purposes of the lip pads are threefold: (1) to eliminate the restrictive pressure of the upper lip on the underdeveloped maxilla; (2) to exert tension on the tissue and periosteal attachments in the depth of the maxillary sulcus for stimulation of bone growth; and (3) to transmit upper lip force to the mandible via the lower labial arch for a retrusive stimulus. Admittedly, such force is quite minimal and probably has little effect other than to give a negative feedback signal to false anterior posturing (Fig. 10-47).

The *labial bow* rests against the mandibular teeth and not the maxillary incisors, which are free to move forward. Unlike the maxillary bow, however, there is a positive contact with the lower incisors by the 0.09 mm (0.036 inch) structural wire (Fig. 10-47). It is usually recommended that a very shallow groove be cut across the

labial of the lower incisors to ensure that a slight tension exists in this wire when the appliance is seated in the patient's mouth. The labial bow should cross the lower incisors at the lowest possible level, without impinging on the interproximal soft tissue, to keep lingual tipping of the lower incisors to a minimum.

The *protrusion bow* of the FR III is similar to that of the FR II, passing behind the upper incisors to stimulate slight to moderate forward movement of these teeth (Figs. 10-46 and 10-47). The configuration is much the same as that used in the FR II, with the horizontal component of the wire contacting the teeth just above the cingula of the maxillary incisors. Occasionally the protrusion bow is divided at the midline to give more finger spring action to individual teeth (Fig. 10-46).

The *palatal bow,* a small posteriorly directed loop at the midline, approximates the palatal mucosa in the same manner as is seen with the FR I and II (Fig. 10-46). The difference is that the ends of the bow pass *distal* instead of mesial to the permanent first molar, or the

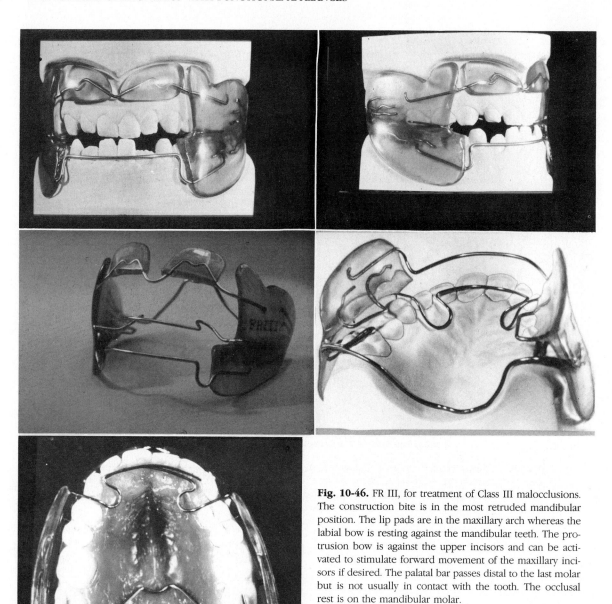

Fig. 10-46. FR III, for treatment of Class III malocclusions. The construction bite is in the most retruded mandibular position. The lip pads are in the maxillary arch whereas the labial bow is resting against the mandibular teeth. The protrusion bow is against the upper incisors and can be activated to stimulate forward movement of the maxillary incisors if desired. The palatal bar passes distal to the last molar but is not usually in contact with the tooth. The occlusal rest is on the mandibular molar.

permanent second molar if it has erupted. The lateral extensions then insert into the buccal shields. The palatal bow is thus capable of delivering a slight anterior stimulus to the maxillary dentition by reforming this wire to contact the distal surfaces of the terminal molars on the tuberosities. Normally, however, it stands away from the last maxillary molar. The palatal bow is not a tooth-moving wire but a stabilizing component replacing the acrylic palatal cover of the conventional activator.

The FR III is *not* locked on the maxilla by the cross-wires from the protrusion bow and palatal bow. However, the close adherence of the buccal shields and lower labial wire to the mandibular basal bone and lower incisors gives a firm grip on the mandibular dentoalveolar structures.

The *occlusal rests* are on the mandibular first molar, instead of the maxillary molar. In line with the Harvold concept of differential guidance of eruption, the mandibular molars are prevented from erupting upward and forward, while the maxillary buccal segment is free to

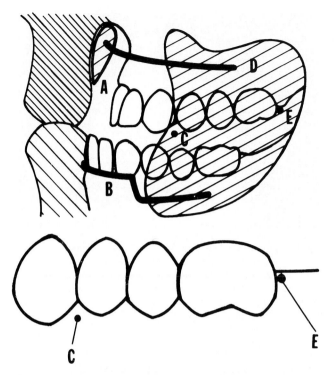

Fig. 10-47. The lip pads *(A)* are in the maxillary labial vestibule for the FR III. The labial bow *(B)* is in contact with the six mandibular anterior teeth, exerting a very slight pressure on them. The protrusion bow *(C)* is in contact with the lingual surfaces of the upper incisors, passing interocclusally at the distal of the canines. The palatal bow *(E)* passes behind the last maxillary molar to enter the shield. It can then recurve and exit to form an occlusal rest over the lower molar, or a separate rest can be made. In most instances it does not touch the distal surface of the maxillary molar.

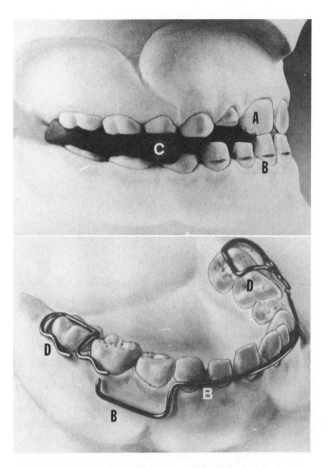

Fig. 10-48. The construction bite for the FR III is taken in the most retruded mandibular position, opening the vertical dimension only as much as is needed to establish an end-to-end bite in the incisors *(A)*. The lower labial wire position *(B)* is marked on the mandibular cast, and a slight groove is notched in the teeth at this line. The wax bite *(C)* must be thick enough to allow the protrusion bow, palatal bow, and occlusal rest wires *(D)* to pass through.

erupt downward and forward, reducing the Class III relationship. The rests thus enhance the mandibular anchorage of the FR III (Fig. 10-48).

The *buccal shields* stand away from the maxillary posterior dentoalveolar structures, similar to the FR I and II, approximately 3 mm, but they are in contact with the mandibular teeth and mandibular apical base (Fig. 10-46). This recognizes that there is an inherent three-dimensional deficiency in the maxilla in most Class III malocclusions, which have buccal as well as anterior cross-bite problems. Any constricting or deforming effect of the buccinator mechanism and orbicularis oris is screened from the maxillary arch and supporting bone. The approximation of the buccal shields to the mandibular arch, however, has a constricting effect on the mandibular dentition. This is aided by the adapted labial wire. The shields and lip pads also exert outward pull

or tension on the maxillary periosteum at the height of the vestibule.

Construction bite. Even though Fränkel recognizes the probable maxillary deficiency and anteroposterior discrepancy in Class III malocclusions, he is fully aware, of course, that it is impossible to posture the maxilla forward to stimulate growth and remove restrictive muscle influences as the FR I and II do for mandibular deficiency in Class II malocclusions. He recognizes that there may be a combined mandibular excess and accommodative forward posturing of the lower jaw, however, which has been the classic analysis of most Class III malocclusions. So the construction bite procedure is done by clinically retruding the mandible as much as possible, with the condyle occupying the most posterior position in the fossa. The vertical dimension is opened only enough to allow the maxillary incisors to move labially past the mandibular incisors for cross-bite correction. The bite opening is kept to a minimum to allow lip closure with minimal strain (Fig. 10-48). Muscle training and lip seal exercises are as important for Class III as for Class II. The typically redundant and everted lower lip of the mandibular prognathism patient can be helped by lip seal exercises. The most retruded mandibular position varies from patient to patient and also depends on whether the habitual Class III occlusion is a true basal relationship or an accommodative anterior mandibular displacement caused by incisor interference. It is likely that the majority of Class III malocclusions are a combination of both sagittal basal discrepancy and adaptive tooth guidance.

The clinical maneuver for obtaining the maximal posterior condylar position is a gentle tapping on the mandible with the flexed knuckles of the clinician's dominant hand while the patient opens a centimeter or so, continuing the tapping gently and then having the patient close slowly and guide the final closure with posterior pressure applied by the thumb against the symphysis and the forefinger under the chin. Before taking the wax registration, it is important to have the patient maintain this position for 1 or 2 minutes so the proprioceptive learning process and feedback to the muscles and tendons will be strong enough to overcome the natural tendency to protrude the mandible when closing into the construction bite wax wafer. The posterior guidance is essential during the actual bite-taking procedure. This position is easier for the patient to hold while the wax sets than for the Class II forward posturing, since it is the registration of a reproducible terminal position. Thus the wax can be softer. The wax is removed, chilled under cold water, and replaced and the bite registration is checked again, as with the FR I and II, before the patient is dismissed.

Deep bite problems require a wider opening of the vertical dimension for the construction bite. This is done so the appliance can be fabricated to stimulate posterior eruption of the maxillary teeth. (Acrylic extensions as well as occlusal rests may be placed over the mandibular molars [Fig. 10-49].) If there is minimal need for vertical development, the occlusal rests are sufficient to hold the lower molars from erupting whereas the maxillary molars are free to move downward and forward to correct the sagittal discrepancy (as has been recommended by Woodside and Harvold). Separating elastics and notching are not necessary for the FR III since the appliance is stabilized on the mandible by the buccal shields, labial wire, and occlusal rests.

Working model pour-up and trimming. The procedure for pouring and trimming the FR III is essentially the same as that already described for the FR I and II.

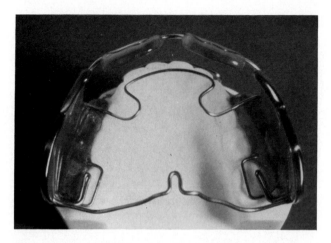

Fig. 10-49. FR III in place on the lower model. It can be modified to allow an acrylic cover over the mandibular buccal segment, providing more stability, since there are no locking wires at the embrasures. This also prevents eruption of the mandibular teeth while freeing selected maxillary teeth to erupt downward and forward. The palatal bow, protrusion bow, and lip pads fit the maxillary arch.

The impressions are poured up immediately in yellow stone, care being taken that there is an adequate base to permit proper carving of the maxillary model. The tuberosity must be faithfully reproduced for the palatal bow extension into the vestibular shield. The excess stone must be trimmed away (as noted previously).

The maxillary cast is trimmed for the lip pads. This is done extensively, after careful inspection of the patient's anatomic structures and palpation of the area in question. The pliable soft tissue of the upper lip will usually accept about a 5 mm deepening of the sulcus. Proper trimming positions the lower margin of the lip pads at a distance of some 7 to 8 mm from the upper incisor gingival border (Fig. 10-47). The pads are more teardrop shaped because of the midline muscle attachment and labial frenum.

The trimming of the model for the FR III buccal shields is the same as for the FR I and II and is also limited to the maxillary cast. Great care must be exercised to prevent creep of soft tissue under the shields at the height of the maxillary sulcus. Proper carving and appropriate wax relief will prevent this undesirable occurrence. No trimming should be done on the mandibular model, although the operator must delineate the muscle attachments to prevent impingement and irritation from the proximity of the acrylic to the mucosa.

Laboratory prescription and fabrication procedure. The wax bite is reinserted and the posterior surfaces of the upper and lower casts are trimmed flush. The bite is then mounted on the fixator, as described previously, before the prescription is written up and the

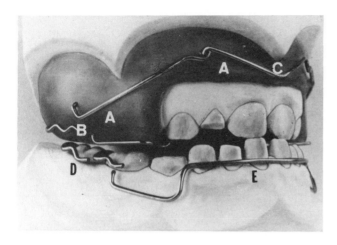

Fig. 10-50. Wax relief *(A)* and labial wire assemblage for the FR III. The lip pad assemblage *(C)* consists of three wires—two side wires parallel to each other that permit uniform advancement of the lip pads later and a central V-shaped wire bent to conform to the frenum attachment. The ends of the palatal bow and protrusion bow wires *(B)* stand about 1.0 mm away from the wax relief. The lower occlusal rest wire *(D)* and labial wire *(E)* will be incorporated in the mandibular portion of the buccal shield. No wax relief is placed on the mandibular arch for the FR III.

models are sent to the laboratory. The laboratory can also mount the models, if requested, but there is less chance of distortion in mailing if it is done beforehand.

Wax relief. The maxillary expansion needs are the same for the FR III as for the other FR variations (with the exception of some Class II, Division 2, problems in which the maxillary arch is broad enough and requires no more expansion). After the areas are outlined in pencil, the buccal and labial aspects of the maxillary teeth and alveolar process are again covered with wax. The thickness of the layer under the shields and pads is 3 mm. Boxing wax that is 3 mm thick works well. No wax is applied to the mandibular arch or teeth (Fig. 10-50). The wax relief discussion (p. 236) should be reread for fabrication of the FR I and FR II.

Wire forming. Both the mandibular labial bow and the palatal bow are formed from relatively heavy 1.0 mm (0.40 inch 18 gauge) stainless steel wire. Because of the demands for flexibility for possible tooth movement, the maxillary protrusion bow requires 0.06 or 0.07 mm wire. Some operators make this wire heavier, however, since they plan to accomplish any tooth movement with pre–Fränkel appliance therapy. This is probably preferable in the long run, reducing breakage of the FR III. All other wires are 0.9 mm (0.036 inch 19 gauge).

For the lower *labial bow* (Figs. 10-46 and 10-48) a shallow groove is carved on the plaster casts across the six anterior teeth, just above the interdental papillae to ensure a close fit. Cutting the groove and keeping the

wire as low on the crown as possible reduce the tendency for lingual tipping of lower incisors, which could occur from a wire position closer to the incisal margin. A 90-degree bend downward at the distal of the lower canine is then made, followed by another horizontal bend approximately 5 mm below the gingival margin. The horizontal leg of the labial bow that is embedded in the acrylic vestibular shield is parallel to the occlusal surface.

The *occlusal rest* originates in the vestibular shield and is adapted to lie snugly in the occlusal fissure of the last mandibular molar. The free ends should be far enough away from the mucosa to be incorporated in the acrylic when it is added on the model (Fig. 10-48). Both ends of the 0.09 mm wire terminate in the shield.

The *palatal bow* also begins in the buccal shields and has a shape similar to that in the FR I and II, but with the midpalatal loop curving posteriorly. It is kept about 0.5 mm away from the palatal mucosa. The wire runs distal to the last molar tooth, as described earlier, giving the molars freedom to erupt and move mesially. If it contacts the last molar, this might interfere with eruption. Where mesial movement of the first molar is the prime objective, however, the wire can be adapted to the distal of the molar, below the distal convexity if possible.

The *protrusion bow* exits from the buccal shields, crossing the interocclusal space at the canine–deciduous first molar embrasure but *not contacting* the opposing teeth. After it is looped on the palatal mucosa it comes forward to contact the lingual surfaces of the incisors just above the cingula, 2 or 3 mm below the incisal margin. If eruption is needed for the particular Class III malocclusion, in contradistinction to the Class II, Division 2, type of problem (in which a depressive force is required), the protrusion bow must not contact the cingula since this would impede incisor eruption (Fig. 10-46). The protrusion bow is always passive at the time of initial appliance placement.

The *lip pad* wiring of the FF III is formed much as that of the FR I and II but on the maxillary arch. Since the maxillary labial frenum attachment is heavier, the central wire **V** must avoid impingement on it. As with the FR I, these wires must be kept away from the relief wax to permit acrylic to cover them completely on the tissue side, even after polishing (Figs. 10-46 and 10-47).

Fabrication of acrylic parts of the FR III. Since the technique for fabricating parts of the FR III is essentially the same as for the FR I and II, the reader is referred to that section. To prevent irritation, the acrylic that contacts the gingival margin of the teeth in the lower dental arch must be ground away; and to prevent tissue damage and actual dehiscence, it is imperative that the maxillary lip pads parallel the slope of the alveolar process. When properly designed, the tear-shaped lip pads will not cause damage as the appliance moves up and down during wear. It is probably easier for the patient to work the FR III up and down with the tongue and when opening the mouth, since it is not locked in the interproximal spaces with crossover wires, even though gravity may help hold the appliance in place on the mandible.

The maximum superior extension of the lip pads is of great importance to Fränkel. He believes it pulls on the "septo-premaxillary" ligament (as described by Latham, Johnston, and Delaire) and the periosteum, enhancing bone deposition as well as freeing the pressure-sensitive membranous bone from adverse lip pressures. A dramatic example of an iatrogenic orbicularis oris effect is seen in repaired cleft lip patients in whom severe maxillary retrusion can be attributed to the tight and unyielding scarified lip.

The FR III may be modified somewhat during the course of treatment. Since maxillary sagittal development is a major goal, any appreciable improvement may lead to mucosal contact with the maxillary lip pads. This can occur in as little as 3 to 4 months after appliance placement. If it happens, the acrylic is cut away from the anchoring tags of the lip pad skeletal wires, which are at right angles to the parallel lip pad wires that emerge from the shields (Fig. 10-51). The straight wires are grasped with an office pliers and are pulled out of the shields to advance the upper lip pads and reestablish the proper distance. Endothermic acrylic can then be added to fill the holes cut in the shields. The appliance is repolished to prevent any irritation. Minor adjustments of the lip pads are usually required to establish a parallel lip pad–mucosa relationship again.

With treatment progress the upper and lower incisors should approach an end-to-end bite. The maxillary protrusion bow may then be activated to stimulate forward tipping of the maxillary incisors. It is important to check that the protrusion bow does not press on the upper incisor cingula at this time, since such action prevents eruption. The slight labial movement of the upper incisors by the protrusion bow prevents jiggling of the incisor teeth by accelerating the "jumping of the bite." When the maxillary incisors are well over their mandibular counterparts, the protrusion bow can be removed to prevent any possible interference with maxillary incisor eruption. The occlusal rests on the mandibular molars should be left intact, however, so the posterior open bite that is usually produced by the sagittal correction closes by virtue of the downward and forward eruption of unimpeded maxillary teeth.

Examples of successful FR III treatment are illustrated in Figs. 10-52 to 10-55.

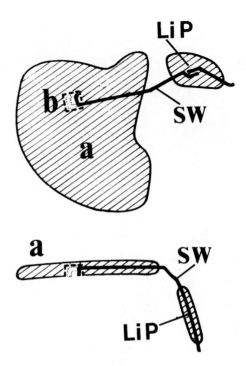

Fig. 10-51. FR III lip pad advancement is done by making a cut in the shield *(a)* and pulling the skeletal wire *(SW)* forward and upward. The cut section of the shield is then filled in with acrylic at *(b)* and polished.

FR IV

The etiology of the open bite malocclusion is not as well delineated as that of Class II, Division 1, problems. How much of the malocclusion is due to morphogenetic pattern, to direction of jaw growth, to abnormal perioral muscle function? Are tongue posture and function primary, perhaps a retained infantile deglutitional pattern, or adaptive to the morphology? What role does finger-sucking play? With a potential multiplicity of contributing factors and considerable individual variation, therapeutic demands vary.

Fränkel designed a deficiency appliance and a muscle-training appliance. If the problem involves something else, the FR alone may not be enough, except in carefully selected cases. There is a school of thought which holds that lip seal exercises are easier to do, with obvious results, when there is a lip trap, as in Class II, Division 1, malocclusions. Training the tongue posture and function, however, is a different matter. A generation of orthodontists (and speech therapists) failed with their "tongue-thrusting" myofunctional therapy in most cases. Thus this modification of the basic Function Regulator appliance used by Fränkel in the correction of open bites primarily is dependent more on careful case analysis and specific case selection (Fig. 10-56). The philosophy of controlling tongue action from the vestibule

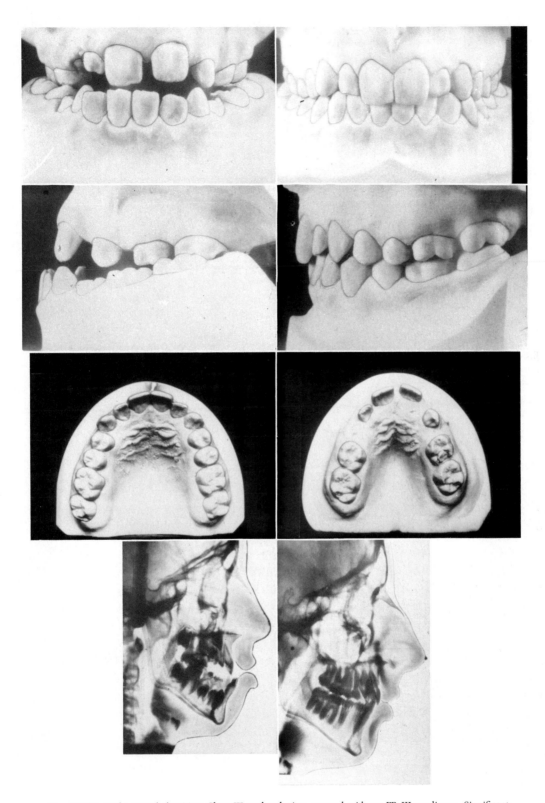

Fig. 10-52. Early mixed dentition Class III malocclusion, treated with an FR III appliance. Significant sagittal improvement and maxillary arch expansion have been achieved.

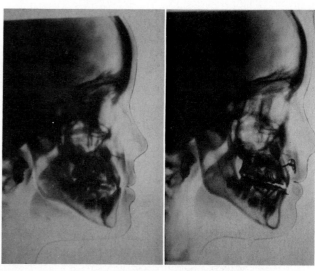

Fig. 10-54. Class III malocclusion in habitual occlusion, **A,** and with the FR III in place, **B.** The construction bite has been taken in the most retruded mandibular position. The lip pads are holding the upper lip away from the maxillary dentition, pulling on the "septo-premaxillary" ligament or fibrous tissues (as elucidated by Latham).

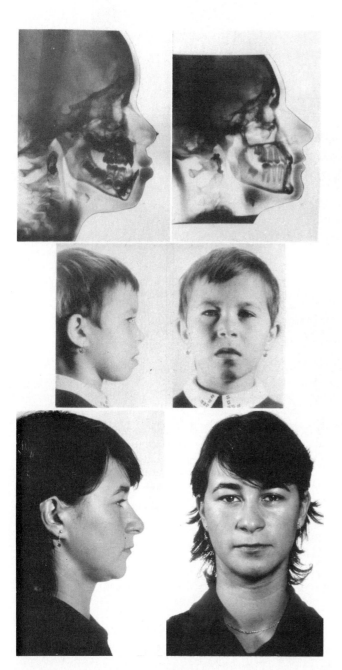

Fig. 10-53. Class III malocclusion, with FR III treatment started in the deciduous dentition. The profile change is a major one, with significant improvement of lip posture. No chin cap therapy was used.

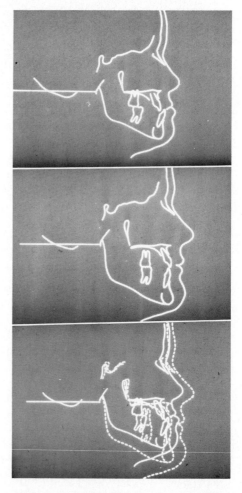

Fig. 10-55. Class III malocclusion before and after FR III treatment. The superimposed tracings show primarily vertical mandibular growth coupled with downward and forward maxillary growth.

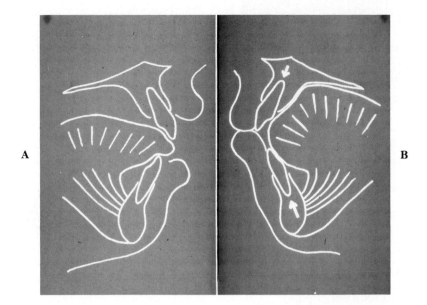

Fig. 10-56. Anterior open bite problems usually show protracted tongue posture, **A,** with incompetence of the lips. The tongue-tooth contact replaces the lip seal during deglutition to create a negative atmospheric pressure. This accentuates the tongue thrusting and enhances the anterior open bite. With the FR IV in place and with lip seal exercises, **B,** lip contact takes over, reducing tongue protrusion and causing the tongue to move back into its normally raised position, in proximity to the palate, during deglutition. Incisors can then erupt normally to close the bite while the tongue reestablishes an interocclusal clearance between the posterior teeth. This allows the mandible to close upward and forward into a more favorable growth direction, reducing the mandibular plane angle. (Courtesy Rolf Fränkel.)

instead of using some sort of screening device within the arch is still not completely accepted, despite a recent article by Rolf and Christine Fränkel illustrating dramatic results. If the cases are chosen properly and if there is optimum patient cooperation, the lip seal exercises are even more important than with the other FR types—if that is possible. The Fränkel report shows that the FR IV is truly a functional appliance, with evidence of significant basal bone change. As much as anything, however, the Fränkel FR IV article shows that aberrant muscle activity can create open bite problems and can redirect growth more vertically. The FR IV reverses the unfavorable growth guidance, so it must be used during an active growth period. Again, the mixed dentition is optimal for its influence, with a longer period of wear usually needed, into the permanent dentition. Not enough American clinicians have had sufficient experience with this appliance in open bite cases to judge for themselves as yet. Diagnosis and case selection, however, along with the compliance of the patient are critical factors.

The FR IV has the same vestibular configuration as the FR I and FR II, but it has no canine loops or protrusion bow (Fig. 10-57). There are four occlusal rests on the maxillary permanent first molars and deciduous first molars to prevent tipping of the appliance (Fig. 10-58). The rests discourage any eruption of posterior teeth—a vital requisite for anterior open bite conditions. The palatal bow is like that of the FR III and is always placed behind the last molar. The occlusal rests often must be adapted to the individual patient. They must not, however, prevent shifting of the appliance in a posterior (or dorsal) direction. Hence the appliance is not locked on either arch by interproximal wires. Occasionally a thin acrylic wafer is interposed between the upper and lower buccal segments; but this cannot be too thick, because lip closure then becomes more difficult. Without the exercises the appliance is doomed to failure. A number of operators use the FR IV in conjunction with extraoral force chin cap therapy, which also helps close down the bite by virtue of a positive depressing action on the buccal segments. At least one modification has incorporated lingual tongue crib spurs to discourage anterior tongue posture and compensatory tongue function, in a manner originally suggested by Frantisek Kraus. A detailed discussion of this appliance and its manipulation is beyond the limits of this book. Figs. 10-59 and 10-60 show a typical treatment result.

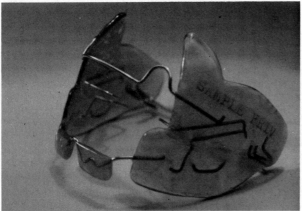

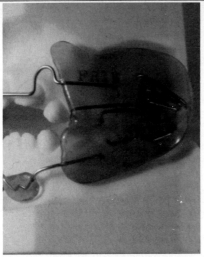

Fig. 10-57. FR IV appliance. There is no maxillary lingual protrusion bow or canine clasp. The maxillary labial arch is usually passive at first although it can be activated to retract the maxillary anterior teeth. Molar and premolar occlusal rests help to stabilize the appliance. Since there is little or no interocclusal clearance, the rests contact both maxillary and molar posterior segments, preventing eruption. A thin layer of interocclusal acrylic is sometimes used for this purpose also, increasing appliance stability and enhancing a depressing force on the buccal teeth.

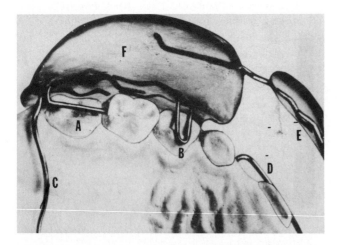

Fig. 10-58. FR IV appliance on the maxillary cast. The rests for the permanent first molar *(A)* and deciduous first molar *(B)* usually contact both maxillary and mandibular occlusal surfaces. The palatal bow *(C)* passes to the distal of the last molar tooth. The maxillary labial arch *(D)*, mandibular lip pads *(E)*, and buccal shield *(F)* can also be identified.

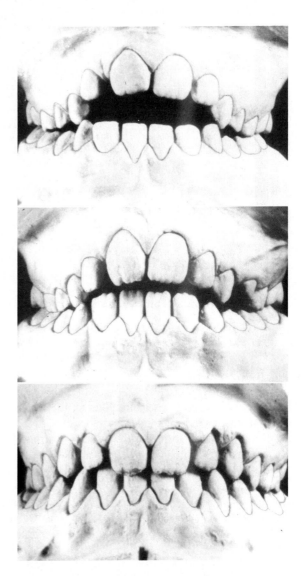

Fig. 10-59. Open bite malocclusion treated with only an FR IV appliance and the prescribed lip seal exercises. Correction is a combination of retardation of posterior segment eruption with unimpeded incisor eruption, under the influence of the established normal lip and tongue function.

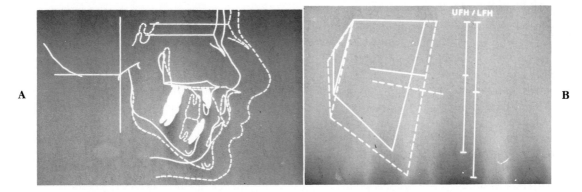

Fig. 10-60. A, Superimposed tracings before and after treatment show elimination of the open bite, enhanced ramus height, a more favorable mandibular plane inclination, and a better posterior to anterior face height ratio. **B,** The polygons show this graphically. Occlusal plane changes are minimal despite the major reduction of the mandibular plane angle under the influence of FR IV therapy and lip seal exercises.

MODE OF ACTION OF THE FUNCTION REGULATOR

The mode of action of the Fränkel Function Regulator is based on its role as a deficiency appliance and its interception of aberrant muscle function. It is not a tooth-moving appliance. Neither is its mode of action the same as that of the conventional activator-type functional appliance. The activator is in contact with the teeth and alveolar bone of both jaws, exerting muscle pressure on these structures largely from within the dental arch. The Fränkel appliance, however, uses the vestibule as its arena of operation and withholds muscle pressure from the developing jaw and dentoalveolar area. Instead of using jackscrews, Coffin springs, finger springs, or selective grinding of acrylic, as is done with the activator, it achieves its effect through the relief of forces exerted by the surrounding neuromuscular envelope. The sagittal posturing to maintain the construction bite relation is also different, since both mandibular teeth and jaws support the propulsive mandibular status in activator-type appliances whereas the lip pads on the labial and the acrylic pad on the lingual form the forward posturing trough for the Fränkel appliance (with no tooth contact). The appliance is entirely tissue borne on the lower arch, since the spring wires behind the mandibular incisors are completely passive and may actually stand away 0.5 to 1.0 mm from the cingula, except when a mild depressing force is desired.

The Function Regulator, with its unique biomechanical design, is capable of achieving the following changes in the orofacial complex:

1. Enlargement of both sagittal and transverse intraoral space
2. Increase of vertical intraoral space
3. Forward posturing of mandible

4. Improvement of muscle tonus and the establishment of proper oral seal, with the development of new neuromuscular patterns

1. *Increase of both the sagittal and the transverse intraoral space* is accomplished primarily through the action of the buccal shields and lip pads. Mechanical pressure of the perioral soft tissue band (buccinator mechanism) is considered an important factor in dentoalveolar crowding and arrested basal bone development. The buccal shields and lip pads eliminate the deleterious mechanical pressures on the responsive membranous bone structures, which then tilts the balance in favor of the forces acting from within the oral cavity (the tongue). This action is particularly true during the multiple deglutitional cycles. Fränkel believes that when the forces of the cheeks are eliminated the teeth move laterally in the direction of least resistance. Our research has shown that under the influence of the vestibular shields the buccal plate exhibits increased external depositive activity, with concomitant resorption on the lingual aspect of the plate, as the teeth move bodily toward the buccal. Thus the alveoli also move buccally. Normally, with buccal crown movement, it is expected to see a tipping of the teeth with lingual movement of the apical portions. However, such movement is resisted by the thick palatolingual plate.

Fränkel hypothesizes that the intermittent outward pull exerted on the connective tissue fibers and muscle attachments in the oral vestibule by the vestibular shields in a dynamic functioning field is transmitted to the contiguous alveolar bone through the fibers which insert into the periosteum and underlying membranous bone. The functional stimulus thus aids in the outward movement of the alveolodental supporting osseous structures. Whether the tissue pull on the periosteum causes actual bone deposition on the underlying contiguous bony surface or not is still open to question. There is clearly more bony activity and actual buccal movement of unerupted teeth, but under the influence of the buccal shields the role of periosteal pull in this reaction has not been completely elucidated. The functional concept is tenable, and research by Enlow, Hoyt, Moffett, and others demonstrates increased bony activity when the periostem is pulled or lifted from the underlying bone. Our histologic studies on primates, however, cannot specifically attribute the increased activity shown in Fig. 10-7 to this. More definitive tissue studies at specific times are needed and are in progress in our laboratory.

Regardless of the ultimate findings of the study, the clinical and histologic results clearly show significant and stable bodily movement of the maxillary posterior teeth by Fränkel appliances in rats, primates, and humans. All this occurs as there is normal vertical development, with the erupted and unerupted teeth moving downward and outward. The net result is that more of a bodily than a tipping movement occurs in the posterior segments during the critical transitional period of development, which is the best time for wearing the FR; and since the FR III is a deficiency appliance, the maxillary lip pads for it (used in the treatment of Class III malocclusions) function the same way, enhancing basal bone development and allowing the incisors to move downward and forward in a more bodily posture. However, if there is a manifest mandibular overgrowth, then the FR III cannot be expected to correct this problem.

Although some clinicians have been claiming significant changes from the Fränkel and other functional appliances in adults, it is important to note that the transverse and sagittal development of the apical base is possible only as long as there is still some natural growth potential remaining. The possibilities of appreciably widening the mandibular base are over by the age of 10 to 11 years, despite the maxillary area's susceptibility to sagittal and transverse stimulation until a considerably later age. This supports the contention that the optimal treatment time for arch form changes is the mixed and transitional dentition period. Some minor adaptive changes surely can be brought about in the adult, even as tooth movement can be done, but this must not be interpreted as "growth guidance"—which, at the same time, is not to say that functional appliances cannot be used in adults. They can, particularly in temporomandibular joint problems, in which forward posturing of the mandible is essential during therapy for many cases. However, claims of major histomorphologic changes are unsubstantiated.

2. *Increase of the vertical intraoral space* is achieved because the forward posturing of the mandible usually requires that the bite be opened. There is greater interocclusal space, allowing the eruption or extrusion of posterior teeth in a manner similar to that seen with anterior bite plates or the conventional activator. An additional advantage of the Fränkel appliance is that the buccal shields prevent invagination of buccal soft tissue into the interocclusal space. Fränkel thinks that the disturbance in vertical development is caused more often by the cheeks than by the tongue. He considers tongue posture and function to be more an adaptive or secondary factor than a primary one, as Ricketts, Garliner, Zickefoose, Straub, and others have thought. According to Fränkel's experience, if there is not a marked arch length deficiency one always observes spontaneous uprighting of the mandibular teeth and leveling of an excessive curve of Spee with the use of buccal shields.

3. *Forward posturing of the mandible,* according to Fränkel, is significantly different with the FR from what it is with a conventional activator. He doubts claims made by activator adherents that their appliances incite condylar growth, when in reality most of the response is due to dentoalveolar changes with the mandibular incisors tipping labially. Bjork, Woodside, and Bimler concur with this observation.

The position of the mandible with the Fränkel appliance is changed through gradual training of the protractor and retractor muscles, followed by condylar adaptation. The lingual acrylic pressure pad and labial lip pads guide the mandible by exteroceptive stimuli to a more mesial position. If the mandible drops back, the pressure sensation on the lingual side of the alveolar process reactivates the protractor muscles, which are gradually conditioned to hold the mandible in the position determined by the construction bite, in the trough between the labial lip pads and the lingual pressure pad. For a variety of reasons it is important not to overactivate or overstretch these muscles. Therefore, in more severe Class II cases the mandible must be postured forward by the construction bite in steps. Fränkel's strong clinical bias for the stepwise forward mandibular movement is supported by animal research from the Petrovic laboratory in Strasbourg, which indicates that each advancement incites a renewed growth stimulation of the condyle.

The Fränkel appliance must accomplish forward posturing of the mandible without tooth contact. It is essential that the lingual pressure pad contact only the tissue and not the teeth. The appliance must be stabilized or locked on the maxillary arch by the interproximal wires, as previously outlined. All too frequently this is not done, and the appliance then moves up and down and distally, causing undesirable sequelae. The maxillary incisors are likely to be tipped lingually by the normally passive labial wire at a time when this is not desired. The lip pads may abrade the gingival tissue in the lower canine and incisor regions, causing actual dehiscence. The lingual pressure pad can then contact the lower incisor teeth, proclining them. Such "floating appliance" activity is to be discouraged by FR I, II, and III patients, even though this was considered by Andresen and Häupl as desirable for the original activator. The key to success for the Fränkel appliance is continuous wearing of a properly made and stabilized appliance (Fig. 10-61).

4. *Improved muscle tone, establishment of proper lip seal, and the development of new neuromuscular patterns* are a major objective of Function Regulator therapy. It is desired to eliminate the deforming influence of the abnormal perioral muscle activity as well as rehabilitate the muscles that have been causing the malformation and malocclusion. The buccal shields and lip pads provide a new and more normal shell or "ought-to-be" arch form for functional matrix adaptation. They massage the soft tissues, enhancing blood circulation. The shields loosen up tight muscles and improve tonicity where it is lacking. This is particularly important in the mentalis region. In the current era of bodily fitness and exercise, it is not difficult to understand why Fränkel calls his appliance an *exercise device* and the exercise regimen oral *gymnastics*. The pads and shields stretch the muscles in distocclusion cases (Fig. 10-62).

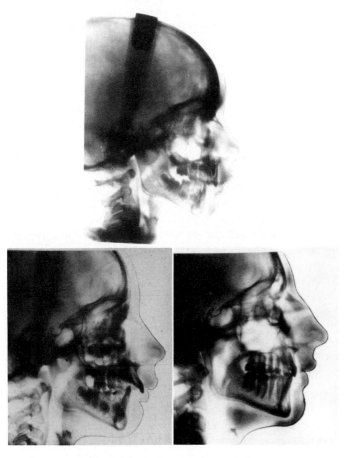

Fig. 10-61. Dramatic results attained by a properly made FR I appliance, worn as prescribed, together with lip seal exercises. A major sagittal change has been achieved.

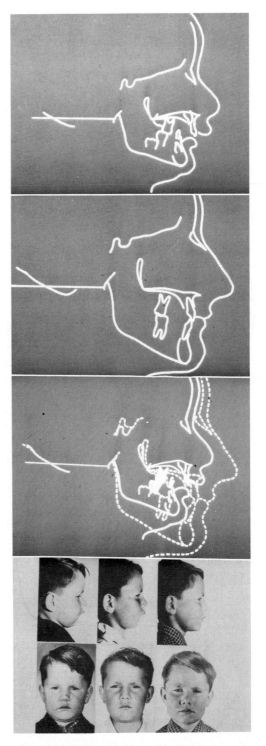

Fig. 10-62. Major sagittal improvement achieved by FR treatment of a severe Class II, Division 1, malocclusion. Almost as dramatic as the basal change is the establishment of normal neuromuscular function, under FR I guidance and lip seal exercises.

The mandibular lip pads also prevent hyperactivity of the mentalis muscle, eliminating the lip trap and helping establish a proper oral seal.

When the FR is being worn properly, all functions—swallowing, speaking, mimic movement—are a form of oral gymnastics. These are not enough to accomplish the retraining and adaptation of the muscles, however. It is imperative that the patient be instructed to keep the lips closed at all times (lip seal) if flaccid or hyperactive oral muscle components are to be corrected. This lip seal function is, in effect, also oral gymnastics. The task can be quite a challenge to the young patient, in whom attention for conscious activity is normally rather limited. It is not easy to reactivate a hypofunctional upper lip and break up a lower lip redundancy and hyperactive mentalis muscle function at the same time. Memory span is short, and volitional attempts at lip seal require constant support. Keeping a piece of paper between the lips when not involved in sports activities or with other children is one good way of constantly reminding the patient of the need to close the lips over the Function Regulator. Isometric exercises, pressing the lips together and against the appliance, also are beneficial when sitting in class, watching television, going to the movies, etc.

An additional exercise is recommended for patients wearing the FR III. In most Class III malocclusions the tongue posture is low. The patient is taught to lift the tongue and force it against the narrowed palate, making "clicking" sounds, for a prescribed period each day at home. Since the Fränkel appliance does not cover the hard palate (as the conventional Andresen activator does), proper proprioception is established, and since there is no appliance restriction, the tongue may exert its normal pressures on the teeth and investing tissues as well as basal bone. The need for this function was recognized a long time ago by Bimler and Balters and their followers, using skeletonized functional appliances.

CLINICAL MANAGEMENT OF THE FRÄNKEL APPLIANCE

The best made appliance will fail unless the operator follows a clinical discipline. This is particularly important for the Fränkel FR, which has more precise demands for fabrication and more exacting tolerances.

At the placement appointment the maxillary arch is checked to ensure that the special heavy spacing separators are still in place. If there still is not enough space or if the clinician has decided to notch the distal of the deciduous second molar and the mesial of the deciduous first molar for seating the crossover wires in the maxilla, a diamond cylinder bur is recommended to make the seating grooves. Stabilizing the appliance on the maxilla at the first visit is absolutely essential. Otherwise the patient cannot adapt to the fully extended shields and lip pads and soreness will develop. Under the best conditions this is an adjustment process that takes time, effort, and constant encouragement. Knowledgeable clinicians make available to parents and patients good descriptive literature on the Fränkel appliance. This should be given to them to read while waiting for appliance placement and to take home for future reference. It should sometimes be given at the time of impression taking so the information can be fully assimilated before appliance placement. Videotapes and slide sequences are also available to give a better idea of patient responsibilities and how to handle the appliance in the critical first days. Showing one of these 7-minute tapes can make the difference between an antagonistic and a cooperative patient.

All margins are checked for smoothness before the appliance is inserted. The appliance is then seated on the maxilla to allow its stability on the dentition to be verified as well as the fit of the shields and the labial and palatal wires. This procedure is repeated for the mandibular arch. The crossover wires must not contact the mandibular teeth, and the lingual wires arising from the acrylic pressure pad, behind the lower incisors, must be passive. The patient then bites into the appliance, and the tissue is checked in the pad and shield area. There should be no obvious blanching of tissue and the peripheral portions should contact sulcular tissue. It is important that the shields be far enough away from the maxillary alveolar mucosa and teeth.

Tissue impingement is the most frequently encountered problem with initial appliance placement and the areas of greatest concern are the buccal frenula and inferior margins of the lip pads. The lip pads must be in a vertical position so their lingual surfaces or margins do not contact the gingival tissue on insertion and removal. If the lower margins are tipped forward, the upper margins will rub against the alveolar and gingival mucosa when the mouth is opened. Improper pad orientation can be corrected by cutting a groove around the wires and rotating the pads to the correct vertical position. Alternately, the support wire can be freed in the buccal shields and moved backward or forward to ensure proper distance from the contiguous soft tissue. Then the slot in the acrylic is filled with self-cure acrylic and polished. Slight modification can be made with pliers, but care must be taken not to distort the shields in the process.

The anterosuperior periphery of the buccal shields, over the maxillary canines, is the next most likely area of irritation. Peripheral margins can be reduced and polished the same as for overextension of the lip pads and shields. If possible, as with a new denture, it is better to await actual tissue reaction than try to anticipate it and cut away acrylic. If there is no blanching of tissue around the periphery of the shields and pads, it is quite safe for the patient to start the breakin period at home. This assumes that the appliance is fabricated properly and that the construction bite is correct. *Tissue redness around the periphery of shields and pads that are properly extended is a normal consequence of proper fit and good patient cooperation.* It is important not to cut away too much acrylic during the first visits. The patient should be told that irritation is possible for the first couple of weeks. Even the experienced clinician should allow ample time for initial FR placement. It is not simply a matter of handing the appliance to the patient, (e.g., a Hawley retainer) and saying "Put it in." A half hour should be set aside for instruction during the first appointment. If the lip seal exercise regimen has not already been instituted at the time of taking the impressions and the construction bite, then this can be started with the appliance placement. Except during meals or when engaging in sports, the patient is instructed to hold a small piece of paper lightly between the lips.

After the patient has grown accustomed to wearing it and can speak intelligibly, the Fränkel appliance will be worn all the time, except for meals. In the beginning, however, it should be worn for only short periods to allow the soft tissues and muscles to adjust to the "foreign body." Generally, during the first couple of weeks, the FR I and II are worn during the day only for 2 to 4 hours. When the patient returns for the first checkup or "control" appointment, the soft tissues are examined carefully and the necessary peripheral adjustments and polishing done. It is emphasized again that the operator should err in the direction of taking away too little rather than too much material. Of course, the appliance must not impinge on the muscle attachments since these areas will not adapt to overextensions.

Before the patient leaves the office with the appliance in place and during the interval between the first and second appointments, it is absolutely essential that the appliance be fully seated on the maxillary arch. If this is not the case, more irritation will occur and more acrylic will be incorrectly removed for irritation that would not exist if the appliance had been locked by the interproximal wires in the seating grooves. Lip pad adaptation, shield extension, and forward posturing all depend on correct stabilization. A frequent complaint is overextension of the lower lingual pressure pad, with resultant irritation of the lingual frenum. Any impingement should be polished away. The experienced clinician knows, however, that until the patient learns to hold the mandible forward there may be ulceration on the inferior margin of the pad. Thus it is vital not to be too hasty in trimming acrylic until it is certain that the appliance

is truly overextended. An astringent mouthwash, warm saline rinses, benzocaine, or Orabase will help control the abrasion and inflammation.

During the interval between the second and third office visits or a period of about 3 weeks, daytime wear is extended to 4 to 6 hours and speaking exercises are encouraged. Normal speech when wearing an FR is one of the most difficult challenges. Speech improvement can be accelerated by having the patient practice reading selected passages into a home tape recorder and listening to the sequence. Some clinicians prefer to wait until this time to initiate the lip seal exercises, making sure first that the appliance fits well and is comfortable.

For the third appointment, after it has been determined that stabilization is good and tissues are not irritated, actual exercises may be prescribed in addition to the lip seal regimen. These oral gymnastics are essentially isometric contractions of the perioral musculature, literally grasping the Fränkel appliance in the vestibule. A speech check should be made with the patient counting from one to ten.

At every appointment, positive reinforcement is needed to maintain a high level of patient compliance. The FR does not do the job by itself, and cooperation lags even in the best 8-to-10-year-old. Showing pictures of the patient with and without the appliance in place and pictures and plaster models of the facial and dental changes achieved in other patients, along with having other Fränkel patients present at the same time for supportive peer pressure, are helpful measures (Fig. 10-63). The management challenge is potent, requiring reinforcement by the home team as well as the office team, and all possible support is given. These early appointments are critical. The gingival mucosa and margins must be inspected for any possible abrasions that might indicate manipulation of the appliance by the tongue in a free-floating status. Full-time daily wear is usually prescribed at the end of the third visit.

For the average FR I or FR II patient it takes about 2 months before the appliance is worn all night. Not every operator will agree with this rule, but Fränkel's experience indicates that nighttime wear should not be rushed. If the patient has only poorly adapted to the constructed forward mandibular posture (even when it is but 3 mm) and is still uncomfortable, the jaw will drop open and back during sleep. Abrasions on the lower lingual mucosa will likely occur. There is then a possible anterior tipping stimulus to the lower incisors as the lingual pressure pad rides on the lower incisors and rests on them for long periods. FR III patients adjust more easily, however, and the appliance can usually be worn all the time after the first 2 weeks. Ulceration and abrasion are possible with this appliance also and should be looked for. Any irritation can be soothed with

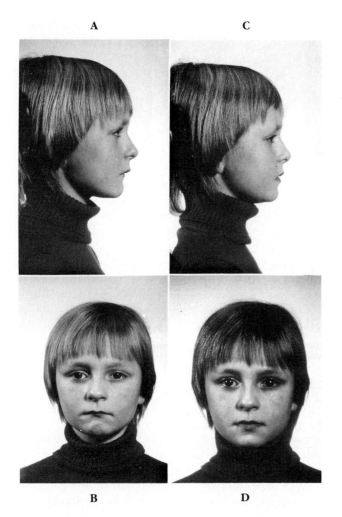

Fig. 10-63. Without the FR II appliance, **A** and **B**, and with it inserted, **C** and **D.** Note the improvement. Such pictures can help motivate beginning patients.

benzocaine or Orabase ointment, which will enhance patient cooperation.

At first, treatment progress and appliance fit should be checked at 4-week intervals. The mucosa of the vestibule and gingivae should be examined at every visit, and (for the FR I and FR II) stabilization of the appliance on the maxillary arch verified. As with the Bionator, minimal changes are necessary during treatment after the patient has grown accustomed to wearing the appliance; and even less must be done, since there is no interocclusal acrylic to worry about for the FR. The visit usually serves more as a motivation stimulus, showing progress and projecting future treatment time. Routinely, although they must be seated interproximally, the canine and molar crossover wires should be checked for possible impingement on the interdental papillae as the deciduous teeth are exfoliated and the canines and premolars erupt. If there is tissue irritation, the FR I canine loops

can be bent occlusally and the molar rests gingivally to relieve the pressure. The canine loops can be modified slightly to guide a buccally erupting canine into proper position. However, interference with normal canine eruption is possible; thus many clinicians prefer the FR II to the FR I. Also any indication of gingival margin abrasion or mucosal irritation must be eliminated, as must any labial tipping of the lower incisors or soreness of the lingual gingival tissue, which could indicate a destabilized free-floating appliance.

As has been pointed out, in a number of cases it is advantageous to have a short pre-Fränkel period of fixed appliance guidance for incisor alignment, space closure, or rotational correction. Hence there is usually little need to activate the labial bow. Minor residual spacing can be closed, however, if done gradually and with care not to retract the incisors too much in Class II, Division I, malocclusions. Too much pressure can cause the archwire to slide gingivally and dislodge the appliance. The FR is not a tooth-moving appliance. The lingual protrusion bow (as it has been called by Fränkel) really does little in the way of protruding anything, except in Class II, Division 2, patients, in whom the maxillary central incisors may be tipped labially; and this can be done much better and more quickly by pre–functional appliance guidance before the FR is placed. Rather, the lingual bow on the FR II helps maintain maxillary stabilization and can also prevent excessive lingual tipping of the maxillary incisors.

Sagittal, vertical, transverse improvement should be apparent after 3 months of full-time wear. Frequently a lateral open bite develops (Fig. 10-64). This is a sign of patient cooperation, since eruption of the lower posterior teeth is usually slower than the change in transverse and sagittal directions. With proper patient compliance, 6 months is all that is required to correct an original cusp-to-cusp Class II malocclusion in the molar region. (The assumption is that case selection has been proper and there is a normal increment of mandibular growth.)

For more severe cases a full distal relationship can be corrected in 9 to 12 months. In these patients, however, it is probable that a staged two- or three-step mandibular protraction approach will be needed to advance the lingual acrylic pressure pad and lip pads as previously described. With advancement of the anterior posturing trough of the appliance, there is a reciprocal distalizing thrust on the body of the appliance. Thus the posteroinferior margins of the shields occasionally must be relieved during the staged mandibular advancement. It is a good office discipline to schedule progress records at 6-month intervals. To assess growth increments and direction and any treatment-induced changes requires a lateral cephalogram.

FR III adjustments are minimal and have been dis-

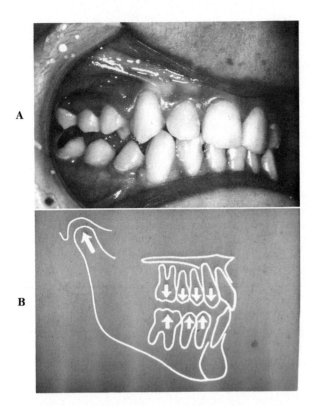

Fig. 10-64. The FR I and FR II usually achieve sagittal correction more rapidly than eruption of posterior teeth. The result is often an incisal contact, with the posterior teeth being out of occlusion, **A.** The open bite that exists is due to condylar growth that propels the mandible downward and forward, **B.** Holding the corrected sagittal relationship with the FR until eruption has been obtained is a normal part of treatment.

cussed in connection with appliance fabrication. Because of the relative ease of handling and the quicker patient acceptance, Fränkel recommends that the neophyte try this appliance first in a mild Class III problem before using the FR I or II.

Although the appliance can be distorted if sat upon, making readaptation to its original shape almost impossible, breakage is usually minimal and confined to the buccal shields or crossover wires. If a fragment of the buccal shield is broken off (and this is usually the antero-superior projection into the canine fossa), immediate repair can be done with cyanoacrylate adhesive. Eirew recommends a double hanger to reduce wire fatigue in this area. The original working models and mounting for the articulator must be saved so repairs or replacements can be made if the appliance is broken or lost.

Treatment timing

The best therapeutic effect of the Fränkel appliance, and of other functional appliances (e.g., Bio-Modulator of Fleischer) as far as *expansion* and *resolution of arch*

length deficiency are concerned, is achieved during the late mixed and transitional dentition period, when both hard and soft tissues are undergoing their greatest adaptational change, with as many as 52 teeth being present in their bony shell. As far as *sagittal* and *vertical* skeletal changes are concerned, growth and development studies and extensive research by Petrovic, Stutzmann, Oudet, Moyers, McNamara, Graber and Graber, and others have shown that maxillary and mandibular growth is essential. The alternative is an accommodative or dual bite, or major dental compensation, that is not likely to be stable. Too many results of this type have already been produced with functional appliances in nongrowing children or improperly chosen cases.

The choice of the optimum Class II treatment initiation time depends on the patient's rate of development. It varies somewhat, but a good sign is when the four upper and lower incisors have erupted (as early as 7½ years, but more likely 8½ to 9 years of age). For arch deficiency problems, with manifest maxillary narrowness, that demand expansion to establish normal arch form placing the FR at the beginning of this stage is better to take advantage of all possible dentoalveolar adjustment. If there is only a sagittal and vertical concern, the appliance can be placed more toward the middle of the mixed dentition period, with the aim of carrying on into the transitional period as far as possible. It is not recommended that the FR be placed in the late mixed or early transitional dentition, when the root resorption is already advanced for the deciduous teeth. Appliance stability and seating on the maxilla are a must, and this is more difficult with loose or missing deciduous teeth. Usually the clinician does not have the choice of when to start treatment. The patient comes in when parents or referring dentists think it is time—and this too often is too late. If too late, it is better to await the eruption of the maxillary and mandibular premolars and canines to provide the proper appliance stabilization. Such prepubertal timing is often more favorable from the standpoint of growth increment and direction for sagittal and vertical changes, particularly in male patients.

Treatment for Class III and open bite cases usually should be started sooner than for Class II problems. This means immediately after eruption of the permanent first molars, even though chin cap therapy may have been employed earlier as a pre-FR phase. The FR appliance effect in Class III problems is not so much a sagittal basal bone adjustment as it is in Class II cases. The construction bite mandibular retrusion is minimal and seldom exceeds 1 or 2 mm. As a deficiency appliance, however, and an exercise device the FR III stimulates anterior maxillary development, relieves abnormal perioral muscle pressures on the upper anterior teeth, and establishes normal lip tone and muscle function. FR III

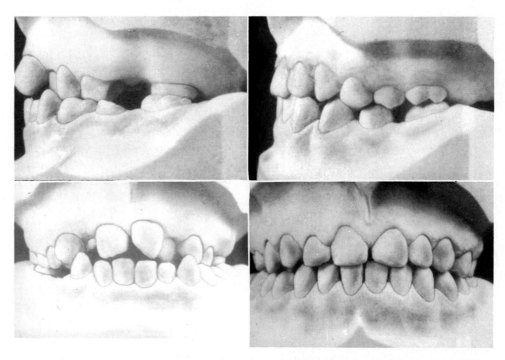

Fig. 10-65. Quite significant maxillary arch expansion and cross-bite correction can be achieved with the FR III appliance, freeing the maxillary dentition from restrictive muscle pressures and stimulating all possible basal bone development. The potential for maxillary arch change is greatest in the transitional dentition.

treatment in the deciduous dentition is usually not advocated because of the patient management and cooperation aspects. Patients at this age are increasingly likely to lose the appliance or to take it out and break it. More is demanded of the FR patient, with full-time wear, care of the appliance, exercises, etc. Another reason for waiting until the lower incisors have erupted is that lateral maxillary arch growth is usually greater at this time and the potential for change per unit time is greater (Fig. 10-65).

Most orthodontists regard Fränkel appliance therapy (and any pre–Fränkel fixed appliance preparation) as a first-phase attack on the malocclusion. Treatment time estimates are difficult; but usually it is advisable to figure 15 to 24 months of guidance, so the patient is in the permanent dentition stage and future treatment decisions can be made. In the average case the active Fränkel treatment is completed and the appliance may then be worn as a retainer, or a Hawley bite plate appliance may be used for the interval between the treatment phase and the permanent dentition time. Fränkel believes that if treatment is started during the permanent dentition a retention phase of 2 to 3 years is needed. A long retention period is especially indicated in Class II, Division 2, Class III, and open bite problems.

Using Fränkel appliances in the treatment of patients with crowding in the permanent dentition is seldom indicated. However, in deep bite sagittal problems, significant improvement can be achieved as one phase of treatment. Use of the Fränkel then requires a depth of experience and a recognition of appliance limitations as well as when to institute other forms of mechanotherapy before, during, or after FR use. Because the Fränkel appliance is not easy to construct or handle, it is advisable for the inexperienced clinician to begin with simpler malocclusions, with patients who are likely to cooperate, and not to treat the more severe skeletal problems in the beginning. End-to-end molar relationships or flush terminal plane cases with an excessive overjet, a deeper than normal overbite, lingually inclined lower incisors, and the pernicious "lip trap" and hyperactive mentalis habit are excellent choices for the neophyte. As indicated earlier, the FR III is the best appliance to begin with for mild Class III problems (Figs. 10-66 and 10-67). Use with a chin cap is permitted *with* the FR III, since it helps hold the appliance in place at night and also exerts a retrusive force on the mandible. This recognizes that many of these problems are combined maxillary deficiencies and mandibular overgrowths.

SUCCESSFUL TREATMENT CONSIDERATIONS

All through Chapter 10 the essential elements for successful Fränkel appliance treatment have been stressed. In addition to the proper impressions, construction bite,

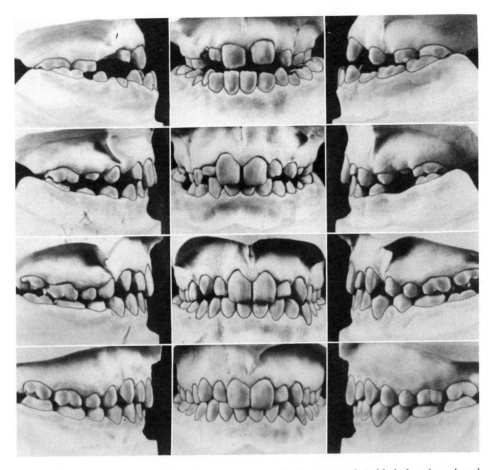

Fig. 10-66. Starting treatment of Class III malocclusions with the FR III is desirable before the pubertal growth spurt. Preferably, it should begin as early as patient compliance can be assured. This may be in the deciduous dentition in some patients, although transitional dentition treatment has shown quite satisfactory results with the exchange of teeth.

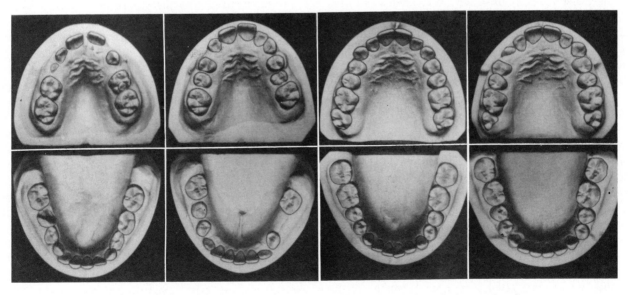

Fig. 10-67. Same patient as in Fig. 10-66. There has been little mandibular arch change other than an uprighting of posterior segments and a rounding out of the arch. The maxillary arch form and dimensional changes, however, are quite significant and stable out of treatment.

appliance fabrication, and patient and appliance management during active therapy, it is appropriate to list three important *preconditions* that should be reemphasized if an optimal result is to be attained.

1. Right indications for treatment
2. Right psychologic introduction of the appliance
3. Cooperation of the patient and parents

Whereas these considerations are requisite for any kind of orthodontic treatment, they are of significantly greater importance for the Fränkel functional appliances, in which the role of the patient is so important.

Despite this admonition, the cooperation of the patient plus a willing compliance encouraged and rewarded by concerned parents is actually easier than one might expect, in view of the appliance's bulk and the necessity of wearing it continuously except during meals. Only minor parts of the FR are inside the dental arches, so the speech impediment should be minimal, even from the beginning, if the appliance is properly made and *stabilized* on the maxillary arch. Some children can speak quite normally right after appliance insertion. Indeed, if speech continues to be a problem, this can be a sign of lack of wear. In all fairness to some of our best patients, however, many children never talk completely normally (though their speech is intelligible).

The proper introduction of the appliance to the patient and parents is important in achieving and maintaining the best possible cooperation. They should be shown the dramatic facial improvement brought about by the changed position of the mandible in "live patients" or photographs of other patients, and then of the patient himself (Fig. 10-63). The elimination of the pronounced mentolabial sulcus by the lower lip pads, the disappearance of the marked nasolabial fold, and the support of the upper lip by the lip pads in Class III malocclusions should be pointed out to the patient and parents. It is vital that the appliance be so made that after insertion the patient's features are actually improved. Making the appliance too bulky would have just the opposite effect on the patient's face and future compliance.

The patient's cooperation in carrying out the aforementioned exercises while wearing the FR is an important part of the treatment regimen. These lip seal and isometric lip closure exercises can really be started as soon as the appliance is placed and comfortable. Some operators believe it is even a good idea to prescribe such exercises before appliance placement, to condition the patient to the need for oral seal and the discipline of oral gymnastics for improved facial appearance. Constant stress of closed lips at all times should be stressed by the "home team" (the parents and siblings of the patient).

Dramatic results achieved by Fränkel appliance therapy have been reported by many clinicians besides Fränkel and the members of the Kieferorthopädisches Institute at Heinrich Braun Hospital in Zwickau, East Germany. McNamara and his associates and Graber and Graber have reproduced similar research results, validating the reports made by Fränkel himself on the amount of stable expansion achieved by the FR.

For an American orthodontic specialty, weaned on nonexpansion extractionist philosophies and the need for multiattachment precision tooth control, the original skepticism was justified; but this is no longer true. Significant sagittal improvement would have to be due to enhanced or optimized condylar growth as well as to beneficial growth direction changes and slight morphologic improvement if the clinical results of Fränkel and the experimental results of Petrovic, Stutzmann and Oudet, McNamara, and Graber are recognized. This does not mean that complete correction is promised or to be expected. Pre–functional appliance guidance with fixed appliances is frequently indicated, and post-FR therapy to settle the canines and improve intercuspation and alignment is desirable in at least 50% of the cases. So often the maxillary canines have a residual Class II or buccal malposition tendency when they erupt. This need for fixed appliances to enhance the FR action and improve final detailing does not detract from the Fränkel success story or from the interceptive guidance and stability of results attained without mass extractions, multiple attachments, anchorage preparation, headgears, etc. Iatrogenic damage is practically nonexistent in properly treated cases. Even when fixed appliances are used before or after FR therapy, the magnitude of the challenge and the treatment time are so reduced that the danger of root resorption, decalcification, etc. with protracted fixed appliances is also reduced.

This chapter can hardly do justice to Fränkel's writings and experiences with the Function Regulator. It omits much of the well-argued and detailed theoretical considerations in his writings, as well as the arguments supporting his concept that have appeared in other publications on orthodontic research and related fields of knowledge. Of particular pertinence is the voluminous and ongoing work of Alexandre Petrovic, Jeanne Stutzmann, Claudine Oudet, and associates in Strasbourg, as well as that of the Center for Human Growth and Development at the University of Michigan. Our own ongoing NIH-sponsored research demonstrates the magnitude of success routinely possible in properly chosen and handled cases. The reading list at the end of this text will enable the clinician to learn more about this truly functional approach to orthodontic mechanotherapy. Courses by Rolf Fränkel, Jim McNamara, Hans Kaufmann, and others will help prepare the orthodontist for the excitement and enthusiasm that disciples of Fränkel share.

CHAPTER 11

COMBINED FIXED AND REMOVABLE ORTHODONTIC APPLIANCES

PHILOSOPHICAL DICHOTOMIES

The great interest in removable appliances in the United States in the past 5 to 10 years has resulted in a melding of both European and American methodologies. Traditionally American orthodontists have looked askance at the use of removable appliances, which are less exact in their accomplishments, offering less control of individual teeth. To many clinicians in the United States, removable appliances were synonymous with socialized dentistry and were derisively labeled, "Poor man's orthodontics." Many European orthodontists were not much more complimentary about the American systems, with their complex wire configurations, heavy forces, high percentage of extractions, all too frequent root resorption, and decalcification, and their lack of understanding of the potential of growth guidance and utilization of the neuromuscular components of the stomatognathic system in the establishment of a normal occlusion.

The "either-or" and "all or none" approaches to mechanotherapy on both sides of the Atlantic failed to recognize that the critical facet of orthodontic care was and should be case selection, diagnostic assessment, and treatment goals, regardless of the appliance used. The strong cultism and dogma that permeated the various systems and the "cookbook" approach reinforced antagonisms towards anything that was different. Discretionary, cognitive, decision-making orthodontics, based on the unique demands of each patient, naturally suffered from this approach.

Despite the great interest in removable appliances in the United States in the recent past and a melding of American and European methodologies, there is still an emotional, unreasoning rejection of biologically based and thoroughly researched technologies in some quarters. It is the purpose of this chapter to show that there is a middle road between fixed and removable appliances. When used properly, with that distillate of diagnostic objectivity and discretion, it is possible to take advantage of the best parts of both appliance philosophies and to reduce or eliminate many of the disadvan-

tages. It is the conviction of the author that the combination or sequential use of removable and fixed appliances for certain malocclusion categories, at specific times in the dental development, can produce results that are superior to either approach alone. Such an approach is based on the acronym KISS, *"Keep it simple, sir!"* This approach has less iatrogenic potential, while offering a superior methodology for correction of problems that should be approached in the mixed dentition. Specifically we are referring to sagittal discrepancy and neuromuscularly induced types of malocclusions, with the bulk of this chapter discussing the management of the Angle Class II problems.

Need for diphasic therapy

A basic tenet of the combined fixed and removable appliance rationale is the realization that there will likely be a need for two phases of therapy, one during the mixed dentition phase of growth and one after the eruption of the premolars and canines. This is particularly true in skeletal Class II and Class III cases, where elimination of sagittal basal malrelationships will probably require harnessing of growth processes. Abundant source material already exists for a variety of appliances. For example, Schwarz's *Das Lehrgang der Gesissregulung* offers many different designs for removable appliances, which are to be used alone or in conjunction with fixed appliances. The new second edition of the book *Removable Orthodontic Appliances* by Graber and Neumann (1984) likewise discusses this combination.

First phase therapy—functional appliances and extraoral force. This chapter concentrates on the combination of functional orthopedic appliances and fixed appliances that utilize extraoral force for the express purpose of guiding the anteroposterior and vertical growth of the maxilla and mandible to a more harmonious relationship and pleasing profile (Fig. 11-1). Although Class I malocclusions are encountered most frequently in the general populace, the greatest number of patients actually seeking treatment have sagittal malrelationships, primarily in the Class II category. This is be-

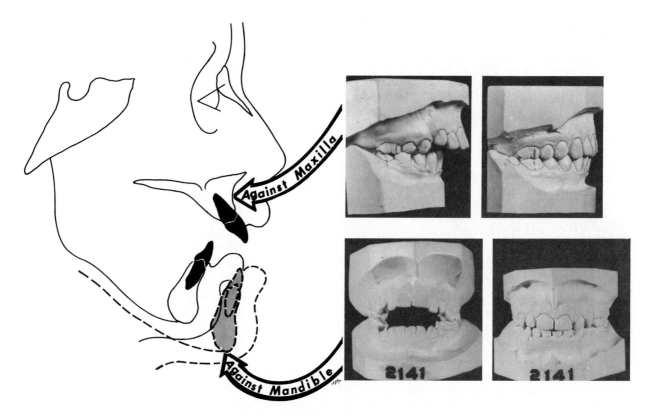

Fig. 11-1. Traditionally extraoral orthopedic force via fixed appliances has been directed against the maxilla and mandible in Class II, Class III, and open bite problems. Both retractive and protractive forces have beem employed in Class III malocclusions.

cause both parents and patients are aware of the relative prominence of the maxillary incisors and the underdevelopment of the lower jaw, as well as the patient's inability to close the lips without strain due to abnormal perioral muscle function. The likelihood of enhancement of the overjet by the deforming muscle activity, if the malocclusion is left unattended until the permanent dentition, is sufficient reason to intercept the problem in the mixed dentition. Added to this, however, is the increased risk of damage to the protruding incisors.

Apical base dysplasia and neuromuscular involvement. A prime requisite of treatment is the reduction of the apical base dysplasia. Paradoxically many American orthodontists have been trained in an appliance regimen that is based on placing full appliances on adult dentition. Only then can gnathologic precepts be implemented. The idea of instituting first phase therapy runs counter to their training and experience. Disregarding the obvious interplay between the three M's—muscles, malformation, and malocclusion—the parent is instructed to bring the patient in when the permanent teeth erupt. Then with full multiattachment fixed appliances, intermaxillary elastics, headgear, and a greater likelihood of tooth sacrifice, the comprehensive treatment is carried to completion. There is no doubt that precise adjustments of arch wires and appurtenances are

capable of correcting individual tooth malpositions and producing the tooth-to-tooth relationships demanded by Angle's "Old Glory" and dyed-in-the-wool gnathologists. Whether the result is completely stable, healthy, and noniatrogenic is sometimes another question. This chapter recognizes that finite detailing is often needed in the second phase of therapy in the permanent dentition, utilizing fixed, multiattachment, light wire mechanotherapy, with its obviously superior tooth position control. This still does not approach the major concern—abnormality of the jaw relationship itself, with adaptive compensatory deforming muscle activity, which makes the whole problem more severe. Too often with the one-shot therapy approach the objective has been to achieve a dental compromise for a skeletal and neuromuscular problem, ignoring the potential of growth guidance directed to the primary areas of concern.

Removable appliance adherents have been no less concerned about malocclusion characteristics. However there has been a greater awareness of the neuromuscular involvement in the malocclusion and the fact that the tooth relationships often reflect basal sagittal jaw malrelationships that are being enhanced by compensatory functional activity. They have turned to the patient's own physiologic processes and to attempts to harness the patient's growth and developmental processes, instead of

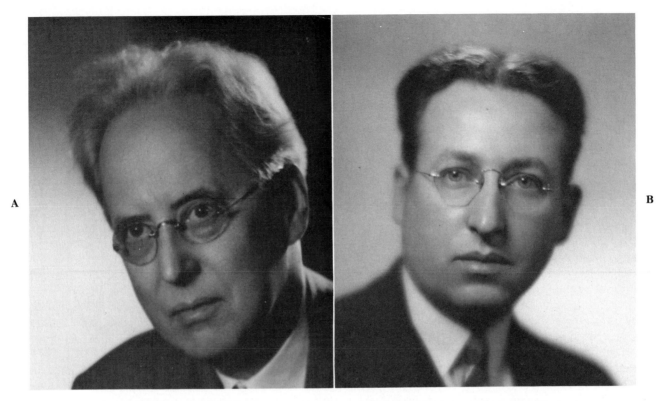

Fig. 11-2. The eminent father and son leaders in biologic aspects of orthodontic therapy. **A,** Frederick B. Noyes, teacher in the Angle School, dean, author, and Professor of Histology and Orthodontics, University of Illinois. **B,** Harold J. Noyes, pediatrician, orthodontist, Professor of Orthodontics, Northwestern University, and Dean of the Dental School, University of Oregon.

trying to make all the corrective maneuvers by shifting teeth into more "normal" relationships and then hoping the bone and muscle components will follow and adapt to the new occlusion.

Functional appliance objectives. Functional appliances, as exemplified by the Andresen activator, Bionator, or Fränkel appliance, attempt to correct the sagittal abnormality by posturing the mandible forward with appliance guidance. The primary objective is to eliminate the deforming neuromuscular activity, which has a retrusive effect on the mandible and a tendency to increase the overjet by tipping the upper incisors further forward. The objectives of functional appliances also include an "unloading" of the condyle, with the research supported expectation of enhanced condylar growth in a more favorable direction and with some evidence of favorable adaptation of the articular fossa itself. The resultant reduction of the anteroposterior dysplasia, the normalization of anterior face height, and favorable local changes in the dentition have also been documented, as other chapters in this book demonstrate.

The treatment challenge—a mixed bag. If all Class II malocclusions were either maxillary protrusions or mandibular retrusions, the challenge would be clearer. The actual situation, however, is often a combi-

nation of both. The major increment of the sagittal discrepancy may well be the relative mandibular retrusion with localized maxillary dentoalveolar compensation, if the cephalometric research of Riedel and McNamara is correct. There is evidence that abnormal muscle function in the classic Class II, Division I, malocclusion may extend to the suprahyoid and infrahyoid group, as well as to the posterior temporalis and deep masseter muscle fibers, which all exert a restricting influence on the mandible itself through the muscle attachments. Permitting these aberrant functional forces to act on largely membranous bones, which are responsive to such forces, is not calculated to enhance normal growth and development or to stimulate corrective compensatory tooth changes in the dental arches.

Historical basis for current concepts. I (T.M.G.) have been fortunate to have been influenced early in my career by a famous father and son team (Fig. 11-2). Harold Noyes, eminent son of an eminent father, was a pediatrician first and then an orthodontist. As head of the graduate orthodontic program at Northwestern University, he looked upon dental problems through the eyes of a physician and gained thereby a broader view of the whole individual. As a great student of growth and development, he would say, "Whenever there is a condition that stands in the way of normal growth and development, it should be corrected!" After completing graduate training and joining practice with Frederick Noyes, Angle teacher, histologist, dean, author (but above all, a biologist), I found that the role of the musculature had become quite clear. In the 5 years of practice with Fred Noyes, I spent many hours in muscle training with patients trying to correct the abnormal functional aspects of malocclusions. Over and over again both father and son preached working with dentofacial growth and development and establishment of a normal neuromuscular environment. I learned a biologic approach.

It is a fact that European dentists, with more of a medical background and training, found this approach appealing before most American orthodontists did. While European orthodontists were trying to implement interceptive orthodontic concepts, Harold Noyes' ideas were a lone cry in the wilderness in Chicago. The prevailing concepts that were emanating from the Edward H. Angle heritage "sanctum sanctorum" across town (Chicago) were well publicized, and a generation of dentists were trained to say, "Don't send in your patients until they are 12 years of age, or until the permanent teeth are in. Then we'll put on 20 bands and two edgewise arches and correct the malocclusion." Paradoxically much of the early cephalometric and growth research was done at this same institution but clinical application was almost nil.

The reception was overwhelmingly negative when I wrote about *dentofacial orthopedics* as opposed to *orthodontics* in the 1960s, about growth guidance for basal sagittal problems as based on my cleft palate growth studies, and about cephalometric assessment of treatment response in these cases as well as in Class II and Class III malocclusions to heavy orthopedic force. This was instead of tooth movement compensations and distal driving of molars with Kloehn headgears. There was a complete denial of the possibility of guiding craniofacial growth and development.

My first report after 10 years of experience was held up for 2 years and then finally turned down by the *American Journal of Orthodontics* with the editorial comment, "The consultants say your interpretations are not possible." It remained for definitive research work in this area by Robert Moyers and his staff at the University of Michigan and by the author and his associates at the University of Chicago to make the growth guidance concepts and techniques acceptable to American orthodontists. How far this has come is evident when the reader looks at the *American Journal of Orthodontics* and sees the subtitle, *A Journal of Dentofacial Orthopedics.* Dentofacial orthopedics was a term introduced by Graber after his early indoctrination by Harold Noyes and his own attempts to correct dentofacial de-

formities created by early and traumatic cleft lip and palate surgery.

This historical aside stresses the development of a broader concept of therapy, away from the overriding concern of interdigitation of upper and lower teeth. It became abundantly clear that the initial elimination of basal bone discrepancies and abnormal perioral muscle function before "tooth-straightening" could significantly reduce the tooth positioning challenge. The perceptive diagnostician must first determine the area of greatest abnormality and then correct the malocclusion, eliminating those deforming neuromuscular factors in the process.

Cephalometrics and growth guidance. Cephalometrics has long permitted us to determine the nature and degree of malrelationship and deficiency in our pretreatment analysis. Yet our treatment objectives have reflected a fundamental compromise, an arbitrary clinical solution, devoid of any suggestion of Popperian philosophy, and a cybernetic appreciation of the total problem, which is so eloquently described in the first chapter of this book by Petrovic. Despite manifest mandibular underdevelopment, many of the multibanded fixed appliance treatment procedures were directed primarily at the maxilla instead of the major area of the abnormality. Distal driving of molars with extraoral force to permit retraction of maxillary incisors to a deficient mandible, or extraction of premolars to make the same dental compromise, was analogous to the or-

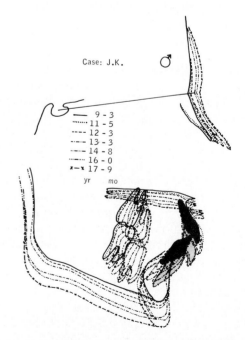

Fig. 11-3. Vertical growth direction of a patient undergoing extraoral force orthopedics. Despite withholding of forward maxillary growth, overjet remained excessive and mandibular retrusion dominated the profile.

thopedic surgeon cutting off the good leg to make it shorter to match the clubfoot. If growth direction was unfavorable for a sagittal correction, extraoral force via a Kloehn cervical gear directed against the maxillary permanent first molars could not cope with the problem nor could Class II elastics (Fig. 11-3). The major mandibular changes were in the dentition, with the lower incisors proclined, intentionally or unintentionally, to correct overjet and overbite. Apical base changes could be shown in the anteroposterior position of point A in the maxilla, but point B in the mandible actually was rocked down and back by many techniques, as the maxillary first molars were extruded by Kloehn headgear treatment.

Role of growth and development

The principles of growth and development must be understood if the clinician is to adapt them to orthodontic treatment. The corrective procedures for Class II malocclusions must have as their objective all possible elimination of the relative mandibular retrusion. Melvin Moss once commented, "Orthodontics is a 6 mm profession." He is correct in his analysis as far as sagittal discrepancy is concerned. This is usually only a matter of 5 to 6 mm. Differential mandibular horizontal growth and

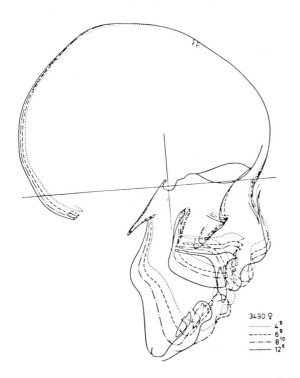

Fig. 11-4. Tracings of lateral cephalograms, showing severe downward and backward path of growth in a muscular dystrophy patient. Both the maxilla and mandible are affected by this abnormal growth vector. Note the great increase in the mandibular plane inclination under the influence of abnormal, selective, and deficient neuromuscular function. (From Kreiborg, S., Jensen, B.L., Møller, E., and Björk, A.: Am. J. Orthod. **74:**207, 1978.)

elimination of functional retrusion are likely to make up only 2 to 3 mm of this increment. The balance comes from fossa change, vertical growth components, selective tooth movement, and alveolar bone compensation. Normally the mandible grows approximately down the Y-axis or in a line from sella turcica to gnathion, as visualized on a lateral cephalometric tracing (see Fig. 4-2). This is accomplished by combined horizontal *and* vertical growth. To maintain equilibrium in the normally growing face requires adjustive and compensatory activity. Posteriorly the combined growth of the mandibular condyle and articular fossa serve to balance the anterior components of maxillary sutural (and septal) growth, plus tooth movement and eruption and dentoalveolar compensation. No one part does it alone. To correct the problem, concentration of therapy on any one part of the dentofacial mosaic is seldom adequate to establish normal, stable, and balanced conditions.

In my doctoral studies on congenital malformations, I learned the truth of the maxim, "From the pathologic, we learn much about the normal." In Kreiborg's study of muscular dystrophy, where there has been atrophy of temporalis and masseter muscles but continuing and adaptive function of suprahyoid and infrahyoid musculature, the dramatic effect of this imbalance and the potential effect of function or malfunction on the mandible is clearly evident (Fig. 11-4). The downward and backward growth pattern and opening of the Y-axis is in marked contrast to the normal downward and forward vector, with a relatively constant Y-axis. Compensatory maxillary and dentoalveolar growth have struggled to maintain some semblance of occlusal relationship, but the challenge has been too great, and the role of the tongue has become a factor, with the result that there is an anterior open bite. Maxillary orthopedics is obviously not going to solve the problem alone.

Yet maxillary growth is a consideration in the ultimate sagittal position of the chin point. If combined maxillary and alveolodental growth provides less vertical growth than the contribution from the downward moving glenoid fossa and the mandibular condyle, the net result will be a more forwardly rotating mandible, a more horizontally placed chin point, and a closing of the Y-axis. This is the converse of the Kreiborg case described above. The maxillary growth can and should be clinically manipulated to either open the Y-axis or close the Y-axis, thus influencing the horizontal position of point B on the mandible through the medium of mandibular autorotation.

Incremental expectations

In growth guidance, the incremental change of the component parts is important. Björk has shown that the maxilla grows downward from the cranial base at a rate of about 0.7 mm per year (Fig. 11-5). Maxillary tooth

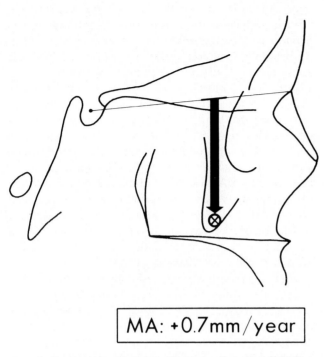

MA: +0.7mm/year

Fig. 11-5. Approximate amount of basal maxillary vertical displacement per year from the anterior cranial base to an implant in the zygomatic process, based on the work of Björk and Skieller. It amounts to less than 1 mm per year. *MA,* Maxillary growth. (Courtesy Paul Stöckli and Ullrich Teuscher.)

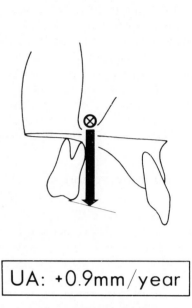

UA: +0.9mm/year

Fig. 11-6. Average annual vertical dentoalveolar growth from an implant in the zygomatic process to the occlusal plane, mesial to the first molars, according to Björk and Skieller studies. It approximates slightly less than 1 mm per year. *UA,* Upper alveolar growth. (Courtesy Paul Stöckli and Ullrich Teuscher.)

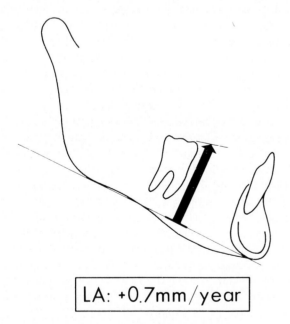

LA: +0.7mm/year

Fig. 11-7. Average annual lower dentoalveolar vertical growth measured from the mandibular plane to the mesial cusp of the first permanent molar, according to Riolo et al. and Teuscher. *LA,* Lower alveolar growth. (Courtesy Paul Stöckli and Ullrich Teuscher.)

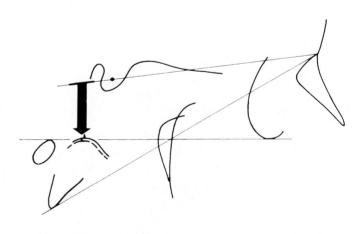

FO: +0.3mm/year

Fig. 11-8. Vertical displacement of the articular fossa averages only 0.3 mm per year, measured from the anterior cranial base line to the superior fossa surface, based on estimates by Björk, Riolo, Teuscher, and others. *FO,* Fossa growth. (Courtesy Paul Stöckli and Ullrich Teuscher.)

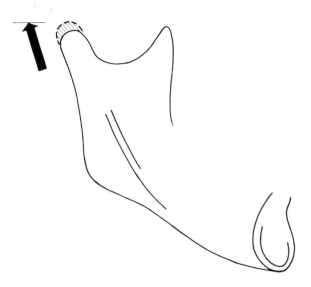

CO: +2.6mm/year

Fig. 11-9. Average annual growth increments expressed at the mandibular condyles, according to Ricketts, Luder, and Teuscher. This is normally about 2.6 mm per year, but the precise vector varies in direction. *CO*, Condylar growth. (Courtesy Paul Stöckli and Ullrich Teuscher.)

eruption increases dentoalveolar height about 0.9 mm per year (Fig. 11-6). Mandibular eruption is about 0.75 mm annually (Fig. 11-7). The nasomaxillary complex thus descends 1.5 to 2.0 mm per year. If eruption of the mandibular teeth is added to this, there is a total vertical development between 2 and 3 mm per year. According to Stöckli and Teuscher, the counterpart development of the glenoid fossa and condyle must be considered. Since the fossa change is minimal (0.25 mm to 0.5 mm annually) (Fig. 11-8), having followed the neural pattern of precipitate growth that is completed early, it is apparent that the condyle must provide the greatest increment of change, approximately 2.5 mm per year (Fig. 11-9). The nasomaxillary complex growth, dentoalveolar growth, and fossa growth are largely membranous, as opposed to a secondary cartilage growth center in the condyle.

Current knowledge, based on the research of Moyers, Stöckli, Petrovic, Graber, McNamara, Carlson, and others is that the most susceptible areas of adjustment are the purely membranous structures (i.e., alveolodental compensation). Condylar growth is also subject to environmental and appliance growth guidance influence, however, even though it is probably the dominant growth center of those units that make up the maxillomandibular growth complex. (See Chapter 2.)

Facial growth equilibrium—a fragile relationship. It is relatively easy to disturb the equilibrium established by the growing dentofacial parts. This can be accomplished by the functional matrix—the normally functioning or abnormally deforming facial, masticatory, suprahyoid and infrahyoid musculature, as shown in the muscular dystrophy case of Kreiborg. It also can be done by orthopedic appliances, such as a Milwaukee brace, or by dentofacial orthopedics, fixed or removable.

Class II elastic traction and Kloehn headgear—a mixed blessing. In an attempt to solve sagittal problems with Class II elastics, the orthodontist finds that vertical changes are also induced by the elevation of the lower molars, with the net effect of rocking the mandible open. This moves point B into a more retruded position and often unfavorably influences anterior face height. The Y-axis angle opens (Fig. 11-3).

Another way to produce this undesirable response is the indiscriminate use of the Kloehn cervical headgear. The maxillary first molars are driven distally into the "wedge," as the molars are actually extruded or tipped down and back. The mandible is rotated down and back, increasing the apparent mandibular retrusion and allowing compensatory alveolodental growth to stabilize this undesirable sagittal change. The maxillary incisors are usually tipped down and back at the same time, restricting forward mandibular growth. This result has become so common that it is now known in orthodontic parlance as the *Kloehn effect*. Instead of a horizontal withholding of the maxilla alone, there is a primary bite-opening tooth movement that exacerbates, instead of correcting, the anteroposterior dysplasia. Even with good torque control and bodily lingual movement of upper incisors, molar extrusion can produce unfavorable sagittal consequences (Fig. 11-10). This lengthens the anterior facial height excessively and enhances undesirable facial esthetics. As there is only a 2.5 mm annual vertical height change normally, it does not take much extrusion of molar teeth to create an unfavorable mandibular rotation, with Class II elastic traction and conventional cervical extraoral force therapy directed against the maxillary first molars with a facebow. Stöckli has demonstrated this change in Fig. 11-11. The eruption of the upper and lower molars by 1.0 mm each will result in opening the Y-axis 2.5 degrees, a retrusion of the chin point and a reduction of the S-N-B angle by 2.5 degrees. As he observes, the claim of a poor growth pattern often is more likely due to an iatrogenic deflection of the natural growth path (Fig. 11-12).

If this reasoning is correct, it would seem that conventional multiattachment, fixed appliance therapy, using Class II elastics and Kloehn cervical gear against the maxillary first molars, primarily attacking the maxilla in

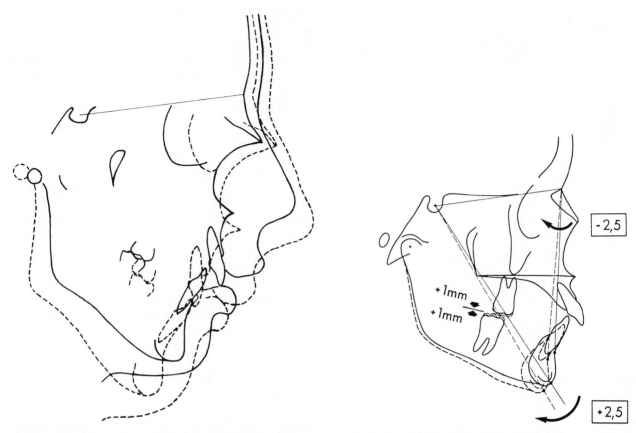

Fig. 11-10. Clinical example of severe downward and backward mandibular growth and rotation due to bimaxillary retropositioning and bodily movement of incisors aided by extraoral force. Note the increased angulation of the mandibular plane. (Courtesy Paul Stöckli and Ullrich Teuscher.)

Fig. 11-11. The effects of a 1.0 mm extrusion of the upper and lower molars during therapy are shown by a 2.5-degree decrease in the S-N-B angle and a 2.5-degree opening of the Y-axis angle. This can be interpreted as vertical growth, when in reality it is a bodily mandibular rotational translation. (Courtesy Paul Stöckli and Ullrich Teuscher.)

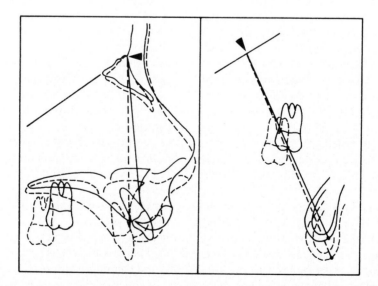

Fig. 11-12. Rotational displacement of the maxilla alone with extraoral force can elongate maxillary molars also, and the net result is to move the symphysis down and back, increasing the Y-axis angle, as shown by Stöckli. (From Ricketts, R.M., et al.: Bioprogressive therapy, Denver, 1979, Rocky Mountain/Orthodontics.)

Class II and ignoring the basal mandibular retrusion, is not likely to produce the best possible results (Fig. 11-13). Nor will it provide optimal growth guidance, even though the mandible outgrows the maxilla by as much as 5 mm, as claimed by Lysle Johnston (1983). How mandibular growth potential is controlled is the key to proper sagittal correction.

Can functional appliances alone provide the answer? Can they enhance the most favorable amounts and direction of growth? This is a primary objective of functional jaw orthopedics. A common maneuver of all modifications of the Andresen activator, including the Fränkel and Herbst appliances, is the forward posturing of the mandible by the appliance, moving the condyle forward in the glenoid fossa.

Laboratory research versus clinical results. The research of Breitner gave hope to the concept that condylar growth could be influenced. Perhaps this could occur, along with some favorable fossa changes, as seen in the primate studies, and sufficient basal maxillary, maxillary dentoalveolar, as well as some mandibular dentoalveolar adjustments, all needed to establish a normal and stable occlusion.

In spite of rather conclusive qualitative and quantita-

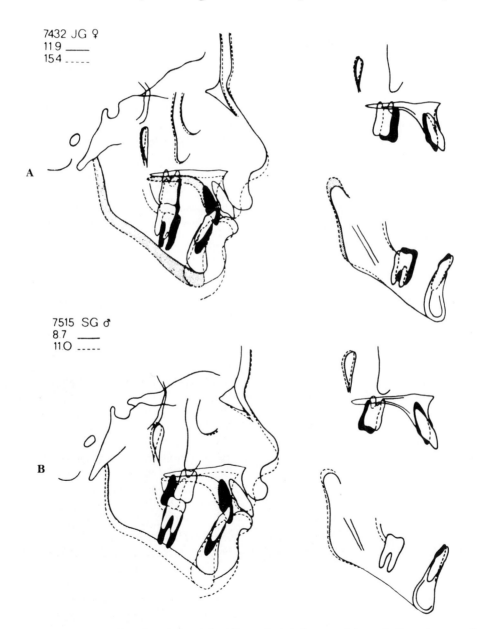

Fig. 11-13. Another clinical example of the effects of cervical extraoral force. **A,** Extraction case; **B,** nonextraction case. In both these patients the direction of change expressed at the symphysis is vertical as the mandibular plane is rocked open. (From Meikle, M.C.: Am. J. Orthod. **77:**184, 1980.)

tive laboratory evidence of enhanced prechondroblastic proliferation in the condyle, of a changed angle of trabecular alignment after mandibular advancement (the Stutzmann angle), of increased mandibular length, and of forward remodelling of the glenoid fossa from the laboratories of Petrovic, Moyers, McNamara, Graber, and others, there is still controversy over what actually takes place in the human patient (see Chapter 2). The skeptic asks, "How can we extrapolate from the rat or monkey to the human?" Most of the skepticism, however, is based on cephalometric measurements, which are suspect at the outset. We start with an infinite variety of malocclusions. The astute observer learns to recognize the multifaceted nature of malocclusions grouped together under a single heading, such as Class II, Division 1, when the primary qualifying factor is molar relationship. Treatment response is no less variable. Since the patient cannot be treated twice—once without condylar protraction and once with protraction—and compared, the clinician uses statistical means or so-called norms and standards. Samples are small and methods of posturing vary with different types of appliances, different techniques, and different clinicians; some have larger horizontal increments in the construction bite and some have larger vertical openings. So no definitive answer is forthcoming. However, based on rather ample samples, McNamara, Dierkes et al., and Graber et al. do show greater condylar growth increments per year than the means given by the computerized data-processing companies. Mandibular length also appears to be enhanced. Carefully done studies such as those cited above confirm the measurements and observations of Rolf Fränkel et al. (1983) at Heinrich Braun Hospital in Zwickau.

The right case and the right appliance, at the right time

The devil's advocates from both the fixed appliance multiattachment and the removable functional appliance school point out that alveolodental compensations and maxillary reaction are largely responsible for skeletal and occlusal changes. There is little doubt that this is partly true. It would seem, however, that case selection is critical for optimal success. The most dramatic changes shown are patients with forward rotating mandibular growth and deep bite problems. Many of these cases show clear evidence of functional retrusion, tied in with mandibular overclosure, excessive posterior temporalis and deep masseter muscle activity, and tooth guidance. Posterior displacement can amount to 1.5 mm in the average patient. So a particular case may well have a postural change in many Class II, Division 1, malocclusions, even as there is in 50% of Class II, Division 2, patients.

In downward and backward rotating facial patterns,

functional appliances are less likely to be successful. Untoward sequelae may occur, such as proclination of lower incisors, excessive anterior face height, poor facial esthetics, lack of lip seal, lack of stability, and a dual bite. (See Chapters 4 and 5.) In these cases of unfavorable growth direction, the functional orthopedic concept alone is as inadequate in correcting the sagittal malrelationship as are fixed appliances that direct their attention primarily to distalizing the maxillary dentition. Optimal response can be achieved only by a combined orthopedic withholding of the maxilla and all possible forward positioning of the mandible. Orthodontic treatment must be directed towards relative depression of the maxillary alveolodental components in cases that start with excessive anterior face height, as well as towards the greatest possible retardation of vertical basal maxillary growth. Success in these endeavors will permit autorotation of the mandible, bringing the chin point upward and forward to improve the S-N-B relationship to S-N-A. High-pull extraoral force directed at the entire maxillary dentition is far more likely to accomplish these objectives than any functional appliance alone.

Growth guidance—what is the potential? Functional appliances are not capable of routinely making major changes in the nasomaxillary complex, as McNamara and associates (1982) have shown. However, animal experiments by Droschl, Graber, Cederquist, McNamara, Moyers, and others have shown significant retropositioning of the nasomaxillary complex. Both major sutural activity and dentoalveolar compensation are seen. Voluminous clinical material is available from the same sources. Delaire (1972) has shown dramatic success in forward protraction of the maxillary complex with fixed orthopedic appliances. Continuous heavy orthopedic force against the maxilla has produced posterior rotation of the whole complex, as shown by Droschl (1973). Delaire shows anterior maxillary rotation around the frontonasal suture with protraction. However, Cederquist (1976) produced major orthopedic maxillary retraction on primates with no maxillary rotation, when heavy intermittent forces were used along the occlusal plane (Fig. 11-14). Nevertheless, with conventional extraoral force, particularly from the cervical direction, downward rotation of the maxilla is a distinct likelihood, as shown by Wieslander. So the *direction* and the *method* of delivery of orthopedic force to the maxilla are important. Otherwise the increased anterior vertical dimension offsets the sagittal gain, rotating the mandible down and back, as discussed earlier in this chapter. All efforts must be made to reduce both horizontal *and* vertical maxillary growth in these unfavorable growth patterns. The combination of functional and dentofacial orthopedics provides the necessary

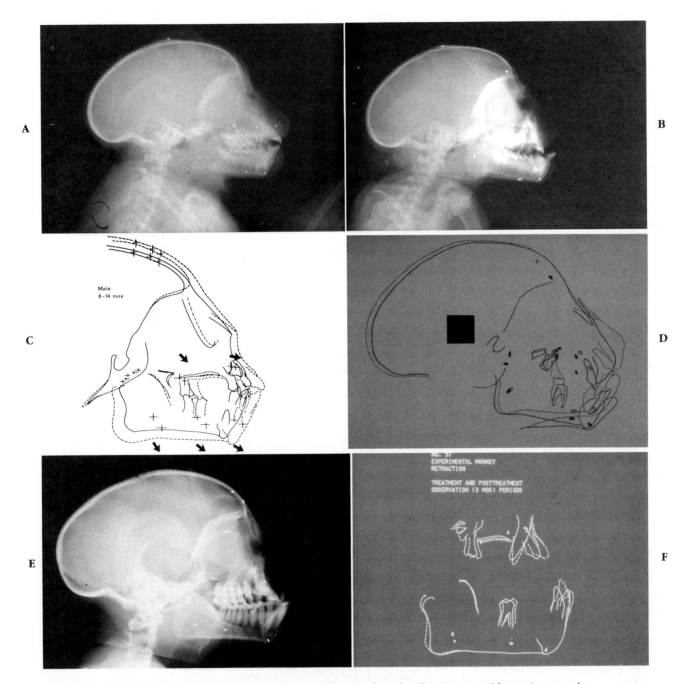

Fig. 11-14. Orthopedic changes produced in the squirrel monkey *(Saimiri sciureus)* by continuous and intermittent forces in the Droschl and Cederquist studies. **A** and **B,** Severe maxillary retraction over a 3-month period with continuous orthopedic guidance. Superimposing on implants, contrast the normal pattern, **C,** with the tracings of the two top head films, **D.** Note the maxillary rotation around a point near the frontonasal suture with a rocking open of the mandible. Intermittent forces in the Cederquist research produced a marked maxillary retraction, **E** and **F,** but no maxillary rotation, with resultant minimal mandibular rotational compensation. (Courtesy Robert Cederquist.)

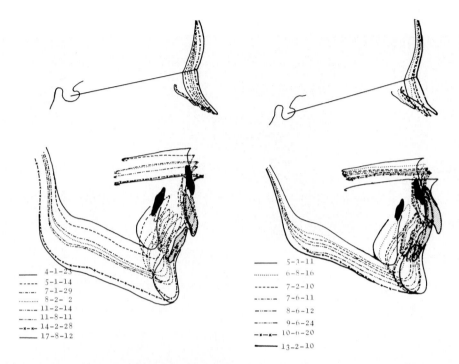

Fig. 11-15. Extraoral orthopedic growth guidance against the entire maxillary arch, not just the first molars, as with the Kloehn appliance. The maxilla has descended vertically, but the mandible has grown in a downward and forward direction. These patients also wore a maxillary biteplate, which unlocked the occlusion and freed the mandible from any retrusive maxillary effects, as seen in Figs. 11-12 and 11-13. There was no maxillary first molar extrusion, as shown in Fig. 11-11.

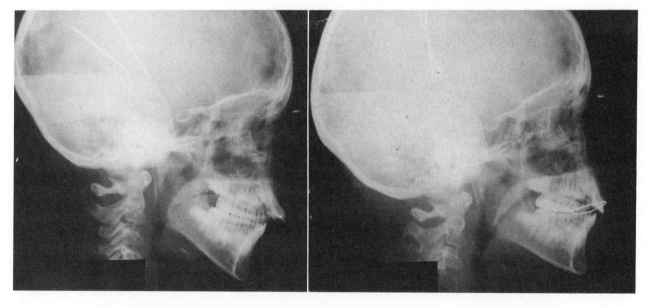

Fig. 11-16. Correction of a Class II relationship and anterior space closure, coupled with good mandibular growth, over a 6-month period. Maxillary orthopedics was directed against the entire dental arch. Because of the initial open bite tendency, no biteplate was needed.

force magnitude and vectors in such cases. Combination therapy may be extended to all Class II, Division 1, and Class II, Division 2, problems with significant benefit. Correction of the malocclusion by direct assault on the dysplastic relationships is the most desirable form of therapy.

Our studies of heavy intermittent force on primates, on humans, and in cases of cleft lip and palate show the viability of the technique for withholding both horizontal and vertical maxillary growth vectors. The appliance need be worn only 10 to 12 hours at night or as an at-home appliance (Figs. 11-15 to 11-19). Maxillary rotation is almost nil, as the Mills et al. (1978) survey has shown. Continuous heavy force does produce maxillary rotation, as does conventional Kloehn-type headgear against the maxillary molars (Wieslander, 1974); but if the force is directed against the entire dentition, as in the Cederquist and Virolainen (1976) and Mills et al. (1978) studies, minimal extrusive tipping of the maxillary first molars occurs even though the force is delivered from the cervical region. Our experience in using a cast Vitallium maxillary splint demonstrates that heavy intermittent orthopedic force can be employed with removable appliances (Fig. 11-20). However, functional appliances cast in acrylic that posture the mandible forward at the same time can be used as the "handle" on the maxilla and can simultaneously remove any growth restrictions on the mandible (Fig. 11-21). Even conventional retainers can be modified to accept high-pull orthopedic extraoral force (Fig. 11-22).

Accepting the challenge—functional appliances plus extraoral force. In skeletal Class II, Division 1, problems, with a more vertical growth direction and excessive anterior face height, the cast acrylic splint incorporates a mandibular acrylic component that postures the mandible forward, unloading the condyle. In addition, concomitant maxillary orthopedic force via high-pull headgear, attached to the acrylic activator, exerts a retarding force on horizontal and vertical maxillary growth vectors. This modified activator approach has

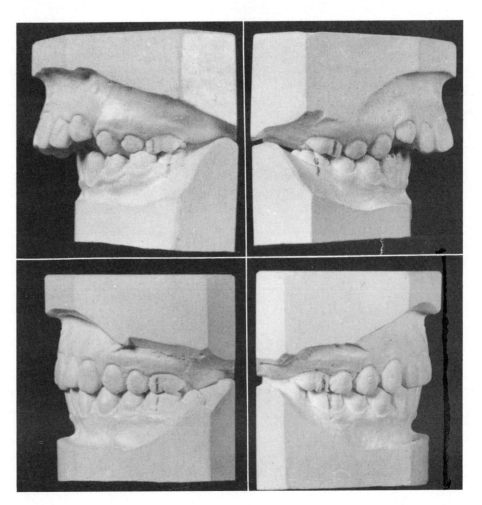

Fig. 11-17. Dentoalveolar changes produced by maxillary extraoral orthopedics directed against the entire dentition, not just the permanent first molars. No appliances were worn on the lower arch.

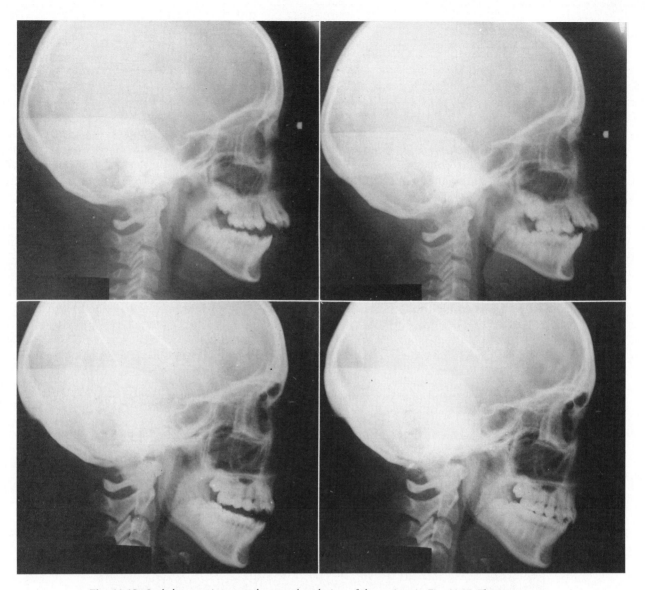

Fig. 11-18. Cephalograms in postural rest and occlusion of the patient in Fig. 11-17. There was some reduction of the excessive interocclusal clearance, as well as a sagittal correction. The change was effected by withholding horizontal maxillary growth, together with unimpeded mandibular growth and favorable upward and forward mandibular dentitional eruption.

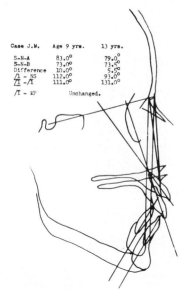

Case J.M.	Age 9 yrs.	13 yrs.
S–N–A	83.0°	79.0°
S–N–B	73.0°	73.5°
Difference	10.0°	5.5°
/1 – NS	112.0°	93.0°
1̄ – /1	111.0°	131.0°
1̄ – MP		Unchanged.

Fig. 11-19. Cephalometric tracings of before and after lateral cephalograms in occlusion for Figs. 11-17 and 11-18. The maxillary plane was not tipped down anteriorly, as is often the case with Class II elastic traction and Kloehn headgear. This result was confirmed by the Mills, Holman, and Graber longitudinal study of 120 treated patients.

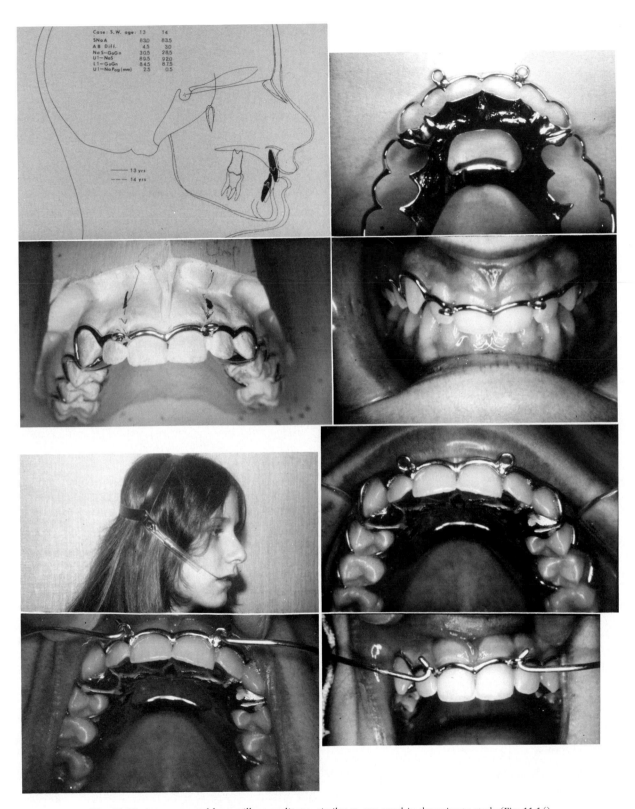

Fig. 11-20. A cast removable maxillary appliance, similar to one used in the primate study (Fig. 11-14), provides good anchorage on the maxilla and attachment for extraoral orthopedic force directed along the Y-axis. No palatal plane or mandibular plane rotation occurs. The primary effect is to withhold horizontal and vertical maxillary downward translation, as well as eruption of the maxillary teeth. This permits some favorable autorotation of the mandible, which is desirable in vertically growing faces. Acrylic may be added behind the maxillary incisors as a biteplate or slightly inclined plane to unlock the occlusion and to prevent inhibition of mandibular growth and positioning by maxillary retraction. This is recommended in deep bite problems.

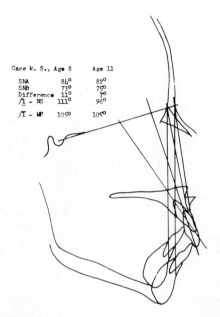

Case M. S., Age 8		Age 11
SNA	84°	82°
SNB	73°	75°
Difference	11°	7°
/1 - NS	111°	96°
/T - MP	105°	105°

Fig. 11-21. Class II, Division 1, malocclusion treated with an activator. Slight maxillary horizontal withholding is combined with optimal mandibular growth increments, unrestricted by maxillary retractive and incisal forces.

been used successfully by a number of clinicians (Hasund, Pfeiffer and Grobety, Stöckli and Teuscher, Hickham, Stockfisch, Graber, and others. The bulkiness of the original *monobloc* acrylic, or Andresen activator, can be reduced and still maintain the dual effectiveness of the appliance. A transpalatal Coffin spring shaped wire can be used, as with the Bionator or Fränkel appliance. Even buccal shielding wires and lip pads can be incorporated, if indicated, to break up abnormal perioral muscle function and the well-known lower lip trap (Figs. 10-39 and 11-47). It is then possible to attack the orthodontic problems at the source of the abnormality. Trying to do it all with fixed appliances, by putting the teeth in proper occlusion, at the expense of a correct tooth to basal bone relationship, often compromising for uncorrected basal jaw dysplasias and neuromuscular problems, is more mechanical than biologic, no matter how efficient the appliances are. When root resorption, sheared alveolar crestal bone, and possible decalcification are also among the hazards of treatment, it is no wonder that some observers have asked "Does the punishment fit the crime?"

COMBINATION THERAPY
Maxillary retraction splints and extraoral force combinations

Margolis ACCO. Fixed appliances have no monopoly on the use of extraoral force. Clinicians like Margolis and Spengeman have incorporated extraoral force with removable appliances for a long time for Class II malocclusions, using them in combination in both active

and retention phases of treatment. Spengeman devised several varieties of removable appliances to hold back relapsing maxillary arches (Fig. 11-22). Margolis has also realized that the removable appliance–headgear combination could be used effectively in active treatment where withholding of maxillary horizontal growth was desired. The Margolis appliance is called ACCO (*AC* for acrylic, and *CO* for cervicooccipital anchorage). Hundreds of orthodontists on the east coast of the United States have used this appliance in one form or another, particularly as a means of active retention. Tennenbaum and Gabriel of Argentina have modified the appliance for treatment of both unilateral and bilateral Class II malocclusions and claim a high degree of success (Fig. 11-23). The adaptation of acrylic over the labial wire of the Hawley-type retainer lends added stability and better retention (Fig. 11-24). Elimination of mild incisor irregularity is possible with these appliances. The teeth are cut off the working model and rearranged in wax before forming the labial wire and adding the acrylic, much like the Harry Barrer spring retainer. Interproximal stripping is used in conjunction with wearing the appliance to effectuate the alignment. Margolis uses the ACCO to hold the torque correction already achieved by fixed appliances; the broad labial acrylic surface holds the incisor inclination better than the conventional round labial wire of the Hawley retainer. The regular removable upper retainer also is not capable of maintaining the sagittal correction that has been achieved. Actually the slight closing of the vertical loops of the labial wire to close incisor spaces left from active treatment can actually offset the torque adjustment already achieved. This tendency is reduced with the labial acrylic construction of the ACCO, which exerts a greater bodily force on the incisors.

Margolis has also modified the appliance further by adding 1.0 mm buccal tubes to the labial wire, soldering them vertically at the canine-lateral incisor embrasure, to receive the J-hook extraoral force arms. An inclined plane may be incorporated to eliminate functional retrusions and to free the mandible for all possible forward growth.

An unwanted retrusive force on the lower jaw is created sometimes by tipping maxillary incisors lingually through the use of a conventional Hawley-type upper retainer; thus the use of an acrylic table behind the maxillary incisors provide bite opening, which prevents this undesirable consequence. Acrylic can be carried over the occlusal surfaces of the posterior teeth to give added support for reception of extraoral force arms, if no tooth movement is contemplated in this area. Occlusal cover may be needed also to prevent overeruption of the posterior teeth and the creation of an open bite. Such a splint is sometimes used in TMJ therapy.

The use of a bite plane alone, engaging only the

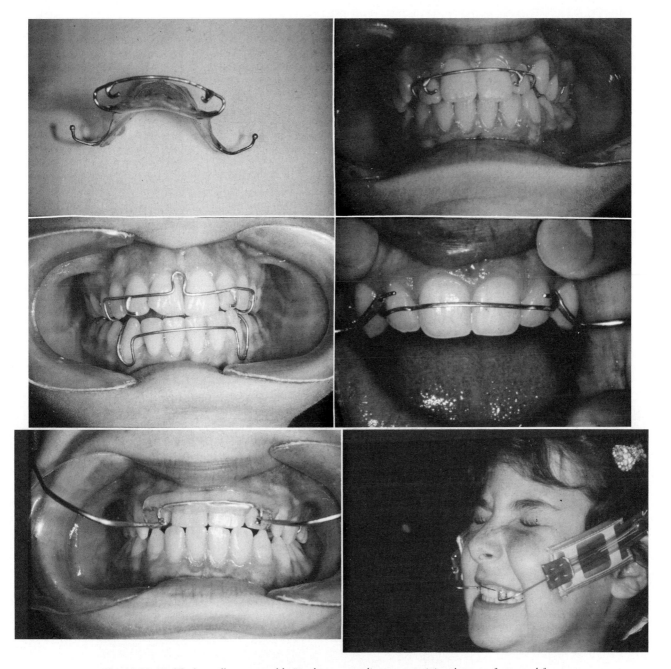

Fig. 11-22. Modified maxillary removable Hawley-type appliances, permitting the use of extraoral force against the maxillary dentition. Multiple ball clasps or occlusal cover can increase the resistance to dislodgement by extraoral traction. (From Graber, T.M., and Neumann, B.: Removable orthodontic appliances, ed. 2, Philadelphia, 1984, W.B. Saunders Co.)

lower incisors, with no posterior occlusal cover, keeps the upper and lower posterior teeth apart, stimulating eruption of the molar teeth. The appliance can be modified to provide differential eruption, as recommended by Harvold and Woodside, by keeping the lower posterior teeth out of occlusion but covering maxillary posterior teeth with a thin acrylic layer, in addition to the anterior biteplate. This method, or the use of metal spurs that act as occlusal rests, reduces the curve of

Spee while allowing for both vertical and horizontal movement of the lower buccal segment teeth. When indicated, acrylic is cut away from the lingual side of the maxillary posterior teeth to permit fingersprings to distalize molar and premolar teeth (Fig. 11-23). With the Margolis ACCO, one side is distalized at a time. Ball clasps or a passive fingerspring on the other side enhance retention of the appliance. A new ACCO is made after extraoral force and fingerspring adjustments have

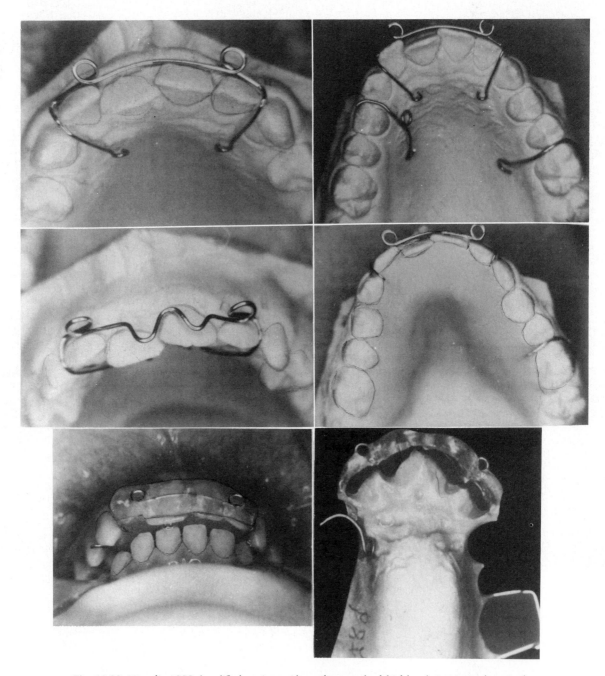

Fig. 11-23. Margolis ACCO (modified retainer with acrylic over the labial bow). Loops are bent in the labial bow to receive J hooks from the extraoral appliance. The labial bow can be notched or undulated for better retention of the adapted acrylic. The teeth can actually be moved distally to a mild degree by cutting away contiguous palatal acrylic and using finger springs. This is usually done on one side at a time. (From Graber, T.M., and Neumann, B.: Removable orthodontic appliances, ed. 2, Philadelphia, 1984, W.B. Saunders Co.)

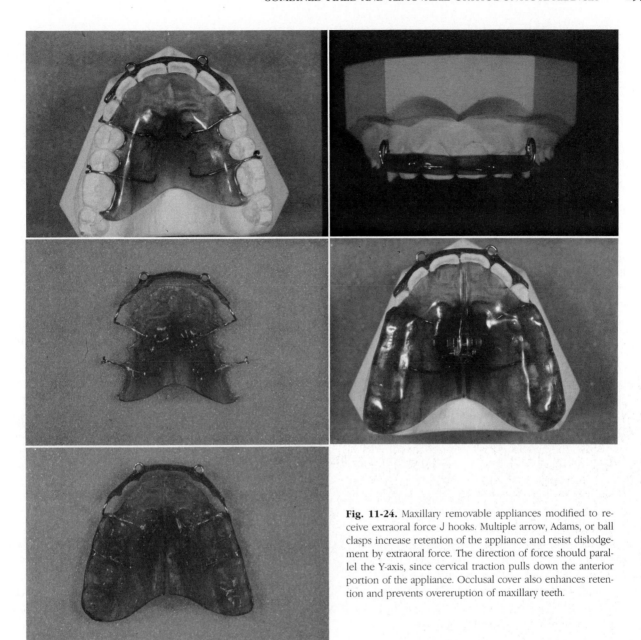

Fig. 11-24. Maxillary removable appliances modified to receive extraoral force J hooks. Multiple arrow, Adams, or ball clasps increase retention of the appliance and resist dislodgement by extraoral force. The direction of force should parallel the Y-axis, since cervical traction pulls down the anterior portion of the appliance. Occlusal cover also enhances retention and prevents overeruption of maxillary teeth.

created a Class I on one side. The new acrylic configuration and clasps on the completed side provide anchorage to correct residual Class II tendencies for the other side of the arch, a maneuver that is completed with combined extraoral force and distalizing fingersprings.

The ACCO should be worn both day and night, with a minimum of 12 hours of nocturnal extraoral force. Fixed appliances are often used as a pre-ACCO phase to correct individual tooth malpositions, much as with other functional appliance procedures. A short period of fixed appliance mechanotherapy may also be needed,

using direct-bonded attachments and flexible arches for incisor rotation and depression. Auxiliaries are possible to provide a very limited degree of axial inclination control or torque. The ACCO can continue to be used as a retainer after the treatment objectives have been achieved. For any residual sagittal abnormality or tendency to return to the original Class II relationship, extraoral force can again be applied to the ACCO, as indicated.

ACCO modifications. I have used a modification of the ACCO for some years as an active retainer in Class II, Division 1, cases, where there is a tendency of relapsing overjet, primarily due to the original maxillary protraction. The initial therapy is accomplished with multi-attachment fixed appliances and whatever auxiliary appliances needed, in addition to extraoral force. Then the ACCO is placed, with or without a jackscrew for transverse control, depending on the need for expansion (Fig. 11-24). The occlusal surfaces of the maxillary posterior teeth are covered for retention and for the added stability needed when extraoral force arms are attached to the labial wire and acrylic assemblage. The acrylic cover for the posterior teeth serves to free the intercuspal interdigitation in Class II cases and to eliminate any retrusive action of anterior or posterior tooth guidance. The appliance may also continue to be used as a biteplate to reduce any excessive overbite. This is done by allowing only the lower incisors to contact the bite plane on the anterior aspect of the palatal acrylic. The lower buccal segments are free to erupt while the upper posterior teeth are prevented from doing so by the acrylic cover. This allows differential eruption, if it is desired, and the sagittal relationship is also improved. If eruption of both upper and lower posterior segments is desired, then the acrylic is cut away from the upper posterior teeth as well.

Jacobson splint. Jacobson has used a splint similar to the ACCO for correction of mild Class II problems or for first-phase therapy or pre–fixed-appliance guidance, with some success. The reduction of overjet and the sagittal discrepancy reduce the deforming action of abnormal perioral muscle function. It eliminates sagittal overjet problems that enhance abnormal perioral muscle function (Figs. 11-25 and 11-26).

The force magnitude with this type of removable maxillary appliance of necessity cannot be too great or the appliance is dislodged. Fig. 11-26 shows that the direction of pull should coincide roughly with that of the Y-axis or of a line extending from the symphysis to a point 1.5 cm in front of the external auditory meatus. This reduces the potential for unfavorable basal maxillary tipping or extrusion of teeth, as noted earlier. The orthopedic potential is thus limited.

Graber soft acrylic appliance. The original use of the Graber soft acrylic appliance of the late 1940s was to cause orthopedic changes in cleft palate patients. Graber used various configurations in his appliance research. Early designs carried the soft acrylic and positioner type of elastoplastic material into the vestibule, with an appliance configuration much like the Mühlmann propulsor, in an effort to have some therapeutic effect on the basal maxillary structures. The rationale was that the operated lips of cleft lip patients exerted a retarding effect on the maxillary horizontal development. By screening off the effect of the lip, as Frantisek Kraus was doing in Czechoslovakia, it was hoped to al-

low the maximum maxillary growth possible. The appliance did work to some degree, but the nonelastic nature of some of the repaired cleft lips made it more difficult for the mucosal tissue to adapt to the appliance. The increased tonicity tended to displace the appliance.

The most successful version of the Graber appliance incorporated a labial bow and extraoral force arms directly into the palatal or labial acrylic. The arms could be bent to control the direction of force and to prevent dislodgement. The Graber appliance (Fig. 11-27) was a modification of the clear plastic and occlusal coverage appliance designed by Robert Ponitz. It has since been copied and is sold commercially (Fig. 11-28). This type of appliance works well as an active retainer for Class II cases, holding individual tooth positions also. Recently unjustified commercial claims have been made for a similar appliance, which ostensibly corrects three-dimensional malocclusions by merely resetting the teeth and ignoring sagittal base and neuromuscular control, using no extraoral force nor protractive mandibular posturing. This has not been supported by our longtime use. The appliance is limited in its accomplishments and cases must be chosen carefully. Generally it is used in two stages.

For minor irregularities, when arch length is adequate, the teeth on the working model are cut off carefully and reset, as with a positioner. Then the appliance is fabricated to the corrected wax setup in a positioner type of plastic and worn by the patient. If there is a minor arch length deficiency, judicious stripping of the interproximal areas will be needed to effect the rotational changes of the anterior teeth.

After the initial alignment stage is completed, a new appliance is fabricated with extraoral force arms to receive the elastic traction from the headcap. The direction of pull is as high as the appliance will tolerate without being dislodged. The occlusal cover helps retain the appliance in place. Ball clasps can be used to increase retention, if desired.

An alternative is to do a quick alignment with direct bonded attachments and a flexible wire (e.g., Nitinol), and then place the occlusal coverage splint as described earlier. Extraoral force arms are incorporated for assistance in a mild Class II correction, or when there is a flush terminal plane relationship, or for preventing a relapsing Class II interdigitation.

Mills-Vig modification. Mills and Vig have demonstrated a comparable and similarly designed appliance with a labial bow for extraoral force that is also incorporated in the acrylic. No accommodation is made for resetting the teeth but merely for the appliance to serve as the handle on the maxilla by virtue of close adaptation to the maxillary teeth (Fig. 11-29). Extraoral face-bow arms may either be incorporated in the palatal

Text continued on p. 298.

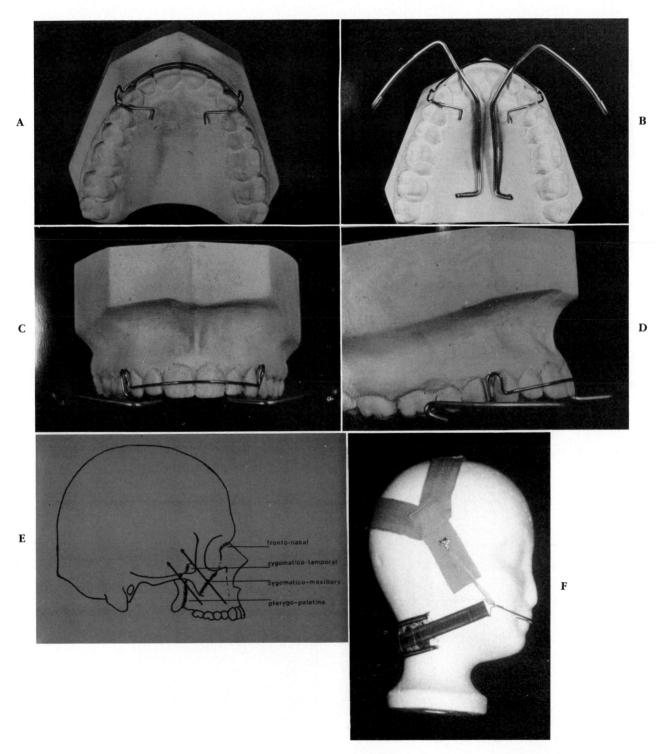

Fig. 11-25. The Jacobson craniomaxillary appliance. **A** to **D,** Extraoral force arms are incorporated directly in the palatal acrylic. A conventional labial bow is used. Retention of the appliance can be increased with arrow, ball, or Adams clasps. The direction of extraoral force is shown in **E** and **F.** According to Sicher, this should have a direct effect on the maxillary sutures. (From Joffe, L., and Jacobson, A.: Am. J. Orthod. **75:**54, 1979. Courtesy Alexander Jacobson.)

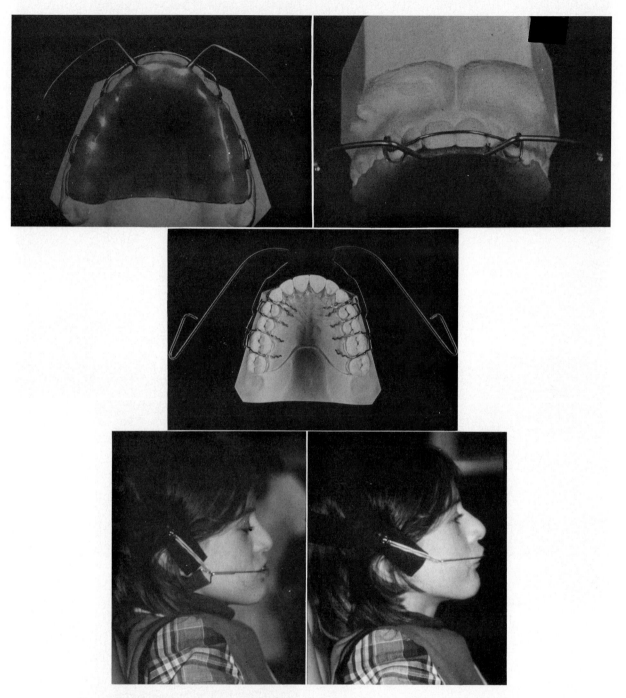

Fig. 11-26. The Jacobson craniomaxillary splint with occlusal cover to enhance retention and prevent maxillary eruption while allowing unimpeded upward and forward eruption of the mandibular buccal segment teeth to assist in sagittal correction. The extraoral force arms can also be soldered to molar clasps. A combination of cervical and occipital force can be used or only occipital traction. (From Joffe, L., and Jacobson, A.: Am. J. Orthod. **75:**54, 1979. Courtesy Alexander Jacobson.)

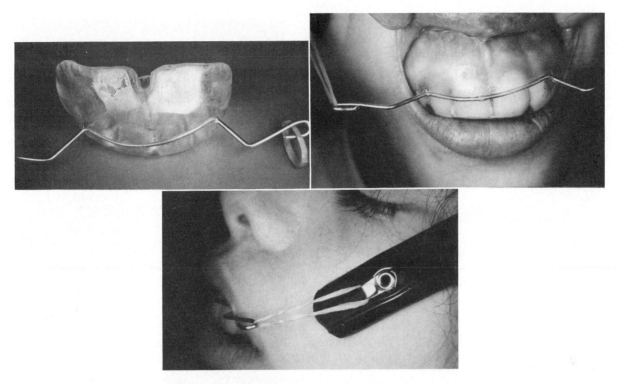

Fig. 11-27. An original soft acrylic plastic palatal appliance (vintage 1949), developed by Graber, similar to the propulsor of Mühlmann or a modified positioner utilizing the same material. The plastic is carried up into the vestibule to influence the basal as well as alveolar structures. The extraoral force arms are incorporated directly into the labial acrylic.

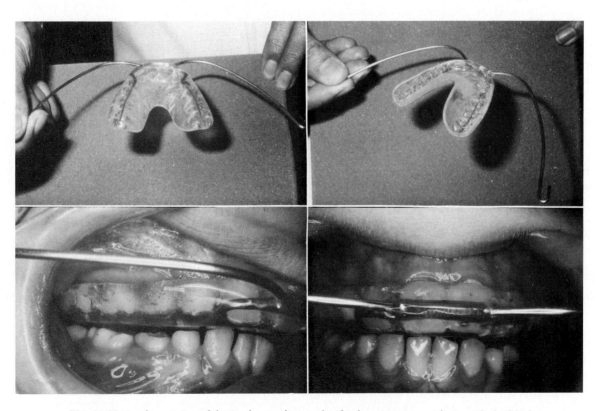

Fig. 11-28. Another version of the Jacobson splint, made of soft positioner-type plastic, with the labial bow anchored differently in plastic. (From Joffe, L., and Jacobson, A.: Am. J. Orthod. **75**:54, 1979. Courtesy Alexander Jacobson.)

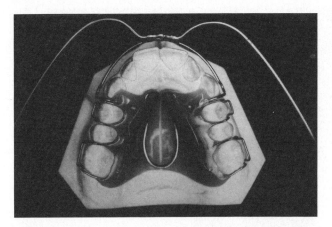

Fig. 11-29. Maxillary removable appliance with the labial bow incorporated and a split palate and Coffin spring for expansion. Adams clasps enhance retention of the appliance, anchoring it on the maxilla. If the occlusal cross-over wires actually fit into the molar/canine interproximal spaces, as with the Fränkel appliance, stability is increased and there is less tendency for appliance displacement. (From Graber, T.M., and Neumann, B.: Removable orthodontic appliances, ed. 2, Philadelphia, 1984, W.B. Saunders Co. Courtesy J.R.E. Mills.)

acrylic and be bent to extend out past the corners of the mouth, or horizontal 1.0 mm buccal tubes can be soldered to the molar Adams clasps, and a conventional facebow may then be used with occipitally directed extraoral traction (Figs. 11-30 to 11-32).

This type of appliance was described by McCallin over 20 years ago and has been widely used in England for some time. It has been copied and described in the American literature and has been dressed up with new names such as craniomaxillary orthopedic appliance, headgear splint, orthopedic functionator, etc. The principle is essentially the same: integral arms are built into the appliance or buccal tubes are soldered on the molar clasps (or combined molar and premolar clasps) for the reception of a conventional facebow.

Verdon combination appliance. Verdon has had demonstrable success with a design of appliance that is similar to the Mills-Vig combination just described (Figs. 11-33 and 11-34). The basic appliance of choice is usually a modified active plate, but it can just as easily be a modified activator, as subsequent illustrations demonstrate, if mandibular protraction is desired. As with other purely maxillary splints, though, the major objective of the Mills-Vig or Verdon splint is to effect a change through a distalizing influence on the maxillary arch, leaving the mandibular arch alone. The magnitude of force is moderate at best, for fear of dislodging the appliance, despite the excellent retention provided by the Adams-type clasps. Yet a surprising amount of force can be used, if the direction of the force is sufficiently high, toward an occipital headcap. As Stöckli and Jacobson point out, this is the best direction, roughly paralleling

Text continued on p. 302.

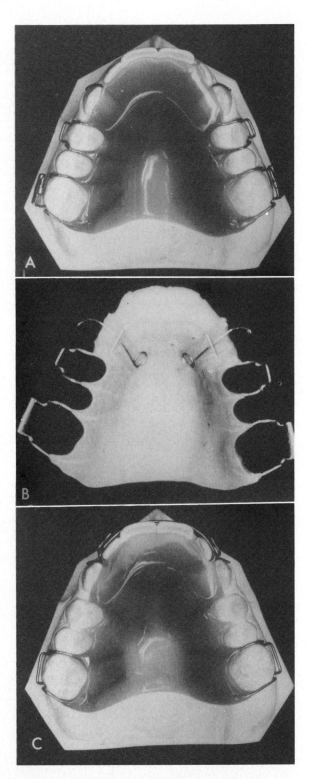

Fig. 11-30. A, Maxillary removable appliance with horizontal buccal tubes soldered to molar clasps for the extraoral facebow. In addition, canine springs **B,** are incorporated to retract these teeth. A maxillary bite plane frees the mandible from any maxillary retractive influence and allows the mandibular posterior teeth to erupt in an upward and forward direction while inhibiting eruption of the lower incisors to reduce the excessive curve of Spee. The acrylic "noses" must be cut away distal to the canines, **C,** if these teeth are to be moved distally. (From Graber, T.M., and Neumann, B.: Removable orthodontic appliances, ed. 2, Philadelphia, 1984, W.B. Saunders Co. Courtesy J.R.E. Mills.)

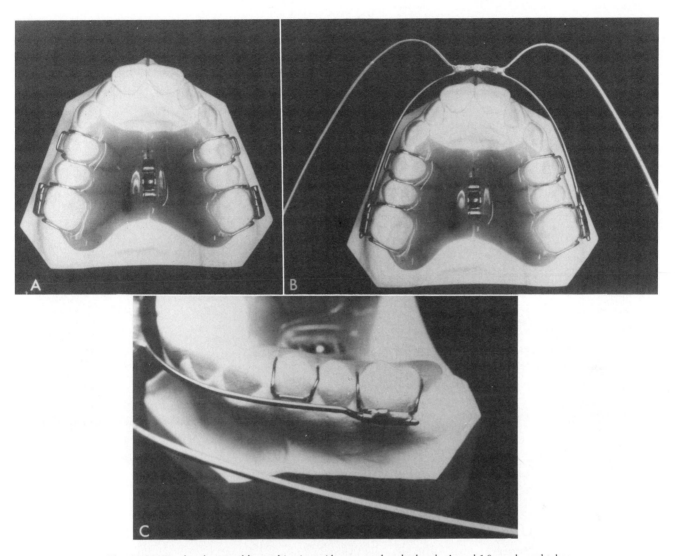

Fig. 11-31. Fixed and removable combination with cemented molar bands, **A,** and 1.0 mm buccal tubes to receive the facebow, **B.** The palatal appliance may be varied by using a flat bite plane or an inclined plane for slight forward mandibular posturing, by adding a jackscrew or Coffin spring for expansion, or by using fingersprings for selected tooth movement. Occlusal cover, **C,** can also be added to enhance stability. (From Graber, T.M., and Neumann, B.: Removable orthodontic appliances, ed. 2, Philadelphia, 1984, W.B. Saunders Co. Courtesy J.R.E. Mills.)

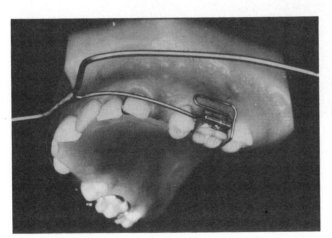

Fig. 11-32. Facebow inserted into buccal tubes on the molar clasps of a combined removable extraoral force appliance. A jackscrew is incorporated for slow palatal expansion. (From Graber, T.M., and Neumann, B.: Removable orthodontic appliances, ed. 2, Philadelphia, 1984, W.B. Saunders Co. Courtesy J.R.E. Mills.)

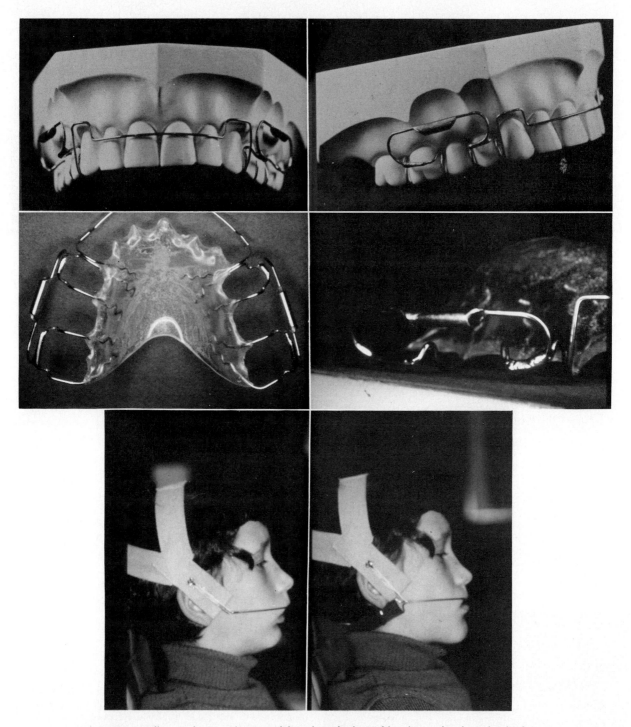

Fig. 11-33. Maxillary appliance with extraoral force buccal tubes soldered to molar clasps for the face-bow. Either occipital or combined occipital-cervical extraoral anchorage can be used. (Courtesy Pierre Verdon.)

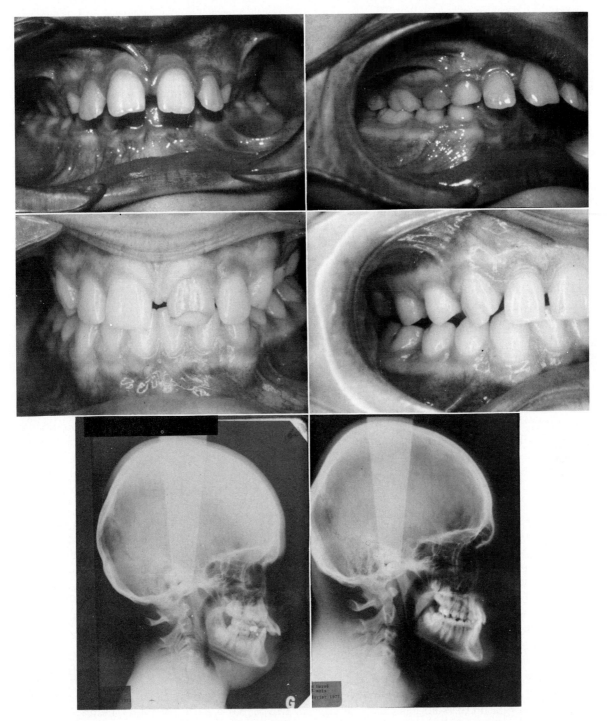

Fig. 11-34. Extraoral force and removable appliance in a Class II maxillary protraction case. The final appliance incorporates an anterior bite plane to allow for eruption of the mandibular posterior teeth. (Courtesy Pierre Verdon.)

the Y-axis, to prevent tipping down the anterior end of the palatal plane. A cervical strap can be used, but the force amounts are significantly less, implying more dentoalveolar and less basal effect.

Cast maxillary splint. Another modification suggested and used by Graber is first to align the maxillary teeth with fixed attachments and flexible archwires for correct arch form and tooth position and then to make a Vitallium casting to receive the extraoral force arms (Fig. 11-20). The loops for the J hooks are actually a part of the labial casting. Conventional cast partial type of construction is done with the cast clasps fitting over the interproximal areas and wrapping around the buccal surfaces of selected teeth. Cast molar tubes can be placed on the first molar cast clasps, if a conventional facebow is preferred to the anterior J-hook attachment. The overjet problem is then attacked with extraoral force either as an active appliance or as a working retainer in Class II malocclusions where there is an unfavorable growth direction or a relapse tendency.

A biteplate is incorporated in deep bite cases to unlock the mandible from any retrusive extraoral force. Placing this acrylic on the lingual of the maxillary incisors gives some differential vertical control, inasmuch as maxillary teeth are prevented from erupting by the casting while the mandibular teeth are free to erupt upward and forward, helping to correct the sagittal discrepancy as well as the vertical deficiency. If the lower incisors are lingually inclined, an inclined plane may be used instead of a flat bite plane in a design similar to the Hotz *Vorbissplatte*. This has a slight forward posturing effect on the lower arch and lower incisors, as the patient attempts to get the teeth into maximum occlusal contact.

Cast splint use in TMJ problems. This appliance, with slight modifications, has been used for some years by the author as a semipermanent splint in TMJ disturbances and for chronic bruxism and clenching patients. If the patient clicks in habitual occlusion but not on incision, the guideplane that is lingual to the upper incisors moves the mandible forward enough to prevent riding over the posterior margin of the articular disk onto the retrodiskal pad. This condition is often seen in patients with Class II tendencies and deeper than normal overbites. When worn at night, it is an effective appliance for preventing damage to the retrodiskal pad and posterior disk periphery that results from bruxism and clenching activity. Care must be taken not to procline the lower incisors. Initial tooth inclination, direction of growth, guide plane angle, type and degree of parafunctional activity at night, and amount of wear are factors that must be considered with this appliance. Extraoral force can be used as indicated for the Class II type problems, but any sagittal effect is minimal in adult TMJ patients. Careful periodic assessment with lateral cephalograms, panoral radiographs, etc. is recommended.

Miscellaneous modifications. A variety of fixed-removable appliance combinations and usages have been suggested to permit incorporation of extraoral force use. Hasund, in a paper before the European Orthodontic Society in 1969, pointed out the importance of preparatory activator treatment for Class II, Division 1, malocclusions in the mixed dentition. He showed how extraoral force could be combined with the activator. Growth amounts, growth direction, amount of time worn, and magnitude of the original insult conditioned the results that might be expected. Subsequent multiattachment fixed appliance therapy and possible tooth sacrifice were usually considered necessary by Hasund. This is only the forerunner of a number of modified activators used in conjunction with extraoral force and fixed appliances by orthodontists in both Europe and America. Some of these modifications will now be described.

Treatment considerations. Usually two or three appliances are required if the clinician wants to make full correction of a Class II, Division 1, malocclusion using only removable maxillary appliances of this type.

Sagittal considerations. After the correction of arch form, spaces, and minor irregularities, it is usually necessary to make a new appliance. Acrylic coverage of the labial wire is added to stabilize the appliance and to add bodily control of movement to the anterior segment. Both the buccal and occlusal aspects of the posterior teeth may also be covered by acrylic to further enhance stability. A facebow may be incorporated directly (Fig. 11-29) or 1.0 mm buccal tubes may be soldered to the molar Adams clasps, care being taken that the tubes are parallel, and sufficiently to the buccal to allow easy insertion and removal of the facebows (Figs. 11-30 and 11-31).

Since the mandible routinely outgrows the maxilla, (as much as 5 mm during puberty), the clinician may utilize this catch-up growth by retarding maxillary forward progression. With a retractive extraoral force inhibiting the horizontal maxillary growth component, the resultant expression of maxillary positional change is primarily vertical. This allows the more horizontally growing mandible to reduce the anteroposterior discrepancy and to establish a more harmonious sagittal relationship. A properly designed splint has the potential for retardation of some maxillary vertical growth. This allows a more favorable autorotation of the mandible, reducing the sagittal discrepancy somewhat as the chin point comes upward and forward 1 to 2 mm.

Beware of counterproductive forces. In Class II malocclusion correction, whatever the appliance of choice, it is a valid treatment objective to prevent elongation or distal driving of the maxillary molars if the net effect is to rock the mandible down and back. This is exactly what happens with conventional cervical extraoral force therapy, increasing the mandibular retrognathism. As will be discussed later in this chapter, the use of appliances that guide both maxillary and mandibular growth is generally more effective in faces that are growing downward and forward in a normal manner.

Thus before selecting the appliance, it should be reemphasized that as clear a picture as possible of the inherent morphogenetic growth pattern should be established by an analysis of pretreatment records, hereditary pattern, and any mechanism that is likely to yield information of value in this area. The direction and intensity of maxillary and mandibular growth are of prime concern. Significant growth increments are important; but they must be in the right direction, lest the sagittal dysplasia not be corrected. The design of the appliance to receive the optimal amount of extraoral force for the longest possible wear is an additional factor to be considered. Retardation of maxillary vertical growth is surely a valid treatment objective in patients with unfavorable anterior-to-posterior face height ratios, open bite tendencies, and vertical or downward and backward growth patterns. However, a combined effect appliance that controls both maxilla and mandible may well be the implement of choice for optimum results in a normally growing face.

Anchorage problem. The greatest problem with removable maxillary splint appliances is the potential for dislodgement. Clasp design, acrylic coverage, and palatal anchorage all help; but even cast appliances are limited in the amount of force they can receive. Critical to force magnitude is the direction of the force. Force directed along the Y-axis is usually more desirable and also better tolerated before the appliance is displaced. Greater stability and resistance to displacement of the maxillary removable appliance are attained if the appliance is kept completely passive, with no springs or screws for tooth movement. The neophyte should guard against the temptation to do too many things at the same time with the same appliance. Reciprocally disadvantageous forces should be kept to a minimum.

Pretreatment fixed appliance alignment. A short period of fixed attachment therapy before placing this type of appliance is quicker, more effective, and enhances the utilization of a passive orthopedic device. The appliance should be fabricated to stabilize the result already achieved as well as prevent future undesirable tooth movement, such as lingual tipping of the maxillary incisors. For this reason acrylic should cover as much as possible of the labial, lingual, buccal, and occlusal surfaces of molars and incisors. If a casting is used, it should be adapted into the interproximal areas, with broad labial incisal coverage. The treatment objective is

to be able to direct the orthopedic force toward the sutures, with the teeth and investing tissues serving as "the handle on the maxilla," so to speak.

Analysis of treatment response. The actual effects of treatment with this type of therapy are hard to assess. How much change is due to normal growth and developmental processes? How much has growth direction been changed? Have growth amounts been influenced? How much of the change is due to distalization of teeth (dentoalveolar) and how much is basal effect? What would have happened if nothing had been done? Obviously precise answers to such questions are not possible. The best projections are approximations, even with a massive data bank to serve the computer.

The probabilities are overwhelming, however, that if any growth does occur the direction of maxillary growth under combined maxillary splint and extraoral force guidance should be more vertical than if no orthopedic force had been applied to the maxilla at all. The occlusal coverage should actually retard total vertical maxillary dentitional change, based on ample evidence that eruption can be restricted with relatively light forces. This should permit some mandibular autorotation to a more favorable ultimate growth direction. Together with the favorable mandibular growth differential alluded to earlier, the sagittal discrepancy can be diminished, even if growth direction was not previously as horizontal as desired. Considerable evidence also exists that the final mandibular growth increments tend to be more horizontal in many cases, even when the growth vector has been dominantly vertical. This is particularly true in boys. While no single component is likely to produce dramatic change, the net effect is sufficient to make up that 6 mm amount needed to eliminate the Class II relationship.

A unilateral response to any form of Class II therapy with headgear or elastics is not at all uncommon. Frequently the magnitude of the sagittal problem is greater on one side than the other. So it is a distinct possibility that a unilateral response will be encountered with combination removable–extraoral force therapy. If such is the case, modifications of the maxillary removable appliance are possible. As noted earlier, fingersprings may be used, as with the ACCO. A unilateral headgear is not usually feasible with a completely removable appliance. The obvious recourse here is fixed appliances, with unilateral elastics or a unilateral headgear directed at the incompletely corrected side. This can be done with the Mills type of appliance, but with the molars banded and the palatal removable device opening the bite sufficiently to prevent occlusal interference with the treatment objective (Fig. 11-32). Tooth sacrifice is always a possibility.

Hygiene problems. Proper oral hygiene is of greater

concern with appliances that cover most of the teeth. They tend to trap plaque and caries-producing debris. Fastidious brushing of both the appliance and the teeth is essential. Optimal patient compliance requires continual motivational assists by both the orthodontist and parents. Soft tissue health is less of a problem than with fixed appliances but still demands attention.

Cemented molar band–removable appliance combination. The use of cemented first molar bands is to be recommended in combination appliance therapy, whether it is only a maxillary orthopedic splint of the type just described (Fig. 11-32) or a bimaxillary appliance like an activator. Since preliminary tooth alignment is often required, with the prospect of some post-activator–extraoral force appliance treatment always present, double buccal tubes are usually placed on the bands. The edgewise tube may also have a small hook soldered on it for future intramaxillary or intermaxillary traction.

Extraoral force transmission to entire maxillary arch. If pretreatment fixed appliances are used, it is a simple matter to fabricate the removable appliance, even leaving incisor attachments in place. The retention of the removable appliance is materially improved as the circumferential clasps snap above the buccal tube assembly on each side. If the clasps are passed distally to the first molars, they can prevent undesirable tipping and elongation of the first molars. Part of the orthopedic philosophy is to *prevent* distal driving of first molars, which is so often seen with the Kloehn appliance. Rather the extraoral force is transmitted to the entire maxillary dentition as a whole and bolstered by some palatal anchorage from the removable appliance. For dentofacial orthopedics, the teeth and supporting tissues serve as the handle on the maxilla. The desired tooth movement is accomplished either in pretreatment or posttreatment phases. Because the extraoral orthopedic force is applied to the entire dentition, not just the maxillary first molars, a greater magnitude of force is needed to produce a basal growth guidance effect. The removable appliance is not in danger of being displaced, however, since the molar bands are cemented. They receive the extraoral force arms or inner bow of the headgear appliance. Without a concern for appliance dislodgement, the direction of force also is less of a problem. A cervical source of extraoral force anchorage is possible more frequently. Better control of horizontal and vertical growth vectors is possible.

Transverse movement and habit control. As noted earlier, if a transverse increase in maxillary arch width is needed, an expansion screw may be built into the removable appliance with or without molar bands (Fig. 11-31). Tongue posture and function problems as well as finger habit or lip habit problems are frequent se-

quelae of Class II malocclusion and excessive overjet. Appliance control is relatively easy with the incorporation of a palatal crib in the removable appliance (Fig. 11-35). Since the anti–tongue thrust loops may also serve as guiding loops to posture the mandible forward 1 to 2 mm, a wider part of the dental arch opposes the maxillary counterpart. There is always the possibility of some slight distal movement of the maxillary molars. Hence it is necessary to place a slight amount of expansion in the facebow or to expand the bimolar distance in the upper arch a certain amount with the jackscrew in the removable appliance.

Vertical control. For vertical control, or in cases where there is a sagittal problem that is to be corrected by maxillary orthopedics only, no forward posturing device is needed. A simple maxillary biteplate will help in reducing the curve of Spee as the posterior teeth erupt. Generally maxillary teeth are prevented from eruption, and the mandibular teeth are allowed to erupt, since they also come forward as they move vertically, reducing the sagittal discrepancy, as noted by Harvold. This differential alveolodental compensation has been pointed out several times, since it is one of the adjustive areas for correction of sagittal malrelationships. The same mechanism is a routine part of Harvold-Woodside, Herren, and L.S.U. activator therapy.

Bimaxillary combination appliances

Without and with fixed appliances. The previous part of this chapter has dealt with maxillary splints only, as combined with extraoral force. Some mandibular guidance has been possible by virtue of biteplates for selective eruption of mandibular posterior teeth, inclined planes to posture the mandible forward slightly as the lower incisors glide upward and forward in an attempt to reach full posterior occlusal contact, and guiding loops built into the palate to engage the lingual mucosal tissue beneath the lower incisors as a proprioceptive trigger, eliciting 1 to 2 mm of forward posturing to avoid the contact. The major emphasis, however, has been on the use of the maxillary splint as a "handle" on the maxilla, receiving extraoral force to restrict horizontal and vertical dentomaxillary development.

Maxillary splint–extraoral force combinations are indicated primarily for maxillary protraction malocclusions, although the withholding of horizontal maxillary growth has the net effect of allowing the mandible to "catch up" and reduce the sagittal discrepancy. The potential for incremental change is limited, however, to 2 to 3 mm, unless there is a functional mandibular retrusion to be eliminated. In this case 1.0 to 1.5 mm of additional sagittal correction is possible. To get the total sagittal correction of a full Class II, Division 1, malocclusion, it is advisable to enlist all possible contributions from the area where the greatest deficiency lies—in the mandible. This is easy to understand when we realize that there is 2.5 mm of condylar growth per year. By eliminating any restriction of this growth from neuromuscular environmental assaults, by optimizing the direction of condylar (and mandibular) and fossa growth, and by enlisting differential upward and forward mandibular dentitional eruption of the lower buccal segments, it is possible for sagittal correction to be increased to 6.0 mm in the average case. Forward posturing of the mandible not only can accomplish

these treatment objectives but also can eliminate the functional retrusion and overclosure problem and the attendant TMJ sequelae.

Posturing the mandible forward. In many cases postural hyperpropulsion alone may be sufficient to achieve the sagittal and vertical correction needed. The posturing appliance may be modified to accomplish the necessary transverse correction.

A generation of European orthodontists thought this was all that was needed, as functional orthopedics dominated the therapeutic scene; but orthodontic research and experience have shown that all Class II, Division 1, malocclusions are not the same and do not grow the same amounts, in the same direction, and with the same expectations of treatment success. There is no Procrustean bed appliance into which all malocclusions can be forced. Morphogenetic factors, functional factors, growth potential, growth direction, tooth size and shape, anterior and posterior face height proportions, and patient compliance are just some of the conditioning factors. The orthodontist must have an armamentarium at his command that permits him to modify his therapeutic efforts to take into account this multiplicity of factors before and during the actual treatment regimen. Even as maxillary splints or extraoral force alone against the maxilla may prove inadequate in attaining a full correction, so may functional appliances. The logical conclu-

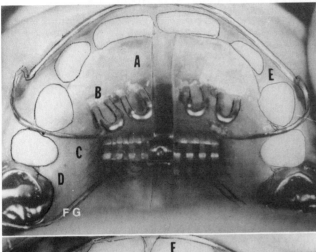

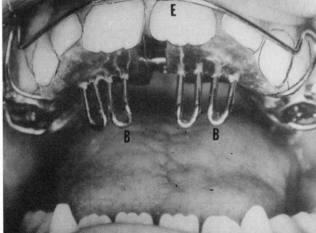

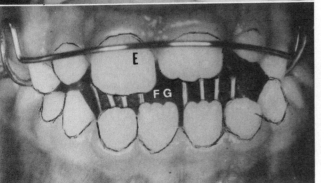

Fig. 11-35. Combined fixed and removable Graber appliance. In this early mixed dentition Class II, Division 1, malocclusion with a narrow maxillary arch, anterior open bite, and compensatory tongue posture, full metal crowns *(D)* are cemented on the maxillary deciduous second molars, with double buccal tubes soldered for reception of a facebow now and possible limited alignment of the incisors in the future. The removable appliance is made of acrylic *(A)*, with vertical guiding and anti–tongue thrust loops *(B)*, jackscrew *(C)*, molar C clasps *(FG)*, and labial bow *(E)*. The guiding loops contact the lower lingual mucosal tissue lightly and trigger a 1 to 2 mm forward posturing from the exteroceptive contact. They also serve to prevent forward tongue posture and thrusting during deglutition. A similar device is shown by Tränkmann in Fig. 11-36. If more then 2.0 mm of advancement is desired from the vertical palatal loops, then to prevent irritation, a lower lingual horseshoe acrylic appliance is needed for the loop contact. The molar clasps pass distal to the crowned molar teeth to prevent their distal movement. This transmits the orthopedic force from the forward-posturing loops and the extraoral force to the entire maxillary dentition, since the labial bow *(E)* contacts the maxillary incisors at the gingival margin, preventing posterior displacement of the palatal appliance. The acrylic may be cut away from the lingual of the maxillary incisors as desired to permit eruption and lingual movement, but it is maintained interproximally in the posterior region to give maximum transverse control and some retardation of eruption of the maxillary posterior teeth. This posterior stability may be enhanced by full occlusal cover, with a more definite restriction of maxillary buccal segment eruption and the establishment of a normal interocclusal clearance in open bite problems.

sion, then, is a bimaxillary assault on the three-dimensional problem. This can be with bimaxillary intraoral appliances alone or with intraoral and extraoral combinations.

Tränkmann approach. Depending on the morphogenetic pattern and severity of the initial malocclusion and on the role of environmental compensations, different appliances may be selected. For less severe problems, it may be quite enough to use conventional removable appliances that have been modified to achieve the treatment objectives. Orthodontic "overkill" via a multiplicity of attachments, loops, elastics, and extraoral force is not always necessary or indicated. This is particularly true when the iatrogenic potential is considered.

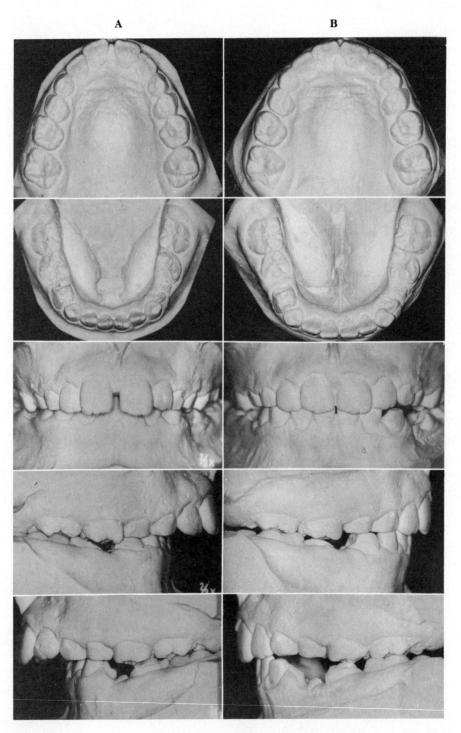

A **B**

Fig. 11-36. Class II, Division 1, malocclusion, treated with removable appliances. **A,** Before and, **B,** after therapy. (Courtesy Joachim Tränkmann.)

Fig. 11-36 shows a mixed dentition Class II, Division 1, malocclusion treated with simple removable appliances (Fig. 11-37). The use of forward posturing loops on the maxillary appliance, which engage the lingual acrylic surface of a lower removable appliance, served to eliminate any functional retrusion and also provided an initial activator effect as the maxillary and mandibular arches were slightly expanded by jackscrews to correct the minor space deficiency. A functional appliance was then placed to complete sagittal and vertical correction with the aid of local fingersprings. If this had not been sufficient to provide the anteroposterior and vertical correction needed, then an extraoral appliance could have been attached to the functional appliance for added maxillary withholding or retraction. Figs. 11-38

and 11-39 show the results achieved without the need for a total assault on the problem. Note that the axial inclination of the lower incisors remains at 90 degrees and the potential proclination of these teeth has not materialized. The spontaneous regression of epipharyngeal lymphoid tissue is a clear sign of restoration of normal nasal breathing and an expected developmental process.

The discretional appliance potential is again illustrated in Fig. 11-40, in a mixed dentition Class II, Division 2, malocclusion complicated by upper and lower arch length deficiencies. The lack of anterior face height is apparent. A well-anchored appliance, judicious use of jackscrews, and exchange of teeth (Fig. 11-41) helped solve the arch length problems; and a simple functional appliance finished the sagittal and vertical correction,

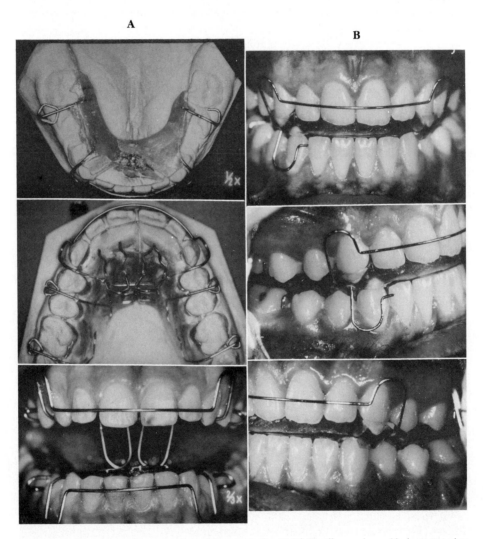

A   **B**

Fig. 11-37. Appliances used in correction of the case in Fig. 11-36. Maxillary and mandibular active plates have expansion screws and efficient arrow clasps for retention. The maxillary appliance has two sagittal guiding loops that engage the lingual mandibular acrylic on closing, protracting the mandible, **A.** Minor arch length problems are corrected by judicious use of the expansion screws. Then a functional appliance is placed to correct the residual sagittal problems. If there is maxillary protraction, horizontal buccal tubes can be added to the molar clasps or incorporated directly into the interocclusal acrylic, **B.** (Courtesy Joachim Tränkmann.)

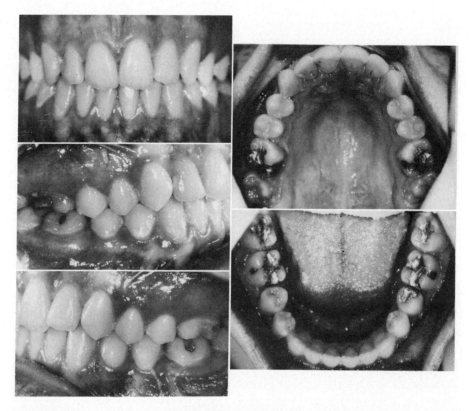

Fig. 11-38. Posttreatment results of this patient. No individual attachments have been used to effect correction of individual tooth malpositions. (Courtesy Joachim Tränkmann.)

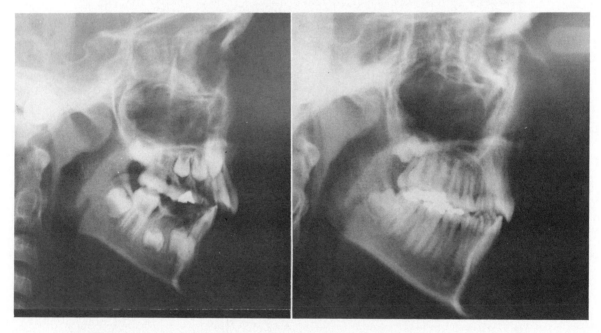

Fig. 11-39. Before and after headplates for the patient in Figs. 11-36 to 11-38. Note that proper incisor inclination has been retained. If sufficient mandibular growth had not been forthcoming, even with the unlocking of the occlusion and positional retraction achieved in the construction bite, then extraoral force could have been used to withhold horizontal maxillary growth. (Courtesy Joachim Tränkmann.)

A   B

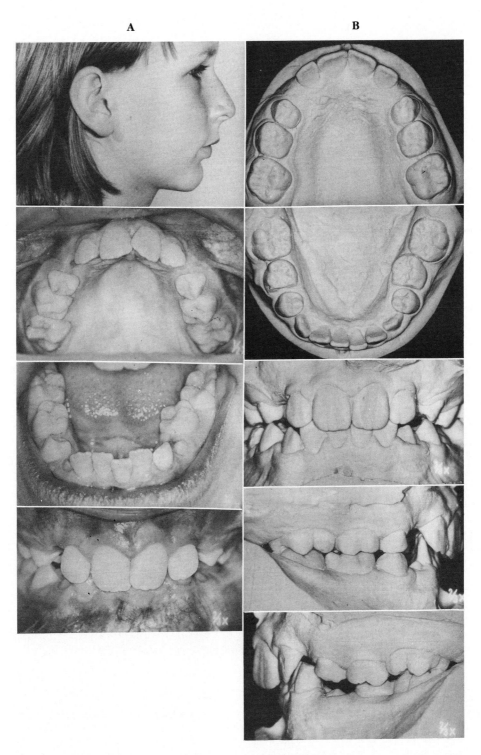

Fig. 11-40. Class II, Division 2, malocclusion complicated by an arch length deficiency. Note the deficient vertical dimension, **A.** (Courtesy Joachim Tränkmann.)

A   B

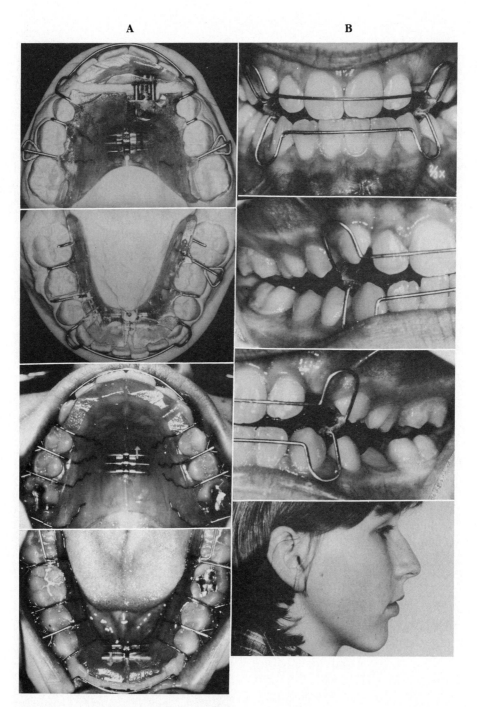

Fig. 11-41. A series of appliances was used for this patient, starting with active plates to expand the maxillary narrow arch and to tip the lingually inclined maxillary incisors labially. This also improved the arch length problem. Then an acrylic anterior bite plane was incorporated on the maxillary appliance to intercept the deep bite and to free the mandible from any possible functional retrusion, **A.** A functional appliance was then placed to assist in the sagittal correction, **B.** Usually, extraoral force is not necessary in this type of problem, where the maxillary relationship is generally normal. The facial profile changes are gratifying. (Courtesy Joachim Tränkmann.)

producing a significant improvement in the facial balance and excellent occlusion (Fig. 11-42). The cephalograms and panoral films taken before and after treatment show the success of the combination of removable appliances (Fig. 11-43). Here again the option of high-pull extraoral force, in conjunction with the activator, was always present in case a strong intrusive maxillary force was desired. Molar bands could have been used for the extraoral force, or the activator could have been modified for reception of the facebow or **J** hooks.

Modifying the activator when used with fixed appliances. The wearing of an activator in conjunction with fixed appliances requires some design modifications. The use of molar clasps has already been mentioned. As Fränkel has stressed, anchoring the functional appliance on the maxillary arch is strongly recommended, whether it be a Function Regulator or a modified activator. There is less likelihood of tipping the lower incisors forward.

In addition, if fixed appliance labial attachments are to remain on the incisor teeth during the wearing of a functional appliance, the labial wire must be bent so as to avoid impingement. The bonded brackets may also enhance the anchoring of the functional appliance on the maxilla. Bonded lugs on the buccal surfaces of the maxillary molars may also be used to enhance retention

of the functional appliance if the molars are not banded or if extraoral force buccal tubes are incorporated directly in the modified activator.

In some deep bite Class II, Division 2, cases, in which there is a greater severity of malocclusion (as in the Tränkmann case just discussed) and when there is excessive "gumminess" as well as overeruption of maxillary incisors, a prolonged vertical-pull orthopedic force is desirable. For these cases fixed appliance combinations with bonded attachments and an archwire with a strong depressing force on the maxillary incisors are preferred. Torque control for axial inclination is also possible, particularly in Division 2 problems. All this may be done concurrently with activator wear. There is, furthermore, the added advantage that the activator unlocks the posterior occlusion and eliminates any functional retrusion tendencies, both of which assist in sagittal correction. These simultaneously fixed and removable appliance adjustments, however, are more difficult to perform without prejudicing the fit of the functional appliance. Hence it is better for the clinician to start with his fixed appliance corrective procedures first and then turn to the combination appliance. After he has gained sufficient experience, the combined adjustments can be done without undesirable side effects.

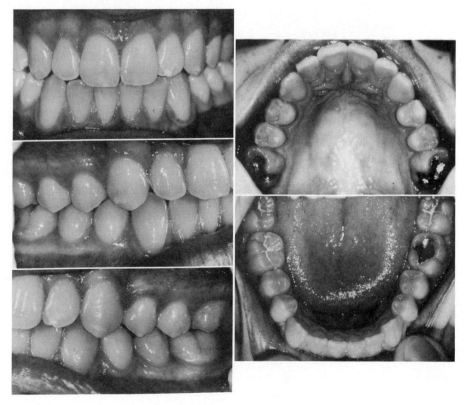

Fig. 11-42. Elimination of vertical and sagittal discrepancies as well as the arch length deficiency. (Courtesy Joachim Tränkmann.)

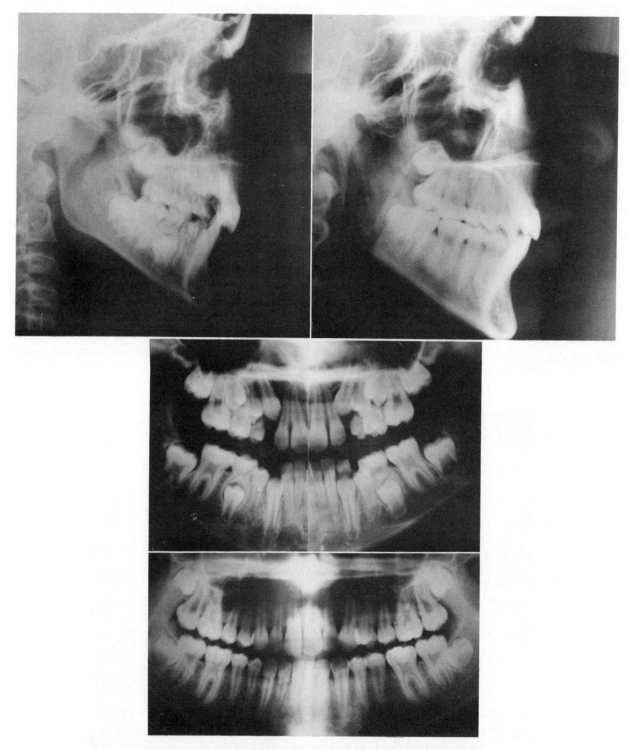

Fig. 11-43. Headplates and panoral radiographs before and after treatment of the patient in Figs. 11-40 to 11-42. Facial balance has been achieved, and the result is stable. (Courtesy Joachim Tränkmann.)

Pfeiffer, Grobety, Stöckli-Teuscher, Stockfisch, Hanson, and Hickham techniques

Dentofacial orthopedic procedures against the maxilla are indicated most in maxillary protrusion problems. Sagittal correction is possible, but any treatment effect is indirect on the mandible, unless a biteplate or Class II elastics are used. It is a fact, however, that most Class II, Division I, malocclusions are primarily mandibular underdevelopment considerations, with localized premaxillary protrusion. It is logical that therapy should call for an attack on the mandibular retrusion. A deficiency appliance is needed. Holding back horizontal growth of the maxilla is not enough. Indeed, as Mills, Holman, and Graber (1978) show, maxillary withholding can transmit the force to the mandible and actually prevent the full accomplishment of mandibular growth; and the mandible may not ever catch up, even after treatment is completed.

Significant growth increments may occur in both the mandibular dentoalveolar areas and the mandibular condyle, as well as in the temporal fossa region. Particularly in Class II malocclusions with a deep bite and premature incisal guidance, there is a frequent postural functional retrusion, which can be restrictive of full mandibular growth pattern accomplishment. A significant factor here is the abnormal retrusive forces of the posterior temporalis, deep masseter, and suprahyoid and infrahyoid musculature.

It is both biologically and therapeutically sound to eliminate restrictive muscle forces early, if at all possible. This means a mixed dentition first phase assault on the problem, or even earlier in the deciduous dentition in carefully selected cases. As Paul Stöckli and Ullrich Teuscher write,*

The prime target of the treatment concept employing the activator-headgear combination is to restrict developmental contributions that tend toward a skeletal Class II and to enhance developmental contributions that tend to harmonize the anteroposterior relationship of maxillomandibular structures. It is of paramount concern that no untoward deflections of growth displacement vectors be introduced when a treatment device is used to interfere with facial growth.

Deflections of growth—favorable and unfavorable. The reference to "untoward deflections of growth" refers not only to the possible restrictive effect of maxillary orthopedics alone when the occlusion is not unlocked but also to the direction of orthopedic force.

As Wieslander, Merrifield, Cross, and many clinicians have observed, the *direction* of extraoral force can and does affect the maxillary or palatal plane. In many cases it is counterproductive to tip the anterior end of the

*In Graber, T.M., and Swain, B.F., editors: Orthodontics: current principles and techniques, St. Louis, 1985, The C.V. Mosby Co., p. 424.

palatal plane down. Yet conventional Kloehn headgear procedures are likely to do that in any protracted therapy, as Stöckli shows (Fig. 11-44). With the facebow directed against the maxillary molars, the combined tipping of the anterior end of the maxillary arch and the posterior tipping and extrusion of the molars produce a rocking open of the mandible, moving the chin down and back. This may be quite acceptable in deep bite, forward rotating growth pattern but is contraindicated in vertical or downward and backward growing faces, as it increases the sagittal discrepancy and mandibular retrusion.

Hence an analysis of the initial pattern and probable growth direction is imperative before arbitrarily placing a cervical extraoral device, with or without the activator combination, in these unfavorable growth patterns. With excessive anterior face height, depression of posterior teeth and all possible efforts to stimulate upward and forward mandibular rotation are indicated. The direction of force should be essentially along the Y-axis, or above, or through the center of resistance of the maxilla. The desirable orthopedic effect on the maxilla would be the restriction of both horizontal and vertical growth increments. As Stöckli and Teuscher show in Fig. 11-45,

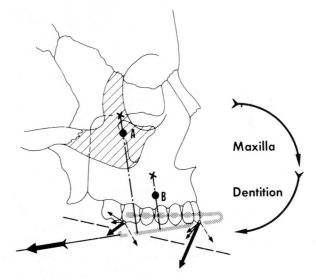

Fig. 11-44. If the teeth are banded and stabilized with an archwire in the maxillary arch, a cervical pull appliance (i.e., Kloehn type) will produce a force direction that is below both the center of resistance of the maxilla (A) and the center of resistance of the dentition (B). The distances of the force vector to A and B will determine the corresponding centers of rotation (x). Thin arrows indicate the reactive movement vectors of the dentition and maxilla at particular points. A posterior rotation of the maxilla and dentition must be expected from the analysis. As the heavier arrows show, the incisors will move down and back more than the molars. This will tip the occlusal plane down, as the interrupted line shows, which blocks open the mandible and moves the symphysis down and back. (Courtesy Paul Stöckli and Ullrich Teuscher.)

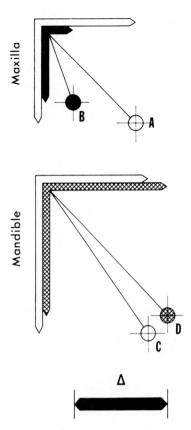

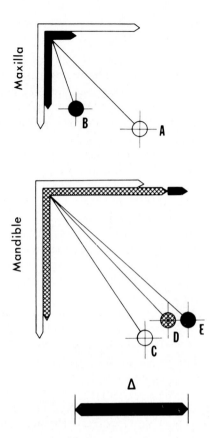

Fig. 11-45. A desirable orthopedic effect on the maxilla would be restriction of both horizontal and vertical growth increments, as recommended by Harvold. If successful, the maxillary position could effectively move from *A* to *B* in the facial profile. With a normal mandibular growth amount and direction *(C)*, reduced maxillary growth would allow favorable autorotation of the mandible to *D*, further reducing the sagittal malrelationship in Class II malocclusions. That such an effect is possible has been shown by Graber et al. (Droschl, Cederquist, Mills, and Holman). (From Stöckli, P.W., and Teuscher, U.M.: In Graber, T.M., and Swain, B.F., editors: Orthodontics: current principles and techniques, St. Louis, 1985, The C.V. Mosby Co.)

Fig. 11-46. As Stöckli and Teuscher show, if the improved sagittal relationship provided by proper horizontal and vertical extraoral orthopedic control (with favorable mandibular autorotation) is further enhanced by a forward-posturing mandibular appliance, condylar growth is optimized and the normal growth vector and amount as exemplified by *C* are changed to a more forward direction and amount by autorotation *(D)*. In addition, there is stimulation of condylar growth *(E)*. Such a reaction is particularly desirable in patients with excessive anterior face height and an unfavorable anterior to posterior height ratio. (From Stöckli, P.W., and Teuscher, U.M.: In Graber, T.M., and Swain, B.F., editors: Orthodontics: current principles and techniques, St. Louis, 1985, The C.V. Mosby Co.)

effective restraint of the maxillary growth and translation would permit a favorable autorotation of the mandible upward and forward, even if no effort was made to interfere with the normal mandibular growth pattern. This is directly counter to the Kloehn effect illustrated in Fig. 11-44. Furthermore, if the favorable autorotation of the mandible is further enhanced by forward posturing of the mandible and optimizing condylar growth increments and direction, the resultant profile improvement potential is even more favorable (Fig. 11-46).

It is not our intent to make Switzerland seem the center for combined activator-headgear therapy. Nevertheless, many of the most important advances in this technique have come from there, because a number of Swiss orthodontists had specialty training in both Switzerland and the United States. Although the emphasis is on removable appliances, to the exclusion of fixed ap-

pliances, in most of Europe, this was not the case at the Department of Orthodontics of the University of Zurich, under Rudolph Hotz, or now under Paul Stöckli. So it was easy for the concept of combined appliance therapy to develop.

Pfeiffer and Grobety combination therapy. Pfeiffer and Grobety* have also had great experience in this approach. They write,

Since 1967, we have combined the action of these two appliances (Activator and headgear), thinking that one would not be detrimental to the other. To our great surprise, we discovered that not only were their actions complementary but also their respective effects increased until they represented a highly efficient combination of therapies.

*In Graber, T.M., and Neumann, B.: Removable orthodontic appliances, ed. 2, Philadelphia, 1984, W.B. Saunders Co., p. 601.

Treatment goals. The treatment goals of Pfeiffer and Grobety mirror their expectations for the mixed dentition combination approach in Class II, Division I, malocclusions. The activator (1) prevents, intercepts, and, if necessary, corrects pernicious habits (thumb-sucking, lip-sucking, abnormal swallowing, mouth breathing); (2) acts as a space maintainer; (3) expands, if necessary; (4) starts to correct individual positions of teeth; (5) starts to correct the deep bite (within the freeway space limits); and (6) helps to correct the Class II relationship in three different ways: (a) prevents vicious habits, reorients physiologic forces, and thus allows for the normal growth of the mandible; (b) promotes, under the influence of the muscles of mandibular retraction, mesial movement of the lower teeth and distal movement of the upper teeth; and (c) possibly inhibits growth of the maxilla by means of the same muscles, which try to return to rest position. In their opinion, the activator does not incite activation of mandibular growth, since they feel that this is a genetically defined potential that cannot be quantitatively altered.

Recent and clinical research findings. This opinion could have been altered, at least in degree, since their last article appeared in 1975, in light of the overwhelming evidence from the Petrovic laboratory in histologic validation of condylar growth enhancement by the activator. Additional research by Elgoyhen, McNamara, Droschl, Cederquist, Graber, and others on nonhuman and human primates shows the potential of growth direction alteration as well as growth increment change. This important work (and still controversial material, if the work of Gianelly and associates is correct) is covered extensively in the first two chapters of this book (by Petrovic) as well as in the Rakosi chapters (3 to 9).

The concern of Pfeiffer and Grobety with mesial movement of the mandibular teeth as well as distal movement of the maxillary teeth calls attention to another controversial aspect of activator effect. One of the strongest criticisms of these appliances has been their tendency to slide the mandibular teeth forward on the basal bone and to procline the mandibular incisors, as Björk noted in 1952. This is in spite of various appliance modifications to prevent this from happening. Case selection is again a critical factor. Starting treatment on a patient with procumbent lower incisors is different from starting it on one with retroclined lower incisors. A discretionary decision is needed as to whether a functional appliance should be used and, if so, what steps should be taken to prevent further proclination. At best it is hoped that forward movement of the mandibular teeth is minimal in most cases and that the effect of the various construction bites in Class II malocclusions is to stimulate all possible forward mandibular growth, together with any changes in morphology that might assist

in the establishment of a normal sagittal maxillomandibular basal relationship. The restrictive effects of mandibular overclosure, functional retrusion, and excessive activity of retractor muscles of the mandible are now considered significant factors in preventing attainment of optimal growth of the lower jaw. The functional appliance intercepts the effects on the growth pattern, permitting a free expression of the morphogenetic blueprint.

Cervical extraoral effects when used with activator. Pfeiffer and Grobety list the probable effects of the cervical appliance that they use in combination with the activator as follows: it (1) slows down or interrupts growth of the maxilla; (2) initiates distal movement of the anchor molars and, to some extent, the adjacent teeth; (3) tips the anchor teeth either way if desired; (4) extrudes the molars, thereby opening the bite, but also rotating the mandible down and back; and (5) tips the anterior part of the palate down.

As mentioned previously, there is considerable question whether all these effects are desirable. Case selection and growth direction are conditioning factors. Distalizing maxillary molars may impact second and third molars later, as has been shown to be the case with Kloehn type therapy, where there is an increase in maxillary second molar cross-bite. Cephalometric studies indicate that the upper first molar position is essentially the same for Class I, II, and III malocclusions, meaning that the sagittal problem does not lie in the forward positioning of the molar itself, in most instances. The posttreatment stability and permanence of the result have been questioned in cases where molars are driven distally by extraoral forces directed against them primarily. Serial cephalometric studies demonstrate that this is largely a tipping and extrusive reaction, and the net result is a partial relapse, when appliances are removed, with the molars uprighting later by relapsing forward.

Many deep bite problems do need molar eruption to reduce the vertical deficiency, but buccal segment eruption is better served by withholding *maxillary* eruption and stimulating all possible *mandibular* buccal segment eruption. Harvold and Woodside have pointed out repeatedly that this differential eruption also has a favorable mesializing component, which reduces the sagittal discrepancy. Extruding maxillary molars tip the mandible down and back, increasing the anterior face height and facial convexity and the apical base difference. Stöckli and Teuscher (1985) note that as little as 1.0 mm extrusion of upper and lower molars can reduce the A-N-B angle 2.5 degrees and open the Y-axis a similar amount. The more the mandible is tipped down, the more procumbent the lower incisors are to the facial plane. This makes these teeth more susceptible to proclination by the activator itself (Fig. 11-11).

Despite these limitations, the evidence is clear that

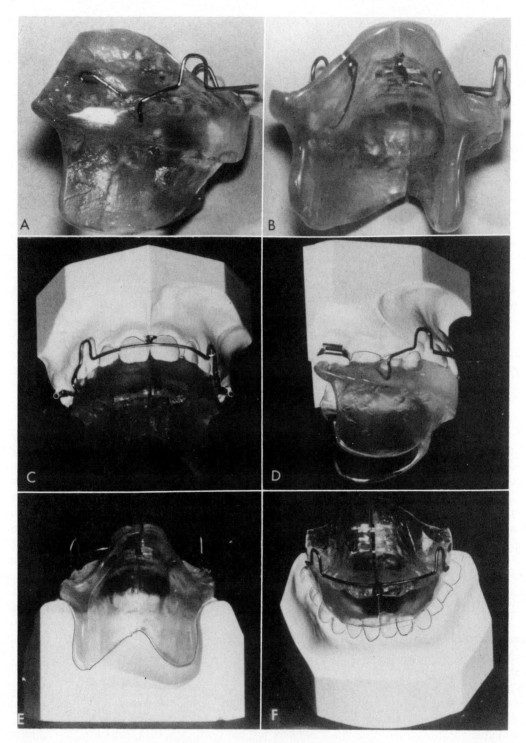

Fig. 11-47. Pfeiffer-Grobety combination technique, using a conventional Andresen-type activator, **A** and **B,** with cemented molar bands and buccal tubes for the extraoral facebow, **C** and **D,** and an orthopedic effect on the maxilla. The lingual flanges are extended as far into the floor of the mouth as possible to give maximum anchorage and a basal bone–guiding effect on the mandible, **E.** Lower incisors are usually capped with acrylic, as are the posterior teeth, to enhance appliance stability and maintenance of the protracted mandibular construction bite, **F.** A jackscrew is incorporated for any needed expansion. The spur on the labial bow serves to control the extraoral facebow position. The occlusal acrylic can be cut to allow differential eruption as indicated. There are no clasps; the appliance is loose and free-floating with this method, unlike the Stöckli-Teuscher approach. (From Pfeiffer, J.P., and Grobety, D.: Am. J. Orthod. **61:**353, 1972.)

significant improvement can be achieved in properly chosen cases, as Figs. 11-47 through 11-51 illustrate. Fig. 11-47 shows six different aspects of the Pfeiffer-Grobety activator. The method of assuring maximum retention and basal bone effect with long and rounded lingual flanges is shown in Fig. 11-48. By distributing the force over a larger basal bone area, the undesirable tooth-tipping effects are reduced. There is a wedging effect on the basal bone supporting the V-shaped buccal segment morphology, so that this area absorbs the pressure from the forward posturing. The proprioceptive feedback from the mucosal tissue transmits a clear message to keep the mandible forward and to reduce any unpleasant sensory responses. Note also the means used for insertion and control of the extraoral facebow with a spur on the labial bow of the activator. No clasps are used in the free-floating Pfeiffer-Grobety activator to retain the appliance on the maxilla, but the maxillary occlusal surfaces are covered with acrylic to prevent their eruption.

The before and after models of a treated severe Class II, Division 1, malocclusion are shown in Fig. 11-49, with the molar bands in place and the activator inserted between the models to show the amount of vertical opening. This follows the concepts of the Herren and Harvold-Woodside activators. With the relatively large sagittal discrepancy, some clinicians would prefer a smaller vertical opening for comfort and ease of patient acceptance; or the advancement might be done as Fränkel recomends in two stages. (See Chapter 14.) The dramatic dental and facial changes are testimony to a successful course of treatment (Figs. 11-49 and 11-50). Fig. 11-51 shows the before and after cephalometric tracings, with a significant reduction of the apical base dysplasia and excessive overbite and overjet and with restoration of normal profile contours.

Stöckli and Teuscher combination therapy. Stöckli and Teuscher recognize the problems of the long misused Kloehn cervical traction and the fact that different types of extraoral force can be used to depress maxillary molars, thus preventing undesirable tipping while still exerting a restrictive influence on the horizontal growth component of the maxilla. Both vertical and horizontal withholding are valid treatment objectives, as the Stöckli-Teuscher activator-headgear combination achieves the desired changes in three planes of space, without some of the disadvantages previously listed. A high-pull headgear can be used for depression but, better still, as they show, if the extraoral force is directed through the potential center of rotation of the maxilla then the maxilla will maintain its position, without tipping the palatal plane down and increasing the anterior face height, as the cervical extraoral appliance is more likely to do. It also will not tip the anterior end of the palatal plane up, which tends to enhance maxillary incisor protrusion and upper lip prominence (Figs. 11-52 to 11-54).*

Stockfisch, Hanson, and Hickham approaches. Stockfisch has been combining his Kinetor functional appliance for some time in a similar manner with the use of extraoral force, banding the maxillary first molars with 1.2 mm buccal tubes to receive the extraoral force facebow. The Kinetor is a skeletonized elastic activator that is easier for the patient to wear during daytime, which is considered desirable. He has incorporated an interocclusal elastic tube arrangement that stimulates functional activity in the construction bite position. He writes, "In about 60-70% of all anomalies, full multibanded therapy can be avoided by combination ther-

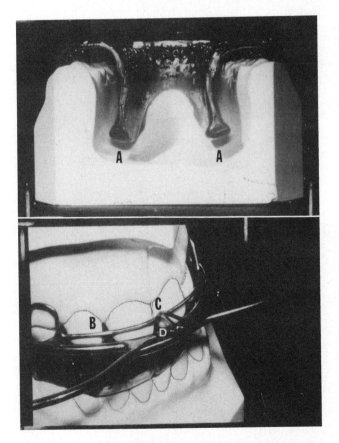

Fig. 11-48. The Pfeiffer-Grobety activator has an unusually long and rolled lower lingual periphery *(A)* to enhance the basal bone effect on the mandible. The labial bow *(B)* has a spur *(C)* to hold the facebow *(D)* and to prevent it from moving up or down and dislodging the activator. (From Pfeiffer, J.P., and Grobety, D.: Am. J. Orthod. **61:**353, 1972.)

*The reader is referred to a comprehensive and beautifully illustrated chapter by Stöckli and Teuscher on the combination activator and extraoral traction approach in Graber, T.M., and Swain, B.F., editors: Orthodontics: current principles and techniques, St. Louis, 1985, The C.V. Mosby Co.

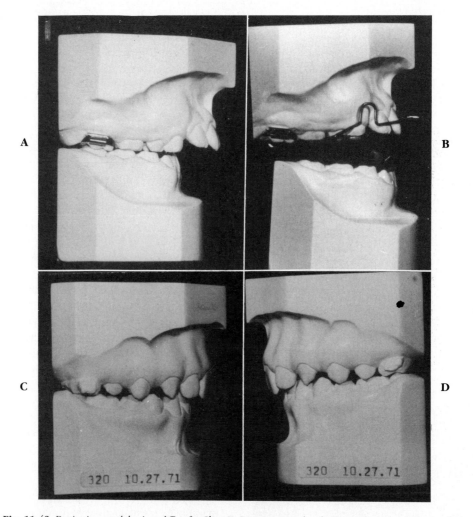

Fig. 11-49. Beginning models, **A** and **B,** of a Class II, Division 1, malocclusion with molar tubes in place and with activator inserted between the upper and lower models. Results after 30 months of treatment, **C** and **D.** Some detailing remains, i.e., space control, axial inclination of the upper incisors, etc. (From Pfeiffer, J.P., and Grobety, D.: Am. J. Orthod. **61:**353, 1972.)

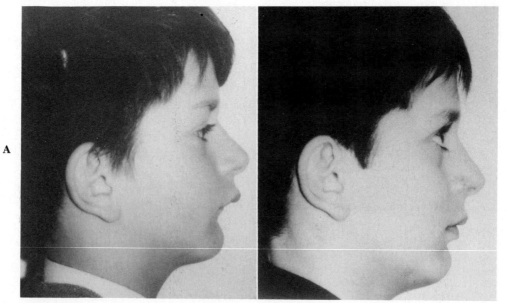

Fig. 11-50. A, Before and, **B,** after treatment. Note the dramatic facial change as a result of combined therapy. In this case cervical therapy was beneficial in that it elongated maxillary molars and tipped the palatal plane down and back, opening the bite in a vertically deficient malocclusion. (From Pfeiffer, J.P., and Grobety, D.: Am. J. Orthod. **61:**353, 1972.)

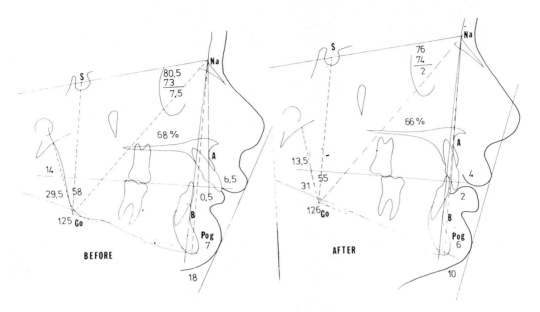

Fig. 11-51. Before and 30 months after removal of combination activator–extraoral force appliances for the patient in Figs. 11-49 and 11-50. There is a 5-degree decrease in the apical base difference and an improvement in the anterior facial height and the relationship of the incisors to the facial plane. The 1.5-degree increase in the mandibular plane inclination is tied to the use of cervical traction, which elongates the first molars as it tips them distally. The whole maxilla usually rotates downward and back with such a force vector. That the molars were moved distally is evident from the residual spacing present in the finished models in Fig. 11-49. (From Pfeiffer, J.P., and Grobety, D.: Am. J. Orthod. **61**:353, 1972.)

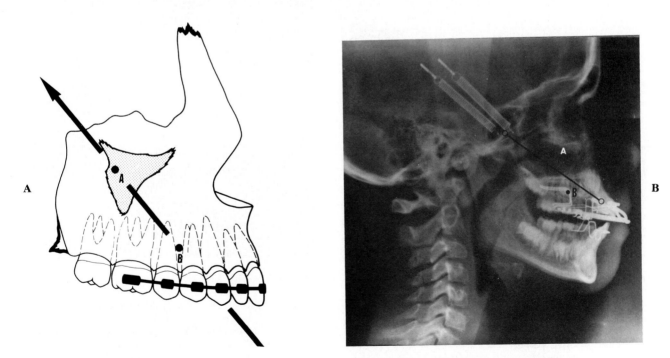

Fig. 11-52. A, Theoretically, to achieve maximum retractive and intrusive mechanics with extraoral force and to prevent the Kloehn effect of molar eruption and downward pull on the anterior end of the palatal plane, extraoral force should be directed as close as clinically feasible through both the center of rotation of the maxilla *(A)* and the center of rotation of the dentition *(B).* **B,** Activator-headgear combination in place. The direction of the occipital pull headgear is between both centers of rotation *(A* and *B).* This will produce a small amount of maxillary posterior rotation and somewhat more anterior offsetting dentitional rotation. From a practical point of view, however, these forces might well offset each other. (Courtesy Paul Stöckli and Ullrich Teuscher.)

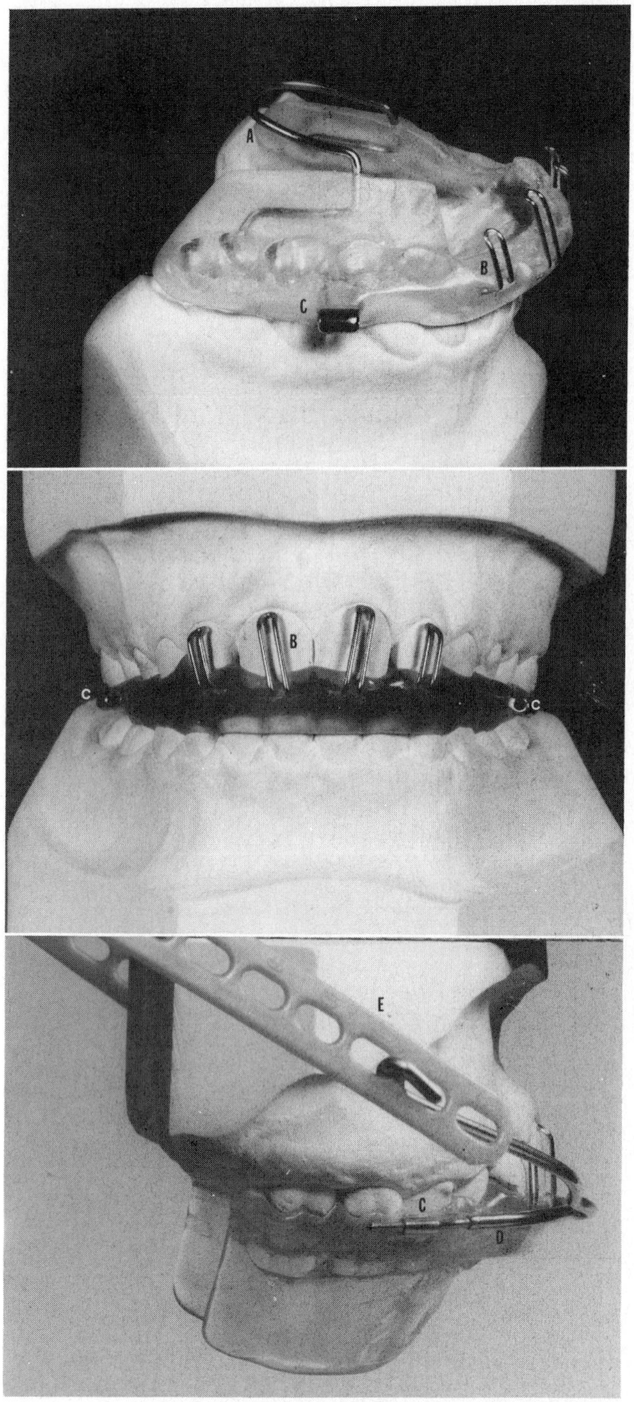

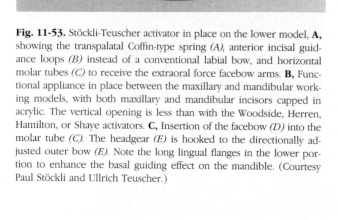

Fig. 11-53. Stöckli-Teuscher activator in place on the lower model, **A,** showing the transpalatal Coffin-type spring *(A),* anterior incisal guidance loops *(B)* instead of a conventional labial bow, and horizontal molar tubes *(C)* to receive the extraoral force facebow arms. **B,** Functional appliance in place between the maxillary and mandibular working models, with both maxillary and mandibular incisors capped in acrylic. The vertical opening is less than with the Woodside, Herren, Hamilton, or Shaye activators. **C,** Insertion of the facebow *(D)* into the molar tube *(C).* The headgear *(E)* is hooked to the directionally adjusted outer bow *(E).* Note the long lingual flanges in the lower portion to enhance the basal guiding effect on the mandible. (Courtesy Paul Stöckli and Ullrich Teuscher.)

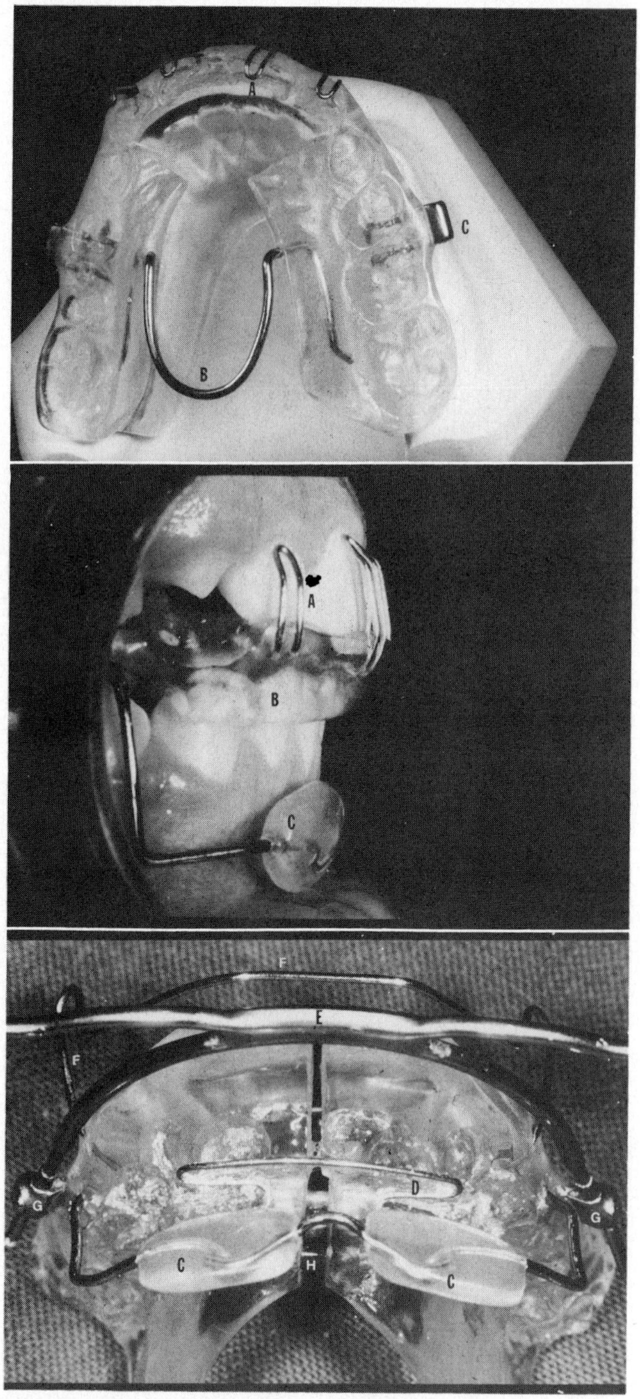

Fig. 11-54. The Stöckli-Teuscher functional appliance, **A,** is quite similar to those with an open palate used by Bionator clinicians. While the transpalatal loop *(B)* is often considered a tongue-control mechanism, it may also be used for expansion by splitting the appliance in the midline between the incisors. Various modifications are possible. Incisor guiding or torquing loops *(A)* can be activated or deactivated, and buccal tubes *(C)* may be incorporated in the interocclusal acrylic whether or not they need to be used. **B,** The acrylic capping *(B)* may be cut away to allow upper or lower incisors to be either proclined or retroclined. With a confirmed lip trap and excessive overjet, Fränkel lip pads *(C)* can be added to enhance establishment of normal perioral muscle function. **C,** Additional modifications besides the lip pads *(C).* A protrusion bow *(D)* may be added to assist in labial tipping of both upper and lower incisors, particularly in Class II, Division 2, malocclusions. The facebow *(E)* is already in place in the buccal tubes *(G).* Instead of labial guiding wires, a conventional labial bow *(F)* can be used, if desired. A jackscrew *(H)* is occasionally added for controlled expansion. (Courtesy Paul Stöckli and Ullrich Teuscher.)

apy—headgear and Kinetor."* Although further fixed attachment guidance is necessary, the first period of combination therapy during the mixed dentition usually reduces fixed appliance treatment time as much as 50%. Stockfisch utilized cemented first molar bands with double tubes for reception of extraoral force facebows and for any future fixed attachment treatment needed for individual tooth malposition correction. The clasp of the Kinetor snaps above the buccal tube assemblage, locking the functional appliance on the maxilla. This is entirely in agreement with Fränkel, who has stressed so often with his FR that it is absolutely essential to anchor the functional appliance on the maxilla to prevent free

*In Graber, T.M., and Neumann, B.: Removable orthodontic appliances, ed. 2, Philadelphia, 1984, W.B. Saunders Co., p. 605.

float, which will produce deleterious effects. The cemented molar bands, with their buccal horizontal tubes, do this very well in these combinations.

Ingrid Janson provides an illustration of her combined approach of functional appliances and extraoral force, following the further development of the Bionator by Ascher. She, too, resolves basal dysplasias and abnormal perioral muscle problems with such therapy in the mixed dentition and then turns to comprehensive fixed attachment edgewise therapy for finishing therapy in the permanent dentition (Figs. 11-55 and 11-56).

A similar combined activator–extraoral force approach to the correction of sagittal problems in mixed dentition Class II, Division 1, problems has been used by Jack Hickham, with consistent success. He also "indexes" or caps the lower incisors, making sure that the

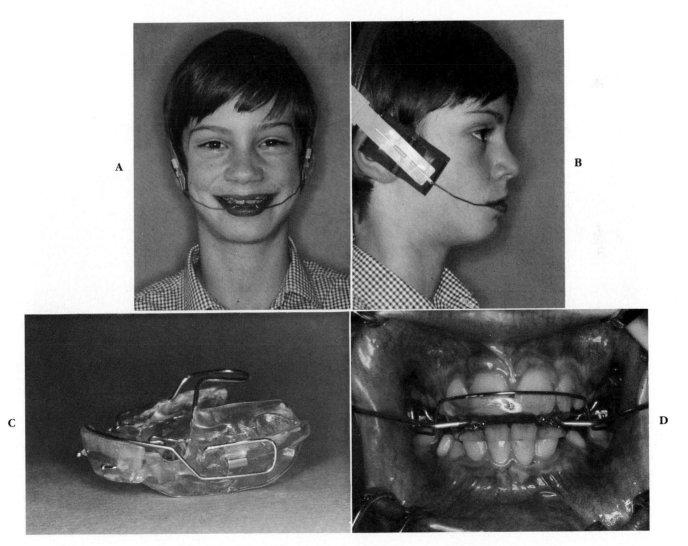

Fig. 11-55. Ingrid Janson has had much experience with the Bionator, as used by Ascher. In a retrospective study of the Bionator alone, she concluded that most of the sagittal change is due to dentoalveolar compensation. However, by incorporating circular loops anteriorly, in the capping acrylic, J hooks may be attached to a headcap to augment maxillary retraction, as the mandible is postured forward and the vertical dimension is opened by the Bionator, **A** to **D.**

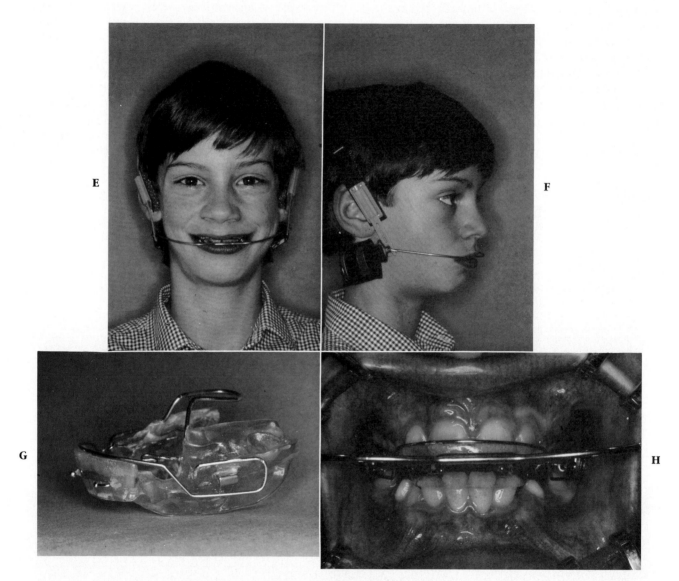

Fig. 11-55, cont'd. Horizontal molar tubes may also be embedded in the posterior interocclusal acrylic to receive the facebow ends, and either a regular oblique-pull headgear or a combination high-pull low-pull type can be used, **E** to **H,** to augment the restrictive effect on the maxillary complex. The operator may alternate anterior or posterior extraoral force attachment, as desired, if both anterior loops and posterior molar tubes are incorporated, **C** and **G.** (Courtesy Professor Ingrid Janson.)

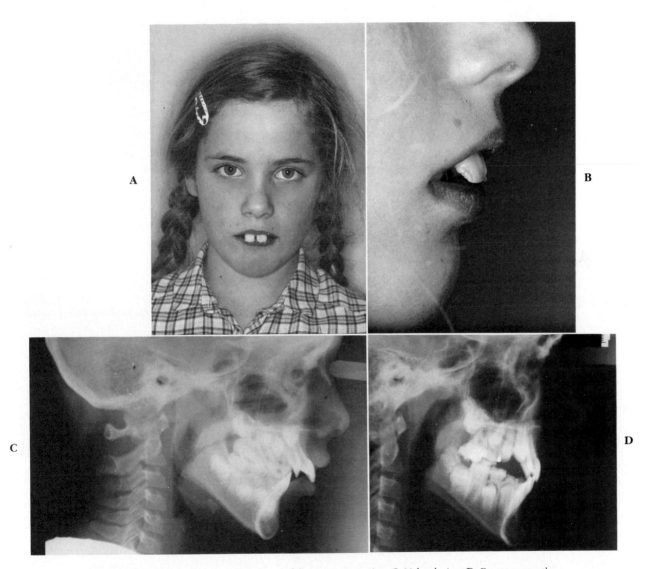

Fig. 11-56. Combined Bionator and extraoral force treatment. **A** to **C,** Malocclusion. **D,** Fourteen months later, after combined headgear is applied to the banded maxillary first molars, plus a Bionator as modified by Ascher.

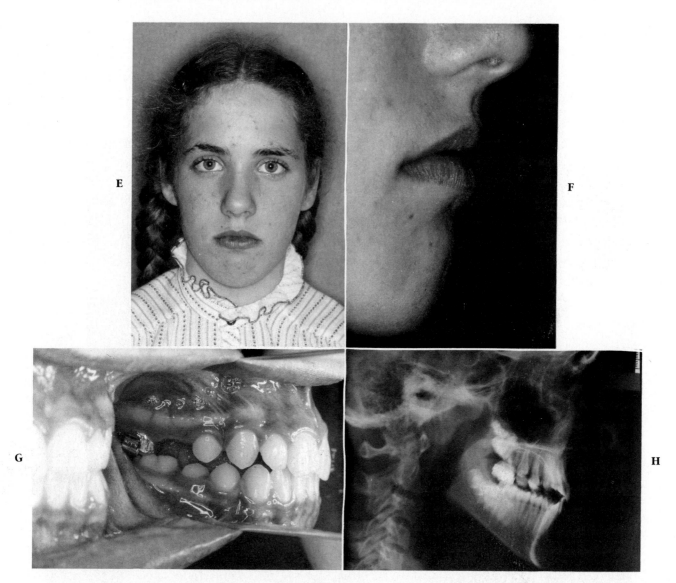

Fig. 11-56, cont'd. E to **G,** Twenty-two months later, in retention, awaiting eruption of the maxillary second premolars. **H,** Result achieved. Note the banded first molars, which help to hold the Bionator in as a retainer and which formerly received the extraoral facebow. (Courtesy Professor Ingrid Janson.)

labial capping of these teeth is extended gingivally enough to discourage all possible labial tipping by the forward posturing of the mandible. Instead of applying the extraoral force to cemented molar bands, he solders hooks to the labial wire of the activator to receive the extraoral force J-hook arms. The same upward and backward occipital direction recommended by Stöckli and Teuscher is used to control maxillary downward rotation. This still permits a restrictive effect on horizontal and vertical maxillary basal and dentoalveolar components. Selective grinding of the activator allows a bite plate effect, which frees the mandibular buccal segments for upward and forward corrective eruption while withholding the maxillary basal and dentoalveolar com-

plexes, or else exerts a slight distal force on them by virtue of the interproximal projections, which engage the mesiobuccal aspects of the maxillary buccal segment teeth.

Shaye–L.S.U. activator headgear combination

Robert Shaye has designed another variation of the activator-headgear combination based on the original Herren-type activator (Fig. 11-57). The modification is called the L.S.U. activator and does not use cemented molar bands for the extraoral force. Rather, small circular wire loops are embedded in the activator acrylic to allow hookup of the extraoral force J-hook arms. An

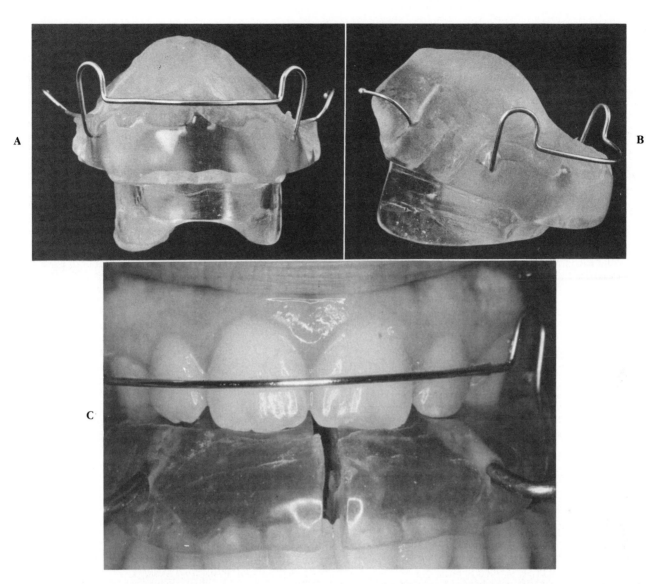

Fig. 11-57. A and **B,** The L.S.U. activator of Robert Shaye. This is a modification of the Herren activator, with clasps fitting mesial to the upper first molars and then curving distally on the buccal surface. The construction bite is taken in a wider open position to enlist the viscoelastic properties of the draping soft tissue. Lower lingual flanges are as long as possible to enhance the mandibular basal effect in the protraction maneuver. The labial bow is anchored in the interocclusal acrylic and is generally passive, after all spaces are closed. Lower incisors are capped in acrylic to reduce the proclination tendency. **C,** The Shaye L.S.U. activator has been modified to receive a jackscrew for needed expansion. The lower incisors are capped in acrylic. Also parallel holes have been cut in the interocclusal acrylic to receive the extraoral force J arms for the high-pull headgear orthopedic force application. The ends of the J hooks are inserted each night and removed in the morning. The combination appliance is worn generally only at night, plus 1 or 2 hours a day. (Courtesy Robert Shaye.)

alternate method is to cut small tunnels in the interdental acrylic and insert the ends of the arms into the activator directly. Shaye also caps the labial of the lower incisors to reduce the tendency toward procumbency. The wider open construction bite espoused by Herren, Harvold, Hamilton, and Woodside is used by Shaye to reduce the tendency for the appliance to deactivate during sleep.

A further modification has been developed by Shaye and Prositioner Laboratories, called the "Reactivator" (Fig. 11-58). An anterior jackscrew is incorporated in the acrylic to permit gradual advancement of the lower jaw in stages, instead of only one 6 to 7 mm of forward posturing, as done by conventional activator techniques. This is in line with Petrovic's research showing a more favorable and continuing tissue response to the new

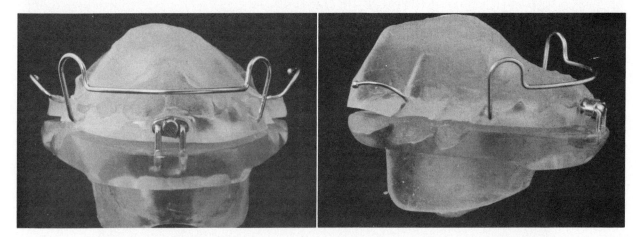

Fig. 11-58. The Shaye L.S.U. Reactivator, a modified Schwarz double-plate. Its purpose is to allow staged advancement of the lower portion of the horizontally split appliance (by adjustment of the specially designed anterior advancement screw). When the final advancement is achieved (usually after 6 to 9 months), self-curing acrylic is added between the two halves to join and stabilize the appliance. Note again that the appliance is locked on the maxilla with the interproximal molar clasps mesial to the permanent first molars. Regular buccal tubes may be embedded in the interincisal acrylic to receive the J hooks from the extraoral appliance, or channels may be cut into the acrylic if maxillary retraction is indicated as well as mandibular protraction. (Courtesy Robert Shaye.)

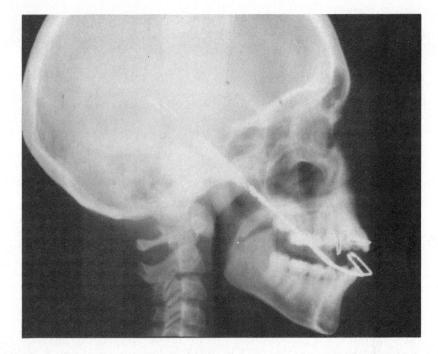

Fig. 11-59. Combination L.S.U. activator and high-pull headgear in place. Note the amount of vertical opening of the appliance and the direction of pull of the extraoral force in an attempt to achieve the most favorable retrusive and intrusive mechanics on the maxillary dentition. (Courtesy Robert Shaye.)

stimuli. As discussed in the first chapters (by Petrovic), this is more desirable from a cybernetic approach as well. Histologic studies of the condylar response show improvement in the incremental and directional reaction to reactivating procedures. Fränkel has also stressed the superiority of this approach with his FR appliance. Fig. 11-59 is a lateral cephalogram showing the extraoral appliance in place with the activator. Note the direction

of pull of the extraoral force and also the amount of vertical opening for the activator.

To illustrate the L.S.U. activator, the following case took only 3 months to "jump the bite," as Kingsley called it 100 years ago.

Fig. 11-60 shows beginning Class II, Division 1, malocclusion intraoral views. After only 1 year of combined treatment, activation was discontinued and the case was

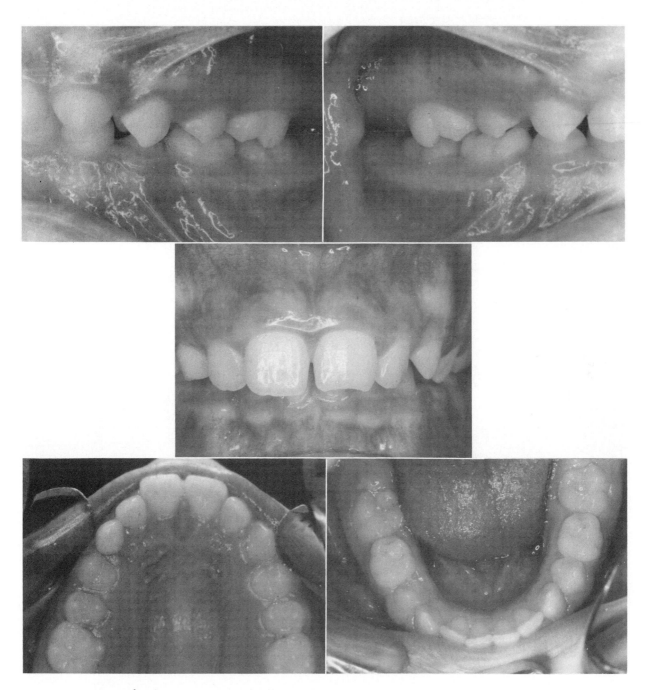

Fig. 11-60. Class II, Division 1, malocclusion in an 11-year-old boy. Significant in this case is the fact that the "jumping of the bite" took only 3 months, with the combined activator-headgear appliance worn only at night. (Courtesy Robert Shaye.)

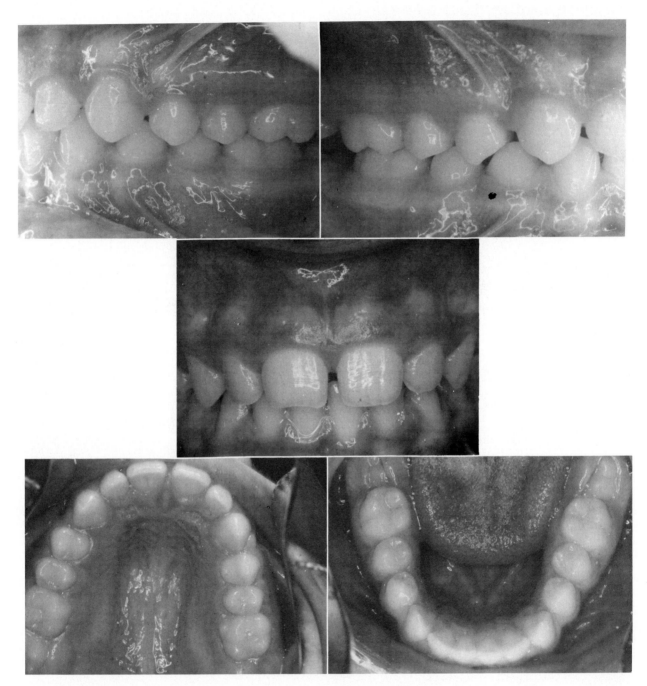

Fig. 11-61. Seven months after appliance placement. The activator was worn every second night as an active retainer to allow settling in of the occlusion. (Courtesy Robert Shaye.)

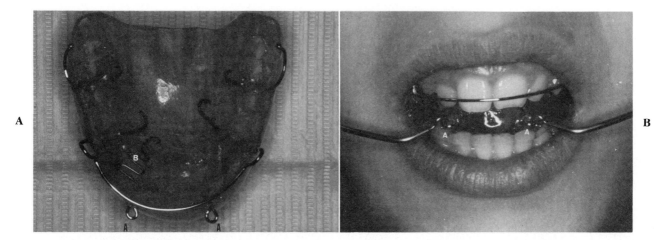

Fig. 11-62. A, Anterior hook-eyes, instead of channels in acrylic, to receive extraoral force J hooks or arms, which can be inserted from above or below. **B,** A small fingerspring has been added to move the upper right lateral incisor labially. (Courtesy Robert Shaye.)

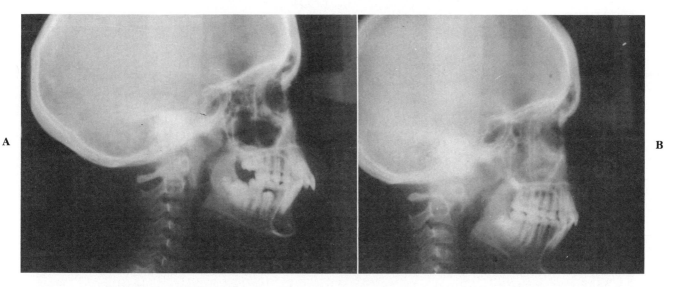

Fig. 11-63. Before, **A,** and after, **B,** treatment of the patient in Figs. 11-60 to 11-62. No lower incisor procumbency or rocking open of the bite has occurred. Normal muscle function has been restored. (Courtesy Robert Shaye.)

retained. Fig. 11-61 shows the results after 7 months of retention, with the activator being worn as a retainer every other night. Extraoral force was actually terminated after 5 months. The high-pull headgear is shown in Fig. 11-62. Cephalograms before and after treatment show the sagittal change (Fig. 11-63).

In a two-phase treatment case that exemplifies the most frequent approach, a 9-year-old girl with a Class II, Division 1, malocclusion with the usual sequelae of ex-

cessive overjet, abnormal perioral muscle function, plus evidence of marked bruxism is shown in Figs. 11-64 and 11-65.

After only 11 months of combined therapy, with the L.S.U. activator and high-pull extraoral traction to buccal tubes on cemented first molar bands, the sagittal malrelationship was largely corrected, abnormal perioral muscle function eliminated, and interdigitation of the posterior teeth improved. Double buccal tubes were

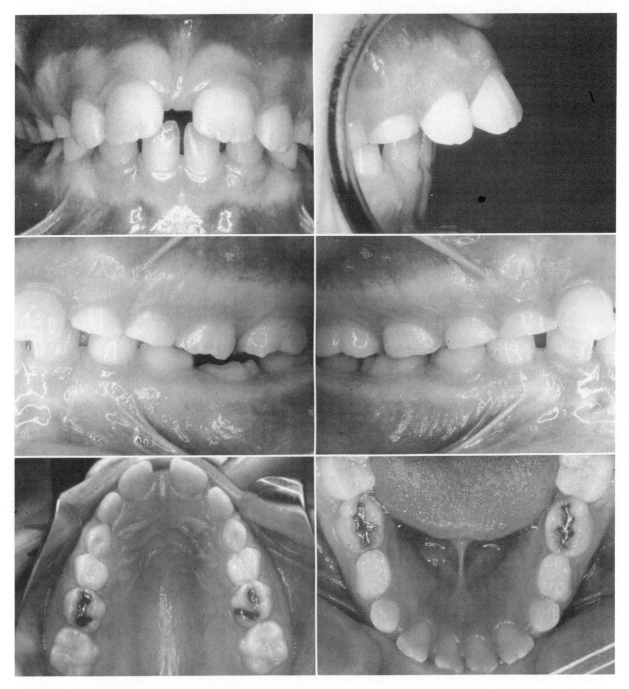

Fig. 11-64. Class II, Division 1, malocclusion in a 9-year-old girl, to be treated with a two-phase approach. First molar bands were cemented for the application of extraoral force via a facebow and high-pull headgear. (Courtesy Robert Shaye.)

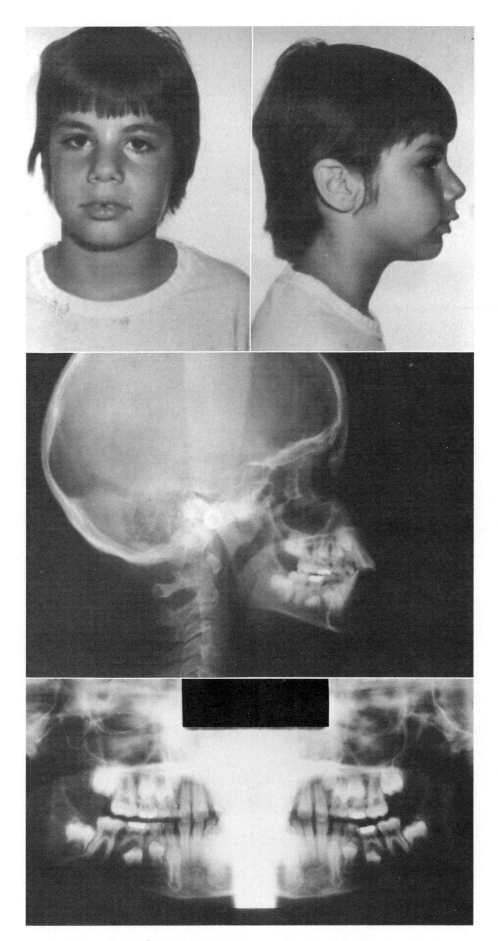

Fig. 11-65. Initial views of this patient. (Courtesy Robert Shaye.)

used, and the bands remained on for the second phase of treatment while serving to retain the activator and the result thus far achieved (Fig. 11-66). The facial and cephalometric changes after only 11 months of combination first-phase therapy are dramatic (Fig. 11-67). The final phase was started after eruption of the permanent canines and premolars and took only 14 months. The intraoral, facial, cephalometric, and panoral radiographic changes are shown in Figs. 11-68 and 11-69, 3.2 years after the end of the second phase of combination therapy.

Hamilton expansion-activator system

David Hamilton combines both the ease of daytime wear of the maxillary splint, with a jackscrew for any needed expansion, with the sagittal correction potential of a modified activator. Although the expansion activator has a jackscrew for transverse correction, the daytime-wear holding plate may augment this as needed. The occlusion is unlocked during the day by the holding appliance, permitting favorable muscle activity that has been initiated by activator wear during the night. Pe-

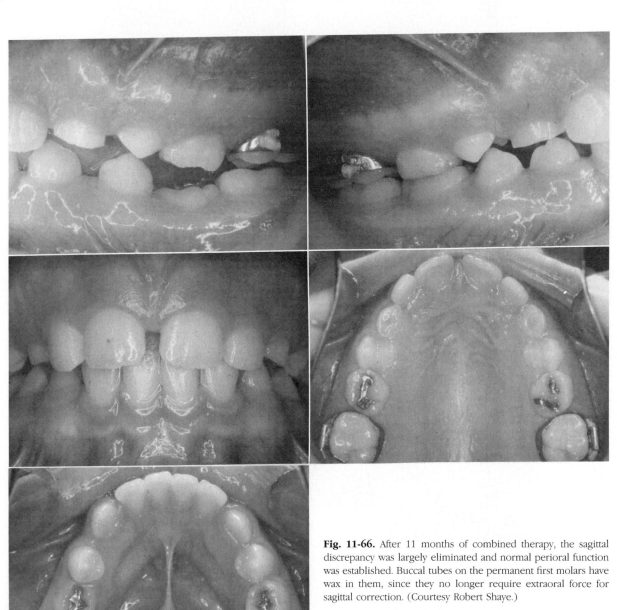

Fig. 11-66. After 11 months of combined therapy, the sagittal discrepancy was largely eliminated and normal perioral function was established. Buccal tubes on the permanent first molars have wax in them, since they no longer require extraoral force for sagittal correction. (Courtesy Robert Shaye.)

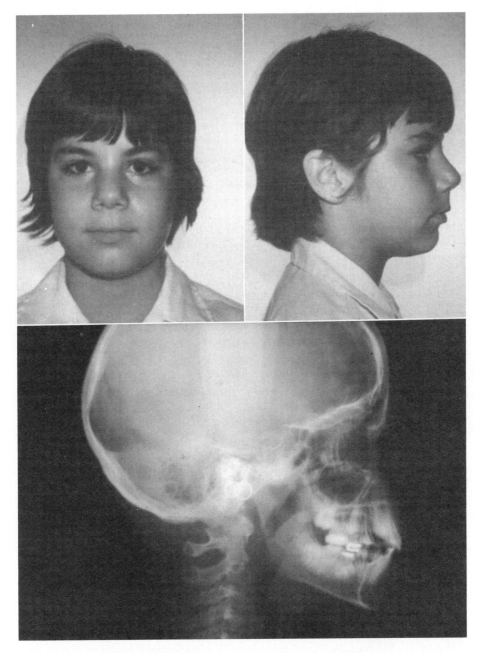

Fig. 11-67. After 11 months of combination therapy. There is significant improvement in the facial balance. Compare with Fig. 11-65. (Courtesy Robert Shaye.)

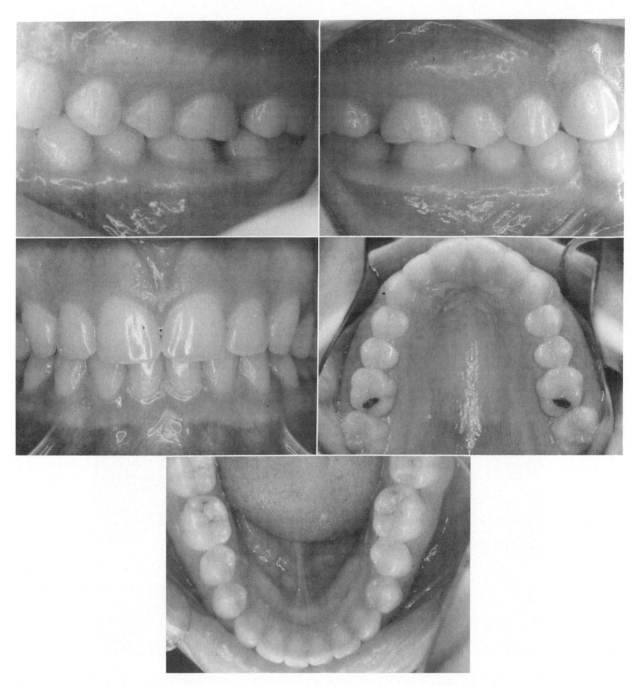

Fig. 11-68. Three years, 2 months, after the end of the second phase of therapy. The final phase of fixed attachment edgewise therapy took 14 months. Compare with Fig. 11-64. (Courtesy Robert Shaye.)

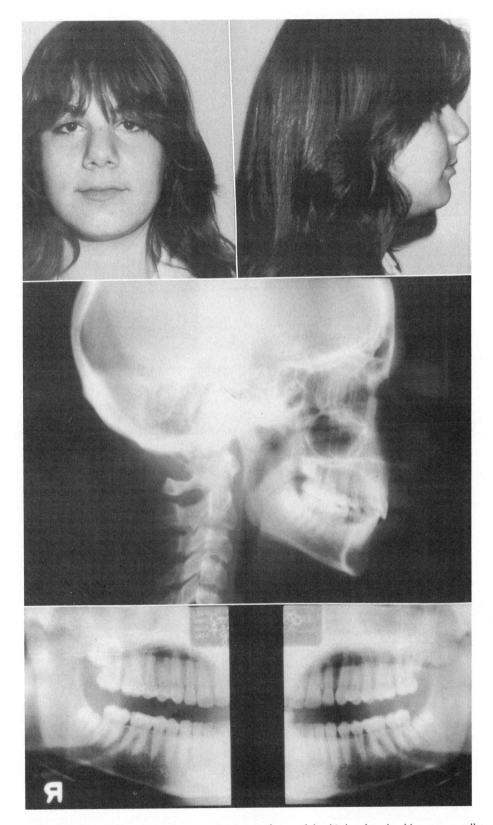

Fig. 11-69. Views of this patient. The correction is complete, and the third molars should erupt normally later on. Compare with Figs. 11-65 and 11-67 for changes effected by the combination fixed-removable treatment. As with most of these cases, there is seldom any iatrogenic response and root resorption is almost never encountered. (Courtesy Robert Shaye.)

trovic has shown (Chapter 2) that nighttime activators continue to have favorable functional effects during the day, even when they are not worn, and that it is the level of functional activity that increases the favorable response at the cellular level. This is similar to the approach of Joachim Tränkmann, who also uses a modified Andresen activator at night with the expansion plate being worn during the day (Figs. 11-36 to 11-43).

The Hamilton appliances are shown in Fig. 11-70. Note the double jackscrews in the holding plate and its innocuous appearance in the mouth during the day. Fig. 11-71 shows various views of the expansion activator, including one with buccal tubes incorporated into the acrylic for application of extraoral force. Note that the upper and lower incisors are capped with acrylic to enhance resistance to proclination and tipping. This is in-

stead of the conventional labial bow. Hamilton makes a concerted effort to anchor the activator on the maxilla, rather than having it float freely, following the logic of Fränkel and others, who maintain that this produces better results during the night when the patient is asleep and the mouth is more likely to drop open. For this reason Hamilton also uses a larger vertical opening in the construction bite.

The expansion activator is illustrated in a patient's mouth in Fig. 11-72. The acrylic capping and wide open construction bite are seen here. Figs. 11-73 to 11-75 show the successful treatment of a severe Class II, Division 1, malocclusion using the Hamilton expansion-activator system. The cephalograms show that the result was achieved without the unfavorable sequelae seen so often with the inept use of functional appliances alone.

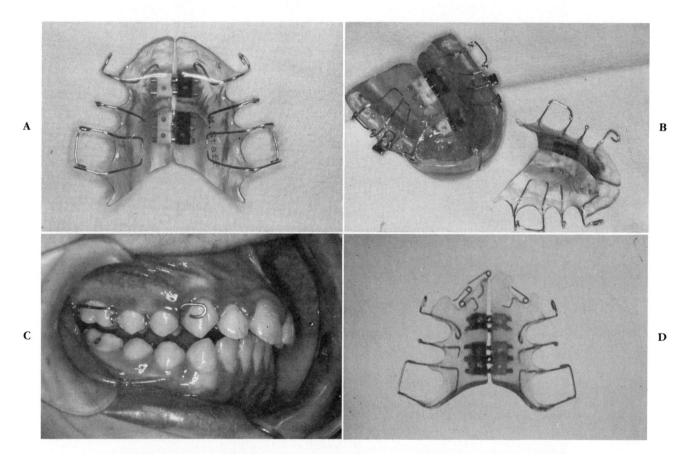

Fig. 11-70. Hamilton expansion activator system. **A,** Daytime holding appliance with twin expansion screws. **B,** Expansion activator for nighttime wear plus a holding appliance for daytime use. Note the horizontal buccal tubes soldered on the molar clasps of the activator to receive the headgear facebow, if needed. Both upper and lower incisor segments are capped by acrylic to minimize any tipping action from the construction-bite forward posturing of the mandible. To help maintain the appliance in place during sleep, and to enlist the viscoelastic properties of the contiguous soft tissues, the vertical opening of the construction bite exceeds the normal interocclusal clearance. **C,** Holding daytime expansion plate in place. **D,** Holding plate with additional fingersprings added for individual tooth movements. Activation is kept to a minimum, however, so as not to dislodge the appliance. (Courtesy David C. Hamilton.)

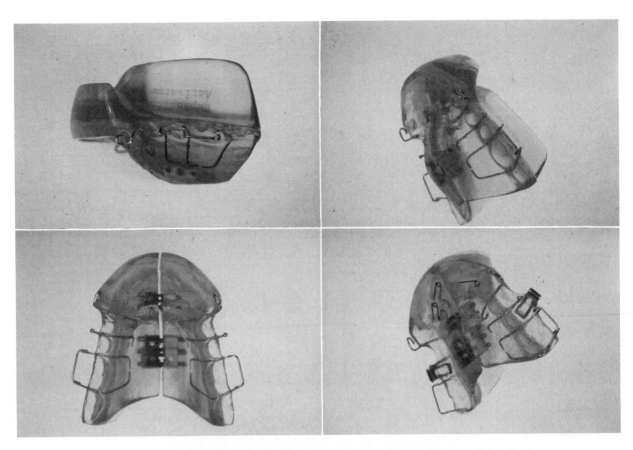

Fig. 11-71. Hamilton activator fingersprings and buccal tubes are added for the extraoral force facebow, if needed. (Courtesy David C. Hamilton.)

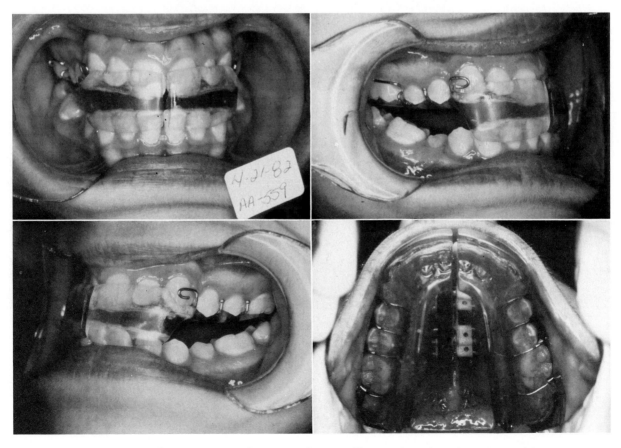

Fig. 11-72. Hamilton activator. Note the capping of upper and lower incisors, the canine springs, and the fit of the appliance on the maxillary arch. (Courtesy David C. Hamilton.)

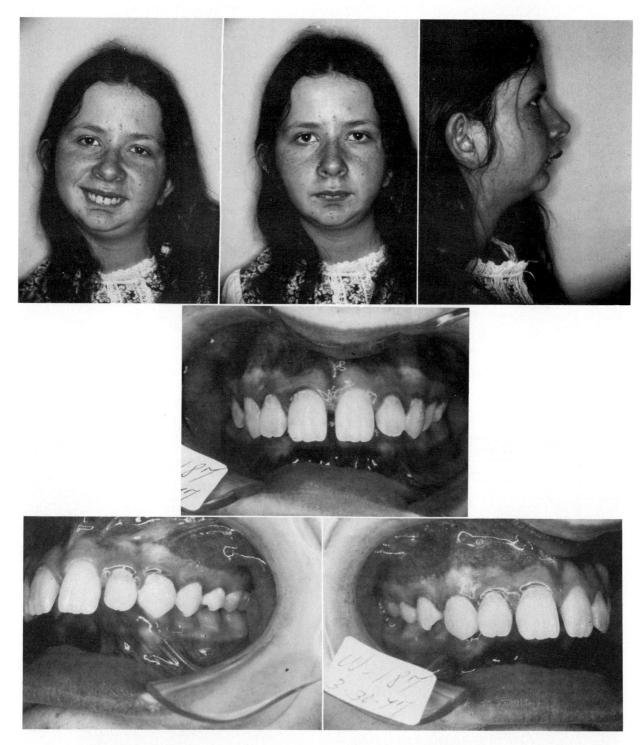

Fig. 11-73. Class II, Division 1, malocclusion treated with the Hamilton expansion activator system. Note the severity of the sagittal and vertical discrepancy and the neuromuscular involvement. (Courtesy David C. Hamilton.)

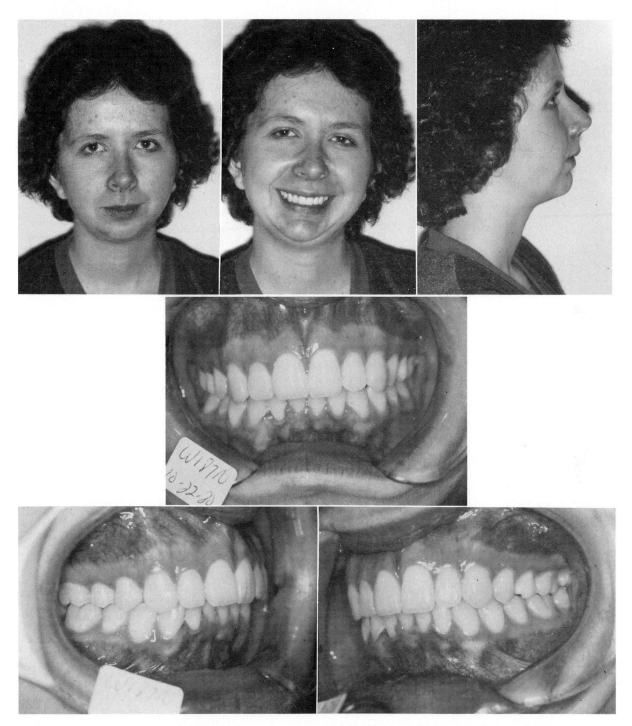

Fig. 11-74. Same patient, treated with the Hamilton expansion activator system. Note the dramatic facial improvement and the sagittal and vertical corrections over the 2-year period. No extraoral force or fixed appliances were used in this case. (Courtesy David C. Hamilton.)

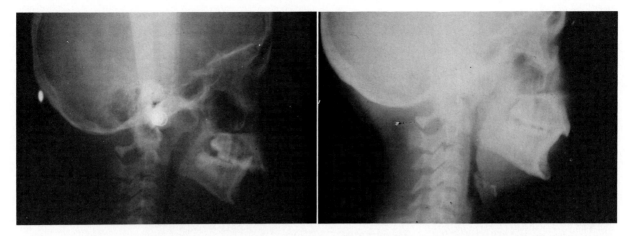

Fig. 11-75. Same patient as in Figs. 11-73 and 11-74. A major correction has been achieved without deleterious proclination of the lower incisors or excessive uprighting of the maxillary incisors. (Courtesy David C. Hamilton.)

Need for final phase fixed appliances. Despite the successful reduction of the apical base dysplasia and the elimination of neuromuscular abnormalities, a final period of fixed appliances is usually needed to achieve the high level of detailing and individualized tooth movement that we have come to expect from American orthodontics. This is not to say that fingersprings and other appurtenances cannot correct some of the individual tooth irregularities; but it is easier, more rapid, and better with a short period of fixed multiattachment mechanics. Such a case that illustrates the potential of this combination therapy well is shown in Fig. 11-76. The patient had a narrow arch, rotations, marked crowding, and excessive overjet and overbite. Treatment was initiated with the expansion-activator approach, as the intraoral views show, with the daytime expansion holding appliance and activator in place for nighttime wear. Facial and dental changes after 15 months of expansion-activator therapy are shown in Fig. 11-77.

Posterior open bite and canine malposition problems. A temporary posterior open bite is frequently seen in functional appliance treatment and is due to the relatively slower eruption of teeth, as compared to the sagittal change (shown in Figs. 11-6 and 11-7). Canine malposition after functional appliance treatment is also a frequent consequence and indicates the need for fixed appliances for final detailing. The patient in Fig. 11-77 is now ready for comprehensive therapy, and Fig. 11-78 shows the appliances in place and achieving the desired tooth positional changes. The facial and dental changes produced by the combination therapy are seen in Fig. 11-79. Total treatment time was 29 months.

Low iatrogenic potential. More important in these cases is the fact that tissue health is excellent, with no evidence of root resorption that might occur from pro-

tracted fixed appliance use. Each element of the appliance is used with the objective it can accomplish best—the expansion-activator system for sagittal, vertical, and transverse changes; the fixed appliances for individual tooth movement. If an extraoral appliance is needed, it can be attached to the activator directly or can be directed against cemented maxillary first molar bands, as illustrated in Figs. 11-62 to 11-66 with Shaye's L.S.U. activator.

Miscellaneous combination appliances

One of the constant problems with any removable appliance is patient compliance; and when extraoral force arms, a headcap, etc. are added to a bulky acrylic activator, patient cooperation is even more of a concern. For this reason, skeletonized activators are used by many clinicians. A favorite appliance is the Bionator, which does not have palatal acrylic coverage and can be worn during the day. Care must be exercised in the utilization of extraoral force so as not to dislodge the appliance. Fixed molar bands are more positive, but the direction of force then becomes a factor, as Stöckli has stressed. Undesirable molar tipping and extrusion, unwanted tipping of the anterior end of the palatal plane, rotation of the mandible down and back to increase a vertical growth direction vector, and equally undesirable labial tipping of lower incisors and lingual tipping of upper incisors should be considered in any design modification. All sorts of variations are possible, such as no use of acrylic capping of the lower incisors if they are lingually inclined; labial capping if resistance to forward incisor tipping is desired; or use of a lower labial bow instead of acrylic capping or maxillary acrylic occlusal cover or spurs and rests, etc. Different horizontal and vertical construction bite registrations are possible, depending on the original malocclusion, the prefer-

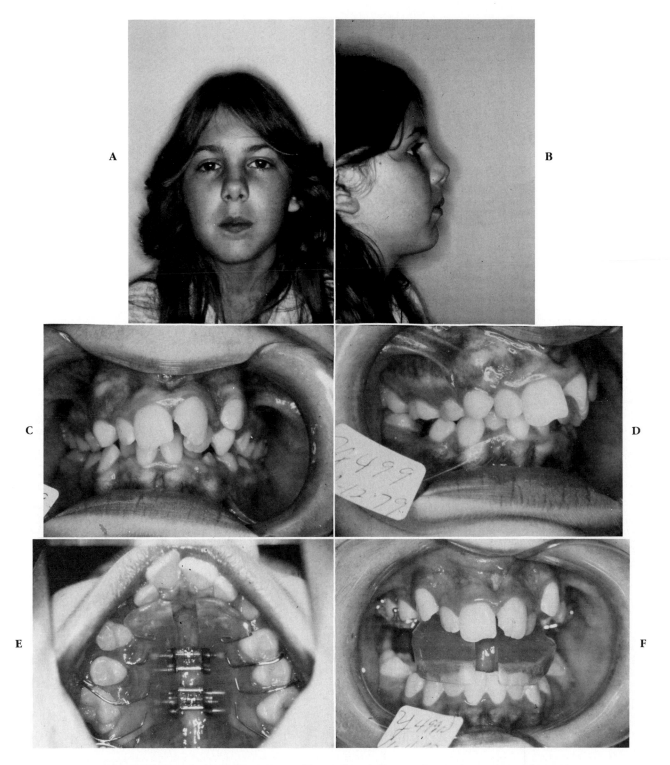

Fig. 11-76. A to **D,** Markedly narrow maxillary arch, crowding, rotations, and excessive overbite and overjet. The patient is to be treated with the Hamilton expansion activator system plus full multiattachment edgewise appliances for the final detailing. The palatal expansion active plate, **E,** is worn during the daytime. The expansion activator, **F,** is in place at night. Note the extent of vertical opening for the construction bite. When there is less forward posturing, the vertical opening can be increased for more effective action. (Courtesy David C. Hamilton.)

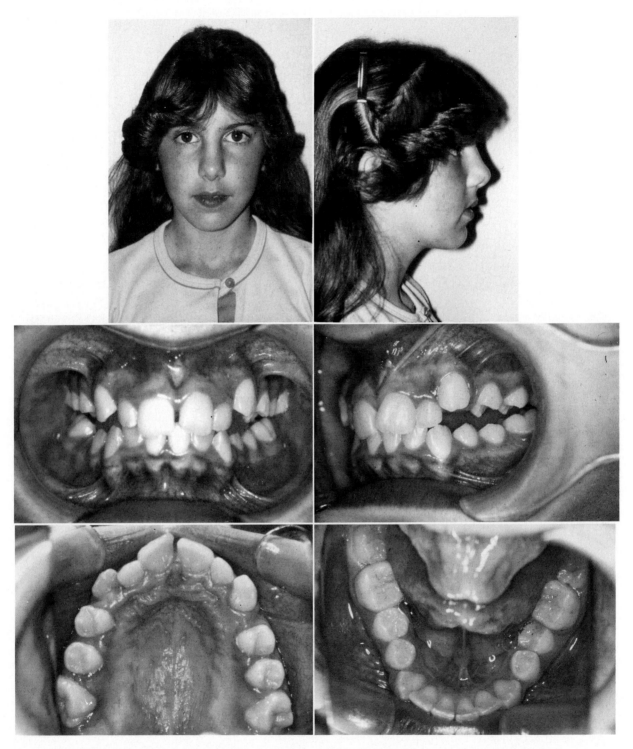

Fig. 11-77. After 15 months of expansion activator treatment, same patient as in Fig. 11-76. A temporary posterior open bite is the usual consequence of functional appliance treatment and, because of the smaller increments of change that normally occur from dentitional eruption (as shown in Figs. 11-6 and 11-7), requires a longer time to correct. Canine malposition after functional appliance therapy is one of the most frequent residual malocclusion characteristics. The patient is now ready for fixed multiattachment appliances. (Courtesy David C. Hamilton.)

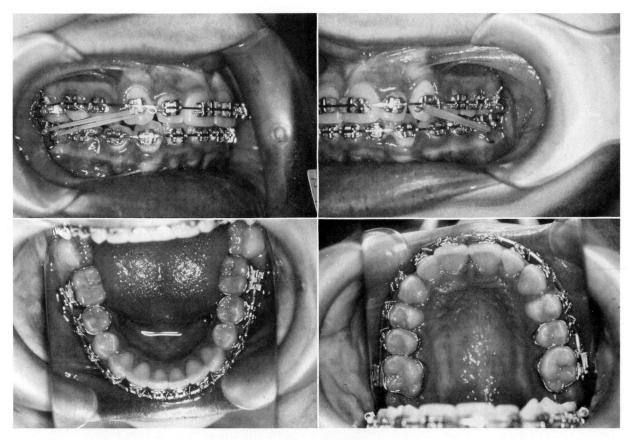

Fig. 11-78. Multiattachment fixed appliances in place, same patient, completing the detailing and settling of the occlusion. Time of fixed appliance wear, 14 months. (Courtesy David C. Hamilton.)

ences of the operator, and the tolerance of the patient. Research by the Petrovic team, reported in the first two chapters of this book, shows that it is better to wear some activators full time and others part-time for optimal tissue response. This section should be read carefully by the clinician who is about to introduce a series of modifications.

POSTSCRIPT

In line with our stated principle of KISS (Keep it simple, sir!), a number of appliances and modifications have been presented to correct sagittal, vertical, and tranverse malocclusion problems. They are consistent with current research in the biomechanical field and depend heavily on careful qualitative and quantitative histochemical studies by Reitan (1984), Rygh (1977), Petrovic and Stutzmann (1972), Petrovic et al. (1982), McNamara (1981), Moyers (1981), Graber (1983), and others on both experimental animals and humans as well as on clinical research by Ahlgren (1979), Bimler (1965), Fränkel, Schmuth (1983), Rakosi (1982), Sander (1983), Stöckli and Teuscher (1982), McNamara, Moss (1981), Shaye (1983), Hamilton (1983), Graber (1984), Björk

(1983), Woodside (1983), and others already quoted in the literature. It is emphasized that the therapy described is not the only approach to achieving similar treatment objectives. It may be simpler, but it most certainly does *not* require less diagnostic study and acumen. Proper case selection is imperative for optimal success with this mechanotherapy as well as any other. Nothing is automatic.

Criteria for case selection are covered in other sections of this book, particularly in Chapters 4 and 5 and 12 to 15; and as is pointed out there, diagnosis is a continuing process, with the patient coming in for routine adjustment and treatment assessment. Growth and development, like "ham and eggs," sounds good, but paying lip service to this developmental phenomenon is not enough. A thorough knowledge of the principles of growth and development is essential before therapy is instituted. A proper means of assessing the actual growth process during treatment is essential. Although it may seem illogical to the untrained neophyte because appliance fabrication and treatment mechanics seem simpler, the best qualified operators for removable appliances are the orthodontic specialists who have the

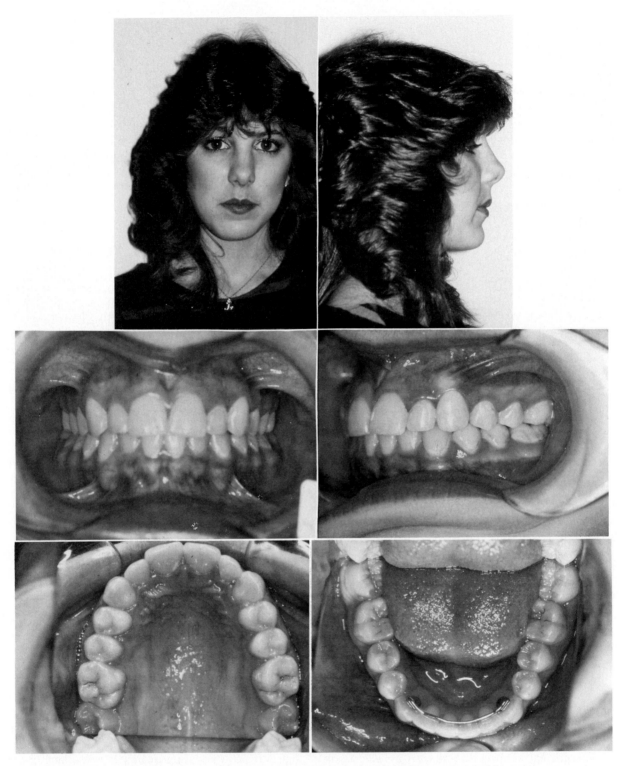

Fig. 11-79. Facial and dental changes effected by combined expansion activator treatment of this patient. Total treatment time, 29 months. Compare with Fig. 11-77. (Courtesy David C. Hamilton.)

sufficient training, experience, and background to know which cases to select, what to do when, how to assess the treatment results, and *when to change direction or appliances.*

No treatment cookbook available

Years of teaching have made me (T.M.G.) aware of the keen desire for a step-by-step set of instructions for therapy. With estimates running from 8 to 64 for the various types of Class II malocclusions and with a multiplicity of factors contributing to the dentofacial morphology at any one time, it does a disservice to the profession and insults the intelligence of our members to describe a neat little package which will permit treatment by the numbers, as if assembling a do-it-yourself kit. It is this constant desire to fit all patients into one treatment mode that has led to the cultism and dogma that permeated orthodontics for the past 50 years. Joseph Johnston exuded supreme confidence as he said of twin-wire, "Don't worry, it is automatic. Put it on and the wires do the rest." The Begg man fitted all his patients into the same mechanical straitjacket, and the Bull man used his own particular bear trap. All three systems were tossed into the historical wastebasket by straight-wire disciples, who disdained any removable appliances because of lack of torque, tip, or in-and-out adjustment potential. Surely we are far enough advanced now to recognize that optimum therapy in regards to tooth alignment, jaw relationship, neuromuscular balance, tissue tolerance, patient compliance, treatment time, and ease of manipulation is not possible with one set of brackets and archwires, no matter how well machined they are or how fantastic the wire memory is. Different approaches and different appliances are needed for different types of malocclusions; and it is abundantly clear now that several appliances for the same patient, at different times in the dental development, may be the best answer. Furthermore, even the best clinician may have to change horses in midstream as one appliance approach has worked (or not worked) for its share of the correction challenge. This cannot always be predicted. Diagnosis is the name of the game—continuing diagnosis at each patient visit. The orthodontist's bag of tricks should include alternate choices all along the way. Combination activator-headgear therapy may look deceptively simple to the neophyte or nonspecialist who is lulled into a sense of false security by traveling salesmen clinicians and orthodontic supply representatives. The appliances *are* simple, and so is their misuse without proper diagnostic assessment at each visit. However, treatment planning is not likely to be so simple.

I would like to end this chapter with a paragraph addressed to this issue from the second edition of *Removable Orthodontic Appliances.**

It is hoped that those who embark on the use of these fixed-removable combinations will have the ethical, moral and professional concerns so that the patient is always served best. Providing less than optimal orthodontic guidance for a child simply because the dentist does not have the skill and training for the job violates the oath of Hippocrates. In addition, weasel-wording and rationalizing about lesser fees and the supposed inability of orthodontic specialists to take care of all the patients will not make the situation any better. The proliferation of orthodontics of all types being done by ill-trained pedodontists and general practitioners whose level of "business" has dropped in other areas is no coincidence. Peer review in this area of dental practice is practically non-existent. Orthodontic consultation from specialists is always available in most cities, but few dentists emulate their medical confreres and seek it out. Only in those instances in which orthodontic specialty guidance or consultation is unavailable, as in many small towns or rural areas, might the dentist feel justified to take on this kind of treatment, even though it is likely to be of a lesser caliber than could be provided by a trained orthodontic specialist. For here, the alternative for the patient is nothing at all. Such a responsibility should not be taken lightly because of the iatrogenic potential of some orthodontic therapy. And we need not wait for the pressures applied by consumer advocacy and a litigious society to do some self-policing. The dentist should educate himself as completely as possible in the fields of craniofacial growth and development and in all aspects of diagnosis, if he plans to embark on orthodontic guidance. Continuing education courses are a must. As a Director of one of the more successful programs of this type in the United States, I am proud to see the number of dentists availing themselves of this type of indoctrination, following the G.V. Black maxim, "The professional man cannot be other than a continuous student."

This, however, is no substitute for a bona fide, 2-year, full-time graduate specialty training. Our ultimate responsibility is to the patient. Our sacred moral duty is to do the best we can for society. If we cannot render the highest level of service, we should make sure that the patient sees someone who can. This is why medical and dental specialties exist.

*Graber, T.M., and Neumann, B.: Removable orthodontic appliances, ed. 2, Philadelphia, 1984, W.B. Saunders Co., p. 614.

CHAPTER 12
TREATMENT OF CLASS II MALOCCLUSIONS

DEVELOPING TREATMENT CONCEPTS

Any description of Class II malocclusions is difficult at best because this arbitrary categorization includes various types of malocclusions. In its original and strictest interpretation, the designation of Class II defines only the sagittal relationship between the upper and lower first permanent molars as propounded by Edward H. Angle. Subsequent clinical experience and the development of more sophisticated diagnostic assessments such as Gnathostatics by Paul Simon and Cephalometrics by Broadbent and a host of workers in the field delineated the broad gamut of types of Class II malocclusion. Particularly important was the recognition of the dysplastic skeletal sagittal relationship of the maxilla and mandible to each other and to the cranial base. Equally important has been the assessment of vertical components and their role in horizontal malrelationships, creating further subclasses of Class II malocclusion. Finally, an essential facet of the differential diagnosis in these cases has been the functional adaptation to the horizontal and vertical dysplasia, which results in posterior (and occasionally anterior) condylar displacement or rocking open of the mandible in an autorotational maneuver, because of excessive anterior or deficient posterior facial height.

The net result has been a malocclusion diagnosed on the basis of the habitual occlusion, first molar relationship. The problem could be a spatial sagittal, abnormality of the maxilla, the mandible, or a combination of both, influenced by a vertical dysplasia of the maxilla, mandible, or both, with a condylar position in the fossa in habitual occlusion that could be normal, posterior, or anterior, depending on occlusal guiding forces and neuromuscular adaptation.

These potentially variable malocclusion characteristics and means of recognizing and relating them are discussed more fully in Chapter 4. This chapter describes the means that are used in coping with the different characteristics, separately or in combination. It is obvious, though, that the many attempts in the past to find a "universal" appliance to treat all Class II malocclusions

could not succeed. Some of the biomechanical treatment procedures were aimed at the mixed dentition and others at the permanent dentition. They can be divided into three broad groups based on the philosophy or working hypothesis espoused.

1. Fundamental to one group of orthodontic therapies has been the concept that bone morphology is presumably inherited and the functional environment adapts to this form. According to this philosophy, growth and development are independent procedures that cannot be influenced. The corrective procedures begin after the eruption of the permanent teeth by moving them to achieve a dentoalveolar correction. The hereditarily linked skeletal pattern cannot be influenced. The only therapeutic possibility is a dentoalveolar compensation of the Class II skeletal relationship (Fig. 12-1). With this philosophy, as exemplified by the Begg technique and some forms of the current straight-wire philosophy, a causal approach to treatment is possible only in dentoalveolar malocclusions. This means that the correction can be done only within the framework of the original

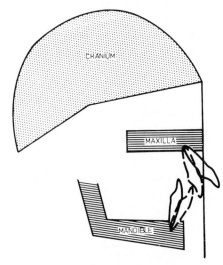

Fig. 12-1. Dentoalveolar compensation of a skeletal Class II relationship. The lower incisors are tipped labially; the upper, lingually.

malocclusion. The mode of therapy is instituted in the adult dentition. The skeletal discrepancy can either be compensated for with the aid of extraction or altered by orthognathic surgery.

2. According to the second concept, every individual has the potential to be perfect. Any deviation from ideal occlusion is attributed to the environment. The first supporter of this hypothesis was Angle. However, the classic edgewise approach as espoused by Brodie and his students was a combination of the hereditary determinism and ideal occlusion philosophies. According to this philosophy, establishing the full dentition in ideal intercuspal relationship would lead to normal function and maintenance of the treated result. A modification of this empiric approach was fostered by Andresen and his followers. The form adapts to function, and the influence of the muscles is considered to be the primary etiologic basis, the primary environmental factor. By altering the environmental factors, it would thus be possible to stimulate mandibular growth, inhibit maxillary growth, and alter growth direction.

Many proponents of a so-called universal appliance were disciples of this doctrine. They were convinced that using the activator, for example, it was possible to stimulate growth of the mandible and to position it anteriorly in all Class II malocclusions.

3. The third and most recent orthopedic-orthodontic philosophy is based on considerable primate research, as well as on clinical experience. It holds that there is a middle ground in the form versus function, heredity versus environment, struggle. Function is not identical with environmental influences. Certain aspects of function can also be inherited, especially the posture and morphology of the muscles and soft tissues. The functional influences conditioned by heredity have been designated as *epigenetic* factors (van Limbourgh). This implies an hereditary influence arising, not from the cells, per se, but guided indirectly by function. According to this hypothesis, there is a range of normal accomplishment. Under the best possible circumstances, it is possible to achieve an optimal growth potential within the scope or range of the individual genetic pattern. This is the basic principle of modern functional orthopedic therapy for the Class II type of malocclusion during the growth period. A prime task of the differential diagnosis is to assess the scope of the genetic pattern in each individual case.

THERAPEUTIC CONSIDERATIONS

The localization of the skeletal dysplasia is decisive in determining the therapy. Not only is the differential diagnosis between the skeletal and dentoalveolar malocclusion characteristics of importance, but an exact determination of the specifics of the skeletal abnormality is essential. The Class II skeletal relationship, for example, can be due to a posteriorly positioned mandible (true, functional, or autorotated open) and/or an anteriorly positioned maxilla (Fig. 12-2).

In simplest terms, growth promotion in the TMJ area is indicated in mandibular retrusion, while growth inhibition is required for maxillary protrusion, directed, if possible, at the sutural hafting zone of the craniofacial complex. These two different objectives require quite different biomechanical treatment procedures. Even the

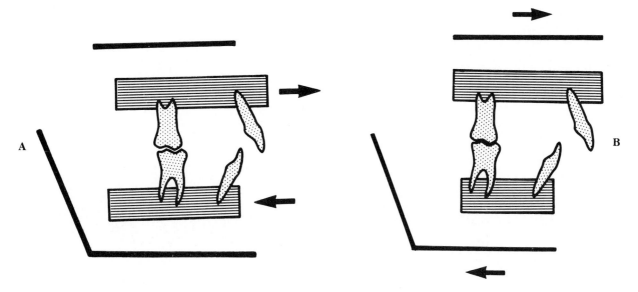

Fig. 12-2. A, Dentoalveolar Class II relationship. The upper dental arch and alveolar process are positioned anteriorly; the lower, posteriorly. **B,** Skeletal Class II relationship. The upper jaw bases are positioned anteriorly; the lower, posteriorly.

limitations imposed by the differential growth accomplishment of the maxilla and mandible require discretionary therapeutic decisions.

Growth stimulation of the secondary cartilaginous condylar growth center is more difficult than for purely membranous bone, because the structures are made to resist compression and other functional stresses. While not as resistant as primary cartilaginous centers such as the epiphysis and diaphysis of long bones, the unique prechondroblast-chondroblast cycle of this growth center is timed in its development so that only certain cells are responsive to external stimuli at precise stages in their maturation. Vascularization is also less efficient than with membranous bone, though recent research by Biggerstaff shows an extensive subcondylar plexus. Therapeutic growth guidance can be performed only during the active growth period (Fig. 12-3).

The membranous bone sutures of the maxilla are quite responsive to external stimuli, with many undifferentiated cells and a high fibroblast turnover in the sutures. Vascularization is quite good, which expedites the local response. Inhibitory action on membranous bone sutures is particularly effective, as fibroblasts hyalinize and die within 4 hours after the application of orthopedic pressures, whereas it takes up to 160 hours for a chondroblast to succumb to even greater pressures. There are clearly different treatment responses in the maxilla and the mandible. Therapeutic inhibition of maxillary growth is not completely limited to active growth spurts, though it is more effective at this time. Some treatment response is possible at a later period when condylar response is minimal or nonexistent.

Mandibular growth alone does not solve all Class II problems. A case in point is a 9-year-old patient with the Class II malocclusion associated with abnormal tongue function. Cephalometric analysis showed no basal skeletal discrepancy and indicated a probable horizontal growth pattern (Fig. 12-4). The maxillary and mandibular bases were short, and the ascending ramus was long. Both upper and lower incisors were procumbent. No orthodontic therapy was performed, and the tongue dysfunction persisted. Three years later, the patient had a definite sagittal discrepancy with a reduced S-N-B angle in spite of a high growth increment of the mandibular base. The lingual tipping of the lower incisors might have been attributed to a change in the perioral dysfunction pattern. There was now a confirmed lip trap with hyperactive mentalis muscle function. If therapy had been instituted during the high growth period, the result would have been good and stable. Lack of treatment meant an enhancement of the skeletal discrepancy and intensification of the adaptive and deforming neuromuscular activity.

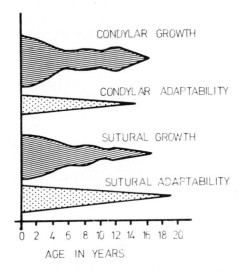

Fig. 12-3. Respective adaptability of condylar and sutural growth, depending on the age of the patient. (According to van der Linden.)

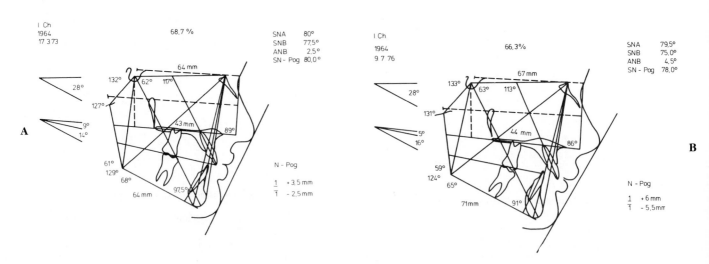

Fig. 12-4. Patient I.C. at, **A,** 9 and, **B,** 11 years of age. In spite of high mandibular growth rates, the skeletal relationship became worse.

TREATMENT PLANNING

Before starting to treat a Class II malocclusion, a number of important facts must be ascertained:

1. Is the malocclusion of skeletal or dentoalveolar origin? Causal therapy of a skeletal malocclusion can be successful only during the growth period.

2. Is the malocclusion a functionally true one, with a normal path of closure from postural rest to habitual occlusion, or is it a functional retrusion, with the condyle moving up and back from postural rest to habitual occlusion? Normally condylar action is primarily rotary in the lower joint cavity from rest to occlusion. Translatory condylar movement not only jeopardizes the normal condyle-disk-eminence relationship but produces a retruded spatial mandibular malposition on full occlusion. A primary treatment objective must be to eliminate the retruded condylar position, harmonizing it with the more anterior postural rest position. This can be done quite successfully by functional orthopedic procedures. If the path of closure is normal, with only rotary condylar function from postural rest to occlusion, and the malocclusion is a true sagittal skeletal discrepancy, the treatment challenge is different. Not only the occlusal position must be changed, but there must also be a neuromuscular adaptation to the new postural position of the mandible, as the condyle grows upward and backward to its correct relationship with the fossa structures. It can be difficult to achieve a permanent neuromuscular adaptation to the appliance oriented mandibular postural position. If the original postural resting position persists, a functional disturbance, "Sunday bite" or dual bite, is the consequence.

3. Forecasting the probable growth direction is very important in the assessment of therapeutic possibilities. With a horizontal growth pattern, therapeutic control of the vertical dimension is difficult, just as control of the horizontal dimension is problematic with a vertical growth vector.

4. Growth increments per unit time are a prime consideration. The questions of how great the growth potential is and when it can be expected are of importance in the choice of the therapeutic method. Treatment timing is critical. The forecast may call for major growth increments in the future; but if appliances are worn during a quiescent growth period, failure to accomplish treatment objectives is likely, even though significant growth increments remain to occur after treatment.

5. The etiologic considerations, differentiating hereditary malocclusions and the consequences of neuromuscular dysfunctions, are of importance in assessing the scope of functional appliances and their efficacy in therapy.

To obtain more detailed and needed information, both the functional and cephalometric examinations are valuable before starting treatment.

Functional criteria

The most important functional criteria for treatment planning for Class II malocclusions are as follows:

1. The assessment of the relationship between rest position and occlusion to differentiate a functionally true and a forced bite malocclusion.

2. The examination of the relationships between overjet and function of the lips. If the lower lip postures and functions in the incisal gap created by the excessive overjet, with hyperactive, adaptive, and exacerbative mentalis muscle function, this deforming activity should be eliminated during the day if the functional appliance of choice is worn only at night.

3. The posture and function of the tongue should be assessed. In some malocclusions the abnormal tongue function needs to be controlled with accessory elements or appliances.

4. The mode of breathing is important because patients with disturbed nasal respiration or enlarged tonsils and adenoids are not able to retain the functional appliance in the mouth as prescribed (Fig. 12-5).

Cephalometric criteria

A complete analysis is necessary before orthodontic therapy. This is no less important for removable than fixed appliances. The following considerations are of particular interest when planning treatment:

1. Relationship of the maxilla to the cranial base. In patients with a prognathic maxilla, usually a maxillary withholding or a distal driving of the 6-year molars is indicated. Functional appliances are not very effective in such cases.

2. Position and size of the mandible. In patients with a retrognathic mandible, the therapeutic require-

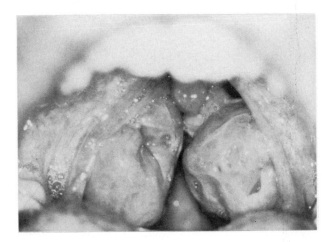

Fig. 12-5. Patients with enlarged tonsils or adenoids have difficulty wearing the activator.

ments are different, depending on the size of the mandible.

3. The axial inclination and position of the incisors is important information before deciding on the mode and amount of movement of these teeth.

4. The growth pattern is decisive for decisions on the design and construction of the appliance.

The cephalometric analysis renders a value judgment as to whether in a specific Class II malocclusion the maxilla is prognathic and/or large or the mandible is retrognathic and/or small. (See Chapter 4.)

CLASSIFICATION OF CLASS II MALOCCLUSIONS
Morphologic classification

There are a number of classifications of Class II malocclusion. One of the simplest divides the malocclusion into the following four groups:

1. Class II dental malocclusions caused only by tooth migration, i.e., dentoalveolar malocclusions.

2. Class II malocclusions with the fault in the mandible; the mandible is retrognathic and the maxilla orthognathic. This category makes up most of the Class II malocclusions encountered in orthodontic practice.

3. Class II malocclusions with the fault in the maxilla; the maxilla is prognathic and the mandible orthognathic. As McNamara's study has shown, this makes up a relatively small percentage of the cases treated.

4. Combinations of 2 and 3. It should be emphasized, however, that both 2 and 3 are likely to have local tooth malpositions in addition to the basal malrelationship, as the incisors adapt sagittally to the perverted perioral musculature. Maxillary arch width is also subservient to such neuromuscular compensations, whether the maxilla is prognathic or orthognathic, in combination with an orthognathic or retrognathic mandible, as long as there is a sufficient basal malrelationship to elicit abnormal buccinator mechanism activity.

Cephalometric classification

A more sophisticated categorization is possible with the help of increasingly detailed cephalometric criteria. When these criteria are used, five basic groups of Class II malocclusions can be recognized.

1. Class II malocclusions based on a Class II sagittal relationship without a skeletal component. The A-N-B angle can be normal. Usually the upper and lower jaw bases both are retrognathic and the S-N-A and S-N-B angles reduced. There is likely to be a labial tipping of the upper incisors; the lower incisors can be tipped either labially or lingually depending on the local neuromuscular compensation for the excessive overjet. Labial tipping of the lower incisors reduces the overjet but makes

orthodontic correction more difficult, because uprighting of the lower incisors is also a necessary treatment objective. This is often quite difficult with no spaces present (Fig. 12-6).

2. Functionally created Class II malocclusions, with a forced mandibular retrusion in habitual occlusion but a normal postural rest relationship. The path of closure is abnormal, or forced, usually in conjunction with an excessive overbite and infraocclusion of the buccal segment teeth. The S-N-B angle is smaller in habitual occlusion but improved in the postural resting position. Usually the mandibular base is of normal size, and there is no growth deficiency. In such cases early interceptive functional therapy is the method of choice (Fig. 12-7).

3. Class II malocclusions with the fault in the maxilla. The profile convexity of the upper jaw can be basal (with a larger S-N-A angle), dentoalveolar (with an increased S-N-Pr angle), or dental (with an increased upper incisor to S-N plane angle, signifying labial incisal tipping) (Fig. 12-8).

Therapeutic mechanisms and possibilities depend on the axial inclination of the incisors and on the type of maxillary prognathism. Simple tipping of the incisors can be corrected with removable appliances, but torque and bodily movement should be done with fixed appliances. Maxillary basal prognathism requires heavy orthopedic force.

The maxillary base can be normal in size and just positioned anteriorly, or it can be too long. When evaluating the maxillary base, its inclination should also be considered. An upward and forward inclination aggravates the maxillary protrusion (Schwarz calls this a pseudo-protrusion). A retroinclination (palatal plane tipped down anteriorly) can actually compensate for a

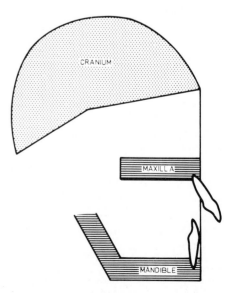

Fig. 12-6. Dentoalveolar Class II relationship with labial tipping of the upper and lingual tipping of the lower incisors.

maxillary prognathism. The control of the vertical dimension in this type of malocclusion is often dependent on the inclination of the maxillary base, especially if it is combined with either a deep overbite or an open bite. A combined type of therapy (headgear and activator) is usually required to influence the maxillary prognathism (Fig. 12-9).

4. Class II malocclusion with fault in the mandible. There is a smaller S-N-B angle with mandibular retrog-

nathism. The retrognathic mandible can be small or normal, but posteriorly positioned in the facial skeleton. If the size is normal, the saddle angle is larger and flatter, with the condylar fossa in a relatively posterior position (Fig. 12-10).

The treatment possibilities depend on the growth increments and growth direction. In cases with horizontal or neutral growth vectors, conventional activator therapy is likely to be successful. With a vertical growth vector, anterior positioning of the mandible is not likely to take place permanently, although in certain cases the so-called vertical activator can be used. Amounts of growth during appliance wear are a consideration, as indicated above.

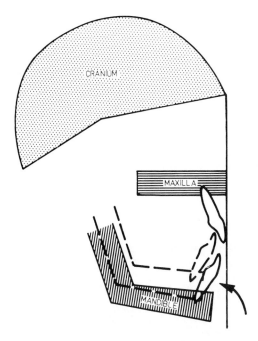

Fig. 12-7. Functional Class II relationship with a distally forced bite. From an anterior rest position the mandible glides into a posterior habitual occlusion usually under the influence of tooth guidance.

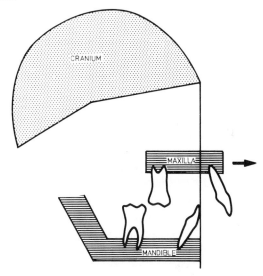

Fig. 12-8. Skeletal Class II relationship with "fault" in the maxilla. The upper jaw base is prognathic; the lower, orthognathic.

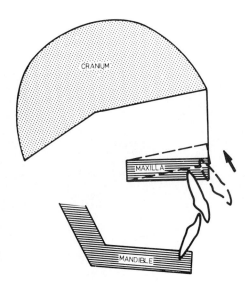

Fig. 12-9. Class II relationship with prognathism and anteinclination of the maxilla (anterior end tipped up).

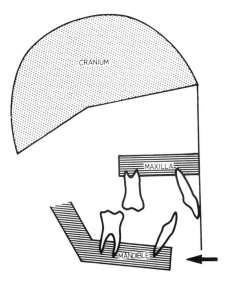

Fig. 12-10. Class II relationship with fault in the mandible. The maxilla is orthognatic; the mandible, retrognathic.

5. A combination of the four previously designated patterns is possible, particularly a combination of 3 and 4. There is also the possibility of a Class II malocclusion with both upper and lower jaws being retrognathic. In such cases treatment is a combined functional and fixed appliance approach, and success is dependent on the growth pattern, direction, and increments during appliance wear.

GROWTH POTENTIAL

As already indicated, growth direction is quite important, but the amount of growth or growth potential is equally so. The size of the jaw bases can be assessed in correlation with the N-Se length, as recommended by Schwarz. The growth rates for the different growth patterns can be evaluated with the help of previously derived tables. (See Chapter 4.) If a particular dimension is too short with respect to the other measurements, higher growth rates can usually be anticipated in the area of apparent deficiency. An exception would be the short mandibular ramus in a vertically growing face.

THERAPEUTIC METHODS

The objectives of mixed dentition treatment for Class II malocclusions vary, depending on the type of malocclusion, as outlined above.

1. The elimination of abnormal perioral muscle function is feasible, using inhibitory therapy. Neuromuscular dysfunctions should be corrected in the first phase of treatment. Most often the lower lip screen can be used in combination with other methods.
2. Anterior positioning of the mandible by elimination of functionally induced retrusions and concomitant growth stimulation is a valid objective with the activator serving as a primary corrective device.
3. Growth inhibition of the maxilla in prognathic maxillary problems, together with distalization of upper buccal segment teeth using extraoral force, is a likely therapeutic method. Active plates can sometimes be used for minor problems in this category.

Experience has shown that a combination of therapeutic tools is necessary to produce the optimum.

APPLIANCES USED IN THE TREATMENT OF CLASS II MALOCCLUSIONS

Different treatment objectives demand different appliances. Appliances for anterior positioning of the mandible are the vestibular screen, for functional retrusion and lip trap problems; the activator and, occasionally, bite planes or guide planes can also be used. The activator and its various modifications are clearly the appliance of choice in most instances.

The bite plane has not yet been described, as it is not a typical functional appliance. However, as Hotz has shown with his *Vorbissplatte,* it can be used in some specific cases where difficulties are likely to arise with use of the conventional activator (e.g., occluded nasal passages, allergic manifestations, mouth breathing) (Fig. 12-11). The appliance looks like a modified Hawley retainer, with acrylic palatal coverage, to which has been added an anterior inclined plane, which engages the lower incisors and causes the mandible to slide anteriorly. Anchorage is obtained with Adams or arrow-type clasps and a labial bow. Prognosis is more favorable with the so-called *Deckbiss,* forced bite type of problem. The postural change potential is adequate, but its growth stimulating potential as far as condylar growth is concerned is clearly less than the activator. The *Vorbissplatte* can be used under the following conditions:

1. At least the first premolars must have erupted to lend good anchorage to the appliance. The use of Adams clasps on the first premolars and first molars is usually recommended. Arrow clasps are often used after eruption of the second premolars.

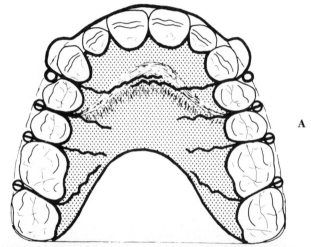

A

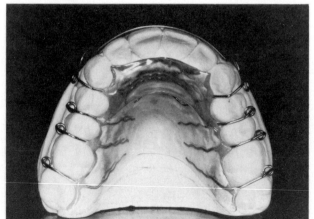

B

Fig. 12-11. Anterior bite plane. **A,** Schematic and, **B,** on the cast.

2. The upper and lower dental arches should be reasonably well aligned. With anchorage a critical matter, additional tooth movement tasks are not feasible, as they would reduce appliance efficiency.

3. The maxillary incisors should not be tipped much to the labial. Appreciable uprighting of these teeth with an intramaxillary appliance such as the biteplate has had only limited success.

4. The lower incisors should be upright or lingually inclined. The appliances tend to tip these teeth labially, which can be beneficial in some instances. However, if these teeth are already labially inclined and are further tipped labially, full correction is not possible because of incisor interference, and the patient will have increased difficulty in wearing the appliance (Fig. 12-12).

Normally the guide plane has an angulation of approximately 45 degrees, with a seating groove for the lower incisors to reduce the labial tipping tendency with the anterior mandibular posturing.

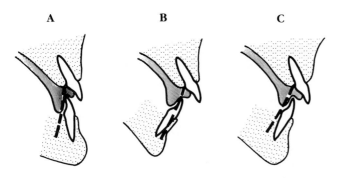

Fig. 12-12. A, With lingual tipping of the lower incisors, construction of the inclined bite plane is difficult. **B,** The plane tips the lower incisors labially. **C,** It guides the mandible anteriorly. (Modified according to Hotz.)

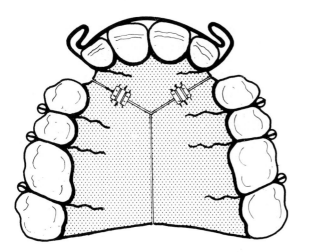

Fig. 12-13. The Y-plate with double jackscrews and arrow clasps for retention.

Appliances for relative distalization or withholding of maxillary buccal segment teeth must be utilized in certain cases. Extraoral force delivered by properly designed headgears can produce both skeletal and dentoalveolar response. After eruption of the permanent dentition, fixed multiattachment appliances can be used with both headgear and elastic traction. Removable Y-plates with jackscrews incorporated for distal movement of the maxillary molars are a possibility in the mixed dentition after eruption of the first premolars.

The Y-plate (Fig. 12-13) is an active removable plate type of appliance that will move teeth under certain conditions. Its appearance is similar to the biteplate, and it is anchored on the maxillary arch with Adams or arrow clasps. The labial bow inserts into the acrylic in the lateral incisor–canine embrasure. The plate has two jackscrews placed in oblique position at the canine areas. The opening of the jackscrews has a distalizing component on the buccal segment teeth, with a reciprocal force being delivered to the anterior palatal contour and maxillary incisors. To reduce the mesial force component, which tends to both tip the incisors labially and dislodge the appliance, the screws are activated alternately and unilaterally. Under the following conditions, the plate can be used to distalize buccal segment teeth:

1. The first premolars have already erupted, giving increased anchorage.

2. The upper incisors are fairly upright so that a slight labial tipping of these teeth is beneficial or at least not undesirable.

3. No extensive bodily movements are required.

4. The second permanent molars have not yet erupted.

Indications for the various treatment methods

No universal method can solve all Class II problems. Various methods and various appliances are required, depending on the malocclusion specifics. Using only functional appliances for all Class II cases would help only those cases with forced bite functional retrusion or retrognathic mandibles, while doing little for problems with prognathic maxillae. Hence fixed appliances and extraoral force are clearly indicated in cases demanding retropositioning of the maxillary base and dentition, but such appliances have a limited influence on the position of the mandible and the elimination of neuromuscular abnormalities.

Dentoalveolar therapeutic measures. The primary objective of functional appliances is the forward positioning of the mandible. However, these appliances can also be used for functional retrusion cases, where there is a forced distal bite, and for some dentoalveolar malocclusions that are the result of abnormal perioral muscle function. Not only the eruption of teeth can be controlled, in deep bite cases for example, but also various tooth movements can be performed. The following is a listing of the possible types of tooth movement that can be attained with the activator:

1. Buccal tipping during transverse expansion adjustments
2. Labial and lingual tipping
3. Extrusion
4. Aligning of abnormally tipped teeth
5. Correction of eccentric rotations

Other types of movement meet with more limited success. These include intrusion and mesial or distal movement. Some kinds of movement cannot be performed with an activator, including bodily movement, centric rotations, and torque. Fixed appliances must be used for these objectives. Together with extraoral force, a distalization of the maxillary teeth is possible, along with an orthopedic effect on the maxilla itself; the withholding of downward and forward growth is a valid and achievable objective in cases of maxillary prognathism. In vertical growth patterns, inhibition of maxillary growth is also a viable treatment goal.

The movement of teeth with an activator also depends on the stage of eruption as well as the nature of tooth movement required. The intraoral eruption process can be divided into two phases or steps (Fig. 12-14).

1. The stage of drift while the tooth is erupting into the oral cavity, when the movement of the teeth is under the influence of contiguous muscle forces.

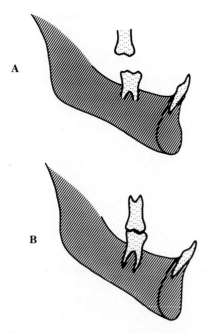

Fig. 12-14. Two stages of the intraoral phase of tooth eruption. **A,** No tooth contact. **B,** Occlusal phase (contact with the antagonists).

This eruption can be guided by using the acrylic planes of the activator itself.

2. The stage of interarch influence, as the teeth contact their antagonists, and some sort of equilibrium is established by the occlusal force. Acrylic guide plane control by the activator is limited in this stage.

The dentoalveolar type of Class II can also be helped using screening appliances, as well as an activator that has been trimmed to provide the acrylic guiding planes. This is in addition to the tried and true use of headgear force applied to the permanent first molars. Purely active nonfunctional removable appliances, as designed by Schwarz, Korkhaus, and others, can be used in simple problems, but skeletal effect from these is minimal. They are all that is needed in dentoalveolar problems.

Skeletal therapeutic measures. It has been emphasized that growth direction is decisive in determining the mode of treatment for skeletal malocclusions. In a Class II relationship, with a horizontal growth pattern during the mixed dentition and a retrognathic mandible, a conventional activator (**H** activator) is recommended. If a prognathic maxilla is the cause of the Class II relationship, as is frequently the case in blacks, then it is not possible to position the mandible anteriorly for a causal correction of the anomaly. Instead growth inhibition is indicated in the midface region. This means that extraoral force is the most likely mechanism, attached to fixed appliances usually, although removable-fixed combinations can be used in properly chosen cases (i.e., in combined basal sagittal dysplasias, with a prognathic maxilla and retrognathic mandible in the same case). If there is also abnormal perioral neuromuscular activity in these combined cases, a lower lip screen may be used simultaneously. In extraction cases the maxillary second molars are often used in this type of pattern, allowing a dental compensation by moving the maxillary buccal segments distally. Only with this method can a deep overbite be opened as the buccal segment teeth are moved distally into the **V**, autorotating the mandible down and backward. Because of the tendency for the chin point to move into a more retrusive position, care must be exercised in such cases, choosing only the more favorable mandibular growth direction cases. Maxillary second molar extraction should be considered only if the developing third molars are normal in size and position. After premolars have been extracted, the posterior segments move mesially to some degree, regardless of appliance efforts to prevent it. This closes down the bite more, so that it is very difficult to correct a deep bite case with such an approach, and even then, the relapse tendency is significant. In the most severe problems, some form of compromise of the result and orthognathic surgery are the only avenues of therapy.

In vertical growth patterns, combined with a retrognathic mandible, a specially designed activator is constructed (the **V** activator). The prognathic maxilla is corrected by high-pull extraoral force or compromised by first premolar extraction. Sometimes both measures are required.

In Class II malocclusions with a vertical growth pattern and a prognathic maxilla, the extraction of only the two maxillary first premolars may be required. The control of the deep overbite in such cases is not difficult due to the vertical growth pattern. A lower lip screen may also be incorporated to eliminate perioral muscle dysfunction. Where maxillary first premolars have been removed, however, multiattachment fixed appliances are usually required.

Functional criteria for determination of mode of therapy. Functional analysis is imperative before choosing a specific type of mechanotherapy.

In functional retrusion cases, where the mandible moves upward and backward from rest position into a forced retrusive habitual occlusion, it is not necessary to attempt to alter the postural resting position of the mandible. In such cases, the Class II relationship is largely of a dental nature caused by improper intercuspation. Screening types of appliances or activators can be used alone with some occlusal equilibration in the later stages of therapy.

In true Class II malocclusions, with a normal upward and forward path of closure from postural rest to occlusion, not only the occlusal position but the postural resting position should be altered by anterior positioning, which is accomplished by proper bite construction. Such neuromuscular adaptation is more difficult and not always successful. In any event such treatment must be done during the growth period.

Occasionally the postural resting position is actually more retruded than the occlusal position in a Class II malocclusion. Tooth guidance slides the mandible forward into what appears to be a less severe skeletal malrelationship than actually exists. It is difficult to treat the sagittal malrelationship in such cases by anterior positioning of the mandible. Dual bite conditions may persist, even after treatment, with consequent TMJ problems during or after active treatment. It is necessary in such cases to exert a distal vector of force on the maxilla and maxillary teeth, usually with the more effective extraoral force methods, either separately or in conjunction with functional appliance therapy.

Treatment of various types of Class II malocclusions

The systematic, definitive methods of treatment just described are possible only in typical cases with the cephalometric and functional criteria elucidated. There are many borderline cases requiring a discretionary combination of the various methods. Such modifications of classic functional appliance therapy are often called *midstream correction* or therapeutic diagnosis. In other words, the response of the patient to a predetermined treatment plan is a major consideration in achieving the ultimate correction. Even similar malocclusions respond differently, and such responses should be continually observed with an eye toward making the necessary therapeutic alterations. We are treating individuals, not malocclusion categories, so exact cookbook procedures do not work for all patients. The perceptive clinician resorts to therapeutic diagnosis and therapeutic modifiability as treatment progresses and is always alert to the need to change treatment plans as treatment response, or lack of response, dictates.

Treatment with the conventional activator.   An 8½-year-old girl with a Class II, Division I, malocclusion and a maternal hereditary pattern is shown in Fig. 12-15. The patient still has a thumb-sucking habit and the retained infantile deglutitional pattern that is so often associated with prolonged finger-sucking.

The growth pattern is average, and the facial type is retrognathic. The Class II relationship is apparently caused by a small mandible (-3.5 mm), short ascending ramus (-3 mm), and larger cranial base angle ($+7$ degrees), which results in a more posterior position of the temporomandibular fossa. The maxillary base is of average length with a slight upward inclination. The A-N-B difference is 5 degrees. The initial pattern shows the lower incisors tipped somewhat labially, which diminishes the overjet. This is often the case in retained infantile deglutitional patterns due to forward tongue posture and function. The path of closure is normal, with a rotary action of the condyle from postural rest to habitual occlusion.

Since the mother's own severe Class II malocclusion provided a strong motivational assist, it was decided to begin treatment as soon as the incisors had erupted. It was felt that the hereditary pattern, plus the deforming perioral neuromuscular activity, would enhance the dysplasia if left alone for a long time. The treatment objectives of elimination of the dysfunction, together with all possible favorable condylar growth stimulation at this early age, had a more favorable prognosis because of the small retrognathic mandible.

A larger growth spurt can usually be expected; and after elimination of the restrictive and deforming perioral malfunction, good sagittally directed mandibular growth is likely. This is due to the favorable morphology of the mandible. With such early and simple treatment guidance, the individual optimum is achieved.

All skeletal relationships were favorable in this case for a conventional activator, but the labial inclination of the lower incisors should have been considered when

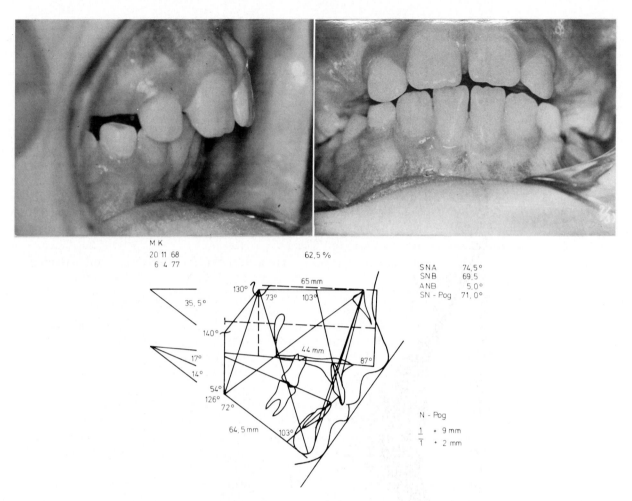

Fig. 12-15. Patient M.K. before treatment.

posturing the mandible anteriorly. Therapy began with a vestibular screen to eliminate the lip trap and hyperactive mentalis function. The activator was constructed 4 months later with a 7 mm mandibular advancement to an end-to-end incisal relationship. The vertical dimension was opened 3 mm.

Both upper and lower labial bows were active, contacting the teeth at the incisal thirds of the labial surfaces. The incisal edges were supported with acrylic. The acrylic was trimmed completely away from the lingual aspect of the lower incisors to help tip the teeth lingually. The acrylic was trimmed away from the lingual side of the upper incisors in the coronal region only, since it was desired to tip these teeth only slightly lingually to partially compensate for the uprighting of the lower incisors. The appliance was trimmed in the buccal segments so as to effect distal movement of the upper molars. Stabilizing wires were incorporated mesial to the permanent first molars. In the lower buccal segments, trimming was performed to stimulate slight extrusion of the lower molars and to assist in achieving a

Class II relationship. The upper molars had a distalizing force against them but were prevented from extrusion.

After 4 years of treatment and retention (also using the activator), the Class II relationship was improved by anterior positioning and growth of the mandible. The retrognathic profile still persisted, despite a reduction of the A-N-B difference to 2.5 degrees. The growth increment of the mandibular base was 7.5 mm, or 3.5 mm over the average values. Maxillary and ramal growth increments were average. The basal difference Ar-Pog to Ar–A point improved from 11 to 18 mm. The growth direction became more horizontal. The lower incisor inclination improved with the anterior positioning of the mandible and pressure from the labial bow (Fig. 12-16). As the illustrations show, early treatment for this patient resulted in elimination of abnormal environmental influences, normalization of function, and an undisturbed growth process. The growth increments of the mandible were quite high. It is conjectural to suggest just what the growth would have been without therapy, but the elimination of the disturbing and restrictive factors and syn-

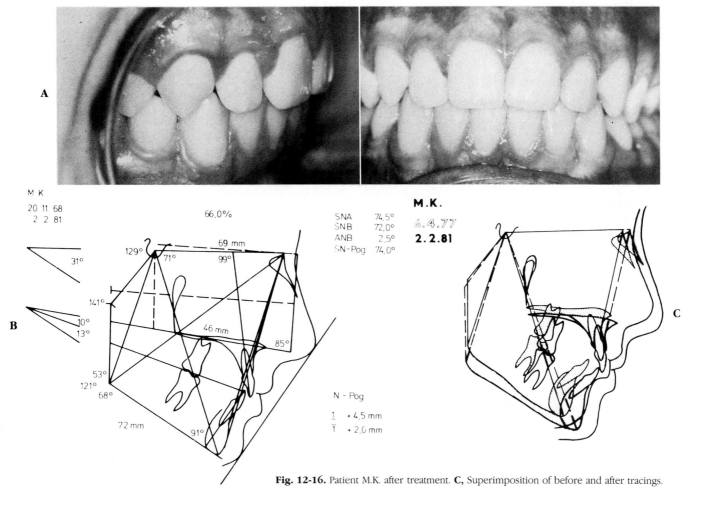

Fig. 12-16. Patient M.K. after treatment. **C,** Superimposition of before and after tracings.

chronization of the growth processes did lead to a harmonious occlusion with no skeletal discrepancy. It is not unreasonable to suppose that the skeletal discrepancy would have increased without treatment, with continuous restrictive suprahyoid and infrahyoid activity, combined with excessive posterior temporalis and deep masseter function, preventing the full accomplishment of pattern. This could have occurred despite growth and would have enhanced the difficulty of causal therapy at a later date.

Compensation of the Class II excessive overjet by labial tipping of the lower incisors. The 9½-year-old patient illustrated in Fig. 12-17 has a Class II skeletal relationship with a retrognathic mandible. The maxillary and mandibular bases are of average length, but the ramus is short (−7 mm). The growth forecast is neutral. The axial inclination of the upper incisors is good, but they are 9 mm in front of the N-Pog line. The lower incisors are tipped labially, decreasing the apparent overjet. The Class II sagittal relationship is more severe in the rest position, and the mandible slides anteriorly into habitual occlusion during the path of closure. This convenience deflection and labial tipping of the lower incisors mask the true severity of the malocclusion. The patient has abnormal perioral muscle function with a lower lip trap and hyperactive mentalis function.

The objectives of therapy here are to eliminate the lip dysfunction and to position the mandible anteriorly to stimulate all possible favorable mandibular growth. Treatment was started with a lower lip screen during the day and an activator at night. The construction bite was taken with the mandible positioned anteriorly 6 mm and the bite opened 5 mm. The upper incisors were held with the labial bow and complete acrylic contact on the lingual and incisal surfaces. The lower labial bow was active, with acrylic in contact on the incisal edges but cut away from the lingual surfaces of the incisors. The acrylic was trimmed in the buccal segments to distalize the maxillary teeth, holding the permanent first molars with stabilizing wires at the mesial embrasure. Since the holding of the forward position of the mandible is difficult in this mesial occlusal guidance type of Class II

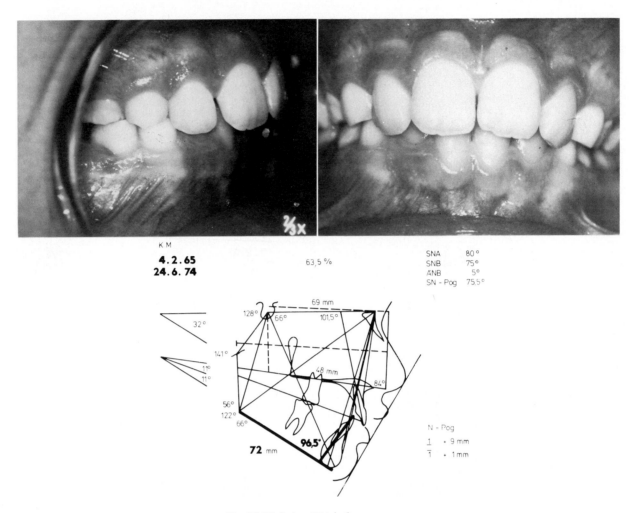

Fig. 12-17. Patient K.M. before treatment.

malocclusion, the acrylic was trimmed in the lower posterior teeth to encourage their mesial movement.

After 3 years, no forward positioning of the mandible could be observed, despite a good growth increment of the mandibular base. There was only slight ramus growth, and the neutral growth pattern persisted. The malocclusion was compensated for by the extreme labial tipping of the lower incisors. A major reason for this tipping was the grinding of the activator acrylic to encourage mesial movement of the lower posterior teeth, plus the fact that these teeth were already labially tipped at the beginning of treatment. The lower lip screen, removing the hyperactive mentalis muscle retrusive effect on the incisors, and eliminating the lip trap also enhanced the labial tipping. Clinical experience shows that it is very difficult to protract and maintain a retrognathic mandible of average base length (to N-Se) in a normal path of closure problem, even when the mandible slides

anteriorly into habitual occlusion. The dental compensation of a Class II problem with labial tipping of the lower incisors is a poor result in the mixed dentition period, except in cases with a vertical growth pattern (Fig. 12-18). In this case, the S-N-B angle remained at 75 degrees and the S-N-A angle at 79 degrees, with an apical base difference of 4 degrees. Since the treatment result was considered unstable, a new activator was made for the retention period. The construction bite was advanced only 2 mm and opened 3 mm. Both upper and lower labial bows were activated. The acrylic was trimmed contiguously to the upper posterior teeth to encourage distalization, while the upper incisors were held with acrylic contact. The lower posterior teeth were held and loaded occlusally, while the lower incisors were relieved of acrylic in the lingual and incisal areas. The appliance was worn for another 18 months. Reexamination 2 years out of retention showed only

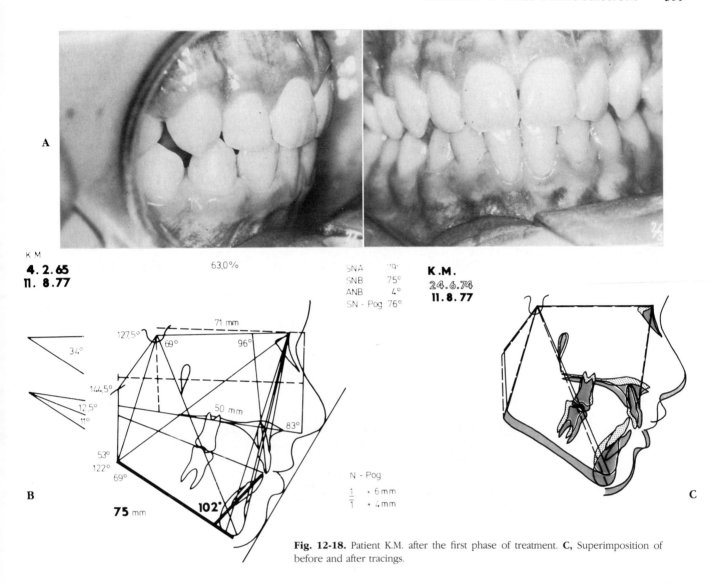

Fig. 12-18. Patient K.M. after the first phase of treatment. **C,** Superimposition of before and after tracings.

slight improvement of the mandibular retrusion, in spite of the high growth rate of the mandibular base and a swing toward a more horizontal growth direction. The axial inclination of the lower incisors improved and ended up at the same value as at the beginning of treatment.

It is stressed again here in this mixed dentition case that the unfavorable functional relationship in the original malocclusion (the anterior guidance into occlusion) made it difficult to position the mandible anteriorly, particularly because the retrognathic mandible was already of average basal length, or longer, in relation to the N-Se length. The only exception is in functional retrusion cases, with abnormal path of closure from postural resting position up and back into a forced habitual occlusion. In cases with a long mandibular base, treatment by attempting to stimulate growth is difficult because of the usual low growth potential and the fact that the mandi-

ble has already achieved its age-dependent individual optimal size. The basic tenet of this working hypothesis is that growth stimulation is possible only in cases of growth restriction or growth deficiency (Fig. 12-19).

This patient had a high incremental growth change in the second period of treatment, together with a more favorable growth direction. The growth increment of the mandibular base, however, was not affected by treatment, because the appliance did not activate the muscles and soft tissues due to the slight forward positioning of the mandible and a low construction bite. The endogenous growth pattern and the change in growth direction to a more horizontal vector were supported by the appliance as it prevented the lower molars from erupting and relieved the lower incisors on the lingual side. Any differentiation of the natural growth processes and those stimulated by treatment is hard to come by. It is possible to stimulate mandibular growth under certain condi-

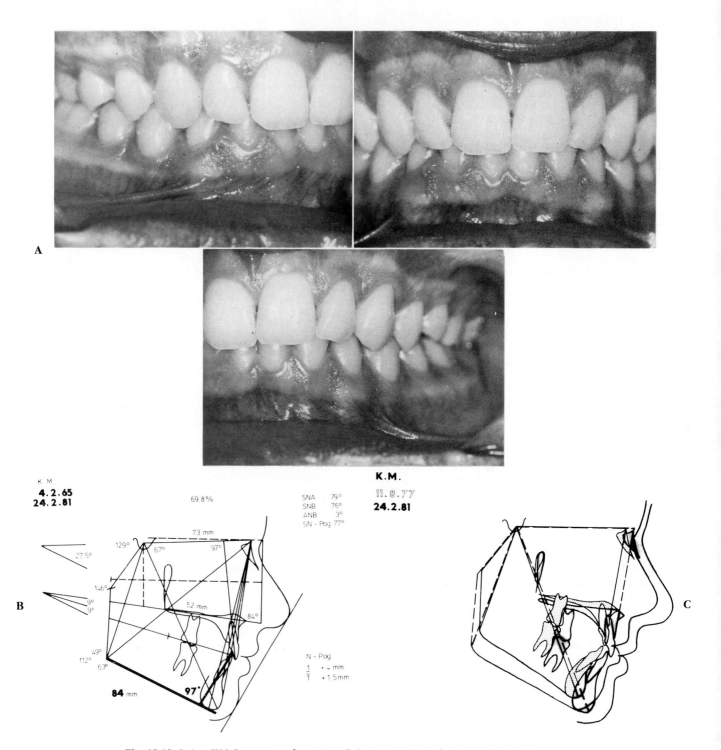

Fig. 12-19. Patient K.M. 2 years out of retention. **C,** Superimposition of tracings after the first treatment phase and after retention.

tions, but not every Class II malocclusion can be treated by growth stimulation of the mandible using an activator. Even in the more difficult cases, though, the abnormal environmental influences can be eliminated and more harmonious occlusal relationships achieved, providing more favorable conditions for optimal and synchronous development of the stomatognathic system.

Treatment of the side effects of extraoral force therapy. Unfavorable or partial response is always possible with any form of orthodontic guidance. The case in Fig. 12-20 illustrates this point. The patient, a 9-year-old girl, demonstrated a Class II malocclusion with a slight maxillary prognathism, combined with a mandibular retrognathism. The maxillary base and ramal height measurements were larger than average, while the mandibular basal length was 2 mm less than the average values. In such cases a higher growth rate of the mandible can usually be expected, resulting in a more favorable horizontal growth direction to help correct the Class II relationship. On the other hand, control of the vertical dimension, correcting a deep overbite, can be difficult.

In the original cephalometric analysis, the upper incisors were labially inclined, 9 mm in front of the N-Pog line, while the lower incisors were well positioned, only 1.5 mm ahead of the N-Pog plane. The patient had a lip dysfunction due to the excessive overjet.

Treatment was started with cervical headgear because

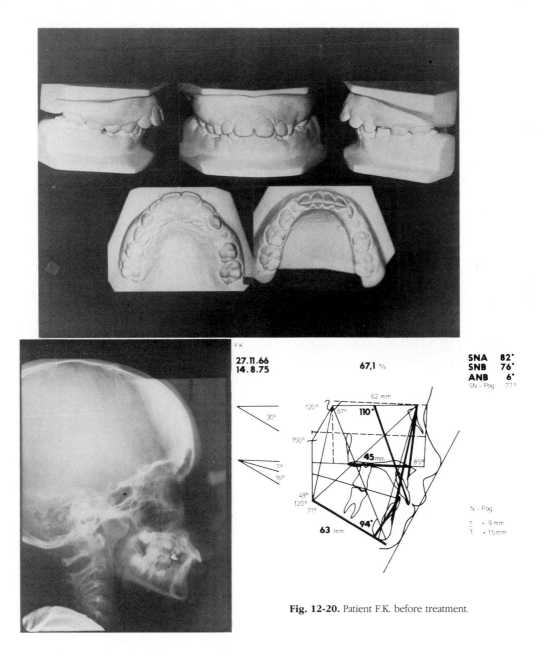

Fig. 12-20. Patient F.K. before treatment.

the maxillary base was slightly protruded, and it was felt that distalization and the extrusive effects of the extraoral force could favorably influence the deeper than normal overbite. Also if the first permanent molars are under headgear therapy before activator treatment, the mesial embrasure is opened and the stabilizing wires readily move into the open contact and continue the favorable eruption guidance of these teeth. A lower lip screen was also used in the initial stages of treatment to eliminate the untoward effects of the lower lip trap.

After 1 year of treatment, the skeletal relationship had improved. There was a growth increment of 3 mm in the mandibular base but no measurable change in the maxillary or ramal area. The S-N-A angle decreased, as the S-N-B angle increased, with a resultant A-B difference of 2.5 degrees. An unexpected finding was the la-

bial tipping of the incisors, particularly the uppers. The original axial inclination of 110 degrees increased inexplicably to 121 degrees. The most probable explanation here is that both the inner labial bow of the headgear and the lower lip screen held off the restraining effect of the labial musculature, while the tongue continued to posture and function in a forward position, exerting a labial vector of force. It is obviously important to check tongue function ahead of time for this possible iatrogenic effect, but compensatory tongue malfunction can also occur during treatment; continual vigilance is essential. In this case both the headgear and vestibular screen were discontinued, and an activator was made with an anterior positioning of 2 mm and an opening of 3 mm in the construction bite to permit the uprighting of the incisors. The objective at this time was to upright the incisors, while guiding eruption of posterior teeth and eliminating the deleterious effects of tongue pressure (Fig. 12-21). Both upper and lower labial bows were activated. The appliance design permitted a lingual sliding of the upper incisors along an acrylic inclined plane, contacting the incisor labial surface, but with the acrylic cut away in the dental and palatal areas. The lower incisors were held on the incisal surface but were allowed to move lingually by grinding away the acrylic from the lingual tooth surfaces.

Two and a half years later, a good axial inclination of the incisors had been achieved. Mandibular growth continued, improving the anterior positioning of the mandible and increasing the S-N-B angle. The articular angle was reduced (Fig. 12-22).

This case is particularly interesting because of the untoward and unexpected side effects of the headgear treatment. Despite favorable initial conditions and projections, with the skeletal discrepancy solved within 1

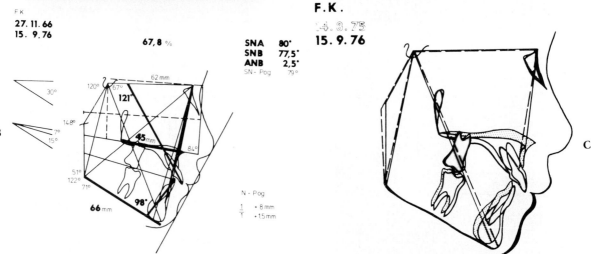

Fig. 12-21. Patient F.K. after the first phase of treatment. **C,** Superimposition of before and after tracings.

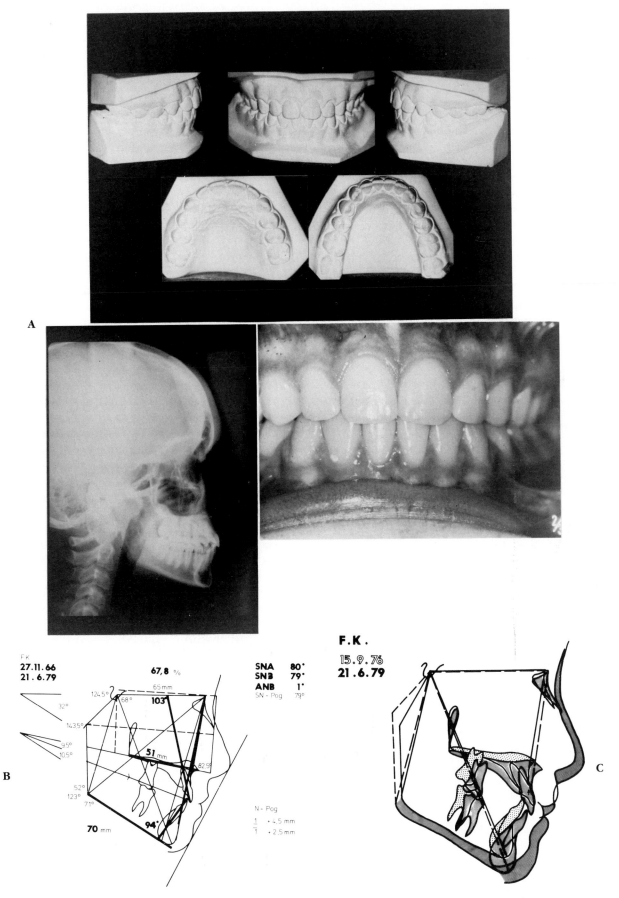

Fig. 12-22. Patient F.K. after treatment. **C,** Superimposition of tracings after the first phase and after completion.

year, the change in muscle balance induced unfavorable axial inclination changes in both upper and lower incisor segments. A good lesson can be taught here, stressing the need for continuing therapeutic diagnosis.

Combined treatment of an incisal biprotrusion.
Fig. 12-23 shows a 6-year-old boy with a Class II skeletal pattern made up of a prognathic maxilla and a retrognathic mandible. The maxillary base was average in length but positioned anteriorly. The distance from sella to pteryerygopalatine fossa was 18 mm larger than average. The mandibular base was short (−4 mm) and the ramus long (+2 mm). The growth pattern was projected as horizontal, with a slight open bite due to an upward tipping of the anterior terminus of the palatal plane. Both upper and lower incisors were tipped labially, and a definite tongue and lip habit could be seen. Despite getting complete diagnostic records, treatment was not started immediately. The patient returned 15 months later and new records were taken. There had been no change in the skeletal discrepancy. Growth increments were slight in both maxillary and mandibular bases. Ramal growth had been significant, however, and the growth direction had become more horizontal. The abnormal perioral muscle function was still present, and the incisors were more labially tipped. Potential lip incompetency was likely (Fig. 12-24).

In spite of the likely need for extraction of the four first premolars later and full multiattachment fixed appliance control if nothing was done until the full permanent dentition, therapy was begun with removable appliances and without extraction because of the persistence of the abnormal deforming muscle forces on both the labial and lingual aspects, which were exacerbating the malocclusion. Also an assessment of the profile showed a relatively normal configuration. Extraction of

the four first premolars had the potential of producing a dished-in face. Only a slight dental discrepancy existed, with spaces present between the upper incisors, and a good relation existed between the lower incisors and the N-Pog line.

The treatment objectives were to eliminate the dysfunction, to distalize the upper posterior teeth and upright the upper incisors, and to achieve a slight anterior positioning of the mandible. It was felt that this treatment approach would harmonize the intermaxillary relationship, even if the incisor protrusion could not be eliminated completely.

Therapy was initiated with a vestibular screen to eliminate, or at least inhibit, the dysfunction. Because of the tongue thrust and incisor protrusion, the screen was constructed with a tongue crib. After reduction of the potential lip incompetence, a distalizing force was applied to the upper molars with extraoral force. The occlusion was then stabilized and retained with an activator. The construction bite moved the mandible anteriorly some 5 mm, and opened the bite 3 mm. The upper incisors were tipped lingually, while the lower incisors were held in place. Incisal edges were supported by acrylic contact; both labial bows were activated.

After 4 years of treatment and retention, the A-N-B angle of 3 degrees showed an improved skeletal sagittal relationship, but the upper and lower jaws both had become prognathic. The jaw bases were of average length, but the ramus length had increased (+7 mm). The incisal protrusion persisted to some degree but the profile was improved (Fig. 12-25).

The message here is that although the patient could have been treated with first premolar extraction later, together with fixed multiattachment appliances, a reasonably good result was achieved by early interception and guidance and no extraction, using relatively simple appliances.

Treatment with a vertical activator. A case report of a 9-year-old boy illustrates the use of the vertical activator (Fig. 12-26). The patient showed a strong vertical growth pattern and a large lower gonial angle measurement on the lateral cephalogram. Both upper and lower jaw bases were retrognathic, with an A-N-B angle of 6 degrees. The mandibular retrognathism was accentuated by the large articular angle. Maxillary and mandibular bases were of average size, but the ramus was quite short (−11 mm). The palatal plane inclination was average, inclined neither upward nor downward. The axial inclination of the incisors was within normal limits, but they were positioned ahead of the N-Pog line. Maxillary incisors were rotated and crowded.

The unfavorable growth direction is a contraindication for conventional activator therapy. Anterior posi-

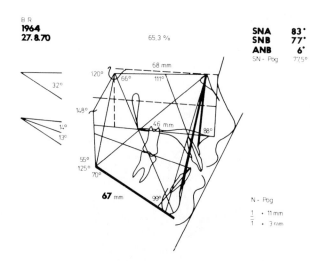

Fig. 12-23. Patient B.R. 1½ years before treatment.

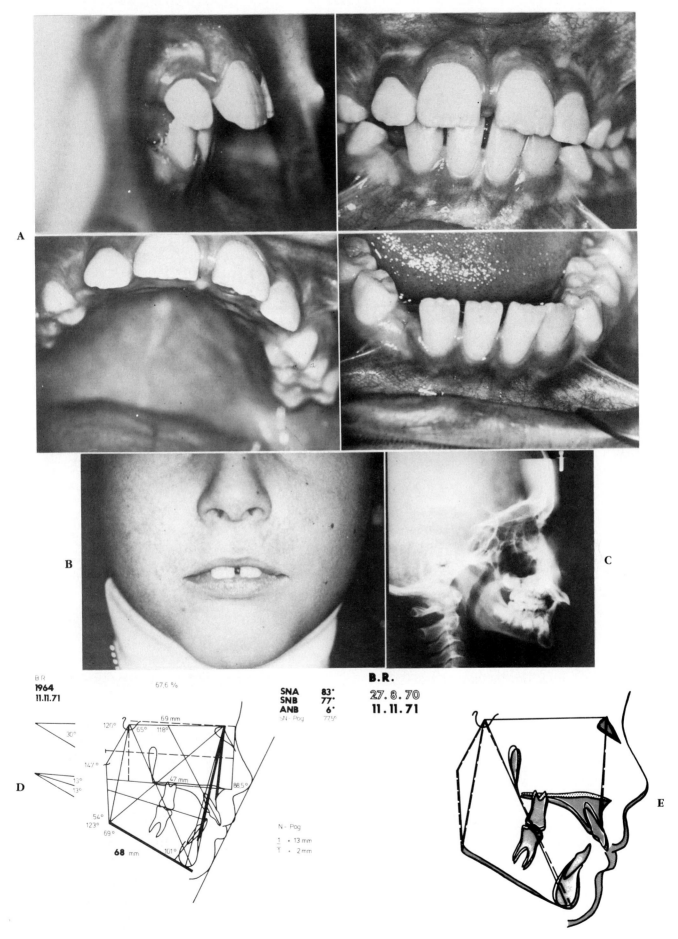

Fig. 12-24. Patient B.R. immediately before treatment. Note the incompetent lip seal, **B,** and the superimposition of tracings 1½ years before and at the initiation of treatment, **E.**

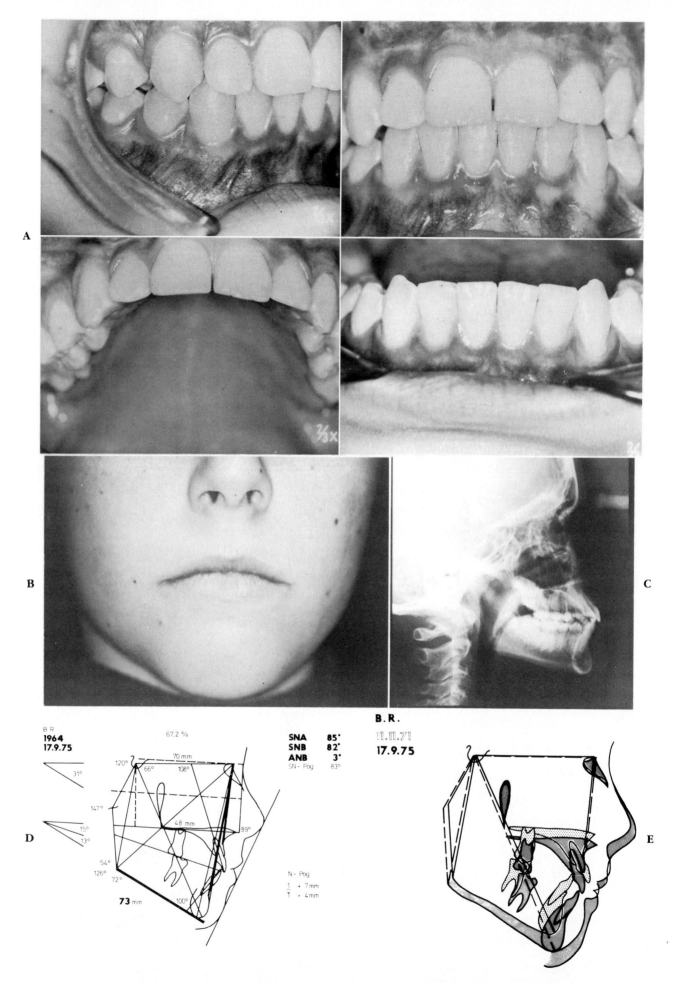

Fig. 12-25. Patient B.R. after treatment. Note the competent lip seal, **B,** and the superimposition of before and after tracings, **E.**

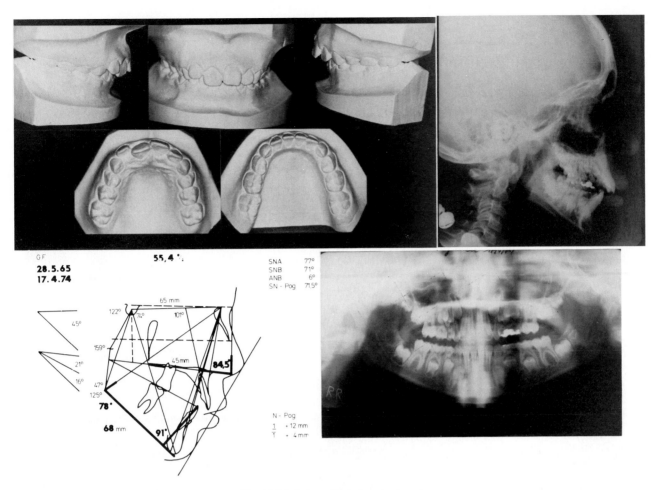

Fig. 12-26. Patient G.F. before treatment.

tioning of the mandible is not possible because of the vertical growth vector. Distalization of the upper molars would rock the mandible down and back, increasing the retrognathism. The following therapeutic alternatives can be considered.

1. Extraction of the upper first premolars and retrusion of the anterior teeth. However, this therapeutic approach is likely to overincrease the retrognathism and to elongate the incisors significantly, yielding a gummy smile.

2. Attempting a slight anterior positioning of the mandible, together with a retroinclination (tipping down) of the maxillary base to compensate for the excessive overjet. Some dental compensation would also be necessary by tipping the upper incisors lingually and the lower incisors labially.

The second method of treatment was chosen. The crowding of the upper incisors was corrected first with an anterior expansion plate (Fig. 12-27). Then a vertical activator was fabricated with a construction bite that positioned the mandible only 2 mm anteriorly but opened

the bite 8 mm. The acrylic was extended labially on the upper incisors to the area of greatest convexity, while an inclined plane was made incisally. The acrylic was ground away on the lingual. The cervically positioned labial bow was activated. The lower incisors were held in their present position with no trimming of the acrylic, although the labial bow was activated. The acrylic was trimmed in the upper posterior regions to distalize the posterior teeth, and stabilizing wires were placed mesial to the upper first molars.

After 3 years of treatment, the Class II relationship had improved. The mandible had been positioned somewhat anteriorly, and there was a high growth increment (+7 mm) with a reduction of the articular angle. However, the S-N-B angle increased to only 73 degrees, leaving the A-N-B angle at 3 degrees. A retroinclination of the maxillary base was achieved (3.5 degrees), indicating an adaptation of the maxillary base to the vertically growing mandible. The upper incisors had been tipped lingually, as planned, to reduce the overjet (Fig. 12-28).

In this case it was possible to treat the Class II vertical

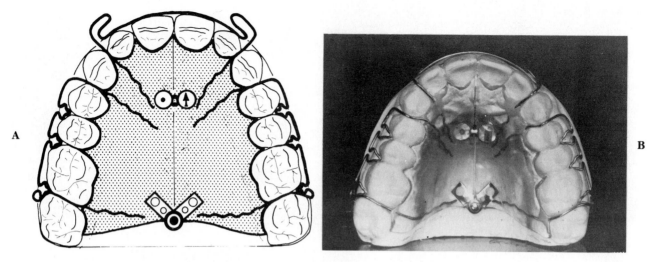

Fig. 12-27. Fan-shaped plate. **A,** Schematic and, **B,** on the cast.

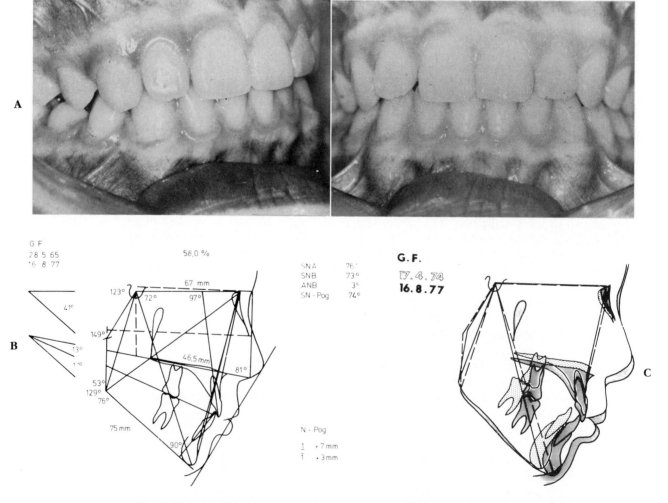

Fig. 12-28. Patient G.F. after treatment. **C,** Superimposition of before and after tracings.

growth pattern successfully with an activator because the inclination of the maxillary base was favorable (at least the anterior portion was not tipped upward) and there was a high growth increment of the mandibular base during treatment. The patient was reexamined out of retention 3 years later. Some growth in the maxillary and mandibular bases could be observed in this postretention phase. The mandibular base was now of average

length, the maxillary base slightly longer (+3 mm), and the ramus still short (−6.5 mm). Both jaw bases were retrognathic. The S-N-A and S-N-B angles were increased, at least partly due to the high maxillary base growth increment. The compensation of the overjet resulted from the labial tipping of the lower incisors. The vertical growth pattern persisted (Fig. 12-29).

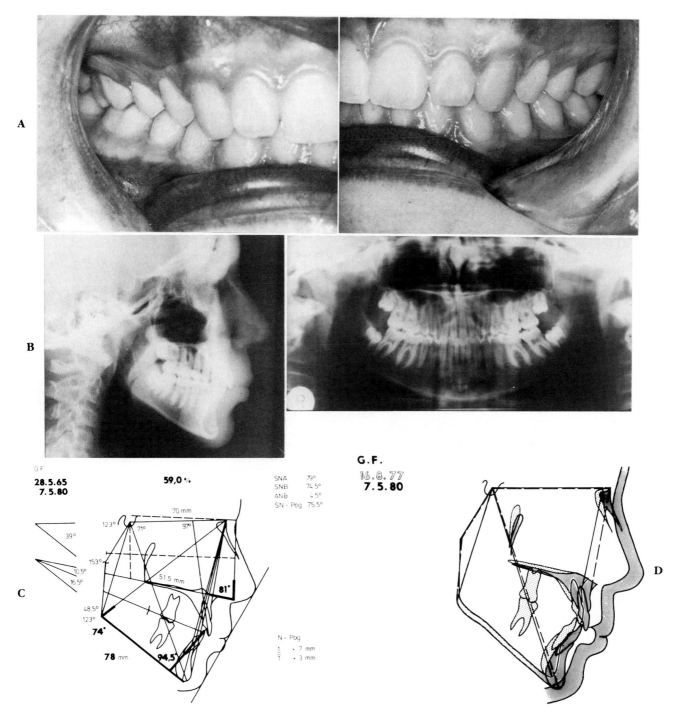

Fig. 12-29. Patient G.F. 3 years out of retention. Note the intercuspation on both right and left sides, **A,** and the superimposition of tracings after the completed treatment and after retention, **D.**

Therapy to effect changes in the inclination of the maxillary base. The tipping up or down of the anterior end of the maxillary base has a significant effect on the ultimate treatment result. The following case of an 8-year-4-month-old girl with a Class II malocclusion caused by a large maxillary prognathism illustrates the problem (Fig. 12-30).

The initial examination revealed a large S-N-A angle and an average S-N-B angle with an A-N-B angle of 6 degrees. The growth projection was average, both saddle and gonial angles were small, and the articular angle was large. Both jaw bases were long, but the ramus was short (−5 mm). The maxillary base was tipped upward anteriorly 6 degrees, and the upper incisors were procumbent. An open bite was present as a result of the tipped palatal plane. There was a prolonged finger-sucking habit present until 6 years of age, and a compensatory tongue malfunction still persisted.

The following treatment plans were considered:

1. Since the Class II relationship was caused largely by the anterior position of the maxilla, with an orthognathic mandible, conventional activator treatment was contraindicated. Distalization of the upper first molars could be attained with extraoral force, but this would tip the mandible down and back, unfavorably influencing the vertical dimension in an original open bite case. Four first premolars could be removed and full multi-attachment fixed mechanotherpay could be done, maintaining maximum anchorage in the maxilla and reciprocal anchorage in the mandible as spaces were closed. However, the patient was too young for this approach, and further enhancement of the malocclusion by abnormal perioral muscle function was likely while waiting for the eruption of the permanent dentition.

2. Because of the worsening malocclusion, a functional approach could be used immediately. At least the deforming effects of the lip and tongue dysfunctions could be eliminated. It was felt that the tipping upward of the palatal plane and the labial inclination of the upper incisors were due to the abnormal perioral muscle function initiated by the longtime finger-sucking habit that had depressed the maxillary anterior segment and allowed overeruption of the posterior teeth.

The treatment objectives were as follows:

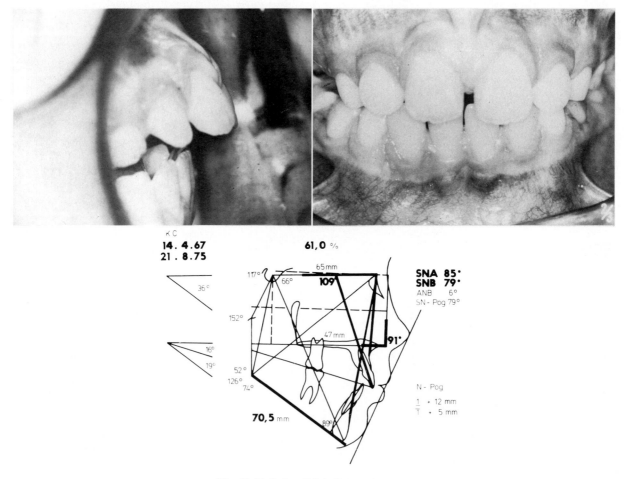

Fig. 12-30. Patient K.C. before treatment.

1. The prognathic maxilla should be adapted to the orthognathic mandible by tipping down the palatal plane and repositioning of the maxilla.
2. In the dentoalveolar region, a compensation could be achieved by lingual tipping of the maxillary incisors.

A vertical activator was constructed, opening the bite 8 mm with no mandibular advancement. The mandibular acrylic portion of the appliance was not trimmed. The lower teeth were held, and the acrylic plate was extended with flanges in the molar region. The acrylic was also extended as high as possible in the labial area of the upper incisors but trimmed away incisally and lingually to permit these teeth to be extruded and move lingually under the influence of an active labial bow. To eliminate the abnormal tongue function, an active plate with a tongue crib was worn during the day during the first months of treatment.

After 4 years of therapy, both sagittal and vertical relationships had been improved, although the maxillary prognathism was still present. The maxillary base had rotated inferiorly in the anterior region some 3 degrees without posterior relocation. The upper incisors had tipped lingually 13 degrees, so that partial skeletal and dentoalveolar compensation existed. Both maxillary and mandibular basal growth increments were high. The ramus remained short, and the projected average growth direction persisted. As indicated previously, the maxillary prognathism was not affected (Fig. 12-31). If headgear therapy had been used, the S-N-A angle could have been decreased; but there also could have been unfavorable bite opening with an accentuation of the open bite and mandibular retrognathism. The vertical dimension was improved by the therapy of choice, even though it was still not quite correct.

A compensation of the malocclusion enables the vertical activator treatment to influence the inclination of the maxillary base. This is especially important in thumb-sucking problems that create deficient midface vertical dimensions. Prognosis for successful therapy is

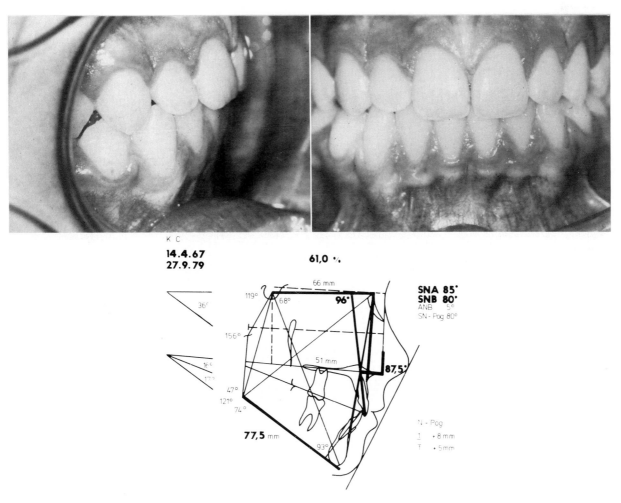

Fig. 12-31. Patient K.C. after treatment.

good in these cases if caught early enough. Cases with an average growth pattern but tipping up of the maxillary base are treated similarly to vertical growth patterns because of the greater need to stress correction of the vertical components of the malocclusion.

Treatment of Class II malocclusions with divergent growth rotation of the jaw bases. These problems, first described by Björk and later elaborated by Lavergne and Gasson, should be recognized early. Yet the 9-year-old patient illustrated in Fig. 12-32 shows a classic contraindication for activator therapy. The girl still sucked her finger when seen and had an anterior open bite. The malocclusion was also due to a skeletal discrepancy, i.e., divergent rotation of the jaws during growth. This type of open bite cannot be successfully treated with screening therapy because of this unfavorable growth process. In addition to the open bite, a maxillary prognathism was present, with an S-N-A angle of 86 degrees. The total discrepancy in the upper arch was 11 mm, divided as follows:

1. A sagittal discrepancy of 8 mm. The upper incisors were 12 mm ahead of the N-Pog line and needed to be moved to about 4 mm ahead of this line. Any anterior positioning of pogonion by future growth increments and proper direction, improving the sagittal relationship as well as the N-Pog line, was not likely in this case because of the downward and backward mandibular growth.

2. The dental discrepancy was 3 mm per quadrant. Spaces existed between the incisors but were inadequate in the canine region. To gain space by distalization of the posterior segments would not be possible because of the divergent jaw bases and the wedging open of the bite. It also was not possible to adapt the mandible to the prognathic maxilla. The mandible was only slightly retrognathic, with no dental discrepancy but with a good relationship of the lower incisors. The maxillary base was relatively long compared to the short mandibular base and ramus length.

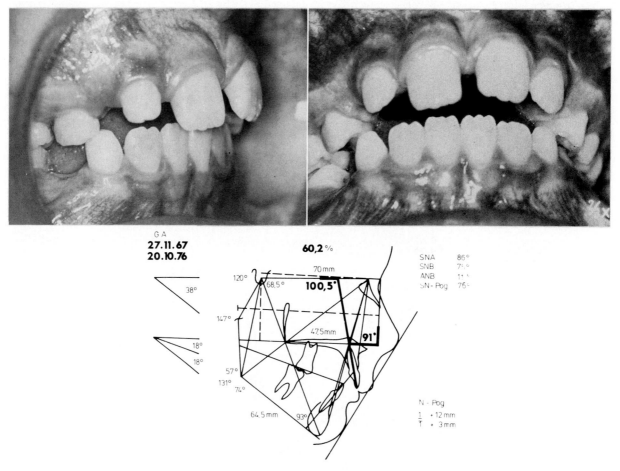

Fig. 12-32. Patient G.A. before treatment.

The treatment decisions were as follows:

1. The correction of the malocclusion should be postponed, because retrusion of the upper incisors and canines was required. The only treatment available was extraction of two upper first premolars followed by fixed multiattachment control.

2. Because of the finger-sucking and perioral neuromuscular compensation and exacerbation, a pretreatment phase of guidance with a vestibular screen was recommended to prevent further deformation and, it was hoped, to eliminate the deleterious environmental influences.

3. The upper first premolars would then be removed at the beginning of the second or active treatment phase, with fixed appliances applying maximum anchorage to the maxillary posterior teeth while retracting and extruding the anterior segment to correct the open bite and excessive overjet.

These approaches were implemented. No lower appliances were used. Three and one half years later the overjet was reduced, but the Class II skeletal and buccal segment relationship remained. The maxillary base and ramus were of average length, the mandibular base was small and retrognathic. The maxillary prognathism had decreased, but the upward tipping of the maxillary base was even more pronounced. The upper incisors had been moved lingually and torqued; the lower incisors had tipped slightly labially. The divergent growth pattern and maxillary prognathism were compensated by the dentoalveolar adjustment (Fig. 12-33).

This type of Class II malocclusion, with a maxillary prognathism and divergent, or at least vertical, growth patterns and a well-aligned lower arch, is probably the only indication for extraction of the two upper first premolars. Functional methods cannot be expected to influence such a skeletal dysplasia much, even though Frän-

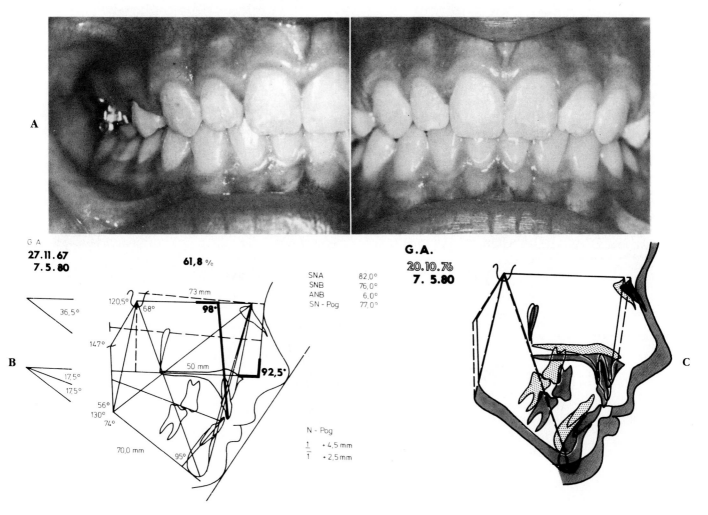

Fig. 12-33. Patient G.A. after the active phase of treatment. **C,** Superimposition of before and after tracings.

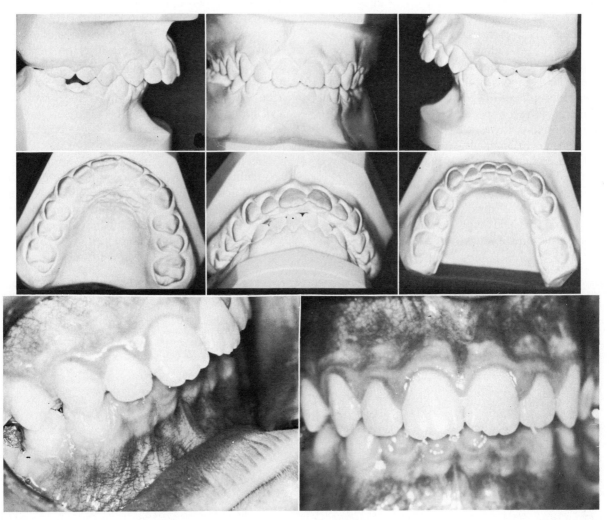

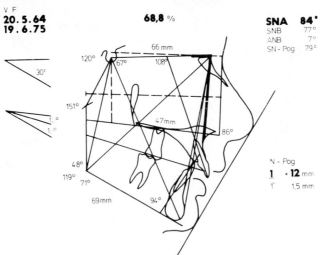

Fig. 12-34. Patient V.F. before treatment.

kel has shown selected cases that seem to indicate a change in growth direction under rigorous FR wear and a stringent exercise discipline. The use of the interceptive vestibular screen in the first phase of treatment reduces only the local neuromuscular deformational potential until full mechanotherapy can be instituted.

Multiattachment treatment after failure of activator therapy. The following case shows the fixed appliance alternatives after unsuccessful early functional appliance attempts.

The patient was an 11-year-old boy with a Class II sagittal relationship, a horizontal growth pattern, and a deep overbite. The boy's developmental age was 12 years, although the permanent second molars had not yet erupted (Fig. 12-34). The patient had a lower lip-sucking habit and a marked mentolabial sulcus. The postural rest position was posterior as the mandible slid anteriorly into habitual occlusion. Despite the deep bite, the interocclusal clearance was small.

Cephalometric evaluation indicated that the Class II relationship was probably due to maxillary prognathism, since there was only slight mandibular retrognathism. The growth direction was markedly horizontal for this age group. The jaw bases and ramus were of average length. The upper incisors were tipped slightly labially and 12 mm ahead of the N-Pog line; the lower incisors were in good position. The slight labial tipping of the lower incisors, despite the confirmed lower lip habit, and no evidence of tongue thrust could be explained by the case history. The patient had been treated with an activator. Unfortunately, no original records were available to assess the original malocclusion. The motivation of the patient seemed to be good, but he was disap-

pointed with the failure of activator therapy. Why had the activator not been successful, despite the horizontal growth direction? The answer seems to be that the morphologic and functional relationships were unfavorable for activator treatment.

In cases with maxillary prognathism, it is better to institute therapy with extraoral force. Even in cases with a horizontal growth pattern, it is not possible to adapt the mandible to a prognathic maxilla. In a reexamination of activator therapy cases that have not been successful, many of them show a larger than normal S-N-A angle. In such cases, particularly with a full Class II relationship, it is advisable to start with a headgear for maxillary retraction.

The functional pattern was not favorable in this case for activator treatment. The posterior rest position was masked by the anterior habitual occlusion, which resulted from cuspal guidance. The small interocclusal clearance was also a contraindication. The lower lip habit increased the excessive overjet.

Treatment was begun with maxillary extraoral force and a lower removable appliance with lip pads to intercept the lip habit. The labial bow of the lower appliance stabilized the lower incisors, while the pads eliminated the perverted function and established normal lip seal. The acrylic lingual to the lower incisors was trimmed away.

After 1½ years of this second phase of treatment, the upper molars had moved distally and were extruded some, opening the bite slightly. The lower incisors had uprighted. The S-N-A angle and the overjet were reduced (Fig. 12-35). An activator might have been used in the second phase, except that the deep bite and func-

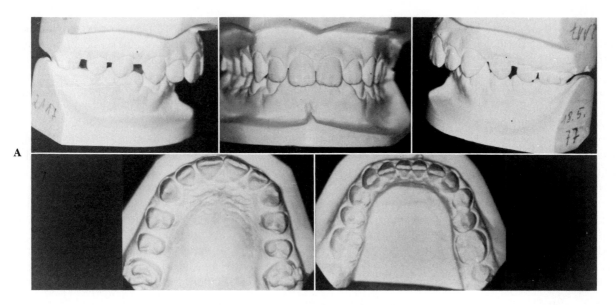

Fig. 12-35. Patient V.F. after the first phase of treatment.

Continued.

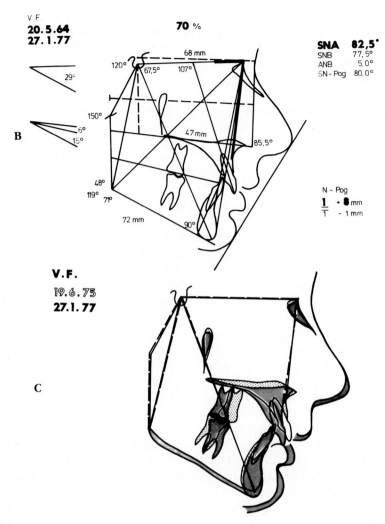

Fig. 12-35, cont'd. B, Before treatment and, **C,** superimposition of before and after tracings.

tional pattern would work against its success. Without leveling of the excessive curve of Spee, the deep overbite could not be completely controlled. After the eruption of the premolars, this type of leveling is not possible with functional methods. Significant extrusion of the lower posterior teeth, together with intrusive forces on the lower anterior teeth, is required for the best possible correction.

After distalization of the upper first molars, spaces were present in the upper buccal segments. Only careful control of fixed appliances allows the proper closure of these spaces by distalization of the remaining buccal segment teeth with torque and intrusion of the incisors. In this case the upper arch was aligned and spaces were closed with elastic traction combined with extraoral force.

After 1½ years of second phase active treatment, the

Class II relationship had been corrected and the overbite and overjet reduced. There was continued mandibular growth and a more anterior position. The S-N-A angle was reduced to 81 degrees. The incisor relationship was partially compensated by a light labial tipping of the lower incisors (Fig. 12-36). Leveling of the curve of Spee (compensating curve) was accomplished as planned. Over the course of treatment the growth increments of the mandibular base and ramus were average, Although the ramus was overly long from the beginning of therapy. Maxillary basal growth was minimal—1 mm.

Hindsight is always better than foresight, but this case might have been treated more successfully in the mixed dentition if therapy had been initiated with extraoral force to reduce the maxillary prognathism. With early correction of the Class II molar relationship, the maxillary buccal segment teeth migrate distally in their erup-

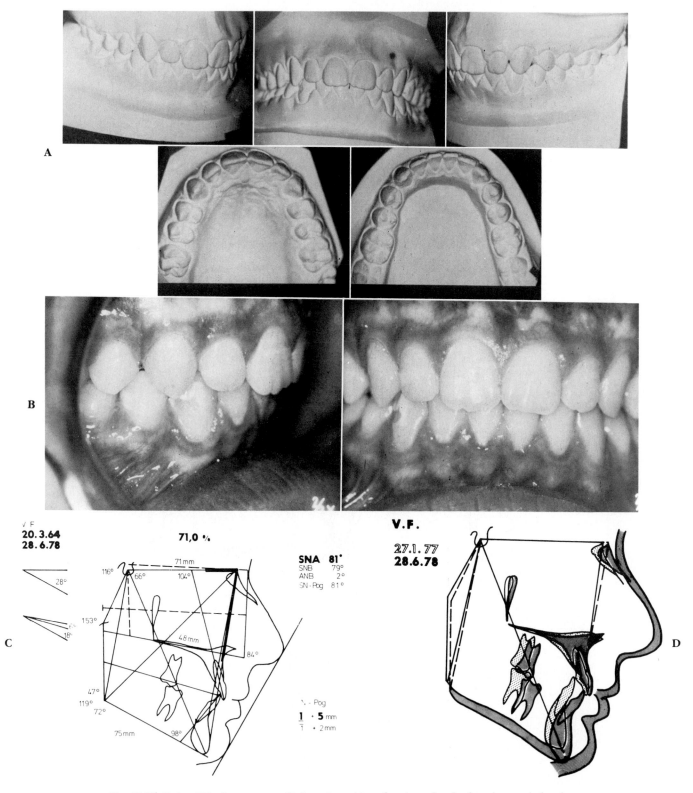

Fig. 12-36. Patient V.F. after treatment. **D,** Superimposition of tracings after the first phase and after the completion of therapy.

tion. This movement can be well guided with an activator. The likely mistake was to begin treatment with an activator instead of a headgear.

Multiattachment fixed mechanotherapy with maxillary second molar extraction, following unsuccessful early activator treatment. There is more than one way to recoup partial activator correction of Class II malocclusions. This is illustrated by a 15-year-old girl with a mature 17-year-old developmental age and a horizontal growth pattern (Fig. 12-37).

Diagnostic records taken at 15 years showed long and prognathic jaw bases in relation to the cranial base. The A-N-B difference was 4 degrees. The incisors were tipped labially. The lower incisors were excellent relative to the N-Pog line, but the upper incisors were still 9 mm

ahead of this plane. The teeth were well aligned in the lower arch but slight crowding existed in the upper arch. The path of closure from postural rest to occlusion was upward and forward, with a normal hinge or rotary condylar movement. The interocclusal space was 3 mm. The patient had been treated between 9 and 12 years of age with an activator. The likely reason for failure was the initial and continuing maxillary prognathism. In retrospect, maxillary withholding and distalization would have adapted the protrusive maxilla to the mandible.

Since the developmental age of 17 years allowed only dental compensation for skeletal malrelationships, and since extensive distalization of maxillary posterior teeth (about 6 mm) was still required, tooth sacrifice offered the only possibility. Premolar extraction was contraindi-

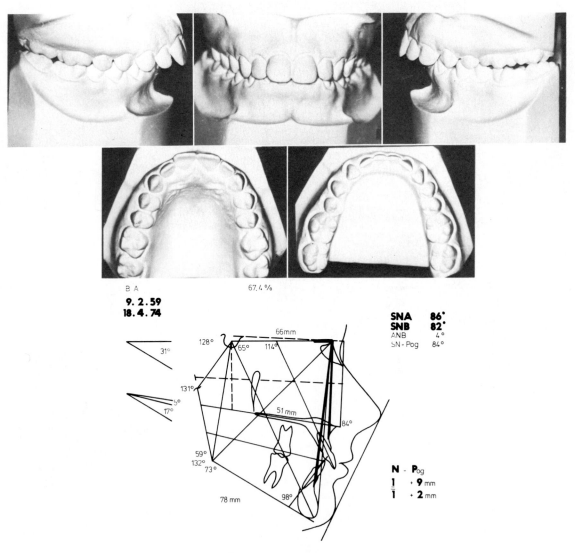

Fig. 12-37. Patient B.A. before treatment.

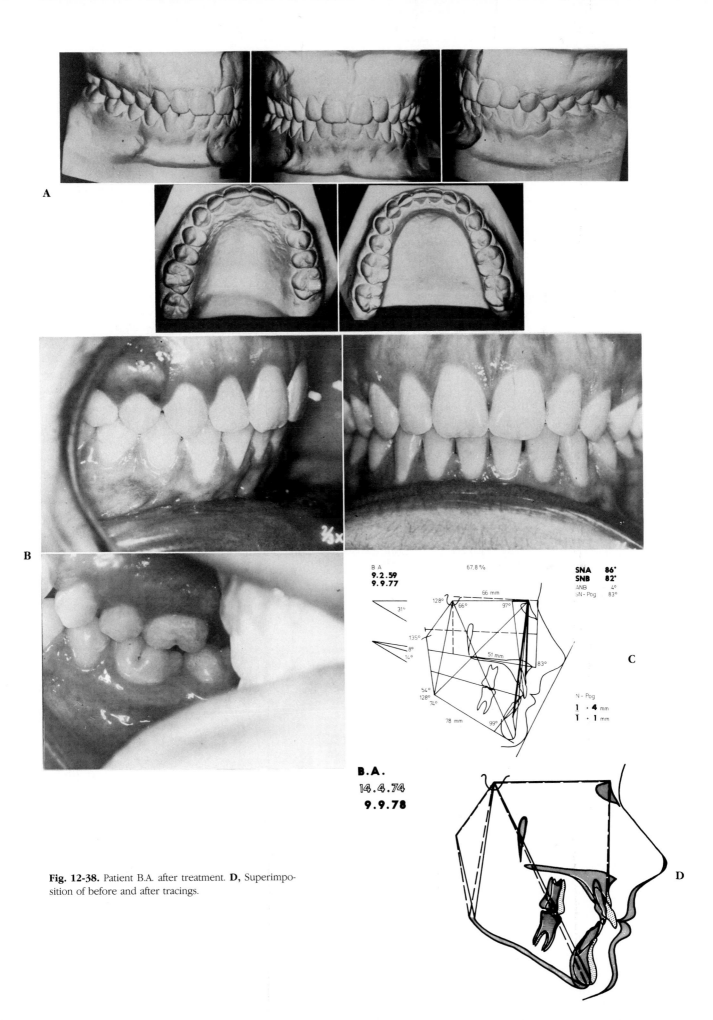

Fig. 12-38. Patient B.A. after treatment. **D,** Superimposition of before and after tracings.

cated because of the horizontal growth pattern and the possibility of residual spacing distal to the canines. Also there was no appreciable help in control of the overbite with such an approach. Only by distalization of all the maxillary buccal segments could the bite be opened and corrected sagittally at the same time. Maxillary incisor intrusion alone would be limited at this stage and would not provide enough correction of the incisor overbite. The only approach left, with third molars present and in good position in the tuberosity area, was to remove the maxillary second molars after being assured of good patient compliance.

In such cases it is quite effective to first distalize the maxillary first molars with extraoral force and then to place the remaining multiattachment appliance to complete the correction. This two-phase approach shortens the treatment time. With continued use of stabilizing headgear to hold the molars in the Class I relationship, distalization of the remaining teeth can be accomplished by intramaxillary elastics and power chains. Retrusive, intrusive, and torque adjustments are necessary to gain the best posible incisor relationship. Class II elastics are also necessary on a part-time basis to assist in this maneuver and to slightly elevate the lower molars for overbite control. Care must be taken not to flare the lower incisors labially. A lower headgear can be used to bolster lower anchorage, if desired.

After 2 years of active treatment, no skeletal change was noted, but the dentoalveolar relationships were improved and the deep overbite was corrected (Fig. 12-38). Profile improvement was also accomplished with an improved lip line. No success had been achieved with the early first phase activator treatment, though early treatment could have prevented the increasing severity of the malocclusion. If extraoral force had been used, the orthopedic changes would have been greater in the area where it was needed most—in retracting the prognathic maxilla. After growth is complete, only dental compensation is possible, as this case illustrates.

SUMMARY

There are a number of ways to attempt the correction of Class II malocclusions. The method chosen depends on a series of factors that must be carefully evaluated before instituting therapy:

1. The developmental age of the patient
2. The localization and etiology of the malocclusion
3. The functional relationship
4. The specific morphologic characteristics in both the skeletal and the dental areas
5. The motivation and likely continuing cooperation of both the patient and the patient's parents

There is no universal appliance or cookbook formula for Class II therapy. All patients cannot be fitted into the same appliance, any more than the fabled Procrustes could fit all his guests into the same bed. Only a careful and complete diagnosis, a continued diagnostic monitoring during treatment, a careful step-by-step accomplishment of the treatment objectives, a number of appliances in the armamentarium, and a willingness to change appliances as changing situations dictate, alone or in combination, assure the best possible treatment.

CHAPTER 13

THE DEEP OVERBITE

In treating a deep overbite, more than the vertical dimension is of concern. It is also necessary to consider the sagittal relationship and the direction and amount of growth to be expected for the particular patient.

Most of the problems concerning treatment objectives have already been discussed in Chapter 12. However, there are some types of Class II malocclusions that have a horizontal growth pattern, in which the correction of deep overbite problems is more difficult than the correction of the sagittal Class II relationship. In many adults, orthognathic surgery is the only answer for complete correction, not because of the sagittal malrelationship as much as because of the vertical dimension deficiency, a deficiency dependent on growth guidance, which is not possible in the adult patient. Excessive overjet can be corrected by the removal of two upper premolars and the therapeutic retrusion of the incisors. In most adults this means an actual deepening of the bite as the incisors are uprighted during space closure.

The overbite problem and the entire vertical dimension should be considered in the treatment of every malocclusion. The vertical dimension is unique in that the growth rate is highest and lasts the longest in this vector. Since growth tends to increase the vertical distance between the jaw bases, it is advantageous to perform the treatment during this period. Yet the vertical dimension is not stable. Even in adults who have never had any orthodontic treatment, significant changes can occur. Abrasion or loss of teeth can close down the vertical dimension. Tooth elongation or overeruption can also occur and can increase the vertical dimension. The stability of the tooth position depends on the eruption or elongation tendency of the teeth on one hand and on the opposing forces on the other. This means that if the occlusal forces are altered the equilibrium is disturbed and the teeth migrate in the direction of the occlusal plane.

ETIOLOGIC CONSIDERATIONS

From an etiologic standpoint, overbite can be differentiated into the developmental deep bite and the acquired deep bite. There are two types of developmental or genetically determined deep overbites.

1. The skeletal deep overbite with a horizontal growth pattern
2. The dentoalveolar deep bite caused by supraocclusion of the incisors. In these cases the interocclusal clearance is usually small, meaning the overbite is functionally a pseudo–deep overbite.

Therapeutic correction of a developmental deep overbite is very difficult and is usually successful only with active mechanical methods.

The acquired deep overbite may be caused by the following factors:

1. A lateral tongue thrust or postural position frequently can produce an acquired deep overbite. This type of dysfunction produces an infraocclusion of the posterior teeth, which in turn leads to a deep overbite. A classic Class II, Division 2, malocclusion is a good example of this type of case. The freeway space is usually large, which is favorable for functional appliance treatment.
2. Premature loss of deciduous molars or early loss of permanent posterior teeth can cause an acquired secondary deep overbite, particularly if the contiguous teeth are tipped into the extraction sites.
3. The wearing away of the occlusal surface or tooth abrasion can produce an acquired, secondary deep overbite.

THE MORPHOLOGIC CHARACTERISTICS OF THE DEEP OVERBITE

The deep overbite can be localized in either the dentoalveolar or skeletal areas. The localization or area affected determines the type of treatment.

Dentoalveolar deep overbite

The dentoalveolar deep overbite is characterized by infraocclusion of the molars and/or supraocclusion of the incisors (Fig. 13-1). The growth pattern usually is average or tends toward the vertical.

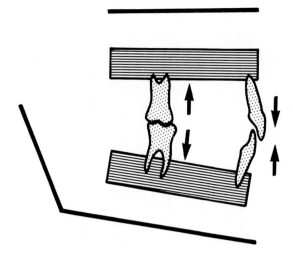

Fig. 13-1. Dentoalveolar deep overbite caused by infraocclusion of the molars and/or supraocclusion of the incisors.

The deep overbite that is due to the infraocclusion of molars has the following symptoms:

1. The molars are partially erupted.
2. The interocclusal space is large.
3. A lateral tongue posture and thrust are present.
4. The distances between the maxillary and mandibular basal planes and the occlusal plane are short.

The deep overbite caused by overeruption of the incisors has the following characteristics:

1. The incisal margins of the incisors extend beyond the functionl occlusal plane.
2. The molars are fully erupted.
3. The curve of Spee (compensating curve) is excessive.
4. The interocclusal space is small.

Skeletal deep overbite

The skeletal deep overbite is characterized by a horizontal type of growth pattern. The anterior facial height is short, particularly the lower facial third, while the posterior facial height is long. While the normal ratio of upper to lower anterior facial height is 2:3, it is reduced in the skeletal deep overbite case to a ratio of 2:2.5 or 2:2.8. The horizontal cephalometric planes (sella-nasion, palatal, occlusal, and mandibular) are approximately parallel to each other. The interocclusal clearance is usually small (Fig. 13-2).

The inclination of the maxillary base is of significance when evaluating the treatment plan for this type of problem. An extreme horizontal growth pattern can be at least partially compensated by an upward and forward inclination of the maxillary base (anteinclination). On the other hand, the combination of a horizontal growth pattern with a downward and forward inclination (retro-

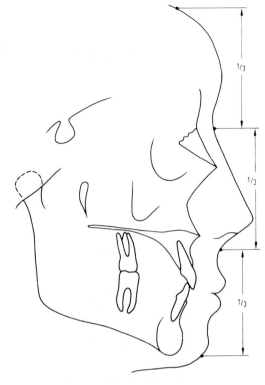

Fig. 13-2. Normal facial proportions are altered in the skeletal deep overbite malocclusions. The anterior lower face height is shorter.

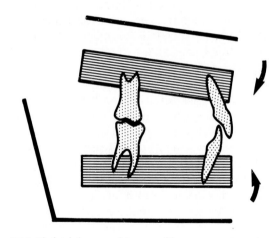

Fig. 13-3. Skeletal deep overbite caused by convergent rotation of the jaw bases.

clination) of the maxillary base results in a more severe skeletal deep overbite (Fig. 13-3).

TREATMENT PLANNING

There are problem-specific therapeutic measures that can be taken, depending on the nature of the deep overbite, either skeletal or dentoalveolar. In skeletal problems therapy should be directed toward enhancement of

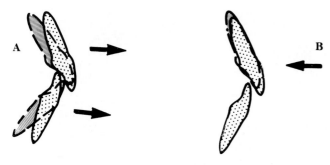

Fig. 13-4. A deep overbite in the incisal region can be treated by labial tipping of the upper and lower incisors, **A,** or distal driving and intrusion of the upper incisors only, **B.**

the divergent rotation of the jaw bases, using whatever appliances that are available, both fixed and removable. In dentoalveolar problems intrusion and labial inclination of the incisors are desirable, as well as extrusion of the posterior segment teeth and a leveling of the occlusal plane to reduce the curve of Spee (Fig. 13-4).

An important consideration is whether the therapy is performed during or after the growth period. During the growth period, tooth eruption can be stimulated in the posterior and inhibited in the anterior segments. The vertical growth component in the condylar and sutural areas is also amenable to favorable therapeutic influence. Extrusion of the molars and premolars also implies a skeletal growth stimulus with vertical rotation of the mandible, rocking the mandible down and back. Such a maneuver, of course, can accentuate the sagittal discrepancy in a Class II malocclusion, increasing the angle of facial convexity.

If treatment is performed in the adult dentition, after all growth has ceased, the extruded molars can create a molar fulcrum, without additional growth or developmental adaptation. The molars thus act as a premature occlusal contact for mandibular rotation (Fig. 13-5). This rotation can occur in either an anterior or posterior direction and has potent TMJ implications.

During anterior rotation, the condylar and TMJ structures can be damaged by subluxation or distraction of the associated ligaments, the retrodiskal pad, the capsule, etc. Subluxation may be needed for acute TMJ dysfunction syndromes, but this should be handled carefully, particularly in light of nocturnal parafunctional activity. TMJ problems can be created by such maneuvers, where they did not exist before, inciting nocturnal bruxism and clenching.

During a posterior rotation the bite will open, creating occlusal interferences and disturbances. While bite opening may be desirable as a therapeutic objective, the clinician must keep in mind that occlusal equilibration will likely be needed, since growth compensation is

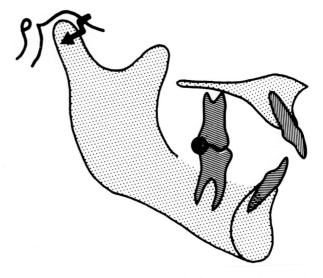

Fig. 13-5. Distal driving of the upper molars can result in a molar fulcrum and premature contact, with levering of the condyles.

minimal or nonexistent. Without constant attention to the establishment of proper exteroceptive and proprioceptive occlusal contact, TMJ dysfunction, with attendant bruxism and clenching, can be created and exacerbated.

Depending on the age or developmental status of the patient and the etiologic basis and location of the malocclusion, a variety of therapeutic measures are available to the clinician. In the growing individual, growth stimulation is a valid treatment objective with functional appliances. In the true deep bite problem, with a large interocclusal clearance, lateral tongue posture and function, and infraocclusion of posterior teeth, functional appliances are valid tools.

In all other types of deep overbite, after the possibility of growth stimulation is gone, fixed or removable mechanical appliances are needed to achieve the optimal treatment response. Causal treatment is possible in the dentoalveolar type of problem by intrusion of the incisors and leveling of the curve of Spee (Fig. 13-6). However, the skeletal discrepancy can be compensated for only by dentoalveolar orthodontic or orthognathic surgical methods.

Treatment of the dentoalveolar deep overbite

Treatment mechanics depend on the specific malocclusion characteristics. In cases of a *true deep overbite,* the goal of treatment is extrusion of the molars and premolars. During eruption of the posterior teeth, the therapy can be performed with an activator to guide the eruption. In cases with extreme lateral tongue thrust, a palatal plate with a lateral tongue crib can be used to discourage the habit. If there is an additional cheek-

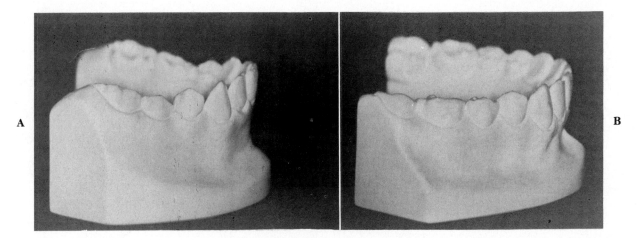

Fig. 13-6. Leveling of the compensating curve is the precondition for correction of a deep overbite. **A,** Before and, **B,** after treatment.

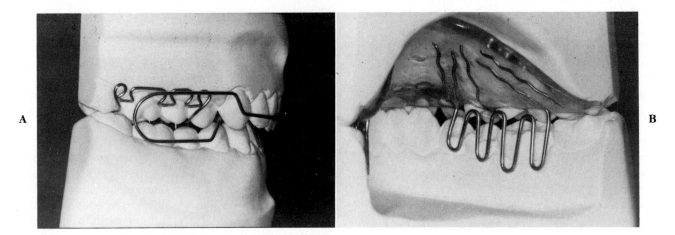

Fig. 13-7. Palatal plate construction for screening of lateral tongue thrust and cheek sucking. **A,** Labial bow with buccinator loops. **B,** The lateral tongue crib permits extrusion of the molars.

sucking habit, this can can be eliminated with a modified labial bow (Fig. 13-7). Similar in construction to the Bionator, the bow has buccinator loops. Use of this type of plate may be alternated with an activator, with the plate being worn during the day and the activator being worn at night.

Elongation or further eruption of the posterior teeth can also be achieved with biteplates. This type of plate loads the incisors for intrusive effect, while the posterior segments are free to erupt, leveling the curve of Spee. Actually intrusion is minimal, but a relative intrusion occurs with the extrusion of the posterior teeth.

The use of the biteplate had not been described yet, since it is not a true functional appliance (Fig. 13-8). However, it can be used in deep bite cases in late mixed, transitional, or early permanent dentitions. The method of anchoring or clasping—arrow, Adams, or crib clasps—depends on the stage of dentitional development. Arrow clasps have the advantage of contacting the teeth at the gingival third of the embrasure, with a wedging effect that stimulates eruption. The labial bow helps to stabilize the biteplate and contacts the teeth at the incisal third. The most important part is the acrylic bite plane or block immediately behind the maxillary incisors. Acting as a premature incisal stop, usually within the confines of the interocclusal clearance, the posterior teeth are freed of occlusal contact and can erupt. To stabilize the position of the mandible where no change is desired, a seating groove is cut for the lower incisors in the acrylic plane. Since the plate is not trying to position the mandible anteriorly, the angle of the plane is 90 degrees to the long axis of the lower incisors. After full eruption of the permanent teeth, treatment usually requires completion with fixed appli-

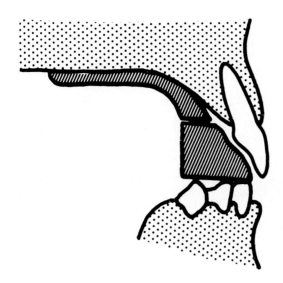

Fig. 13-8. Bite plane for intrusion of the lower incisors and simultaneous extrusion of the molars.

ances, except when the original problem was solely one of dysfunction, a condition that has been corrected by the activator.

The treatment of *pseudo–deep overbite* is more difficult. The prime objective here is the intrusion of the incisor teeth, which can be done with only limited success by an activator or biteplates. It is possible to achieve a slight intrusion in the mixed dentition, along with some labial tipping of the incisors, which has the effect of reducing the overbite. Multibanded control is still necessary in the more severe cases.

The treatment of the *acquired deep overbite* really requires multiattachment fixed appliances for optimal correction, although it can be improved with plates and pullsprings. The uprighting of tipped molars has a significant effect on the reduction of the overbite. Fixed appliances do this best.

The steep compensating curve (of Spee) must be leveled for maximum correction of the deep overbite. This leveling can be done during the eruption of the posterior teeth by eruption guidance with the activator that has been properly ground in the interocclusal area. Again leveling in the permanent dentition requires fixed appliances with individual tooth control and intermaxillary elastic traction or vertical elastic stimulus of eruption.

Treatment of skeletal deep overbite

As pointed out initially in this chapter, the treatment of a skeletal deep overbite requires consideration of the sagittal dimension. Most skeletal deep overbites are combined with Class II sagittal intercuspation.

The treatment of a deep overbite that is combined with a Class II sagittal malrelationship can be handled by several therapeutic approaches. Growth inhibition of the upper jaw and growth promotion in the lower jaw combined with dentoalveolar changes should result in the improvement of a deep overbite. The treatment can be performed by the use of a headgear in combination with an activator. Treatment may proceed as follows:

1. Distalization and elongation of the upper first permanent molars. The eruption of the teeth in the posterior segments can then be guided by a properly trimmed activator.
2. The unfavorable inclination of the jaw bases should be opened, if at all possible, in convergent growth rotation patterns. This can be achieved at least partly with an activator of special design or by the use of extraoral force.
3. Dentoalveolar compensation for a deep bite is needed, especially in skeletal deep overbite when the growth period is completed. This can be performed by extrusion and distalization of the maxillary molars, sometimes aided by second molar extraction. Intrusion and labial tipping of the lower incisors with leveling of the curve of Spee further benefit the dentoalveolar compensation.

Early treatment of deep overbite

Treatment started in the early mixed dentition has the possibility of influencing the skeletal characteristics of the deep overbite malocclusion. A case in point illustrates the potential.

A 6-year-3-month-old patient has a severe overbite with demonstrable gingival impingement (Fig. 13-9). There was evidence of constant traumatic irritation of the impinged gingival margin because of the deep bite. The objective of early treatment was to relieve the gingival impingement and to support the overbite dentally. Treatment of this tissue impingement type of deep bite is indicated later on; but without growth, orthognathic surgery may be the only mode of correction to prevent early loss of incisor teeth.

The growth direction in this patient was horizontal despite a short and retrognathic mandibular base. This retrognathism was accentuated by the posterior position of the temporal fossa (a large cranial base angle). The ramus was long, however, as was the maxillary base. The functional analysis indicated a large interocclusal clearance and lateral tongue thrust and posture symptoms. This malocclusion configuration is usually amenable to correction by functional appliances.

The objectives of treatment were as follows:

1. Distalization of the upper molars to help on both the sagittal and the vertical dysplasia, opening the

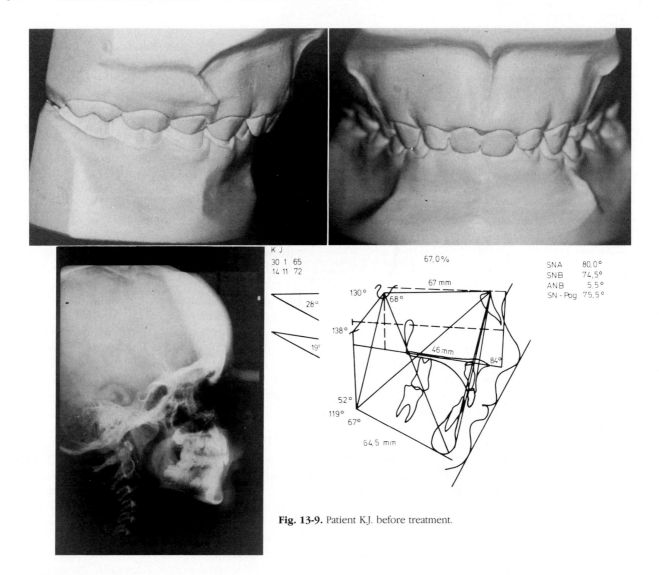

Fig. 13-9. Patient K.J. before treatment.

bite as the teeth were moved posteriorly and extruded into the wedge. This task was to be performed with extraoral force.

2. Extrusion of the partially erupted buccal segment teeth as the second phase of orthodontic guidance. An activator was fabricated and trimmed to stimulate extrusion of the posterior segments, while exerting an intrusive force on the anterior teeth to level out the curve of Spee.

3. Elimination of the lateral tongue posture and thrust, which created much of the problem by preventing full eruption of the posterior teeth. This was controlled by a removable plate–type appliance that incorporated lateral tongue cribs and was worn during the day. The labial bow of the plate incorporated buccal loop extensions similar to those in the Bionator to prevent the cheeks from interposing between the occlusal surfaces.

The period of treatment, including retention, contin-

ued beyond the eruption of the first premolars and lasted 4½ years. An examination made 2 years after retention showed an improvement of both the mandibular retrognathism and the deep overbite. The molars had been extruded while the incisors were intruded (Fig. 13-10). The relationship between the eruption height of the incisors was thus altered favorably. According to Schwarz, the relationship in a normal case should be a ratio of 5:4 for the incisor to molar height (Fig. 13-11). In this particular case, before treatment, the molar infraocclusion resulted in a ratio of 5:3.7 in the upper and 5:3.8 in the lower dental arch. Therapeutic correction changed this ratio to 5:4.4 in the upper and 5:4.1 in the lower jaw.

Early treatment of Class II, Division 2, malocclusion

A Class II, Division 2, problem in an 8-year-old boy is used to illustrate early treatment. The initial habitual oc-

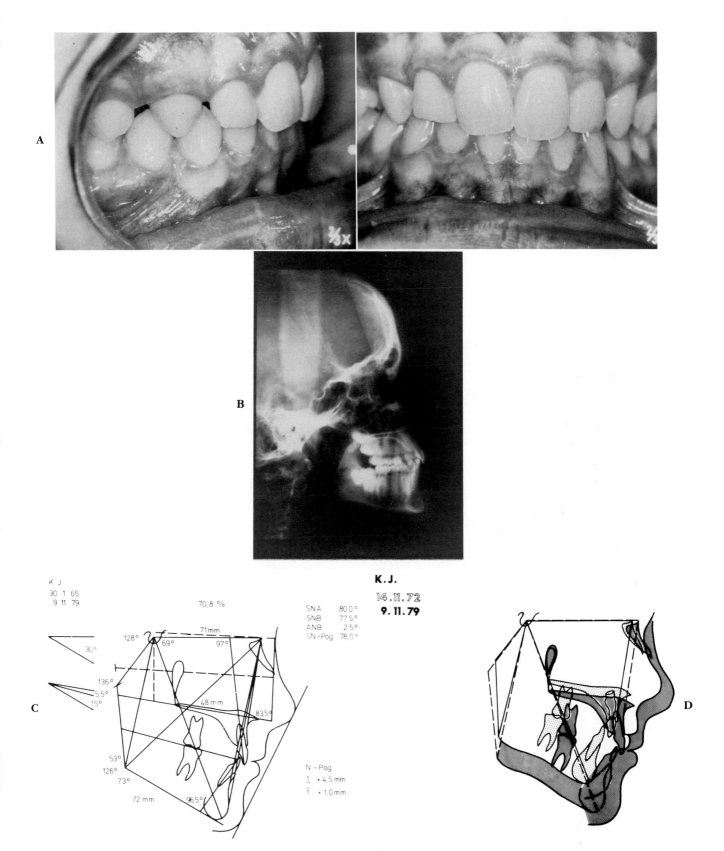

Fig. 13-10. Patient K.J. after treatment. **D,** Superimposition of before and after tracings.

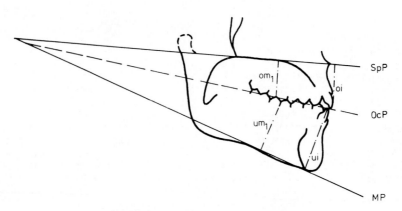

Fig. 13-11. Measurement of anterior and posterior alveolar heights. *o.i.,* Upper incisal; *o.m.,* upper molar; *u.i.,* lower incisal; *u.m.,* lower molar. Planes are represented by *SpP* (palatal), *OcP* (occlusal), and *MP* (mandibular). (According to A. M. Schwarz.)

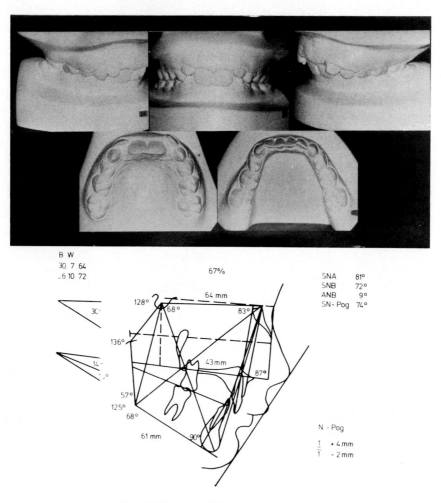

Fig. 13-12. Patient W.B. before treatment.

clusion relationship involved a deep, gingivally imping-ing overbite (Fig. 13-12). Despite this deep bite, the in-terocclusal clearance was not overly large, and there was a normal path of closure from rest to occlusion. The growth projection was markedly horizontal, but the mandibular base was short and retrognathic, while the ramus height and maxillary base were both of average size. The maxillary central incisors were lingually tipped, and the lateral incisors were labially tipped. The upper molars had migrated mesially. The first priority in treatment was to distalize the upper molars, using ex-traoral force. For the second phase of treatment, an ac-tivator was placed to fulfill the following treatment ob-jectives:

1. Anterior posturing of the mandible
2. Intrusion of the incisors and extrusion of the buc-cal segments
3. Protrusion of the upper central incisors

The reciprocal force from the last adjustment was

transmitted through the acrylic stabilizing projections at the mesial embrasure of the upper first molars, enhanc-ing the distalization of these teeth. The alignment of the maxillary incisors in these cases is often done in the initial stage while using extraoral force, particularly if there is a functional retrusion present. This requires only a short period of direct-bonded attachments on these teeth. Double buccal tubes on the upper first mo-lars permit the use of a light wire for tooth alignment and the reception of the inner bow of the headgear facebow at the same time.

Five years later, out of retention, the deep overbite and Class II relationship had been improved. To in-crease the chances of stability, a change in the inclina-tion of the maxillary base, tipping the anterior end up or withholding it while the posterior end continued to descend, and opening the Y-axis all were important. The change in the dentoalveolar region was not as ex-tensive as in the previous case (Fig. 13-13). The incisor

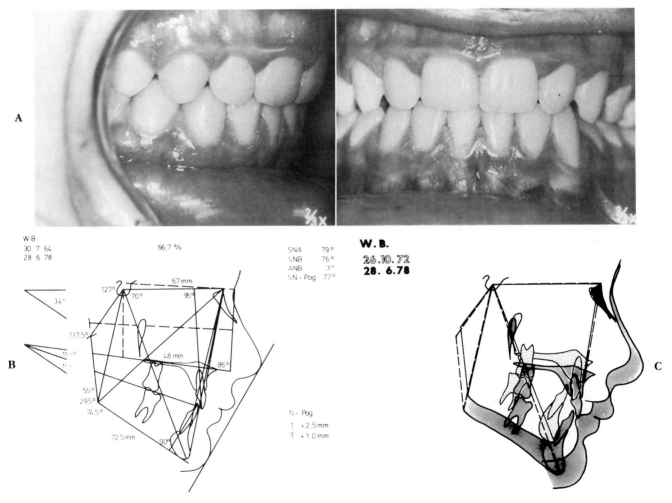

Fig. 13-13. Patient W.B. after treatment. **C,** Superimposition of before and after tracings.

to molar height ratio was improved in the upper arch from 5:3 to 5:3.6, and in the lower arch from 5:3.8 to 5:3.9. The relatively normal overbite at the end of treatment was due to skeletal alteration during the growth period.

Most deep overbite malocclusions are combined with a Class II relationship and horizontal growth pattern.

The treatment of this group of malocclusions has already been described in Chapter 12. In adults combined therapy is usually needed, with strong reliance on extraoral traction and possible removal of maxillary second molars. The treatment challenge is beyond the capabilities of functional appliances alone.

CHAPTER 14

TREATMENT OF CLASS III MALOCCLUSIONS

The factors creating and influencing true Class III malocclusions are quite different from those in Class II relationships.

While both types of malocclusions may be morphogenetically determined, most Class III problems have a strong hereditary component. This generally implies that the endogenous developmental pattern is dysplastic and becomes increasingly so from infancy to maturity. Functional influences play only a secondary or adaptive role in the etiology of Class III malocclusion.

The differentiation of the various types of Class III malocclusion is important; some types can be successfully treated in the early stages with functional appliances, while other Class III skeletal relationships can be corrected only by orthognathic surgical procedures. The limitation of activator therapy is reached much sooner in Class III cases than in mandibular retrognathism patients.

ETIOLOGIC CONSIDERATIONS

As indicated already, environmental factors are of less importance in the genesis of the malocclusion. Regardless of functional activity, the progressive severity of the maxillomandibular malrelationships can usually be observed. This dysplasia is thus linked to age. In a study

by the author (Fig. 14-1), mandibular length was correlated with the nasion-sella distance on the lateral cephalogram in patients between the ages of 6 and 19 years. In patients younger than 7½ years, the mandibular base length was relatively short. After this age the base length became progressively longer in relation to the average values. This curve expresses the genetically linked development of the Class III relationship.

Functional factors and soft tissue can also have some influence on these inexorable malocclusion patterns. A flat, anteriorly positioned tongue that lies low in the mouth is considered by van Limbourg and others to be a local epigenetic factor in Class III malocclusion. This should be eliminated during therapy, if possible. Whether tongue posture is a compensatory, adaptive phenomenon or a primary etiologic factor, inherited as are bone size and shape, is controversial. Some patients have a compulsive habit of protruding the mandible, which seems to support the development of mandibular prognathism. This phenomenon has been observed with some types of mental disease. As pointed out by Moyers and others, enlarged tonsils and nasorespiratory difficulty may also result in anterior tongue posturing, with the tongue dropping down and flattening out, as this strong reflex action maintains a patent airway. Linder-

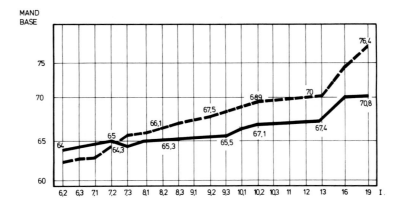

Fig. 14-1. Increments of mandibular base length between 6 and 19 years of age in patients with a Class III malocclusion. Broken line denotes average length.

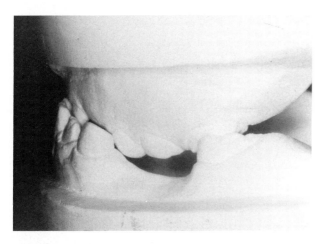

Fig. 14-2. Frontal cross-bite arising after preliminary loss of deciduous teeth.

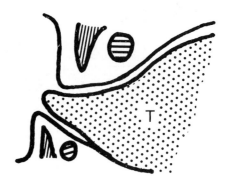

Fig. 14-3. Persistence of embryonic prognathism in the neonatal period associated with the suckle-swallow function. (According to A. M. Schwarz.) *T,* Tongue.

Aronson has alluded to the compensatory tongue position change with excessive epipharyngeal lymphoid tissue and the autonomous improvement observed over a 5-year period after the removal of the occluding mass.

Occlusal forces created by abnormal eruption may also produce unfavorable incisal guidance and promote a Class III relationship. The anterior displacement of the mandible by incisal guidance produces what is called a functional or pseudo–Class III malocclusion. If this is left unattended, in many cases it can become a functionally and skeletally true Class III malocclusion in the later dentofacial developmental stages (Fig. 14-2). Premature loss of deciduous molars may also cause mandibular displacements with occlusal guidance from maloccluded teeth or lingualized maxillary incisor teeth. If the mandible loses its posterior proprioceptive and functional support in habitual occlusion, it may be extended anteriorly to attempt to establish full occlusal contact during chewing. Such neuromuscular compensation can result in a permanent prognathic mandibular position and subsequent eruption of teeth into positions that support this malrelationship (i.e., labially tipped lower incisors, lingually tipped maxillary incisors, and interference with the full eruption of the maxillary teeth). Indeed, lack of eruption of maxillary buccal segments, which is sometimes caused by tongue thrusting or postural activity, permits the mandible to close through an excessive interocclusal space, autorotating into a Class III malocclusion because of the abnormal vertical development. In open bite problems, this autorotational maneuver is sometimes created to close down the bite by removing teeth, letting the mandible close further and reducing what might be a Class II tendency. Overclosure can thus accentuate a Class III malocclusion, even as it can enhance a Class II problem under tooth guidance. It is a

fact that maxillary vertical height is usually deficient in Class III cases.

FREQUENCY OF CLASS III MALOCCLUSIONS

The frequency of Class III malocclusion is only 1% to 3%, which is quite low in comparision to Class II problems. This figure is dependent on ethnic and geographic factors as well as age. The midface deficiency so often seen in oriental societies results in a high percentage of Class III malocclusion problems. Scandinavian percentages for Class III problems are higher than, for example, for the Italian populace. There is a lesser incidence of Class III malocclusion among blacks (and more bimaxillary protrusion). Occasionally in isolated geographic areas, where inbreeding exists, the frequency can rise significantly. One age-dependent Class III relationship, for example, is neonatal mandibular protrusion. This embryonic conditions occurs during the second month and usually disappears after the fifth month. In isolated cases, however, especially in premature births, it can persist (Fig. 14-3).

An age conditioned growth characteristic is the great mandibular growth spurt between 2 and 6 years of age, when the mandible literally emerges from its seemingly retruded position at birth. Some observers attribute this early growth spurt to the suckling or nursing posture, the mandible being thrust forward constantly to grasp the nipple. This infantile suckle-swallow pattern usually disappears by 2 years of age.

Most Class III malocclusions become apparent during or after the eruption of the deciduous teeth. Before 6 years of age there is an increase in the frequency of the Class III malocclusion, especially in dentitions abraded by nocturnal bruxing associated with anterior positioning of the mandible. Since the malocclusion is progressive, it should be treated early. One study of 2000 preschool children done in Germany reports that the frequency of Class III malocclusion is 18% of all malocclusions before the exfoliation of the deciduous teeth. This number decreases to 3% during the first phase of the mixed dentition period. One third of these cases result in the development of severe dysplasia, which are treated in conjunction with surgery (orthognathic procedures) or by surgery alone.

MORPHOLOGIC AND FUNCTIONAL CONSEQUENCES

The sequelae associated with this malrelationship are varied:

1. Incorrect loading of the teeth
2. Disturbances in the functional equilibrium
3. Impairment of chewing and speech functions
4. Difficulty of prosthetic restoration
5. Cosmetic and occasional psychologic considerations

These manifestations may occur singly but are usually associated with varying degrees of severity, depending on dentofacial and behavioral compensation.

Initial symptoms of Class III malocclusion

Beginning signs of a true, progressive mandibular prognathism occasionally can occur in infancy. A protruded mandible with an anteriorly positioned tongue can be seen only in cases of very severe dysplasia before the eruption of the incisors. In the first months of life, a sequential development of the Class III condition may be observed. This step-by-step progression is described as follows (Fig. 14-4):

1. Eruption of the maxillary central incisors in a lingual relationship and the mandibular incisors in a forward position with no overjet
2. Development of an incisal cross-bite during the eruption of the lateral incisors into a normal relationship
3. Full incisor cross-bite some weeks later
4. Flattening of the tongue as it drops away from palatal contact and postures forward, pressing against the lower incisors
5. Habitual protraction of the mandible by the child into the protruded functional and morphologic relationship

It has been estimated that about 10% of all Class III cases actually originate during infancy. This mode of development is of interest for several reasons. The etiology of the malocclusion determines or should assist in outlining the corrective treatment procedures. The skeletal growth pattern and growth centers of the maxilla and mandible are not the sole interest. The functional environment is also quite important. As indicated previously, most Class III malocclusions become apparent during or

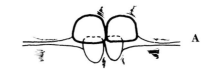
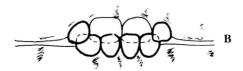
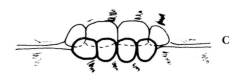

Fig. 14-4. Step-by-step development of a Class III relationship during eruption of the deciduous incisors. **A,** Eruption of the centrals. **B,** Incisal cross-bite of the centrals. **C,** Cross-bite of all incisors.

after eruption of the deciduous teeth or during eruption of the permanent incisors.

In evaluating the Class III relationship during the deciduous dentition period, the question arises whether the problem will progress or simply correct itself. The possibility of therapy at this time must be weighed carefully for certain cases. To make a proper determination, a careful analysis of all possible signs for future development must be undertaken. In the deciduous dentition these include looking for such symptoms as a scissors bite with facets of wear on specific teeth, spaces between the teeth, or tooth buds in the mandible and underdevelopment of the maxilla.

In the mixed dentition other possible signs may exist (cross-bite of individual teeth, minimal overjet, lower incisors lingually inclined to reach back to achieve a normal overjet, and selected skeletal symptoms that are apparent from a cephalometric examination; see Chapter 4).

DIAGNOSTIC CONSIDERATIONS

As with any type of dentofacial abnormality, the diagnostic assessment should be thorough and complete. It comprises a clinical examination, a functional analysis, a radiographic examination, a cephalometric analysis, a

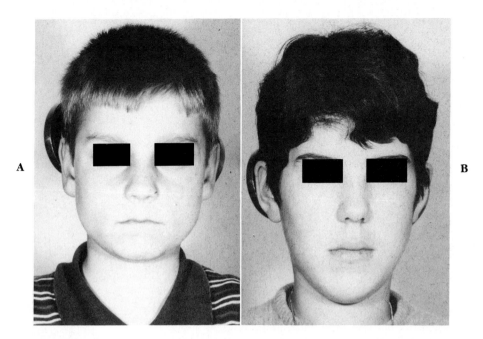

Fig. 14-5. The shape of the face should be considered before an expansion treatment. **A,** Mesoprosopic and, **B,** leptoprosopic faces.

study model analysis, and the soft tissue examination. Since these are covered in detail in other chapters, only the most salient factors will be discussed here for treatment planning for Class III malocclusions.

Clinical examination

The clinical examination comprises the usual general medical and dental background details, anamnestic information that might demonstrate a predisposition to malocclusion, plus specific dentofacial details associated with a particular problem. Blood dyscrasias might jeopardize future surgery and should be noted. Juvenile diabetes and some other diseases increase surgical preparation time and also the general risk if surgery is indicated.

The general examination. The general examination comprises the following:

1. An assessment of general physical attributes
2. Height and weight comparisons with normal standards
3. Visual and digital examination of the morphology of the face and head
4. Evaluation of the biologic age of the patient
5. Projection of the growth potential

As noted above, the shape of the face and skull can be of value in predicting future dysplastic relationships (Fig. 14-5). The skull can be dolichocephalic, brachycephalic, or mesocephalic. The face can be leptoprosopic, euryprosopic, or mesoprosopic. The dolichocephalic

and leptoprosopic configurations are accompanied by a long face syndrome and have a dominant vertical growth pattern. Tooth extraction is likely to be more frequently indicated in these cases, and rapid palatal expansion is regarded as more likely to be feasible. In the brachycephalic and euryprosopic combination, there is a short face with a more horizontal vector of growth. Expansion treatment is possible but extractions are seldom indicated.

To evaluate the age and growth potential, it is necessary to consider not only chronologic but also biologic age, which depends on skeletal maturation, morphologic evaluation, and an estimate of the likely onset of puberty. The prepubertal and pubertal growth peaks must be considered. The adolescent growth potential often causes difficulties for retention procedures in the corrected Class III malocclusion. Assessment of biologic age helps determine if the major increments of growth have been accomplished or still lie ahead. If the developmental age of the patient is younger than the chronologic age, higher growth rates lie ahead and surgery should be postponed. Retention is easier in a developmentally mature patient after treatment; surgery, if necessary, can be performed earlier. The hand and wrist x-ray films may provide information on the relative maturity, with specific concern for whether growth has ceased or will continue in significant amounts.

The dental age of the patient should be determined. Depending on the number of erupted teeth, the growth

BOYS								
Inc. centr.	6:08	6:10	7:00	7:11	*)	*)	6:08	7:04
Inc. lat.	7:04	8:04	8:10	9:00	6:11	7:03	7:11	8:06
Caninus	10:08	11:06	12:02	12:06	10:00	10:07	11:02	11:10
Praemolaris I.	10:05	10:08	11:10	12:00	9:01	9:08	10:04	11:01
Praemolaris II.	10:10	11:11	12:05	13:00	10:01	10:07	11:02	11:10
Molaris I.	6:00	6:04	6:08	6:10	*)	*)	*)	*)
Molaris II.	12:09	12:10	13:06	14:00	10:09	11:02	11:09	12:05
GIRLS								
Inc. centr.	6:06	6:10	7:04	7:08	*)	*)	*)	7:01
Inc. lat.	7:05	7:08	8:06	8:07	6:07	7:00	7:05	8:00
Caninus	9:10	10:02	11:03	11:08	9:02	9:10	10:05	11:02
Praemolaris I.	9:02	10:02	10:05	11:03	8:11	9:04	9:11	10:05
Praemolaris II.	10:05	11:01	11:05	12:02	9:10	10:02	10:09	11:03
Molaris I.	6:03	6:03	6:08	6:10	*)	*)	*)	*)
Molaris II.	11:11	11:11	12:10	13:05	10:05	10:10	11:04	12:00

Data in years and (after the colon) months

*) Eruption took place earlier than could be determined with our cases.

Fig. 14-6. Assessment of the dental age. (According to Maticka and Lukášová, modified by Adler.)

rate varies. With more teeth still to erupt, a greater growth rate can be expected, and greater potential treatment changes are possible than if the developmental age is precocious with regard to chronologic age (Fig. 14-6). The cephalometric examination can also help in forecasting the growth potential. Thus the clinical growth projection is based on the relation between chronologic, developmental, and dental ages, together with the parental and sibling history. If there is growth acceleration or retardation in the genetic pattern, the likelihood of this being repeated in the patient is considerable.

The specific clinical examination. The specific clinical examination is the same as for other malocclusions, with assessment of the craniofacial and oral soft tissues and dentition.

The configuration and form of the forehead and nose in relation to the lower face are of significance for the esthetic evaluation and prognosis. A well-formed nasolabial angle is important for the esthetic improvement. When the angle is acute, the premaxillary segment can be retracted; with an obtuse angle, the segment must be protracted to improve facial esthetics (Fig. 14-7). The soft tissue chin can compensate for or accentuate a skeletal Class III relationship, depending on its thickness. Gingival retraction or dehiscence can often be seen in an early Class III malocclusion. This damage is irreversible and is an indication for early treatment (Fig. 14-8).

The next step is examination of the dentition, i.e., the morphology and number of teeth. Congenital absence in the maxilla (e.g., missing canine or first premolar teeth) will make treatment more difficult (Fig. 14-9). When evaluating the axial inclination of the teeth, there are certain irregularities that are disadvantageous, e.g., labial tipping of the upper incisors and lingual tipping of the lower incisors still in anterior cross-bite. A concavity of the lingual alveolar structure in the·mandible

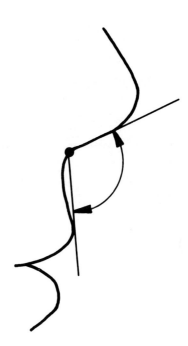

Fig. 14-7. The nasolabial angle.

also is a clue to future difficulties for correction of the Class III malocclusion (Fig. 14-10). Crowding of maxillary teeth also enhances treatment problems, as they may require extraction of the counterpart teeth in the lower arch, with great difficulty in closing spaces and maintaining proper incisor axial inclination. To make treatment easier when mandibular extractions are required, they should be done ahead of those in the maxilla. Depending on the state of development, enucleation or germectomy may be feasible for the lower first premolars. The molar occlusal relationship is usually Class III, but the plane of occlusion should also be evaluated as correction may be necessary before surgery.

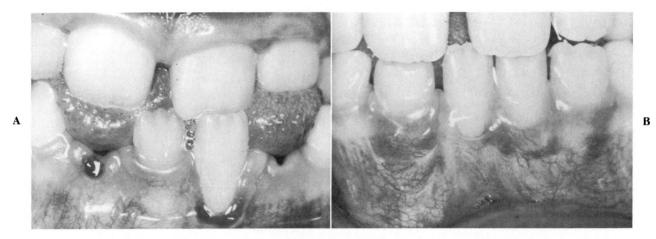

Fig. 14-8. A, Gingival damage following eruption of the central incisors in a cross-bite relationship. **B,** Even after correction of the relationship, the gingival retraction remains irreversible.

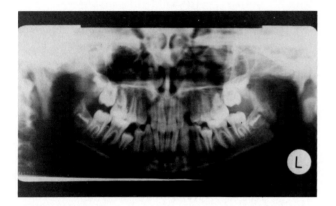

Fig. 14-9. Anodontia of the upper canines makes treatment of a Class III relationship more difficult.

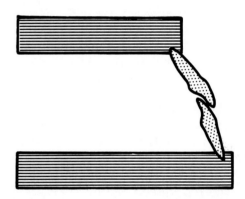

Fig. 14-10. Labial tipping of the upper and lingual tipping of the lower incisors indicate dental compensation in a Class III skeletal relationship. An orthodontic treatment of this condition is difficult, for the condition cannot be corrected with removable appliances.

Functional analysis

Functional analysis is obviously an integral part of the assessment. The path of closure from the postural rest position to occlusion must be carefully studied. The mandible may slide anteriorly into a forced protrusion, because of premature contact and tooth guidance, when the jaw closes into full occlusion. Such anterior displacements have a more favorable prognosis. By contrast, problems with an anterior rest position, with respect to habitual occlusion, are difficult to treat and usually require orthognathic surgical teamwork for correction (Fig. 14-11).

In addition to the true Class III poor prognosis and functional Class III good prognosis cases, there is a pseudo–forced bite category. This is a skeletal Class III malocclusion with a dental compensation comprising labial tipping of the upper incisors on a deficient maxillary base and lingual tipping of the lower incisors on an excessively long mandible. Orthodontic presurgical treatment must decompensate these malpositions before

surgical procedures are performed. Preorthodontic and postorthodontic treatment assistance is almost always necessary to attain the achievable optimum result that requires surgical adjustment of the apical bases.

TMJ assessment. Examination of the temporomandibular joints is also important. Some Class III characteristics predispose patients to future TMJ problems (e.g., premature contacts; traumatic occlusion; mandibular functional displacement, particularly asymmetric opening; and tongue malfunctions). With the condyle occupying the most posterior position in the temporal fossa, the likelihood of its riding over the posterior periphery of the articular disk is increased, with concomitant clicking and later crepitus. Impingement on the retrodiskal pad may produce undesirable objective symptoms. However, it is difficult to predict future TMJ problems in asymptomatic Class III patients because of the variable circumstances. Their age distribution may be the same as for other TMJ patients, but Class III pa-

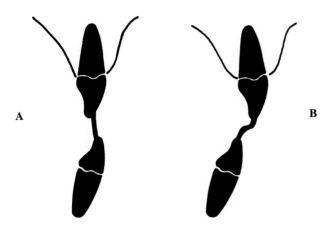

Fig. 14-11. Fuctional relationships in Class III malocclusion. **A,** True malocclusion and, **B,** forced bite.

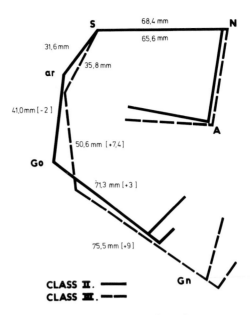

CLASS II. ———
CLASS III. ━ ━ ━

Fig. 14-12. Comparison of the linear relationship in a group of 50 patients with Class II and Class III malocclusions.

tients have usually undergone years of orthodontic-orthopedic treatment, and the surgical treatment does not always produce correct bilateral condylar function. These are predisposing causes, but TMJ patients often seem better able psychologically to adjust to their chewing problems because of their long history of functional difficulties.

Abnormal tongue function, size, shape, or posture must be considered at all ages. Whether the abnormality is a primary etiologic factor or a compensatory secondary characteristic is controversial and often hard to ascertain. The possibility exists that it is a combination of both. The tongue may be postured low in the mouth, flat and elongated, especially in cases of mouth breathing. In cases of macroglossia the tongue is not contained within the dentition, and the scalloping effect of tooth contact may be visible.

Radiographic assessment. In addition to the clinical examination of tongue size, a cephalometric evaluation is important. The tongue position can be examined palatographically both before and after treatment to determine the effectiveness of the therapeutic measures. It is quite important to differentiate tongue position problems. These involve tongue shape. If the tongue is too big, it can have an influence on the dental arch, with both tooth impressions on the tongue and spacing in the dental arches a concern. Active tongue thrusting may be noted during swallowing and should be checked. Such activity may be associated with the so-called infantile or visceral swallow. This is frequently a retained infantile pattern that has not matured, but it can also be a compensatory activity.

Lip function and morphology assessment. Finally lip size, posture, and function should be assessed. A short hypotonic upper lip is often seen in combination wtih a heavy, redundant, everted lower lip. Correction of the skeletal and dental aspects of the mal-

occlusion is not guaranteed to correct soft tissue abnormality.

Cephalometric examination

The goal of the cephalometric examination is the same for any skeletal malocclusion such as a Class II: it is to evaluate the facial type, the relationship of the jaw bases, the growth pattern, the dentoalveolar relationship, the localization of the malocclusion, the soft tissues and their relationship to the etiologic and prognostic considerations, the functional relationships, and the scope of the therapeutic possibilities.

The facial type is completely different for the Class III patient when compared to a Class I or Class II problem. In a study by the author, Class II and Class III malocclusions were compared (Fig. 14-12). In Class III cases the prognathic pattern began in the cranial base area. It was not possible to localize the Class III malocclusion in one craniofacial area alone. The sella angle and the articular angle were smaller in the Class III problem, moving the mandible anteriorly in relation to the cranial base. The gonial angle was not large in all Class III malocclusions. The study also showed that the mandibular bases in both classes of malocclusion were larger than normal. However, the amount was 3 mm in the Class II group and 9 mm in the Class III sample. Coupled with the anterior positioning of the mandible in the face, this created the sagittal discrepancy. Soft tissue changes also were different. These were amenable to significant change after orthognathic surgical intervention, both clinically and cephalometrically. It is of interest to note how a small alteration in the soft tissue proportions is able to change the whole facial image impression of observers. In patients in whom orthognathic surgery has been done on the ascending ramus to correct the prognathism, the face appears larger. Measurements, however, show that the face is not larger following the Class III surgery; only the facial length is shortened. This shortening averages only 2% and is mostly in the lower third of the face. If the osteotomy is done in the mental region, the distance between subnasion and the oral commissure appears larger. This may be due to the lengthening of the lip, following the upward rotation of the mandible. If the orthognathic surgery involves setting the maxilla forward, the visual impression is again different, depending on what has been done in the mandible. These potential changes in profile should be studied carefully before choosing a particular surgical technique.

Cephalometric classification of the Class III malocclusion

The scope and possibilities of treatment depend on the localization of the malocclusion characteristics in the skeletal and/or dentoalveolar area. The following possibilities exist in categorizing the Class III sagittal relationship:

1. Class III malocclusion due to a dentoalveolar malrelationship
2. Class III malocclusion with a long mandibular base
3. Class III malocclusion with an underdeveloped maxilla
4. Class III skeletal maloclusion with a combination of an underdeveloped maxilla and a prominent mandible (The growth pattern can be either horizontal or vertical.)
5. Class III skeletal malocclusion with tooth guidance (a pseudo–forced bite)

Class III malocclusion due to a dentoalveolar malrelationship. In the dentoalveolar Class III malocclusion (Fig. 14-13) there is no basal sagittal discrepancy. The A-N-B angle is within normal limits. The problem is primarily concentrated in the incisal relationship, with the maxillary incisors tipped lingually and the mandibular incisors tipped labially.

All that is usually needed in these patients is correction of the incisal malrelationship. This is a simple procedure that may be performed at any age. Most Class III malocclusions are in this category in their initial stages. However, during the eruption of the permanent teeth, the problem can become more severe. Some observers feel that prolongation of this malrelationship can actually exacerbate the sagittal discrepancy with an activator-like function effect that enhances the mandibular prognathism and may retard the maxillary horizontal development. This would be more likely in the anterior cross-bite or forced bite category, however. Hence it is advisable to institute treatment early, establishing a nor-

mal functional engram and stimulus in the developing face.

If a dentoalveolar Class III malocclusion is encountered in the adult, it can still be successfully corrected with orthodontic procedures alone, providing the symptoms are purely local. It is not easy to predict at an early age which cases will maintain the primarily dentoalveolar discrepancy and which will become more progressive, involving the basal structures. Hereditary pattern is a strong clue, however. Early detection is sometimes possible by looking at the lateral cephalogram. In some cases a long mandibular base with spaces between the developing unerupted teeth can be a clue to future prognathism. The maxilla is a critical area in these cases. If it adapts to the strong mandibular growth, the relationship can remain harmonious; if not, the facial skeleton will show an apparent mandibular overgrowth. It should be emphasized that all Class III malocclusions are not the fault of the mandible. Particularly in some oriental strains, there is manifest midface underdevelopment, which is a major factor.

Class III malocclusion with a long mandibular base. As Fig. 14-14 shows, both the mandibular base and the ascending ramus are large. The S-N-A angle is normal, but the S-N-B angle is larger than normal, creating a negative A-N-B difference. The gonial angle is usually large and the articular angle small, but not always so. The mandible is not only longer but is also usually anteriorly positioned. The tongue morphology is flattened, while the tongue is postured forward and lies lower in the mouth. Often a cupping out of the lingual alveolar bony support below the lower premolars is seen in association with this postural adaptation.

The axial inclination of this type of Class III is the opposite of the dentoalveolar Class III problem. The upper incisors are tipped labially and the lower incisors are inclined lingually. This kind of relationship is an in-

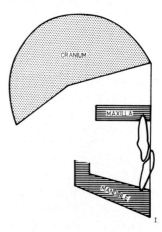

Fig. 14-13. Class III dentoalveolar malocclusion. The bases are normally related.

dication of a partial dentoalveolar compensation and limits the therapeutic possibilities. In these cases there is often a lateral cross-bite, as the maxillary arch appears to be narrowed. Actually part of the problem is that a wider part of the mandibular dental arch has been moved anteriorly to relate with a narrower maxillary width dimension. Many malocclusions in this group can only be treated in the early mixed dentition period. In older patients, or where the dysplasia is severe, orthognathic surgery combination treatment is the best answer. This type of malocclusion can be designated as one with the fault lying in the mandible.

Class III malocclusion with an underdeveloped maxilla. In some Class III malocclusions the maxillary base is small and retrognathic (Fig. 14-15). There is a smaller than normal S-N-A angle combined with a normal S-N-B angle. Cleft palate patients are a good example of this category as are certain oriental groups with midface deficiencies. Early treatment can be successfully performed by growth guidance during the eruption of the maxillary incisors or in cases with favorable initial lingual inclination of the upper incisors, which permits their labial tipping. Actual growth stimulation or a change in maxillary growth direction in the middle face can be accomplished by extraoral orthopedic protraction procedures, using appliances such as the Delaire mask (Fig. 14-16).

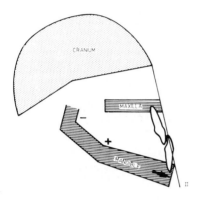

Fig. 14-14. Class III skeletal relationship with large mandibular base.

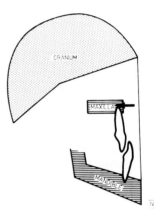

Fig. 14-15. Class III skeletal relationship with underdeveloped maxilla.

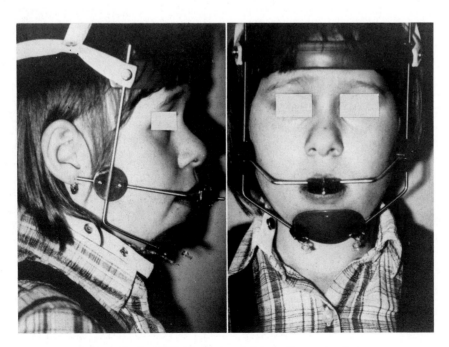

Fig. 14-16. Modified Delaire mask for maxillary protraction.

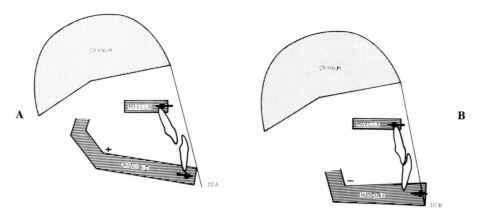

Fig. 14-17. Class III skeletal relationship with underdeveloped maxilla and prominent mandible. **A,** Vertical and, **B,** horizontal growth patterns.

Class III malocclusion with a combined underdeveloped maxilla and a prominent mandible. In the retrognathic maxilla–prognathic mandible combination, the S-N-A angle is small and the maxillary base is short (Fig. 14-17). The S-N-B angle is large and the mandibular base is long. The ramus can be short or long. Depending on the ramal length, it is possible to differentiate the two variations in this category.

In cases with a short ramus, the growth pattern is vertical, and the gonial angle is large. There is often a Class III sagittal relationship combined with an open bite. Sometimes there is also crowding in the upper arch that may require extraction during correction. Treament is possible in the more moderate cases, usually only with four first premolar extraction and fixed multi-attachment appliances. If the problem is severe, orthognathic surgery is the only answer.

In cases with a long ramus, the growth pattern is horizontal, the gonial angle is small, and there is a reversed overbite. In early treatment, it is possible to correct the overbite and to control mandibular development in many cases by the use of occlusal force. However, the maxilla may also become prognathic if treatment is performed during the eruption of the incisors. In other cases the overbite may remain stable, but the mandible becomes more prognatic. Prediction is more difficult in these problems.

Class III skeletal malocclusion with a pseudo–forced bite or anterior displacement. Pseudo–forced bite or anterior malocclusions (Fig. 14-18) have already been discussed in Chapter 5. The condition known as Class III skeletal dysplasia is partially compensated by the labial tipping of the upper incisors and lingual inclination of the lower incisors. This tooth malposition results in additional anterior guidance of the mandible on the path from postural rest to habitual occlusion, as the lingual of the lower incisors rides on the maxillary incisor margins after initial contact. While the

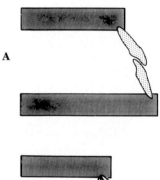

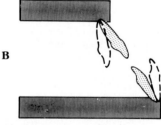

Fig. 14-18. Class III skeletal relationship with pseudo–forced bite. **A,** Compensation of a Class III relationship. **B,** Uprighting of the incisors.

full occlusal relationship makes it appear that the mandible is even further forward than it is, this type of case is very difficult to treat orthodontically because of the unfavorable axial inclination of both upper and lower incisors and the true sagittal basal malrelationship. In these cases therapy consists mostly of uprighting the incisors and then instituting an orthognathic surgical regimen to correct the anteroposterior basal jaw relationship.

TREATMENT PLANNING FOR CLASS III MALOCCLUSIONS

The therapeutic possibilities are dependent on the developmental age of the patient and the exact nature of the malocclusion. For example, dentoalveolar Class III malocclusions and forced bite, anterior displacement

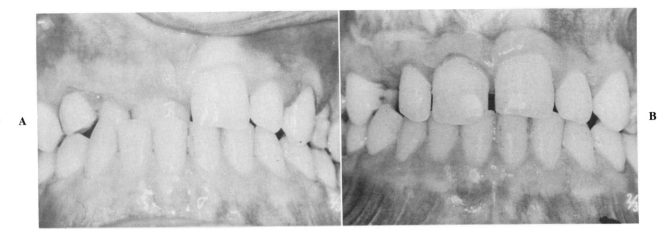

Fig. 14-19. A 31-year-old patient with forced bite of the incisors. **A,** Before and, **B,** after treatment.

cases without skeletal involvement, may be treated at any time. The treatment objectives include uprighting labially tipped lower incisors and lingually inclined upper incisors. Expansion is sometimes also necessary in the upper arch. This kind of treatment can be performed easily with active plates (with jackscrews, fingersprings, etc.), inclined planes, or activators, without multiattachment fixed appliances in the mixed or permanent dentition. For example, Fig. 14-19 shows a 31-year-old patient who had an incisor cross-bite corrected with an inclined plane before prosthetic rehabilitation. The malocclusion here is dentoalveolar.

The skeletal Class III malocclusion may be divided into three groups with regard to therapy.

1. The malocclusion "fault" is in the mandible; the mandible is prominent, with a long body. The treatment is concentrated primarily on the mandibular base. A posterior repositioning of the mandible is possible during the growth period with functional or extraoral orthopedic procedures. However, growth can only be effectively inhibited or redirected in cases treated during the deciduous dentition or early mixed dentition.
2. The malocclusion fault is in the maxilla; the maxillary base is retrognathic and short. Stimulation of maxillary development is possible. Treatment is more effective, particularly during the eruption of the upper incisors. As with the mandible, maxillary growth can be redirected only during the growth period.
3. The malocclusion fault is in both the maxilla and mandible; this type of dysplasia requires a combined approach, often leading to ultimate orthognathic surgical correction.

Investigations show that the actual difference in jaw base length in maxillary retrusion and mandibular retraction is not so significant in the permanent dentition as in the deciduous or mixed dentitions. In the group

where the mandible is at fault, a maxilla of normal size can be retarded in its further development, while in a malocclusion where the fault lies in the maxilla, an average size mandible can become large with increasing age (Fig. 14-20).

The length of the maxillary base can be increased with treatment; the younger the patient, the more significant is the potential for correction. Clinical research demonstrates that the length of the upper jaw base can be influenced with treatment up until 10 years of age. In older age groups, the maxillary base no longer shows any appreciable change during treatment (Fig. 14-21).

Scope and limitation of treatment in the various dentitional periods. As the age of the patient increases, the amount of growth to be expected decreases, and the skeletal Class III relationship becomes more permanent. As has been pointed out before, it is advantageous to influence the growth process and tooth eruption as early as clinically feasible in the initial stages of the dysplastic relationship. Treatment is possible in the different stages of dentitional development, but early treatment is more likely to be successful.

Treatment in the deciduous dentition. Early malocclusion symptoms are usually apparent in the deciduous dentition. The patient will often posture the mandible habitually in an anterior relationship, with the tongue also posturing low and forward as the dorsum flattens out. If these symptoms are observed, orthopedic control via a chin cap may be the method of choice to hold the mandible in a posterior position. Treatment can be started as early as 1 year of age and can be continued until the age of 4 or so as the only growth guidance procedure. Combination treatment is usually necessary later on, with an intraoral appliance. Only treatment done on the deciduous dentition has the potential of being completely successful in most cases when there is any significant degree of potential mandibular prognathism. Treatment begun later is more likely to have resid-

Dentition	Mean duration of treatment in months	Extent of mandible in mm			Ascending ramus in mm		Extent of maxilla in mm	
		Ideal	Found, before treatment*	Found, after treatment**	Found, before treatment*	Found, after treatment**	Found, before treatment*	Found, after treatment**
Primary dentition								
Fault in mandible	7	61.6±1.1	+2.0±1.0	+0.9±1.8	0 ±2.3	+2.6	+0.2±1.0	+0.5
Fault in maxilla	18	65.7±1.9	−4.2±2.4	+1.5±1.2	−2.7±1.3	+2.0	−5.0±1.0	+4.21±1.2
Together	13	64.0±1.7	−1.4±2.1	−0.9±2.0	−1.5±1.8	+2.2	−2.8±1.2	+2.8±1.4
Mixed dentition								
Fault in mandible	6.2	64.0±2.2	+4.9±2.3	+0.6±1.0	−0.4±1.5	+1.4	−0.3±1.4	+0.7
Fault in maxilla	10	67.6±2.6	−2.1±2.2	+1.0±1.0	0.0±1.6	+0.7	−3.0±2.4	+0.7
Together	9	65.7±2.1	+1.4±2.4	+0.6±1.0	−0.4±1.5	+1.4	−1.4±2.0	+0.7±2.3
Permanent dentition								
Fault in mandible	15	66.2±1.2	+6.4±3.4	∅	+6.5±3.2	+0.6	0.0±1.0	∅
Fault in maxilla	8	70.5±3.1	+0.5±3.0	∅	+4.6±3.6	∅	−2.0±2.2	∅
Together	14	68.5±3.5	+0.5±3.0	∅	+6.0±2.5	∅	−1.5±1.5	∅

* Relative to 'ideal' values.
**Relative to 'found' values prior to treatment.

Fig. 14-20. Extent of the mandibular base, maxillary base, and ascending ramus in cases of mandibular prognathism.

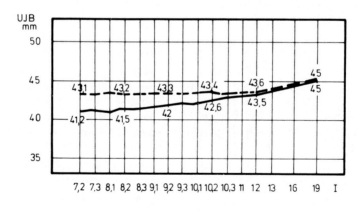

— UJB – LENGTH BEFORE TREATMENT
-- UJB – LENGTH AFTER TREATMENT

Fig. 14-21. Increments of maxillary base length between 6 and 19 years of age in patients with a Class III malocclusion. Broken line denotes average length.

ual signs of mandibular prognathism or maxillary retrusion, even though the dental result can be quite successful. Obviously the magnitude of the original insult and the dominance of the morphogenetic pattern are qualifying factors.

After eruption of all the deciduous teeth, three types of Class III relationship can be differentiated.

FUNCTIONAL CLASS III RELATIONSHIP. In this category no skeletal Class III signs are present. The mandible slides anteriorly into an edge-to-edge or cross-bite relationship. Usually the tooth guidance is in the canine region. Often careful equilibration of these teeth is all that is needed to correct the problem. In other cases decreased intercanine distance, which might be due to chronic nasorespiratory problems, and low tongue posture may be dominant factors in the creation of the morphology that results in tooth guidance. In such cases expansion of the maxillary arch without canine equilibration is indicated. Canines that have been needlessly ground down do not retain well in these cases. It should be remembered, however, that a functional Class III relationship may be the beginning signs of a true Class III malocclusion. Such patients need to be followed continuously, and orthopedic guidance may be needed at any time.

CLASS III RELATIONSHIP WITH THE FAULT IN THE MANDIBLE. A fault in the mandible can become manifest in the deciduous dentition, despite the fact that the mandible appears retrognathic in the early years for most children. In these cases the mandibular basal measurement and the S-N-B angle can be large. However, the mandibular base can be of average length or even short in the deciduous dentition, but the mandible itself is prominent or anteriorly positioned. The maxilla is usually normally developed in these cases. Growth inhibition or redirection and posterior positioning of the mandible is a valid treatment objective here. A chin cap or a reverse (Class III) activator can be used to exert a retrusive force on the mandible in patients who fall in this group.

CLASS III RELATIONSHIP WITH THE FAULT IN THE MAXILLA. Patients with the fault in the maxilla show a retrognathic maxilla or midface, even though the mandible is orthognathic or essentially normal. The tooth buds of the upper incisors are often rotated and crowded. Treatment can usually be accomplished with an activator or Fränkel appliance in mild cases, though extraoral orthopedic protractive force using a Delaire-type face mask is required in severe problems. It is advantageous to treat this type of problem during the eruption of the incisors before the maxillary incisors become locked behind the mandibular counterparts. Loading the palatal area behind the upper incisors, while at the same time relieving the labial muscle forces with lip pads, as recommended by Frantisek Kraus, Rolf Fränkel, and others, is often effective.

A combination of these two types of Class III malocclusions (retrusive maxilla and protrusive mandible) of course is possible and logically requires therapeutic control of both areas via maxillary protraction and mandibular retractive growth guidance.

To illustrate treatment in a case that employs these principles, Fig. 14-22 shows a 6-year-old boy with a developmental age of 5 years. His mother had a severe Class III malocclusion. She had come for a prognostic evaluation of the problem in the boy's deciduous dentition because of her concern. Clinically the patient already exhibited an edge-to-edge incisal relationship and a prominent symphysis. The cephalometric examination showed prognathic tendencies in both jaws, more in the upper than in the lower jaw. The growth pattern was projected as horizontal, but the upward and forward tipping of the maxillary base (anteinclination) was opening the bite anteriorly. The maxillary base was 1.5 mm longer than average, the ramus 3 mm shorter, and the mandibular body 4 mm above average, which is extremely large for this age. It is a good sign of a genetically determined mandibular prognathism. Assessment of the axial inclination of the incisors is not of much value at this time because these teeth are naturally quite upright in the deciduous dentition.

Treatment was postponed for 1½ years until the eruption of the incisors. In the meantime, the prognathism, especially in the mandible, increased. The A-N-B angle was now −3 degrees. Both the mandibular base and the ramus height were now large, while the maxillary base was of average length. The horizontal growth pattern and the anteinclination of the maxillary base persisted. Comparison of the serial cephalograms showed increasingly severe malocclusion. The functional analysis showed a normal path of closure with no tooth guidance, making this a true Class III problem.

Treatment was started with a Class III activator. The construction bite was opened 4 mm to achieve an edge-to-edge relationship after all possible retrusion of the mandible. A tongue crib was used in the lower anterior region instead of the usual acrylic material. The lower incisors were guided lingually with a labial bow. Lip pads were incorporated in the appliance in the upper anterior segment to hold off any pressure from the contiguous musculature, while the upper incisors were guided labially by adding successive thin layers of self-curing soft acrylic. Therapy was continued in this manner until all incisors had erupted.

After 1½ years of mechanotherapy, a good overbite had been achieved (Fig. 14-23). The prognathism of the maxillary base had increased, while the mandibular prognathism was decreased, resulting in a posterior positioning of the mandible, despite a high growth rate of the maxillary base. The skeletal discrepancy was partially

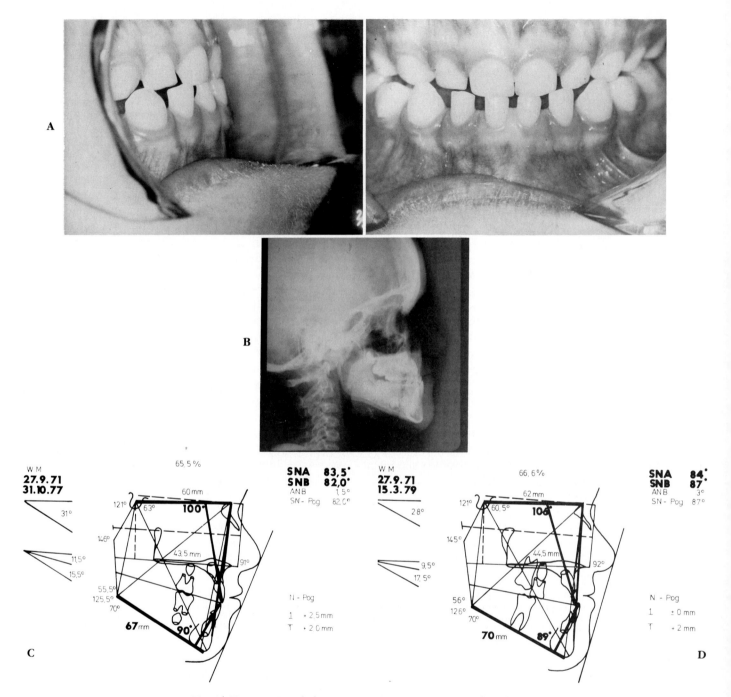

Fig. 14-22. Patient W.M. before treatment. Tracing **D** is 1½ years later than **C**.

compensated for by the labial tipping of the upper and the lingual tipping of the lower incisors. During the course of further development, the intermaxillary relationship remained stable because of the adaptation of the maxillary complex to the prognathic mandible.

Treatment in the mixed dentition. Even in the mixed dentition, a posterior position of the mandible can still be achieved. The goal of early treatment is to gain proper incisal guidance as soon as possible, which can

lead to harmonious growth of the jaw bases if the dysplasia is not severe. Obviously treatment at the earliest possible time, when only minor Class III symptoms are present, is likely to be the most successful and stable.

In this group, in which the problem is primarily dentoalveolar, the upper incisors are tipped lingually initially while the lower incisors are tipped labially. The first objective of treatment is to correct the incisor crossbite and to upright these teeth. As previously noted,

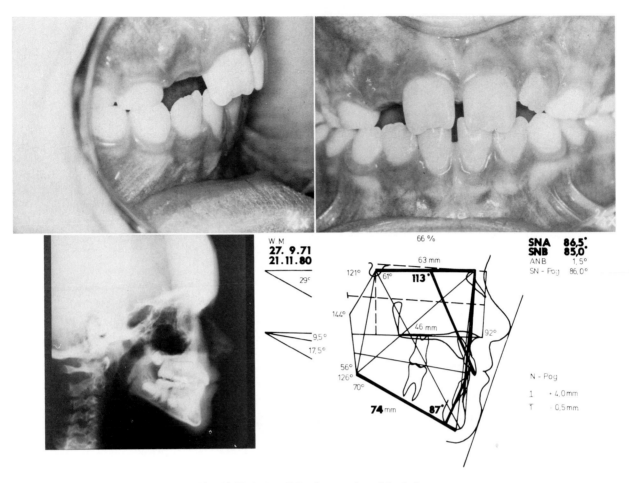

Fig. 14-23. Patient W.M. after eruption of the incisors.

treatment can be performed with variations of the active plate, inclined planes, or activators. During treatment, some skeletal symptoms of the Class III malocclusion often arise, i.e., a long mandibular base or a forward positioned mandible. Continued observation of the developing dentition is necessary in these cases, with long-term follow-up and a readiness to intercede with the proper orthopedic or fixed attachment guidance as indicated. Often an activator can continue to be used as a retainer, or a chin cap may be necessary to control the mandibular prognathism tendency.

Treatment, or at least supervision, is essential in mixed dentition cases until the full eruption of the permanent teeth.

In Class III malocclusions with the fault in the mandible in mixed dentition cases, the same treatment objectives of growth inhibition and posterior mandibular positioning are indicated. An activator can be used to alter the incisal guidance and to attempt to position the mandible posteriorly. Sometimes in the early mixed dentition, extraction of the lower deciduous canines and deciduous first molars can be performed to facilitate the correction of the incisal guidance. In some carefully selected cases, enucleation of the lower first premolars is possible, to decrease lower arch length and to provide a dental compensation for the skeletal problem, as the six lower anterior teeth are retracted into the extraction sites. Germectomy also has the effect of limiting alveolar growth.

Treatment of a Class III malocclusion with a vertical growth pattern is more difficult than with a horizontal pattern. It is difficult to achieve a good overbite with a vertical growth vector. There is excessive anterior face height, which compensates but usually not enough. In these cases a chin cap may be helpful, in addition to a low- or high-pull headgear, to control posterior eruption, depending on the growth direction.

In Class III malocclusions in the mixed dentition, with the fault in the maxilla, all efforts should be made to promote growth and to protract the maxillary complex.

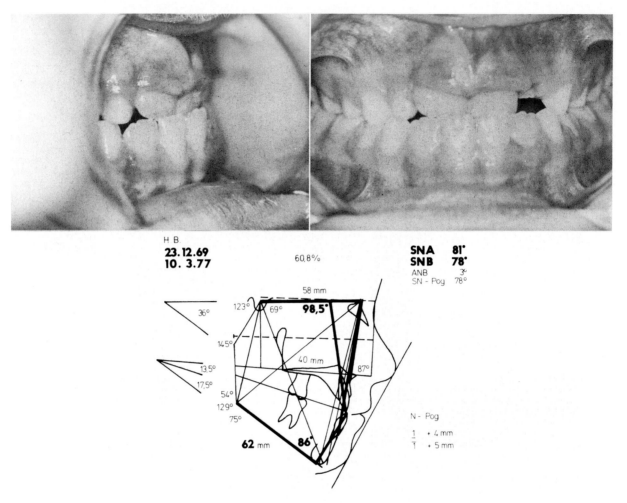

Fig. 14-24. Patient H.B. before treatment.

This means both horizontal and vertical growth, since maxillary vertical deficiency enhances the apparent mandibular protrusion with its autorotation into an overclosed habitual occlusion. Many of these cases have excessive interocclusal clearance so that stimulation of maxillary vertical growth also means enhancement of eruption of the posterior teeth, which has the net effect of rotating the mandible down and back into a more normal sagittal relationship. An improvement in the midface concavity can be seen when treatment is performed during the eruption of the maxillary incisors. The eruption can be channelled as desired by the guiding planes of the activator, with simultaneous relief of labial muscle force provided by the lip pads at the depth of the vestibule. Simultaneously the mandible can be under a retrusive chin cap force to reduce the sagittal discrepancy. An alternate approach is to align the maxillary arch with a short period of direct-bonded attachments or with active plates, while the midface can be favorably influenced by the orthopedic protraction of a

Delaire mask. If the crowding of the maxillary arch is too severe, extraction may be required in the maxillary arch. This means that the lower first premolars must also be removed to allow proper dentitional adjustment. Clearly fixed multiattachment therapy plus possible orthognathic surgery may be the therapy of choice, depending on the severity of the problem and the age-linked expressivity.

To illustrate management of a mixed dentition problem, Fig. 14-24 shows an 8½-year-old girl with an incisor cross-bite. The growth pattern projected was average; the jaw bases of average length for her age; the basal relationship normal, despite a short ramus; and the A-N-B angle was 3 degrees. The upper dental arch was crowded, but the lower arch was well-aligned and wide.

Treatment was started with a Class III activator to guide the upper incisors labially and to move the lower incisor lingually. To assist in this correction, the lower deciduous canines were extracted. After full eruption of the incisors and all four first premolars, the upper arch

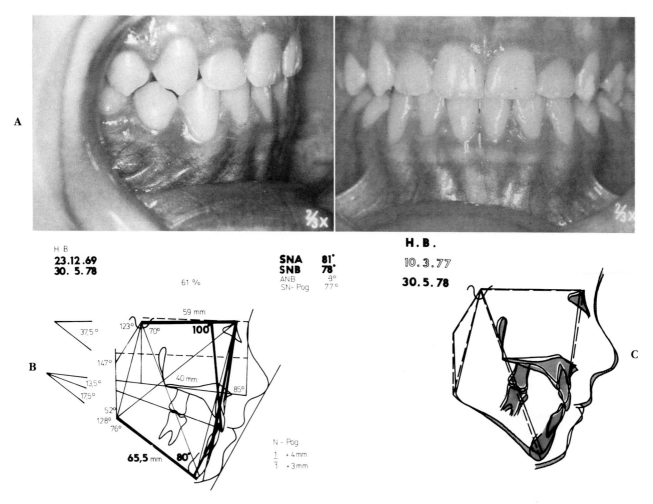

Fig. 14-25. Patient H.B. after activator and fixed appliance treatment. **C,** Superimposition of before and after tracings.

was expanded with an active place. Subsequently the lower arch was also expanded to align and upright the teeth. A good overbite was achieved after 15 months of activator treatment, although the lower incisors were tipped lingually (Fig. 14-25). The basal relationship, as evidenced by the A-N-B angle, remained stable, despite a high growth increment of 3.5 mm in the mandibular base. The maxillary base and ramus height were both short by this time. The growth rate of the mandibular base is characteristic of a morphogenetically dominant Class III pattern. It is postulated that because of early incisal control and development of a normal engram of proper incisor proprioception during the transitional dentition period, the mandible did not slide into a prognathic relationship. What effect there is on the temporomandibular fossa as a result of retrusive stimulus on the mandible is a matter of speculation. However, since this area is membranous bone, it is susceptible to potential morphologic change and adaptation, as primate studies have shown. So the possibility exists that part of the cor-

rection seen in some of these Class III cases under orthopedic influence is due to a distalizing of the fossae themselves as well as to some minimal mandibular change.

In another example, Fig. 14-26 shows a 7½-year-old girl with an anterior cross-bite and maxillary arch crowding. The arch length deficiency was large above with no room for the lateral incisors. Both upper and lower jaw bases were retrognathic in position. The A-N-B angle was almost a straight line at 0.5 degree. The length of the jaw bases was average. The growth pattern was horizontal.

The correction of the incisor cross-bite was not considered a problem because of the lingual inclination of the maxillary centrals, which could be tipped labially. The crowding was so severe, however, that extraction of the first premolars would be necessary later. Because of the early mixed dentition period timing, it was possible to initiate a program of serial extraction and to simultaneously correct the anterior cross-bite.

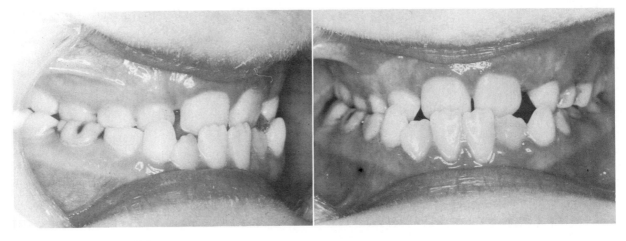

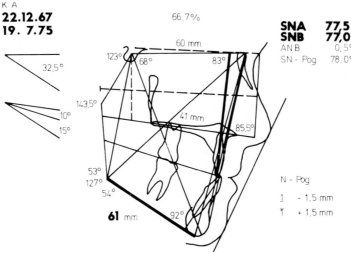

Fig. 14-26. Patient K.A. before treatment.

The treatment was carried out with two activators. With the first activator, the upper incisors were tipped labially while the mandible was held in a retruded position. This was done by adding layers of self-curing soft acrylic on the lingual surfaces of these teeth and the contiguous alveolar process, while the lower incisors had an active labial bow retrusive effect. Serial extraction procedures were carried out with removal of the lower first premolars first and then the upper first premolars as these teeth erupted. It is almost always advantageous in Class III malocclusions to remove the lower first premolars before the upper teeth. The second activator was used for retention and to seat the occlusion.

After 4½ years of treatment and retention, a good incisal and skeletal relationship had been achieved with a normal 3-degree A-N-B angle (Fig. 14-27). The growth increments had been average. The early initiation of therapy allowed the use of functional appliances. Later appliance introduction meets with more severe tooth malalignment, and fixed appliances become the mecha-

nism of choice. They may be necessary, anyway, as a final phase of treatment to align malposed teeth after establishment of a proper skeletal sagittal relationship.

In another pertinent case report, a 9-year-old girl demonstrated a Class III malocclusion with the maxilla at fault and an A-N-B angle of −2 degrees (Fig. 14-28). The growth pattern was projected as vertical. The maxillary base was small and retrognathic. The upper arch had crowding and rotations present.

Treatment was done with multiattachment fixed appliances and extraction of four first premolars. The Class III relationship was compensated for by dentoalveolar adjustment (Fig. 14-29).

Treatment in the permanent dentition. By the time the permanent teeth have erupted, treatment for a Class III malocclusion can be successful only if the problem is primarily dentoalveolar and not a true skeletal malrelationship. The skeletal type of Class III can be compensated for by tooth removal and/or surgery. The method of choice depends on the severity of the prob-

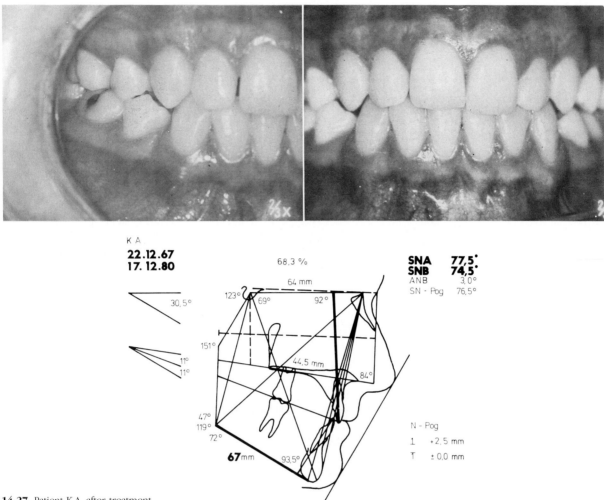

Fig. 14-27. Patient K.A. after treatment.

lem and a projection of residual sagittal growth changes still possible in the terminal developmental period. It is quite important to do a thorough diagnosis and to make a projection based on a likely growth pattern. If the problem is too severe for orthodontic correction alone, with or without extraction, then the proper preparations should be made for surgery. Past history shows many examples of patients wearing orthodontic appliances for 4 to 6 years before a decision is made to resort to orthognathic surgery. In many of these cases a proper diagnosis at the beginning would have provided the necessary information indicating the likelihood of a need for orthognathic procedures.

Sometimes presurgical therapy means decompensating for natural adjustments that have been made. This requires uprighting lingually inclined mandibular and labially inclined maxillary incisors to reduce excessive eruption of incisors and to level the curve of Spee, etc. The patient is treated to regain an anterior cross-bite, since the skeletal change affected by surgery will reestablish a normal overbite and overjet. All these treatment procedures require fixed multiattachment therapy and are beyond the scope of functional appliances, as well as of this book (Figs. 14-30 and 14-31).

The activator can be used for retention after orthognathic surgical correction. The amount of disturbance, the exact mode of natural adaptation to changed muscle pull after surgery, and the functional adaptation are often unknown quantities. The changing of the origins or insertions of muscles during the course of orthognathic surgery calls for adaptation both in these muscles and in the bony tissues in which they insert. Retention is strongly indicated to help guide the posttreatment adaptation in the most favorable direction. An activator is ideal for this muscle training. The appliance is fabricated with the mandible in the most retruded position, with a slight opening of the vertical dimension. The lower incisors are held with an acrylic capping or indexing. The acrylic is not trimmed away in the molar area, since it is supposed to hold the teeth as they are.

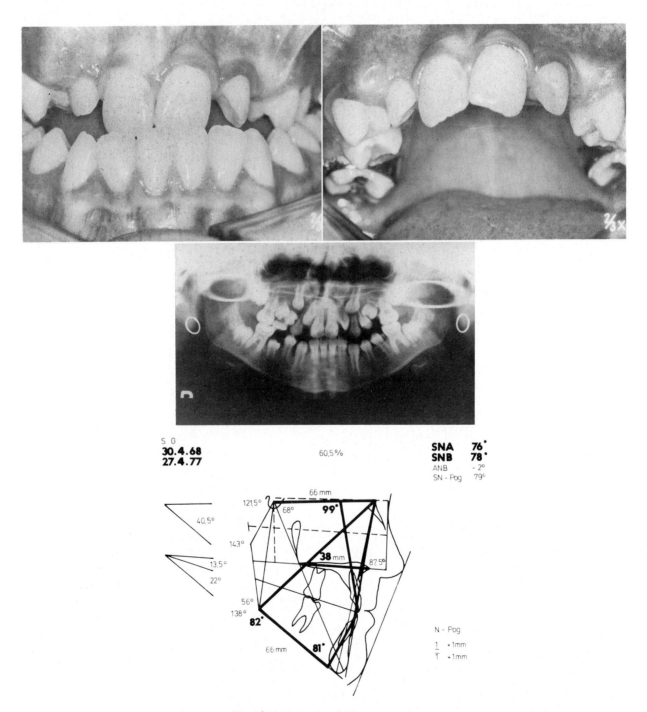

Fig. 14-28. Patient S.G. before treatment.

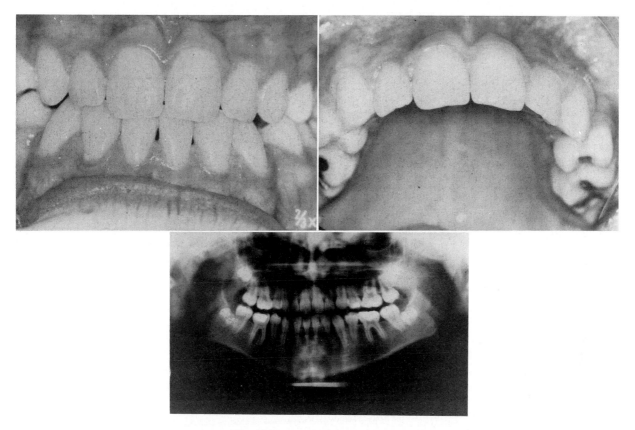

Fig. 14-29. Patient S.G. after treatment.

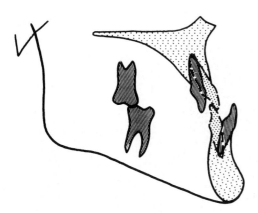

Fig. 14-30. Dental compensation of a Class III skeletal relationship by labial tipping of the upper and lingual tipping of the lower incisors.

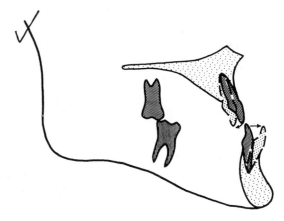

Fig. 14-31. Presurgical decompensation of a Class III relationship by uprighting the tipped incisors.

Removable functional appliances can be used successfully in the treatment of Class III malocclusions if they are introduced early, even in the deciduous dentition of selected cases. Use in mixed dentition, when the incisors are erupting and when the skeletal characteristics are not yet blatantly manifest is highly desirable, and the results attained are more likely to be stable. In all other cases the range of use of functional appliances in the treatment of Class III malocclusions is limited, and these appliances can be used effectively only in conjunction with other fixed appliance methods and/or orthognathic surgery. Use as a retainer is to be recommended in many instances, since muscle adaptation is slower and the activator serves as a training appliance.

CHAPTER 15

THE OPEN BITE MALOCCLUSION

The treatment of an open bite malocclusion is partially covered in Chapter 3. This section deals with the general concepts of open bite therapy.

ETIOLOGIC CONSIDERATIONS

Epigenetic and environmental factors are both of concern in the etiology of open bite.

Under the heading of epigenetic factors are posture; morphology and size of the tongue; skeletal growth pattern of the maxilla and mandible, particularly the lower jaw; and vertical relationship of the jaw bases. These characteristics are genetically determined. There is generally a vertical deficiency in the amount of basal and alveolar bone growth in a specific area.

Of the environmental factors, abnormal function and improper respiration are the most important. Most children (91% in Rakosi's study) have some sort of abnormal functional pattern or potentially deforming habit. The significance of tongue dysfunctions in the etiology of open bite has already been discussed in Chapter 5. Disturbed or occluded nasal respiration can cause a change in the posture or function of both the tongue and the mandible, which can lead to an open bite malocclusion.

ESTHETIC CONSIDERATIONS

The dentoalveolar open bite malocclusion is esthetically unattractive, particularly during speech when the tongue is pressed between the teeth and lips. In evaluating the esthetics, the following relationships are of special interest:

1. The balance between the nose, lips, and chin profile.
2. The nasolabial angle. If this angle is small or acute, a retraction of the upper incisors is likely to improve the esthetics after a premolar extraction. Where the nasolabial angle is obtuse or large, proclination of the upper incisors could enhance facial appearance. This assumes that the change is not due to changes in the nasal contour but rather in the draping of the lip itself.

3. The configuration of the lips, meaning the space between the lips at rest as well as the relation of the lip line to the underlying teeth and gingival tissue. A short upper lip that reveals excessive amounts of maxillary gingival tissue is not esthetically appealing.
4. The length of the lower third of the face (Fig. 15-1) and the relative prominence or retrusion of the chin. Of particular concern is the distance between stomion and subnasale, which is often short (see 3 above) with respect to the total maxillo-mandibular profile height.

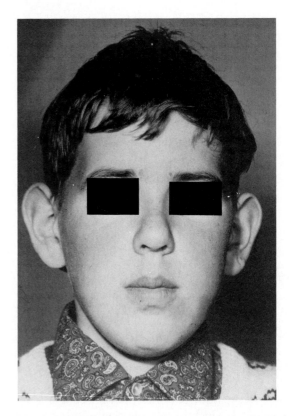

Fig. 15-1. The lower facial third is enlarged in patients with a skeletal open bite.

FUNCTIONAL CONSIDERATIONS

Tongue posture and tongue function should be a prime consideration in open bite problems. It is necessary to differentiate primary causal and secondary adaptive or compensatory tongue dysfunction. The functional analysis also must assess the magnitude of force, i.e., simple pressing versus strong protractive action. Cephalometric analysis can localize the nature of the open bite, i.e., skeletal or dentoalveolar. Hence it is necessary to correlate the functional and cephalometric analyses when making a determination of the role and effect of tongue activity.

According to Bahr and Holt, it is possible to differentiate four varieties of tongue thrust activity:

1. Tongue thrust without deformation. Despite the abnormal function, no deformation ensues.
2. Tongue thrust causing anterior deformation, i.e., anterior open bite, sometimes coupled with bilateral narrowing of the arch and a posterior crossbite. Moyers terms this a *simple open bite.*
3. Tongue thrust causing buccal segment deformation with a posterior open bite. A lateral tongue thrust activity can also be responsible for a functional deep bite, which is a variation of the posterior open bite (Fig. 15-2). Some Class II, Division 2, malocclusions fit this category. Invagination of the cheek into the interocclusal space may also be a factor.
4. Combined tongue thrust, causing both an anterior and posterior open bite. This is called a *complex open bite* by Moyers and is more difficult to treat.

It should again be stressed that tongue posture is as important as tongue function. The retained infantile deglutitional pattern usually has a forward posturing tongue as a vestige of the nursing posture. Finger-sucking habits often serve to prolong this infantile pro-

tractive tongue posture, with the tip of the tongue between the anterior teeth. In the normal maturational cycle, the tip of the tongue drops back as the incisors erupt. Once the anterior space is created by interference with normal incisor eruption, compensatory function is evident during deglutition, as the individual tries to effect a seal during the swallowing cycle.

CLINICAL CONSIDERATIONS

There are various forms of anterior open bite, depending on the severity of the malocclusion.

1. Cases with an overjet combined with an open bite of less than 1 mm can be designated as pseudo–open bite problems.
2. A simple open bite exists in cases where there is more than 1 mm between the incisors, but the posterior teeth are in occlusion.
3. A complex open bite designates those cases where the open bite extends from the premolars or deciduous molars on one side to the corresponding tooth on the other side.
4. The compound or infantile open bite is completely open, including the molars.
5. The iatrogenic open bite is the consequence of orthodontic therapy, which produces atypical configurations due to appliance manipulation or adaptive neuromuscular response.

In the mixed dentition period, various therapeutic measures may cause an open bite:

1. An open activator with a high construction bite can cause a tongue thrust habit and resultant anterior open bite. During intrusion of the posterior teeth, a posterior open bite may also be created, especially in the deciduous molar area.
2. In expansion treatment, the buccal segments can be tipped excessively buccally, with elongation of the lingual cusps. This creates prematurity and effectively opens the bite.
3. In distalization of maxillary first molars with extraoral force, the molars are often tipped down and back, elongating the mesial cusps. This creates a molar fulcrum that can open the bite and is of particular concern in downward and backward growing faces that already have excessive anterior face height.

CEPHALOMETRIC CRITERIA

A proper cephalometric analysis enables a classification of open bite malocclusions to be achieved.

In the dentoalveolar open bite the extent of the open bite depends on the extent of the eruption of the teeth. A supraocclusion of the molars and/or infraocclusion of the incisors can be a primary etiologic factor. In a vertical growth pattern, the dentoalveolar symptoms are

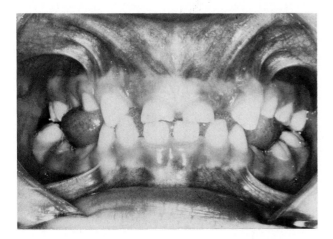

Fig. 15-2. Bilateral open bite in the deciduous dentition in which the tongue was a factor.

usually a protrusion in the upper anterior teeth combined with lingual inclination of the lower incisors. In a horizontal growth pattern, tongue posture and thrust may cause proclination of both upper and lower incisors.

A lateral open bite may be considered dentoalveolar in combination with infraclusion of molar teeth. Contributing causal factors may be abnormal muscle activity such as cheek-sucking, lateral tongue thrust, or lateral postural tongue spread in the postural resting position. Interruption of the abnormal function with appliances (screening therapy) can bring about significant improvement.

An example is shown in Fig. 15-3. A 14-year-old boy had a severe cheek-tongue dysfunction that was eliminated with therapy and the posterior open bite also eliminated.

In cases of skeletal open bite the anterior face height is excessive, particularly the lower third, while posterior face height (ramus height) is short. The mandibular base is usually narrow, and antegonial notching is often present. The symphysis is narrow and long and the ramus is short. The gonial angle, particularly the lower section, is large, and the growth pattern is vertical. Depending on the inclination of the maxillary base, or palatal plane, the following variations may be observed:

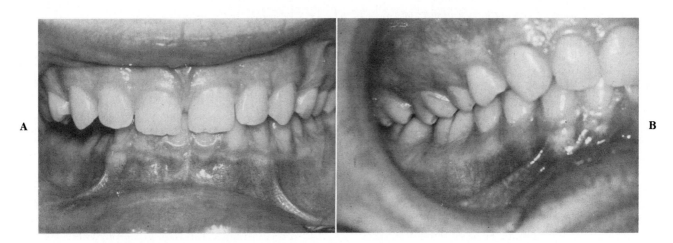

Fig. 15-3. Lateral open bite in a 14-year-old patient with nonocclusion of the right premolars. **A,** Before and, **B,** after screening of the dysfunction.

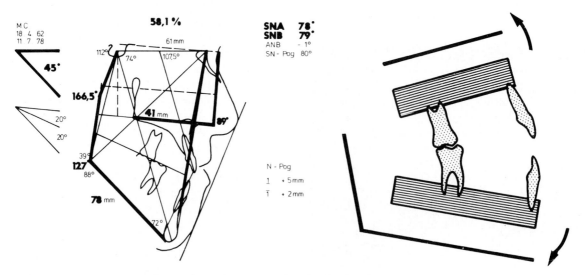

Fig. 15-4. Vertical growth pattern combined with anteinclination of the maxilla.

1. A vertical growth pattern with upward tipping of the forward end of the maxillary base. This can provide a condition in which unfavorable sequelae complement each other to cause a severe skeletal open bite (Fig. 15-4).
2. A vertical growth pattern with downward tipping of the anterior end of the maxillary base. This can combine with an offsetting relationship to compensate the open bite (Fig. 15-5).
3. A horizontal growth direction with an open bite caused by the upward and forward tipping of the maxillary base (Fig. 15-6). This type of problem is designated a decompensated deep overbite.

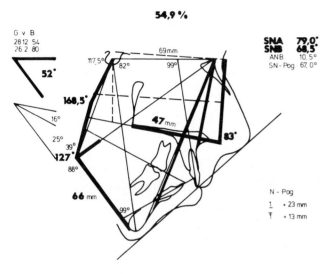

Fig. 15-5. Vertical growth pattern, partially compensated by a slight retroinclination of the maxilla.

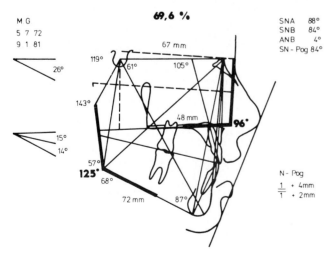

Fig. 15-6. Horizontal growth pattern with anteinclination of the maxilla. This is the cause of the open bite.

THERAPEUTIC CONSIDERATIONS

Therapy depends on the localization and etiology of the malocclusion. Habit control and the elimination of abnormal perioral muscle function are causal therapeutic approaches in the dentoalveolar open bite problem. In skeletal open bite problems a redirection of growth is possible during the active growth period. Later only compensatory therapy with extraction and tooth movement or orthognathic surgery are possible.

In addition to the dentoalveolar and skeletal open bite categories, there is possible a combined skeletodental type that requires a combined therapeutic approach. Even in a dentoalveolar treatment approach the growth pattern should be considered because of the different reactions of individual growth patterns to various neuromuscular abnormalities and vice versa. In the latter case a bimaxillary protrusion can occur in a horizontal growth pattern, while lingual tipping may result in a vertical growth pattern.

The proper time to institute treatment depends on the etiology of the malocclusion. If the causal factor can be eliminated, early interceptive therapy is indicated, because dysfunctions should be eliminated as soon as feasible. On the other hand, skeletal problems can be solved or at least compensated for at an older age.

Various treatment regimens are possible during the various developmental periods of the dentition. Many of these problems are discussed in Chapter 3. Only a summary of the different treatment approaches is given here.

Open bite treatment in the deciduous dentition

Control of the abnormal habits and elimination of dysfunctions should be given top priority in this stage. In many instances the open bite improves as soon as the habit is stopped. Autonomous improvement can be expected only when the deforming muscle activity is terminated, and the open bite is not complicated by crowding of the upper arch or cross-bite. Treatment with screening appliances or activators is indicated in such open bite cases.

A skeletal open bite is seldom observed in the deciduous dentition. Habit control is of only secondary consideration in these cases, retarding the increasing severity of the dysplasia. To redirect growth, extraoral orthopedic appliances such as chin caps can be used effectively.

Treatment of open bite in the mixed dentition

It is possible to differentiate among three types of open bite malocclusion in the mixed dentition period.

1. *Dentoalveolar* open bite malocclusion as a consequence of various dysfunctions. In the early mixed dentition period, screening therapy (as described in Chap-

ter 3) is indicated. In the late mixed dentition, however, with a severe tongue thrust or posture problem, screening therapy may be unsuccessful. In such cases the open bite may respond favorably to multiattachment fixed appliances, but a long posttreatment retention phase is necessary until the abnormal perioral muscle function can be reduced. Swallowing exercises (i.e., swallowing without thrusting, putting the tip of the tongue behind the upper or lower incisors) may reinforce the establishment of a mature deglutitional and functional pattern for the tongue, both during treatment and during retention.

The example shown here is an 8-year-old girl with a developmental age of 9½ years. There was an open bite with a tongue posture-dysfunction problem (Fig. 15-7). The maxillary and mandibular bases were prognathic, the maxillary base of average length, and the mandibular base and ramus long. Interocclusal space was minimal or nonexistent. The growth pattern was extremely

horizontal, as might be expected from the skeletal configuration. The tongue thrust had apparently caused a double protrusion. Because of the abnormal function and the small size of the incisors, generalized spacing existed between the teeth. The open bite was complicated by the upward and forward inclination of the maxillary base. An inhibitory treatment was initiated, using a double screen, but with no success. The severe tongue pressures prevented uprighting the incisors and closing the spaces. The open bite was corrected with fixed appliances, intermaxillary elastics, etc. after eruption of the canines and premolars. Even with the closure of the open bite, a slight protrusion of the upper incisors persisted (Fig. 15-8). This protrusion was also a compensation for the Class III basal relationship tendency, as shown by the A-N-B angle of 0 degrees. Growth increments were predictably high in the mandibular base as opposed to average increments in the maxilla.

The inhibitory treatment failed in this case because it

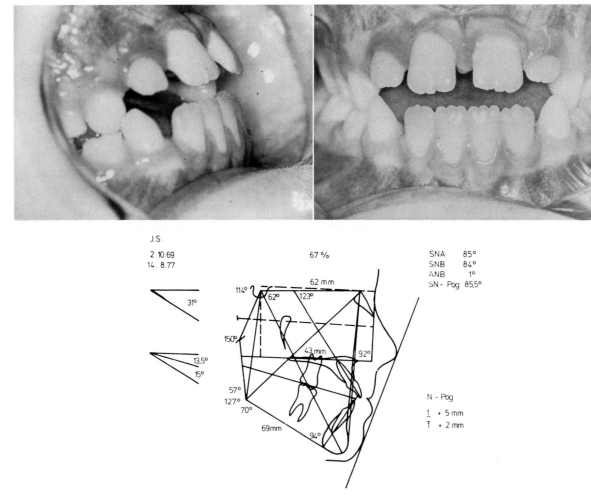

Fig. 15-7. Patient E.S. before treatment.

is difficult to correct a double protrusion using screening appliances alone; the tongue problem cannot be completely eliminated. Complementary active force was required to upright the incisors, although the growth vector was horizontal. The bite was open because of the strong anteinclination (upward and forward tipping) of the maxillary base. Lack of a normal freeway space probably indicates overeruption of the posterior teeth.

2. *Skeletal* open bite malocclusion. Treatment of skeletal open bite is dependent on at least two factors—the severity of the malocclusion and the possibility of dental alveolar compensation.

The growth pattern in this type of problem is almost always vertical. Not only the extent of this vertical growth pattern but also the inclination of the maxillary base is decisive in treatment planning. If the rotation of the jaw bases is divergent, the prognosis is poor. If the maxillary base is tipped downward and forward (retroclined), functional therapy may sometimes be successful.

In addition to intrusion of buccal segments and extrusion of the incisors, mesial movement of the posterior teeth is also a beneficial dentoalveolar measure to help close the bite. Moving teeth forward in the V by the removal of the four first premolars often makes it possible to close the bite, despite the skeletal nature of the problem. Treatment can be undertaken with activators combined with extraction and/or extraoral force application. In extreme cases, with divergent rotation of the jaw bases, removal of four premolars and fixed appliance therapy constitute the best approach to treatment. Severe cases still will require orthognathic surgery, with impaction of buccal segments and even sagittal split osteotomy, in some cases, to close the bite and provide stable correction.

Fig. 15-9 shows an 8-year-old girl with a long face syndrome, extremely vertical growth pattern, but only a slight anterior open bite. Her jaw bases were retrognathic and short, with an A-N-B difference of 4 degrees and reduced ramus length (−13.5 mm). The posterior to anterior height ratio was 49%, which is quite low. The lower gonial angle was large at 93 degrees. Crowd-

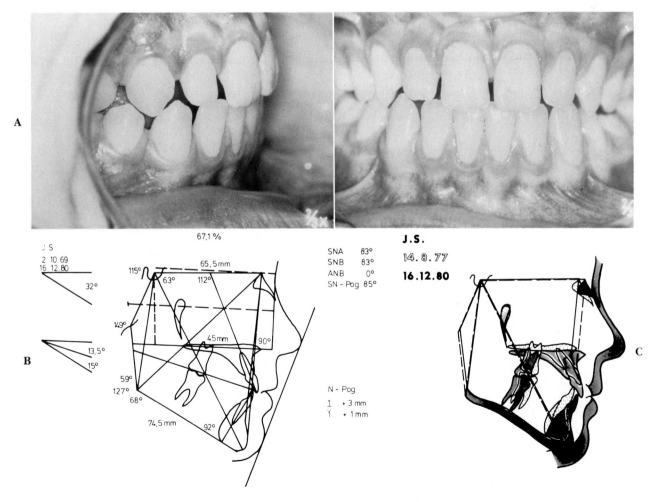

Fig. 15-8. Patient E.S. after treatment. **C,** Superimposition of before and after tracings.

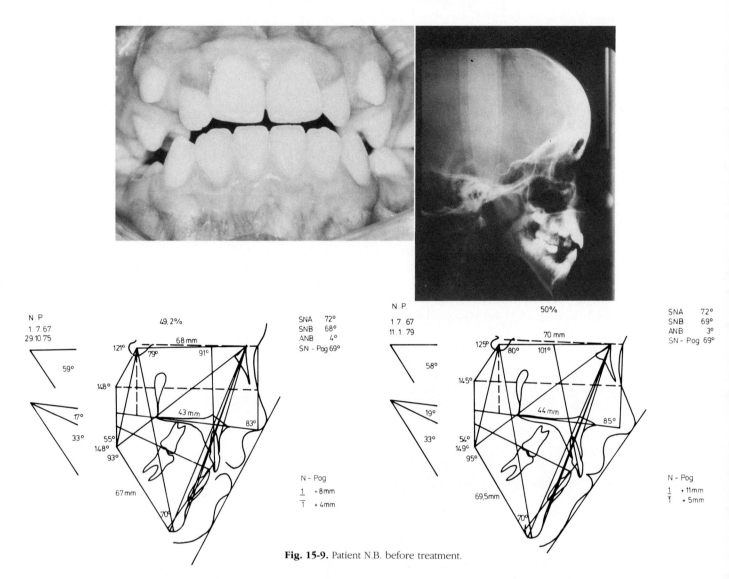

Fig. 15-9. Patient N.B. before treatment.

ing was present in the upper arch. The slight open bite was considered secondary. The maxillary base was retroclined at an angle of 83 degrees, which was considered favorable for therapy. Four premolars were removed, and fixed appliances were planned for later, in hopes of preventing the need for surgical correction at a later date. Since habit control was not deemed necessary, therapy was postponed to 11½ years of age. In the interim the upper incisors had uprighted some, possibly due to acquired abnormal lip function. The growth pattern persisted in a vertical direction, with the ramus remaining short (− 10 mm).

After 2½ years of multiattachment mechanotherapy, the dental arches were aligned and the open bite was closed, but there was no improvement of the skeletal relationship (Fig. 15-10). A study of three siblings showed the hereditary nature of the long face syndrome that dominated the family facial pattern. Since the malocclusion was not caused by a functional aberration, function appliance therapy was not justified.

In some cases of extreme vertical growth patterns lip sealing ability is significantly disturbed. To achieve a better neuromuscular environment, a surgical resection of the mentalis muscle can be done to reduce the "golfball chin" effect (Fig. 15-11). This operation is indicated in the mixed dentition period after eruption of the lower canine teeth, according to Schilli. Following the growth period, cosmetic plastic surgery of the chin area may be necessary (Fig. 15-12). This type of transposition of the mentalis muscle attachment, permitting greater extension of the lower lip to effect a lip seal, can enhance the stability of the treatment result and bite closure.

3. *Combined* open bite. In actual practice, it is likely that most skeletal open bite cases are at least partially attributable to abnormal perioral muscle function. The work of Rolf and Christine Fränkel supports this observation. Because of the dual nature of the etiology, a combined treatment approach is recommended. There are two possible combinations—elimination of abnor-

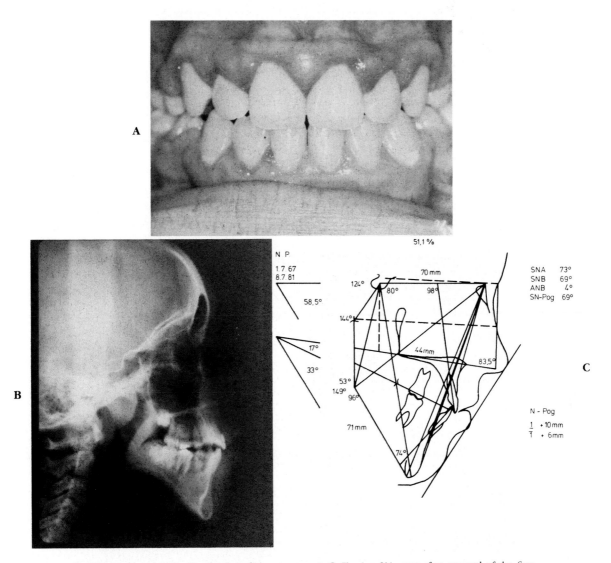

Fig. 15-10. Patient N.B. after fixed appliance treatment. **C,** Tracing 3½ years after removal of the first molars.

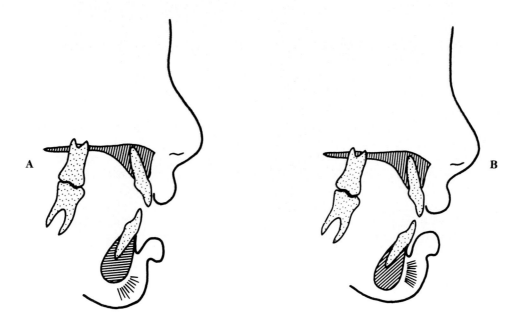

Fig. 15-11. Operative transposition of the lower lip musculature, according to Schilli. **A,** Before and, **B,** after the mentalis resection.

mal perioral muscle function and/or improvement of skeletal relationships.

The abnormal perioral muscle function is eliminated or at least intercepted in the early mixed dentition period, and the required serial extraction procedures, if indicated, are performed. Tooth eruption can be guided and the habit pattern can be controlled fairly well with an activator. After the eruption of the permanent teeth, the remaining malocclusion can be reduced by compensatory tooth movement, usually performed with fixed appliances.

Case report. An example of this combined treatment is shown in Fig. 15-13. The patient, a 7½-year-old girl, had an open bite and a severe vertical growth pattern. The mother and one sibling had the same morphogenetic pattern. Both jaw bases were retrognathic, and the maxillary base and ramus particularly were short (−15 mm). The vertical growth pattern was partially compensated by a downward and forward inclination of the maxillary base. The axial inclination of the incisors was average. Crowding existed in the upper and lower den-

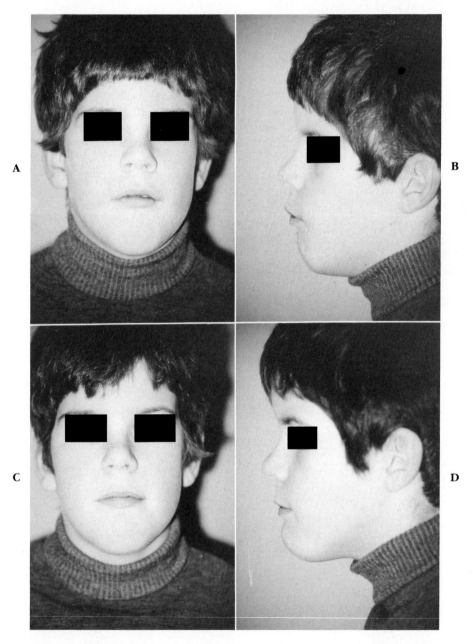

Fig. 15-12. Patient D.S., 10 years old. **A** and **B,** Before mentalis resection and, **C** and **D,** after the transposition of muscle attachment.

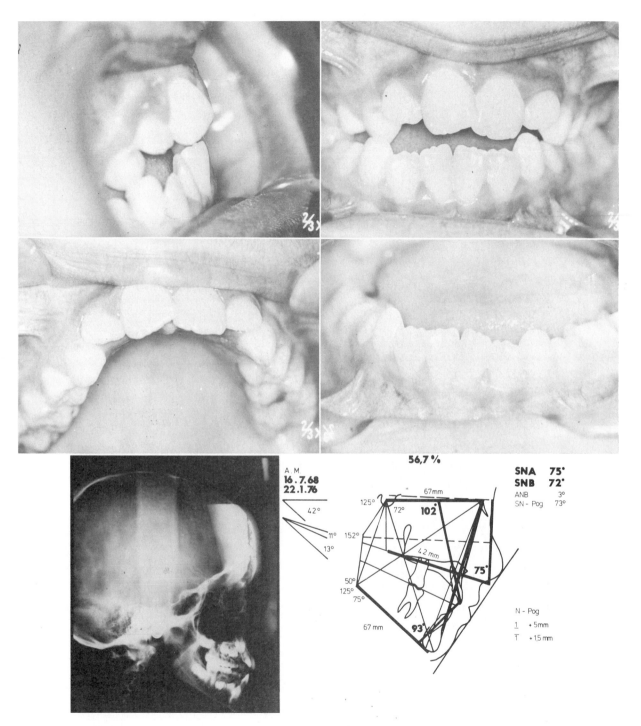

Fig. 15-13. Patient A.M. before treatment. Downward and forward tipping of the palatal plane has partially compensated the open bite.

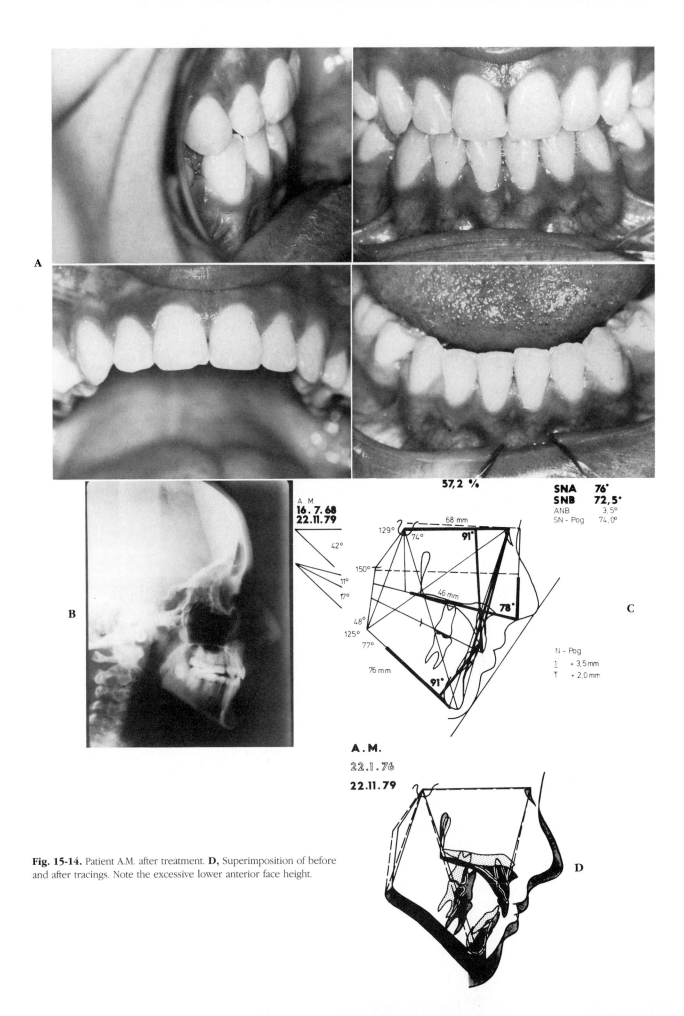

Fig. 15-14. Patient A.M. after treatment. **D,** Superimposition of before and after tracings. Note the excessive lower anterior face height.

tal arches. A tongue problem had existed along with a finger-sucking habit until the age of 6 years.

Serial extraction procedures (including first premolar sacrifice) were instituted, along with concomitant placement of an activator. The construciton bite was established at 5 mm vertically, but the mandible was positioned only slightly anteriorly (2 mm). The treatment objective was to control the neuromuscular malfunction while loading the posterior teeth that had overerupted, freeing the incisors for further eruption, under the guidance of the labial wire of the activator. After the eruption of the canines and premolars, the remaining spaces were closed with fixed, multiattachment therapy and intermaxillary traction for the open bite.

At the end of active treatment 3½ years later, despite the dentoalveolar improvement, there was only a slightly better skeletal relationship. The growth rate of the mandibular base was high, but the ramus remained short (−13.5 mm). The maxillary growth increments were average. The retroclination of the maxillary base persisted and aided the alveolodental compensation for the original malocclusion (Fig. 15-14).

The achievable optimum of therapy was possible in this case only because of the favorable inclination of the maxillary base and the compromise decision of tooth removal, allowing dentoalveolar compensation. The early interceptive habit control at least prevented exacerbation of the malocclusion by the potentially deforming abnormal function.

Another example of this combined treatment might be to try to achieve some skeletal improvement and correct the dental malrelationships in the second phase.

To illustrate this approach, an 11-year-old girl with an open-bite malocclusion, severe tongue dysfunction problems, and a double protrusion of incisors is shown in Fig. 15-15. The maxilla was prognathic, but the mandible was orthognathic. Although the growth pattern was horizontal, the upward and forward inclination of the

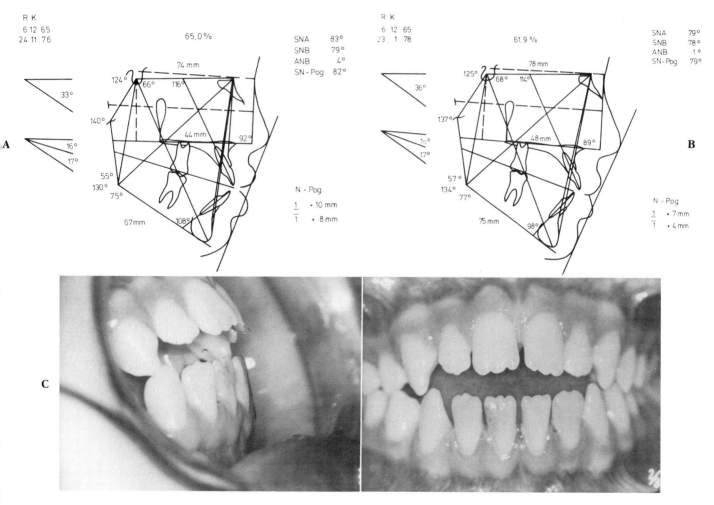

Fig. 15-15. Patient R.K. **A,** Before therapy. **B,** After treatment with functional appliances. **C,** Before fixed appliance therapy.

maxillary base contributed to the open bite relationship. Treatment was started with an activator, with the following objectives:

1. To intercept and control the abnormal neuromuscular influences
2. To influence the unfavorable upward tipping of the maxillary base and, at the same time, to reduce its relative prognathism

The treatment of the double protrusion and the final correction of the open bite were planned for a later treatment phase. A vertical activator was constructed that extended the acrylic over the labial surfaces of the upper and lower incisors (indexing) and was trimmed away from the acrylic linguoincisally. The posterior teeth were loaded and an occlusal acrylic cover interposed for a depressing action, inasmuch as the interocclusal clearance was minimal and the viscoelastic properties of the muscle and the stretch reflex action could be enlisted. After 14 months of activator treatment, the

protrusion and upward inclination of the maxillary base were reduced. The labial tipping, of the lower incisors in particular, also was reduced. Posterior segment eruption was thereby withheld.

A second phase of this combination approach required fixed appliances to achieve the final adjustments; it took less than 7 months (Fig. 15-16).

Treatment of open bite in the permanent dentition

The use of functional methods is limited in the permanent dentition. Usually multiattachment fixed mechanotherapy is the method of choice, together with guided extraction procedures to correct the dentoalveolar problems and to compensate for any skeletal problems that exist. If the dysfunction persists, functional therapy can play only a subordinate role.

Actually some minor improvement in the dentoalveolar region can be achieved, e.g., closing a posterior open

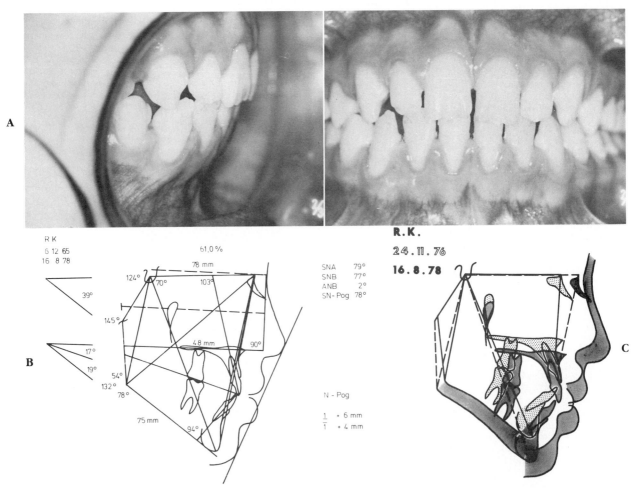

Fig. 15-16. Patient R.K. after fixed appliance therapy. **C,** Superimposition of tracings, before activator and after fixed appliance therapy.

bite by screening the tongue from interposing between the occlusal surfaces. A slight anterior open bite may be reduced also, if there is no crowding. Using a combination of screening and some active extrusive force on the incisors, with a tongue crib on a palatal plate together with an active labial bow, for example, will reduce the open bite. Needed intrusion of posterior teeth is very difficult, however, although initial success with repelling magnetic force appliances appears promising.

Functional appliances are helpful in the retention phase of therapy. Interocclusal cover of the posterior teeth prevents relapsing overeruption of the buccal segments, while aberrant neuromuscular activity is effectively screened from deforming the dentoalveolar region.

Diagnosis is still the major challenge in these open bite problems. The correct indication of any mode of therapy should be determined ahead of time. Both functional and cephalometric analytic assessments are needed before treatment planning is done. The therapy for some open bite malocclusions is very simple, with self-improvement after the elimination of abnormal perioral muscle function. The diagnostic assessment will determine if the particular case satisfies the criteria for such screening therapy. Cases with unfavorable morphogenetic pattern, unfavorable growth vectors, or unfavorable patient ages will not respond adequately to functional appliance treatment. Indeed they are likely to become progressively worse despite appliance wear, disappointing both the patient and the operator. However, the fault does not lie with the appliance but with improper diagnosis.

CHAPTER 16

THE FUTURE OF FUNCTIONAL APPLIANCES

This book cannot be finished without a look at the future. For the past century, orthodontic therapy, including functional appliances, has been mainly a mechanical activity. It is likely to remain that way. Yet there is no doubt that functional appliances will be further improved conceptually, technologically, and operationally. We are witnessing this phenomenon every day. New findings on the cellular and biologic levels will transform the orthodontic specialty by introducing biochemical, bioelectrical, and other physical procedures. These will be designed to have an amplifying effect on some elements of the causal chain located between the mechanical appliance and the reestablishment of the normal intermaxillary relation and occlusion. The contemporary orthodontist also must always be prepared intellectually for the transformation of his specialty. This book was devised to help him achieve such an ambitious goal.

Tomorrow's orthodontics is not only therapy and interception. It is also prevention. Certainly genetic engineering is not in the immediate future; but there are other methods of prevention. It is worthwhile to report a recent animal experiment by Stutzmann and Petrovic that may be of interest in upbringing of babies (breast-feeding versus stiff nipple or soft nipple bottle-feeding).

In the first experimental group, newborn male rats were exposed to different feeding modalities. When sacrificed at the age of 20 days, the following observations were made:

1. The growth rate of the condylar cartilage was highest in the breast-fed and lowest in the gavage-fed rats (Table 16-1).
2. Stutzmann angle (direction of condylar growth) was highest (more vertical) in gavage-fed rats and lowest (more horizontal) in those breast-fed (Table 16-2).
3. The length of the mandible was about the same in the stiff nipple–fed and ultrasoft nipple–fed rats and in gavage-fed rats; but all three mandibles were significantly shorter than in the breast-fed rats (Table 16-3).

In the second experimental group, the four above-mentioned categories (breast-fed, stiff nipple–fed, ultrasoft nipple–fed, and gavage-fed rats, from birth to the age of 20 days) were exposed after the age of 20 days to the usual feeding (Tables 16-4 to 16-6). In each category, one half of the animals were exposed to a postural hyperpropulsor (construction bite, 2 mm forward positioning of the mandible for 12 hours daily) while the other half served as controls. Some treated and nontreated rats of each category were killed at the age of 48 days (puberty period) and at the age of 180 days (adult animals). The results concerning the mandible (Table 16-4 to 16-6) may be summarized as follows:

1. Regardless of the age of sacrifice (48 or 180 days), there was little difference, if any, between breast-feeding and stiff nipple–feeding. However, the growth of the mandible was obviously impaired by ultrasoft nipple–feeding and, in a more pronounced manner, by gavage-feeding. Although the growth of the condyle had been more posteriorly

Table 16-1. Total number of tritiated thymidine labeled cells in the condylar cartilage (fifteen 20-day-old male rats in each group)

Treatment	Mean	Standard error
Breast-feeding	472	
Stiff nipple–feeding	419	
Ultrasoft nipple–feeding	396	±7.02
Gavage-feeding	378	

Analysis of variance

Source of variations	Sum of squares	Degrees of freedom	Mean square	F ratio
Way of feeding	74 784	3	24 298	33.71
ERROR	41 402	56	739	p < 0.01
TOTAL	116 186	59		

Smallest significant difference at 5% level between two means: 14 (number of ^{3}H-thymidine–labeled cells)

Table 16-2. Angle between the growth direction of the condyle and the mandibular plane (Stutzmann angle) (fifteen 20-day-old male rats in each group)

Treatment	Mean	Standard error
Breast-feeding	137.8	
Stiff nipple–feeding	141.0	± 0.64
Ultrasoft nipple–feeding	143.4	
Gavage-feeding	144.1	

Analysis of variance

Source of variations	Sum of squares	Degrees of freedom	Mean square	F ratio
Way of feeding	366.85	3	122.28	20.03
ERROR	341.73	56	6.10	$p < 0.01$
TOTAL	708.58	59		

Smallest significant difference at 5% confidence level between two means: 1.3 degrees

Table 16-3. Length of the mandible equals the distance between the posterior border of the condylar cartilage and the mental foramen (fifteen 20-day-old male rats in each group)

Treatment	Mean	Standard error
Breast-feeding	7.83	
Stiff nipple–feeding	7.39	± 0.0903
Ultrasoft nipple–feeding	7.28	
Gavage-feeding	7.30	

Analysis of variance

Source of variations	Sum of squares	Degrees of freedom	Mean square	F ratio
Way of feeding	2.9349	3	0.9783	7.99
ERROR	6.8569	56	0.1224	$p < 0.01$
TOTAL	9.7918	59		

Smallest significant difference at 5% confidence level between two means: 0.18 mm

Table 16-4. Number of tritiated thymidine–labeled cells in the condylar cartilage (12 male rats in each group)

Birth to day 20	Day 20 to sacrifice	Age at sacrifice	
Feeding modalities	Usual feeding, no appliance (H_o) or postural hyperpropulsor (H)	48 days	Standard error
Breast	H_o	878	
	H	1499	
Stiff nipple	H_o	906	
	H	1513	
Ultrasoft nipple	H_o	787	± 36.75
	H	1227	
Gavage	H_o	675	
	H	932	

Analysis of variance*

Source of variations	Sum of squares	Degrees of freedom	Mean square	F ratio
Way of feeding	2 575 497	3	858 499	53.25
Postural hyperpropulsor effect	5 556 031	1	5 556 031	344.65
Interaction	525 113	3	175 038	10.86
ERROR	1 148 623	88	16 121	
TOTAL	10 075 264	95		

*Smallest significant difference at 5% confidence level between two means = 73

Table 16-5. Angle between the growth direction of the condyle and the mandibular plane (Stutzmann angle): mean values (degrees) and standard error calculated for the whole population (12 male rats in each group)

Birth to day 20	Day 20 to sacrifice	Age at sacrifice		
Feeding modalities	Usual feeding, no appliance (H_0) or postural hyperpropulsor (H)	48 days	180 days	Standard error
Breast	H_0	128.9	131.9	
	H	140.5	133.9	
Stiff nipple	H_0	128.2	131.2	
	H	138.2	132.6	±0.4991
Ultrasoft nipple	H_0	134.1	137.0	
	H	140.3	142.5	
Gavage	H_0	137.6	138.6	
	H	140.5	145.6	

Analysis of variance*

Source of variations	Sum of squares	Degrees of freedom	Mean square	F ratio
Feeding modality (F_m)	2083.90	3	694.64	232.13
Postural hyperpropulsor (H)	1633.33	1	1633.33	545.82
Duration of hyperpropulsion (T)	20.02	1	20.02	6.69
Interactions				
$F_m \times H$	20.42	3	6.81	2.27
$F_m \times T$	233.22	3	77.74	25.97
$H \times T$	168.75	1	168.75	56.39
$F_m \times H \times T$	388.17	3	129.39	43.24
ERROR	526.67	176	2.99	
TOTAL	5074.48	191		

*Smallest significant difference at 5% confidence level between two means = 0.98 degree

Table 16-6. Length of the mandible (distance between the posterior border of the condylar cartilage and the mental foramen): mean values (mm) and standard error calculated for the whole population (12 male rats in each group)

Birth to day 20	Day 20 to sacrifice	Age at sacrifice		
Feeding modalities	Usual feeding, no appliance (H_0) or postural hyperpropulsor (H)	48 days	180 days	Standard error
Breast	H_0	13.93	20.05	
	H	15.44	22.57	
Stiff nipple	H_0	13.83	20.23	
	H	15.80	22.70	±0.1465
Ultrasoft nipple	H_0	13.17	18.67	
	H	13.86	19.73	
Gavage	H_0	12.52	17.59	
	H	13.00	18.20	

Analysis of variance*

Source of variations	Sum of squares	Degrees of freedom	Mean square	F ratio
Feeding modality (F_m)	264.12	3	88.04	341.74
Postural hyperpropulsor (H)	95.47	1	95.47	370.59
Duration of hyperpropulsion (T)	1738.88	1	1738.88	6749.78
Interactions				
$F_m \times H$	24.47	3	8.16	31.67
$F_m \times T$	3.04	3	3.04	11.81
$H \times T$	19.68	1	6.56	25.47
$F_m \times H \times T$	1.29	3	0.43	1.66
ERROR	45.34	176	0.26	
TOTAL	2192.29	191		

*Smallest significant difference at 5% confidence level between two means = 0.29 mm

oriented, the length of the mandible was significantly shorter.

2. Regardless of the age of sacrifice (48 or 180 days), the responsiveness of the mandible to the stimulating effect of the functional appliance was of the same order of magnitude in breast-fed and in stiff nipple–fed rats; however, it was greatly reduced in ultrasoft nipple–fed and gavage-fed rats.

It can be dangerous to extrapolate from the animal to the human situation, but these experiments again demonstrate the interrelationship between form and function, extending well beyond the dentoalveolar region for the orthodontist. Neither entity is mutually exclusive, but each depends on the other. The results of this research again substantiate a long-term clinical study by Graber (unpublished) on 600 children with thumb- and finger-sucking habits and retained infantile deglutition. When these habits persist beyond 4 years of age, the malocclusion characteristics are more likely to be permanent. Specifically, the relative mandibular retrusion, the more vertical growth direction (smaller Stutzmann angle), and the narrow maxillary arch occur with significantly greater frequency in these children than in children with no abnormal sucking habits and with normal deglutitional maturation. One observation in the Graber study was that breast-fed babies were increasingly likely to discard finger- and thumb-sucking habits earlier, before any permanent damage had occurred, and that deglutitional maturation and tongue function were more likely to be normal. It also appeared that the gratificational aspects of breast-feeding were responsible for significantly less parafunctional activity (bruxism and clenching) in the birth-to-4-year-old group than in bottle-fed babies, most of whom had been given soft nipples or poorly designed pacifiers to suck on.

The choice of orthodontics or dentofacial orthopedics clearly depends on early developmental and environmental factors. The orthodontist of the future must take these considerations into account and become involved at an earlier age with simple functional appliance adjuncts that prevent or intercept developing malocclusions, which demand extensive mechanotherapy at a later date. Working with the pediatrician, the orthodontist will be able to remove any roadblocks to optimal dentofacial development. As the above cited research shows, the methodology may include dietary, endocrine, functional, and simple interceptive appliance guidance. Our patient service horizons will expand as the clinical approaches are subjected to searching scrutiny by researchers in cell biology and oral physiology.

ANIMAL EXPERIMENTATION, DOES IT REPLICATE CLINICAL SITUATIONS?

The question arises, are concepts and theories established from *normal* animals (irrespective of the species) valid, and, if so, to what degree for the human *orthodontic patient?* To be more specific, why do various orthodontic patients react to the same functional appliances in a different manner?

According to research investigations on condylar cartilage, as well as on mandibular basal and alveolar bone, in growing animals and in children by one of the authors (Petrovic), almost all orthodontic patients (excluding general craniofacial anomalies) display, not qualitative, but merely *quantitative* variations involving a number of elements of the morphophysiologic organization of the face. Findings at the cell and molecular level may be summarized as follows:

1. No significant difference with reference to either the cytosolic concentration of Na^+, Ca^{++}, and H^+ or the intracellular pH could be detected in skeletoblasts and prechondroblasts—whatever the origin of the human condylar cartilage, Class I, II, or III.

2. In children without respiratory or allergy problems, the following correlation has been identified: The greater the turnover rate of the mandibular alveolar bone, the greater will be the magnitude of the variation—e.g., the reaction to an appropriate standardized pressure on the condylar cartilage that has been placed in organ culture—in the cytosolic concentration of Na^+, Ca^{++}, and H^+, as well as in the intracellular pH. Consequently there is a corresponding decrease in the cell multiplication rate. In this connection, the highest responsiveness to biomechanical factors in the condylar cartilage was discovered in skeletoblasts about to differentiate into prechondroblasts.

3. The correlation in paragraph 2 is of uppermost interest to orthodontists for the following two reasons (Petrovic and Stutzmann, 1979; Stutzmann and Petrovic, 1980): First, a high turnover rate of the mandibular alveolar bone is most often associated with a low angle (anterior growth rotation) whereas a low turnover rate of the mandibular alveolar bone is usually associated with a high angle (posterior growth rotation). Second, the greater the turnover rate of the mandibular alveolar bone and the higher the dividing cell index in the vestibular subperiosteal area of the mandible, the greater will be the clinical effectiveness of a functional appliance, whatever its type (L.S.U. activator, Fränkel FR, postural hyperpropulsor, Bionator, etc.). Everything happens as if there were a direct proportionality between the alveolar bone turnover rate, the dividing cell index in the vestibular subperiosteal area, and the responsiveness of the condylar cartilage and posterior border of the mandible to growth stimulation induced by a functional appliance.

4. In a child with strong facial asymmetry, the magnitude of the variation as a reaction to the appropriate standardized pressure on the condylar cartilage placed in organ culture—of the cytosolic concentration of Na^+, Ca^{++}, and H^+ as well as the intracellular pH—was considerably less in skeletoblasts and prechondroblasts originating from the condylar cartilage on the hypoplastic side. As a matter of course, the variation in cell multiplication rate was reduced.

According to these findings, the difference between a child with normal occlusion (Class I) and a child with a skeletal malrelation (Class II or III) seems to reside *mainly* in the decreased (Class II) or increased (Class III) responsiveness of the condylar cartilage and of the posterior border of the ramus to the agents (hormones, local mediators, local regulators, biomechanical factors, etc.) stimulating the growth. Hence the deviations giving rise to the variations in the responsiveness to growth-stimulating agents should be searched for primarily in the *inter*cellular signals regulating the multiplication rate of the organized cell population forming either the condylar cartilage or the subperiosteal area of the ramus posterior border.

It is absolutely clear from this research that the difference between the normal occlusion and a malocclusion is not qualitative but quantitative in nature. Nevertheless, at crucial moments of facial development, very small fluctuations around a so-called bifurcation point in the intercuspal relationship (Fig. 1-5) can result in either of two very different types of occlusal pattern (Petrovic, 1982; Lavergne and Petrovic, 1983).

Along these lines, the pathogenesis of interjaw malrelations should be sought, as a matter of course, at all levels of biologic organization. Recent cell and molecular biology advances are a supplemental research tool to elaborate conceptually fruitful and therapeutically helpful concepts and theories in dentofacial orthopedics. No sector of dentistry has been so totally revised conceptually as orthodontics. Several scientific and biomedical disciplines have been brought together. New research approaches have been added. Whether the clinician likes it or not, the progress of our knowledge about functional appliances will, in the near future, unavoidably depend to a large extent on further advances in highly sophisticated image-processing, microscopic, physiologic, biophysical, biochemical, and genetic engineering research procedures.

However, these scientific and biomedical achievements, marvelous as they may be, will not take the place of clinical observation. They will solely promote understanding of why and how malocclusions and interjaw malrelations appear and can be treated. They will develop the field of craniofacial growth mechanisms to a degree beyond the imagination of present-day orthodontists. Forward-looking clinicians will ceaselessly be obliged to upgrade their knowledge in this increasingly complex field, without relying on an information that is only a few years old. Time-honored clinical procedures will be dropped into disuse—a challenging and inspiring situation! The clinical orthodontist will enjoy the benefits that arise from a permanent contact with new biomedical discoveries.

REFERENCES AND
SELECTED READINGS

Adams, C.P.: An investigation into indications for and the effects of the function regulator, Eur. Orthod. Soc. Rep. Congr. **45**:293, 1969.

Adams, C.P.: The design and construction of removable appliances, ed. 5, Bristol, 1984, John Wright & Sons, Ltd.

Adran, B., and Kemp, F.: A radiographic study of the movement of the tongue in swallowing, Dent. Pract. **5**:252, 1955.

Ahlgren, J.: An electromyographic analysis of the response to activator (Andresen-Häupl) therapy, Odontol. Rev. **11**:125, 1960.

Ahlgren, J.: The neurophysiologic principles of the Andresen method of functional jaw orthodontics. A critical analysis and new hypothesis, Svensk Tandlak. Tidskr. **63**:1, 1970.

Ahlgren, J.: A longitudinal clinical and cephalometric study of 50 malocclusion cases treated with activator appliances, Eur. Orthod. Soc. Rep. Congr. **48**:285, 1972.

Ahlgren, J.: Tongue function during activator treatment. A cephalometric and dynamometric study, Eur. J. Orthod. **55**:1251, 1979.

Ahlgren, J., and Posselt, U.: Need of functional analysis and selective grinding in orthodontics, Acta Odontol. Scand. **21**:187, 1963.

Andresen, V.: The Norwegian system of functional gnatho-orthopedics, Acta Gnathol. **1**:5, 1936.

Andresen, V.: Funktions-Kieferorthopädie, ed. 2, Leipzig, 1939, Hermann Meusser.

Andresen, V., and Häupl, K.: Funktions-Kieferorthopädie, Leipzig, 1936, Hermann Meusser.

Andresen, V., and Häupl, K.: Funktionskieferorthopädie. Die Grundlagen des norwegischen Systems, ed. 4, Leipzig, 1945, Johann Ambrosius Barth.

Andresen, V., Häupl, K., and Petrik, L.: Funktionskieferorthopädie. VI. Umgearbeitete and erweiterte Auflage von K. Häupl und L. Petrik, Munich, 1957, Johann Ambrosius Barth.

Andrew, R.J.: Evolution of facial expression, Science **142**:1034, 1963.

Andrews, L.F.: The six keys to normal occlusion, Am. J. Orthod. **62**:296, 1972.

Ascher, F.: Praktische Kieferorthopädie, Vienna, 1968, Urban & Schwarzenberg.

Auf der Maur, H.J.: Elektromyographische Befunde am musculus pterygoideus externus während der Distalbisstherapie mit dem Aktivator, Schweiz. Monatsschr. Zahnheilkd. **88**:1085, 1978.

Baker, J.: The tongue and the dental function, Am. J. Orthod. **40**:927, 1954.

Ballard, C.F.: A consideration of the physiological background of mandibular posture and movement, Dent. Pract. **6**:80, 1955.

Ballard, C.F.: Some observations on variations of tongue posture as seen in lateral skull radiographs and their significance, Eur. Orthod. Soc. Trans. **35**:69, 1959.

Ballard, C.F.: Variations of posture and behaviour of the lips and tongue which determine the position of the labial segments: the implications in orthodontics, prosthetics and speech, Eur. Orthod. Soc. Rep. Congr., p. 67, 1965.

Balters, W.: Ergebnis der gesteuerten Selbstheilung von keiferorthopädischen Anomalien, Dtsch. Zahnaerztl. Z. **15**:241, 1960.

Balters, W.: Eine Einführung in die Bionatorheilmethode: ausgewählte Schriften und Vorträge, Heidelberg, 1973, K. Herrmann Verlag.

Baron, R.: Remaniements de l'os alvéolaire et des fibres desmodontales au cours de la migration physiologique, J. Biol. Buccale **1**:151, 1973.

Baume, L.J.: The post-natal growth activity of the nasal cartilage septum, Helv. Odontol. Acta **5**:9, 1961.

Baume, L., and Derichsweiler, H.: Is the condylar growth center responsive to orthodontic therapy? Oral Surg. **14**:347, 1961.

Baume, L.J., Häupl, L., and Stellmach, R.: Growth and transformation of the TMJ in an orthopedically treated case of Pierre Robin syndrome, Am. J. Orthod. **45**:90, 1959.

Baumrind, S.: A reconsideration of the propriety of the "pressure-tension" hypothesis, Am. J. Orthod. **55**:12, 1969.

Baumrind, S., and Buck, D.L.: Rate changes in cell replication and protein synthesis in the periodontal ligament incident to tooth movement, Am. J. Orthod. **57**:109, 1970.

Bay, R., and Rakosi, T.: Fernröntgenologische Untersuchungen von zwei ethnischen Gruppen mit Distalbiss, Fortschr. Kieferorthop. **32**:161, 1971.

Benninghoff, A.: Architektur der Kiefer und ihre Weichteilbedeckung, Paradentium **6**:48, 1934.

Bimler, H.P.: Indikation der Gebissformer, Fortschr. Kieferorthop. **25**:121, 1964.

Bimler, H.P.: Stomatopedics in theory and practice, Int. J. Orthod. **2**:5, 1965.

Björk, A.: The principle of the Andresen method of orthodontic treatment. A discussion based on cephalometric x-ray analysis of treated cases, Am. J. Orthod. **37**:437, 1951.

Björk, A.: Facial growth in man studied with the aid of metallic implants, Acta Odontol. Scand. **13**:94, 1955.

Björk, A.: Variations in the growth pattern of the human mandible: Radiographic study by the implant method, J. Dent. Res. **42**:2, 1963.

Björk, A.: Sutural growth of the upper face studied by the metallic implant method, Acta Odontol. Scand. **24**:109, 1966.

Björk, A.: Prediction of mandibular growth rotation, Am. J. Orthod. **55**:585, 1969.

Björk, A.: Cited in Graber, T.M.: Orthodontic principles and practice, ed. 3, Philadelphia, 1972, W.B. Saunders Co.

Björk, A.: Facial development and tooth eruption, Am. J. Orthod. **62**:339, 1972.

Björk, A., and Skieller, V.: Normal and abnormal growth of the mandible. A synthesis of longitudinal cephalometric implant studies over a period of 25 years, Eur. J. Orthod. **5**:1, 1983.

Bluestone, C.D.: The role of tonsils and adenoids in the obstruction of respiration. In McNamara, J.A., Jr., editor: Nasorespiratory function and craniofacial growth, Monograph 9, Craniofacial growth series,

1979, Ann Arbor, Center for Human Growth and Development, University of Michigan.

Blume, D.G.: A study of occlusal equilibration as it relates to orthodontics, Am. J. Orthod. **44**:575, 1958.

Boman, V.R.: Research studies on the temporomandibular joint, Angle Orthod. **22**:154, 1952.

Bookstein, F.L.: Comment on "Issues related to the prediction of craniofacial growth," Am. J. Orthod. **79**:442, 1981.

Brauer, J.S., and Holt, T.V.: Tongue thrust classification, Angle Orthod. **35**:106, 1965.

Breitner, C.: Experimentelle Veränderung der mesiodistalen Beziehungen der oberen und unteren Zahnreihen, Z. Stomatol. **28**:134, 1930.

Breitner, C.: Bone changes resulting from experimental orthodontic treatment, Am. J. Orthod. Oral Surg. **26**:521, 1940.

Brigham, G., Scaletta, L., Johnston L., and Occhino, J.: Antigenic differences among condylar, epiphyseal, and nasal septal cartilage. In McNamara, J. A., Jr., editor: The biology of occlusal development, Monograph 7. Craniofacial growth series, Ann Arbor, 1977, Center for Human Growth and Development, University of Michigan.

Brodie, A.G.: Some recent observations of the growth of the face and their implications to the orthodontist. Am. J. Orthod. Oral Surg. **26**:741, 1940.

Brodie, A.G.: On the growth pattern of the human head from the third month to the eighth year of life, Am. J. Anat. **68**:209, 1941.

Burstone, C.J.: Lip posture and its significance in treatment planning, Am. J. Orthod. **53**:262, 1967.

Cederquist, K.R., and Virolainen, K.: Craniofacial growth in the squirrel monkey *(Saimiri sciureus),* Am. J. Orthod. **69**:592, 1976.

Celestin, L.A.: La thérapeutic bionator de Wilhelm Balters, Paris, 1967, Librairie Meloine Sa.

Charlier, J.P., and Petrovic, A.: Lack of independent growth potential of rat mandibular condylar cartilage, as revealed in organ culture. Presented at the eighteenth annual meeting of the Tissue Culture Association, Philadelphia, 1967a.

Charlier, J.P., and Petrovic, A.: Recherches sur la mandibule de rat en culture d'organes: le cartilage condylien a-t-il un potentiel de croissance indépendant? Orthod. Fr. **38**:165, 1967b.

Charlier, J.P., Petrovic, A., and Herrmann, J.: Déterminisme de la croissance mandibulaire: effets de l'hyperpropulsion et de l'hormone somatotrope sur la croissance condylienne de jeunes rats, Orthod. Fr. **39**:567, 1968.

Charlier, J.P., Petrovic, A., and Herrmann-Stutzmann, J.: Effects of mandibular hyperpropulsion on the prechondroblastic zone of young rat condyle, Am. J. Orthod. **55**:71, 1969a.

Charlier, J.P., Petrovic, A., and Linck, G.: La fronde mentonnière et son action sur la croissance mandibulaire. Recherches expérimentales chez le rat, Orthod. Fr. **40**:99, 1969b.

Chateau, M.: Traitement de la retrognatie mandibulaire par l'hyperpropulsion systématique, Orthod. Fr. **36**:637, 1955.

Cleall, J.F.: Deglutition: a study of form and function, Am. J. Orthod. **51**:560, 1965.

Cleall, J.F.: Growth of the palate and maxillary dental arch. J. Dent. Res. **53**:226, 1974.

Craig, C.E.: The skeletal pattern characteristics of Class I and Class II, division 1, malocclusion in norma lateralis, Angle Orthod. **21**:44, 1951.

Dausch-Neuman, U.: Biometgesicht und Kieferheilkunde, Fortschr. Kieferorthop. **32**:353, 1971.

Delaire, J.: La croissance des os de la voûte du crâne. Principes généraux (introduction à l'étude de la croissance des maxillaires). Rev. Stomatol. Chir. Maxillofac. **62**:518, 1961.

Delaire, J.: The potential role of facial muscles in monitoring maxillary growth and morphogenesis. In Carlson, D.S., and McNamara, J.A., Jr., editors: Muscle adaptation in the craniofacial region, Monograph, 8,

Craniofacial growth series, Ann Arbor, 1978, Center for Human Growth and Development, University of Michigan.

Delaire J., and Chateau, J.P.: Comment le septum nasal influence-t-il la croissance premaxillaire et maxillaire? Déduction en chirurgie des fentes labiomaxillaires, Rev. Stomatol **78**:241, 1977.

Delaire, J., Verdon, P., Lumineau, J.P, et al.: Quelques résultats des tractions extra-orales à appui fronto-mentonnier dans le traitment orthopédique des malformations maxillo-mandibulaires de Class III et des séquelles osseuses des fentes labio-maxillaires, Rev. Stomatol. Chir. Maxillofac. **73**:633, 1972.

Demisch, A.: Effects of activator therapy on the craniofacial skeleton in Class II, Division I, malocclusion, Eur. Orthod. Soc. Rep. Congr., p. 295, 1972.

Demisch, A.: Langzeitbeobachtungen über die Stabilität der Okklusion nach Distalbisstherapie mit dem Berner Aktivator, Schweiz. Monatsschr. Zahnheilkd. **90**:867, 1980.

Demner, L.M., and Nassibulin, G.G.: Kiefergelenkumbau bei der Behandlung sagittaler Bissanomalien, Stomatol. D.D.R. **27**:693, 1977.

Dickson, G.C., Grossmann, W., Mills, J.R.R., et al.: Symposium on functional therapy, Dent. Pract. **15**:255, 1965.

Downs, W.B.: The role of cephalometrics in orthodontic case analysis and diagnosis, Am. J. Orthod. **38**:162, 1952.

Droschl, H.: The effect of heavy orthopedic forces on the maxilla in the growing *Saimiri sciureus* (squirrel monkey), Am. J. Orthod. **63**:449, 1973.

Eirew, H.: Dynamic functional appliances, Trans. Br. Soc. Stud. Orthod. **19**:287, 1969.

Enlow, D.: Handbook of facial growth, ed. 2, Philadelphia, 1982, W.B. Saunders Co.

Eschler, J.: Die funktionelle Orthopädie des Kausystems, Munich, 1952, Leonhard Hanser.

Eschler, J.: Die muskuläre Wirkungsweise des Andresen-Häuplschen Apparates, Oesterr. Z. Stomatol. **49**:79, 1952.

Falck, F.: Vergleichende Untersuchungen über die Entwicklung der apical Basis nach kieferorthopädischer Behandlung mit der aktiven Platten und dem Funktionsregler, Fortschr. Kieferorthop. **30**:225, 1969.

Fox, J.: Natural history of the human teeth, London, 1803, Cox.

Fränkel, R.: The theoretical concept underlying treatment with function correctors, Eur. Orthod. Soc. Rep. Congr. **42**:233, 1966.

Fränkel, R.: Funktionskieferorthopädie und der Mundvorhof als apparative Basis, Berlin, 1967, V.E.B. Verlag Volk & Gesundheit.

Fränkel, R.: The functional matrix and its practical importance in orthodontics, Eur. Orthod. Soc. Rep. Congr. **18**:207, 1969a.

Fränkel, R.: The practical meaning of the functional matrix in orthodontics, Eur. Orthod. Soc. Rep. Congr. **45**:207, 1969b.

Fränkel, R.: The treatment of Class II, Division 1, malocclusion with functional correctors, Am. J. Orthod. **55**:265, 1969c.

Fränkel, R.: Maxillary retrusion in Class III and treatment with the function corrector III, Eur. Orthod. Soc. Rep. Congr. **46**:249, 1970.

Fränkel, R.: The guidance of eruption without extraction, Eur. Orthod. Soc. Rep. Congr. **47**:303, 1971.

Fränkel, R.: Technik und Handhabung der Funktionsregler, Berlin, 1973, V.E.B. Verlag Volk & Gesundheit.

Fränkel, R.: The applicability of the occipital reference base in cephalometrics, Am. J. Orthod. **77**:379, 1980a.

Fränkel, R.: A functional approach to orofacial orthopaedics, Br. J. Orthod. **7**:41, 1980b.

Fränkel, R.: Lip seal training in the treatment of the skeletal open bite, Eur. J. Orthod. **2**:219, 1980c.

Fränkel, R., and Fränkel, C.: A functional approach to treatment of skeletal open bite, Am. J. Orthod. **84**:54, 1983.

Freunthaller, P.: Cephalometric observations in Class II, Division 1, malocclusions treated with the activator, Angle Orthod. **37**:18, 1967.

Frislid, G., and Rakosi, T.: Analysen und Ergebnisse nach Headgearbehandlung, Fortschr. Kieferorthop. **37**:184, 1976.

Gasson, N.: Les rotations de croissance des deux maxillaires: étude céphalométrique sur matériel avec implants et confrontation avec les données expérimentales. Doctoral thesis in dental surgery, Strasbourg, 1977a, Université Louis-Pasteur.

Gasson, N.: Utilisation des implants métalliques dans l'étude céphalométrique de la croissance: l'application à l'analyse des rotations de la face. Orthod. Fr. **48:**289, 1977b.

Gasson, N., and Lavergne, J.: Maxillary rotation: its relation to the cranial base and the mandibular corpus. An implant study, Acta Odontol. Scand. **35:**89, 1977a.

Gasson, N., and Lavergne, J.: Maxillary rotation during human growth: variations and correlations with mandibular rotation, Acta Odontol. Scand. **35:**13, 1977b.

Gasson, N., and Petrovic, A.: Mécanismes et régulation de la croissance antéro-postérieure du maxillaire supérieur. Recherches expérimentales chez le jeune rat, sur le rôle de l'hormone somatotrope et du cartilage de la cloison nasale, Orthod. Fr. **43:**271, 1972.

Gasson, N., Stutzmann, J.J., and Petrovic, A.: Les mécanismes régulateurs de l'ajustement occlusal interviennent: ils dans le contrôle de la croissance du cartilage condylien? Expériences d'administration d'hormone somatotrope et de résection du cartilage septal chez le jeune rat, Orthod. Fr. **46:**77, 1975.

Geering-Gaerny, M., and Rakosi, T.: Initialsymptome von Kiefergelenkstörungen bei Kindern im Alter von 8-14 Jahren, Schweiz. Monatsschr. Zahnheilkd. **81:**691, 1971.

Gianelly, A.A.: Force-induced changes in the vascularity in the periodontal ligament, Am J. Orthod. **55:**5, 1969.

Gianelly, A.A., et al.: Mandibular growth, condylar position and the Fränkel appliance, Angle Orthod. **53:**131, 1983.

Graber, L.W.: The alterability of mandibular growth. In McNamara, J.A., Jr., editor: Determinants of mandibular form and growth. Monograph 4, Craniofacial growth series, Ann Arbor, 1975, Center for Human Growth and Development, University of Michigan.

Graber, L.W.: The variability of treatment response in 50 treated Fränkel appliance cases. Presented at the annual meeting of the American Association of Orthodontists, Boston, May 1983a.

Graber, T.M.: A study of the congenital cleft palate deformity. Doctoral dissertation, Chicago, 1950, Northwestern University Medical School.

Graber, T.M.: A critical review of clinical cephalometric radiography, Am. J. Orthod. **40:**1, 1954.

Graber, T.M.: The "three M's": muscles, malformation, and malocclusion, Am. J. Orthod. **49:**418, 1963.

Graber, T.M.: Orthodontics: principles and practice, ed. 3, Philadelphia, 1972, W.B. Saunders Co.

Graber, T.M.: Extrinsic factors influencing craniofacial growth. In McNamara, J.A., Jr., editor: Determinants of mandibular form and growth, Monograph 4, Craniofacial growth series, Ann Arbor, 1975, Center for Human Growth and Development, University of Michigan.

Graber, T.M.: Evolution of the concepts underlying craniofacial growth. In McNamara, J.A., Jr., Ribbins, K.A., and Howe, R.P., editors: Clinical alteration of the growing face, Monograph 13, Craniofacial growth series, Ann Arbor, 1983b, Center for Human Growth and Development, University of Michigan.

Graber, T.M.: Experimental and clinical studies of the effect of the Fränkel FR appliance in primates and humans. Presented at the annual meeting of the American Association of Orthodontists, Boston, May 1983c.

Graber, T.M.: Temporomandibular joint disturbances in the periodontium, Int. J. Periodontics Restorative Dent. **6:**8, 1984.

Graber, T.M.: Functional appliances: an overview. In Graber, T.M., and Swain, B.F., editors: Orthodontics: current principles and techniques, St. Louis, 1985, The C.V. Mosby Co.

Graber, T.M., Chung, D.B.B., and Aoba, J.M.: Dentofacial orthopedics versus orthodontics, J. Am. Dent. Assoc. **75:**1145, 1967.

Graber, T.M., and Neumann, N.: Removable orthodontic appliances, ed. 2, Philadelphia, 1984, W.B. Saunders Co.

Grude, R.: Myo-functional therapy. A review of various cases some years after their treatment by the Norwegian system had been completed, Nor. Tannlaegeforen. Tid. **62:**1, 1952.

Gwynne-Evans, E.: An analysis of the orofacial structures with special reference to muscle behavior and dental alignment, Am. J. Orthod. **40:**715, 1954.

Hamilton, D.G.: The expansion-activator system. Presented at the annual meeting of the American Association of Orthodontists, Boston, May 1983.

Harvold, E.P.: The role of function in the etiology and treatment of malocclusion, Am. J. Orthod. **54:**883, 1968.

Harvold, E.P.: The activator in interceptive orthodontics, St. Louis, 1974, The C.V. Mosby Co.

Harvold, E.P., and Vargervik, K.: Morphogenetic response to activator treatment, Am. J. Orthod. **60:**478, 1971.

Hasund, A.: The use of activator in a system employing fixed appliances, Eur. Orthod. Soc. Rep. Congr. **41:**329, 1969.

Häupl, K.: Gewebsumbau und Zahnveränderung in der Funktionskieferorthopädie, Leipzig, 1938, Johann Ambrosius Barth.

Hauser, E.: Variationskombinationen im Aufbau des Gesichtsschädels, Fortschr. Kieferorthop. **32:**425, 1971.

Hauser, E.: Functional orthodontic treatment with the activator Eur. Orthod. Soc. Trans. p. 427, 1973.

Henry, H.: An experimental study of external force application to the maxillary complex. In McNamara, J.A., Jr., editor: Factors affecting the growth of the midface, Monograph 6, Craniofacial growth series, Ann Arbor, 1976, Center for Human Growth and Development, University of Michigan.

Herren, P.: Die Wirkungsweise des Aktivators, Schweiz. Monatsschr. Zahnheilkd. **63:**829, 1953.

Herren, P.: The activator's mode of action, Am. J. Orthod. **45:**512, 1959.

Heusner, A., and Petrovic, A.: Appareil de culture d'organes en milieu liquide continuellement oxygéné, Med. Electron. Biol. **2:**381, 1964.

Hickham, J.H.: Activators for the fixed appliance orthodontist, J. Clin. Orthod. **14:**529, 1980.

Hickham, J.H.: Combined extraoral force and activator systems, Continuing Education course, Kenilworth Research Foundation, University of Chicago, June 1982.

Hiniker, J.J., and Ramfjord, S.P.: Anterior displacement of the mandible in adult rhesus monkeys. J. Dent. Res. **43**(suppl.):811, 1964.

Hiniker, J., and Ramfjord, S.P.: Anterior displacement of the mandible in adult rhesus monkeys, J. Prosthet. Dent. **16:**503, 1966.

Hirzel, H.C., and Grewe, J.M.: Activators: a practical approach, Am. J. Orthod. **6:**557, 1974.

Hockenjos, C., Komposch, G., Schumann, C., and Rakosi, T.: Fernröntgenologischer und klinischer Befund bei erschwerter Nasenatmung, Fortschr. Kieferorthop. **35:**391, 1974.

Holdaway, R.A.: Soft-tissue cephalometric analysis and its use in orthodontic treatment, Am. J. Orthod. **84:**1, 1983.

Holdaway, R.A.: The "VTO," Houston, 1976, University of Texas Press.

Hopkin, G.B.: Neonatal and adult tongue dimensions, Angle Orthod. **37:**132, 1967.

Hotz, R.: Orthodontia in everyday Practice, ed. 1, Bern, 1961, Hans Huber AG.

Hotz, R.: Application and appliance manipulation of functional forces, Am. J. Orthod. **58:**459, 1970a.

Hotz, R.: Guidance of eruption versus serial extraction, Am. J. Orthod. **58:**1, 1970b.

Hotz, R.: Orthodontics in daily practice: possibilities and limitations in the area of children's dentistry, ed. 5, Baltimore, 1980, The Williams & Wilkins Co.

Houston, W.J.B.: The current status of facial growth prediction: a review, Br. J. Orthod. **6**:11, 1979.

Humphreys, E. An improved method for determining calcium 45 in biological materials, Int. J. Appl. Rad. Isot. **16**:345, 1965.

Jacobsson, S.O.: Cephalometric evaluation of treatment effect on Class II, Division 1, malocclusions, Am. J. Orthod. **53**:446, 1967.

Jann, G.R., and Jann H.W.: Orofacial muscle imbalance, J. Am. Dent. Assoc. **65**:767, 1962.

Janson, I.: Cephalometric study of the efficiency of the Bionator, Eur. Orthod. Soc. Rep. Congr. **54**:283, 1978a.

Janson, I.: Skelettale und dentoalveolare Anderungen durch die Bionatorbehandlung in der vorpubertaren und pubertaren Wachstumzeit, Fortschr. Kieferorthop. **39**:62, 1978b.

Janson, I.: Skelettale und dentoalveolare Anderungen durch die Bionatorebehandlung in der vorpubertären und pubertären Wachstumzeit, Berlin, 1982, Quintessenz Verlag.

Janson, I., and Hasund, A.: Indikation und Grenzen der Funktionskieferorthopädie in der taglichen Praxis. In Deutscher Zahnärztekalender Ketterl, Munich, 1979, Carl Hanser Verlag.

Janzen, E. and Bluher, J.: The cephalometric, anatomic, and histologic changes in *Macaca mulatta* after application of a continuous acting retraction force on the mandible, Am. J. Orthod. **51**:823, 1965.

Jarabak, J.R., and Fizzel, J.A.: Light-wire edgewise appliance, St. Louis, 1972, The C.V. Mosby Co.

Joho, J.P.: Changes in form and size of the mandible in the orthopaedically treated Macaca irus (an experimental study), Eur. Orthod. Soc. Rep. Congr. **44**:161, 1968.

Johnston, L.E.: Jr.: The functional matrix hypothesis: reflections in a jaundiced eye. In McNamara, J.A., Jr., editor: Factors affecting the growth of the midface, Monograph 6, Craniofacial growth series, Ann Arbor, 1976, Center for Human Growth and Development, University of Michigan.

Johnston, L.E., Jr.: Personal communication, 1983.

Jonas, I.: Die Auswirkungen des Übungseffektes auf die Genauigkeit Röntgenkephalometrischer Durchzeichnungen in der Kieferorthopädie, Radiologe **16**:427, 1976.

Jonas, I.: Histomorphologische Untersuchungen über das destruktive und restitutive Verhalten des Ligamentum parodontale unter kieferorthopädischen Zahnbewegungen, Fortschr. Kieferorthop. **39**:398, 1978.

Jonas, I.: Die Reaktionsweise des Parodonts auf Kraftapplikation, Fortschr. Kieferorthop. **41**:228, 1980.

Jonas, I., Debrunner, M., and Rakosi, T.: Wirkungsweise abnehmbarer Behandlungsmittel, Fortschr. Kieferorthop. **37**:277, 1976.

Jonas, I., Mann, W., and Münker, G.: Relationship between tubal function, craniofacial morphology and disorders of deglutition, Arch. Otorhinolaryngol. **218**:151, 1978.

Jonas, I., Mann, W., and Schlenter, W.: Hals-Nasen-Ohren-ärztliche Befunde beim offenen Biss, Fortschr. Kieferorthop. **43**:127, 1982.

Jonas, I., Schlenter, W., and Mann, W.: The effect of the perforated vestibular screen on nasal respiration, Eur. J. Orthod. **5**:59, 1983.

Kingler, E.: Etude de l'ostéoclasie alvéolaire par contrainte. Doctoral thesis in Odontologic Sciences, Faculté de Médecine de Paris, 1971.

Kingsley, N.W.: Oral deformities, New York, 1880, D. Appleton & Co.

van der Klaauw, C.J.: Cerebral skull and facial skull, Arch. Neerl. Zool. **7**:16, 1946.

Klammt, G.: Der offene Aktivator, Stomatol. D.D.R. **5**:332, 1955.

Komposch, G.: Reaktionsfähigkeit temporomandibulären Strukturen auf kieferorthopädische Massnahmen. Eine Tierexperimentelle Studie. Habilitationsschrift zur Erlangung der venia legendi einer Hohen Medizinischen Fakultät der Allbert-Ludwigs-Universität zu Freiburg im Brisgau, 1978.

Komposch, G., and Hockenjos, C.: Die Reaktionsfähigkeit des temporomandibulären Knorpels, Fortschr. Kieferorthop. **38**:121, 1979.

Korkhaus, G.: Die Auswertung des Fernröntgenbildes in der Kieferorthopädie, Dtsch. Zahn. Mund. Kieferheilkd. **3**:714, 1936.

Kortsch, W.E.: The tongue and its implications in Class II malocclusions, J. Wisconsin Dent. Soc. **41**:261, 1965.

Koski, K.: Analysis of profile roentgenograms by means of a new "circle" method, Dent. Rec. **73**:704, 1953.

Koski, K.: Cranial growth centers: facts or fallacies? Am. J. Orthod. **54**:566, 1968.

Kraus, F.: Prevence a náprava vývojových nad orofacialní soustavy, Prague, 1956, Verlag SZN.

Kreiborg, S., Leth Jensen, B., Møller, E., and Björk, A.: Craniofacial growth in a case of congenital muscular dystrophy. A roentgenographic and electromyographic investigation, Am. J. Orthod. **74**:207, 1978.

Kuhn, T.S.: The structure of scientific revolutions, Chicago, 1962, University of Chicago Press.

Kühn, U., and Rakosi, T.: Palatographische Untersuchungen der Beziehungen zwischen Zungenlage und Dysgnathien an 30 Patienten der Angle Klasse II,1, Fortschr. Kieferorthop. **36**:474, 1975.

Kühn, U., and Rakosi, T.: Palatographische Untersuchungen über den Einfluss kieferorthopädischer Apparate auf die Zungenlage, Fortschr. Kieferorthop. **38**:36, 1977.

Kühne, K., Jonas, I., and Rakosi, T.: Weichteilmorphologie bei der Progenie, Fortschr. Kieferorthop. **40**:275, 1979.

Kvam, E.: A study of the cell-free zone following experimental tooth movement in the rat, Eur. Orthod. Soc. Rep. Congr. **45**:419, 1970.

Kvinnsland, S.: Partial resection of the cartilaginous nasal septum in rats; its influence on growth, Angle Orthod. **44**:135, 1974.

Latham, R.A.: Maxillary development and growth: the septo-premaxillary ligament, J. Anat. **107**:471, 1970.

Lavergne, J.: Morphogenetic classification of malocclusion as a basis for growth prediction and treatment planning, Br. J. Orthod. **9**:132, 1982.

Lavergne, J., and Gasson, N.: A metal implant study of mandibular rotation, Angle Orthod. **46**:144, 1976.

Lavergne, J., and Gasson, N.: Operational definitions of mandibular morphogenetic and positional rotations, Scand. J. Dent. Res. **85**:185, 1977.

Lavergne, J., and Gasson, N.: Analysis and classification of the rotational growth pattern without implants, Br. J. Orthod. **9**:51, 1982.

Lavergne, J., and Petrovic, A.: Discontinuities in occlusal relationship and the regulation of facial growth. A cybernetic view, Eur. J. Orthod. **5**:269, 1983.

Lavergne, J., and Petrovic, A.: Pathogenesis and treatment conceptualization of dentofacial malrelations as related to the pattern of occlusal relationship. In Dixon, A.D., and Sarnat, B.G., editors: Second International Conference on Clinical Factors and Mechanisms Influencing Bone Growth, 1985. (In press.)

Lemoine, C.: Remaniements des maxillaires consécutifs aux transplantations dentaires chez le rat. Doctoral thesis in dental surgery, 1970.

Lemoine, C., Charlier, J.P., and Petrovic, A.: Réaction condylienne à la déviation mandibulaire provoquée chez le rat. Nouvelles données sur le rôle des facteurs mécaniques dans la croissance mandibulaire, Orthod. Fr. **39**:147, 1968.

Lemoine, C. and Petrovic, A.: Le marquage á la tetracycline dans les expériences de transplantation dentaires et d'orthodontie chez le rat blanc, Rev. Fr. Odontostomatol. **9**:1191, 1969.

Lemoine, C., Petrovic, A., and Stutzmann, J.J.: Inflammatory process of the rat maxilla after molar autotransplantation, J. Dent. Res. **49**:1175, 1970.

Lieb, L., and Schlagbauer, P.: Möglichkeiten einer Beeinflussung des Gesichtsschädels am Rhesusaffen, Fortschr. Kieferorthop. **33**:113, 1972.

van Limbourg, J.: The regulation of the embryonic development and the skull, Acta Morphol. Neerl. Scand. **7**:101, 1968.

Linder-Aronson, S.: Adenoids—their efforts on mode of breathing and nasal airflow and their relationship to characteristics of the facial skeleton and the dentition, Acta Otolaryngol. (suppl.) **265**:1, 1970.

Linder-Aronson, S.: Naso-respiratory function and craniofacial growth. In McNamara, J.A., Jr., editor: Naso-respiratory function and craniofacial growth, Monograph 9, Craniofacial growth series, Ann Arbor, 1979, Center for Human Growth and Development, University of Michigan.

Linge, L.: Klinische Relevanz tierexperimentelle Untersuchungen (Korreferat zum Vortrag Petrovic), Fortschr. Kieferorthop. **38**:253, 1977.

Logan, W.R.: The vestibular appliance, Trans. Br. Soc. Stud. Orthod. **19**:287, 1969.

Logan, W.R.: The clinical management of the Fränkel appliance. The FR I, Trans. Br. Soc. Stud. Orthod. **21**:205, 1971.

Luder, H.U.: Effects of activator treatment—evidence for the occurrence of two different types of reaction, Eur. J. Orthod. **3**:205, 1981.

Lundström, A., and Woodside, D.G.: Longitudinal changes in facial type in cases with vertical and horizontal mandibular growth direction, Eur. J. Orthod. **5**:259, 1983.

Macapanpan, L.C., Weinmann, J.P., and Brodie, A.G.: Early tissue changes following tooth movement in rats, Angle Orthod. **24**:79, 1954.

Mandelbrot, B.B.: The fractal geometry of nature. San Francisco, 1982, W.H. Freeman Co.

Margolis, H.I.: Personal communications, July 1976, August 1983.

Markostamou, K: Contribution à l'étude des réactions de l'os alvéolaire au cours du déplacement orthodontique expérimental. Doctoral thesis in Odontologic Sciences, Faculté de Médecine de Paris, 1974.

Markostamou, K., and Baron, R.: Etude quantitative de l'ostéoclasie sur la paroi alvéolaire au cours de l'orthodontie expérimentale chez le rat, Orthod. Fr. **44**:245, 1973.

Marschner, J.F., and Harris, J.E.: Mandibular growth and class II treatment, Angle Orthod. **36**:89, 1966.

Martin, J.R.: The stability of the anterior teeth after treatment, Am. J. Orthod. **48**:788, 1948.

Martin, R., and Sauer, K.: Lehrbuch der Anthropologie, ed. 6, Stuttgart, 1957, Gustav Fischer Verlag.

Mason, R.M., and Proffit, W.R.: Myofunctional therapy: background and recommendations, J. Speech Hear. Disord. **39**:115, 1974.

McCallin, S.G.: Retraction of maxillary teeth with removable appliances using intermaxillary or extra-oral traction, Dent. Rec. **74**:36, 1954.

McDougall, P.D., McNamara, J.A., Jr., and Dierkes, J.M.: Arch width development in Class II patients treated with the Fränkel appliance. Am. J. Orthod. **82**:10, 1982.

McEwan, D.C.: Some illusory phenomena of importance in orthodontics, Am. J. Orthod. **44**:46, 1959.

McNamara, J.A., Jr.: Neuromuscular and skeletal adaptations to altered orofacial function, Monograph 1, Craniofacial growth series, Ann Arbor, 1972, Center for Human Growth and Development, University of Michigan.

McNamara, J.A., Jr.: Neuromuscular and skeletal adaptation to altered function in the orofacial region, Am. J. Orthod. **64**:578, 1973.

McNamara, J.A., Jr.: JCO interviews: Dr. James McNamara on the Fränkel appliance, J. Clin. Orthod. **14**:320, 1980.

McNamara, J.A., Jr.: Components of Class II malocclusion in children 8-10 years of age, Angle Orthod. **51**:269, 1981.

McNamara, J.A., Jr., and Carlson, D.S.: Quantitative analysis of temporomandibular joint adaptations to protrusive function, Am. J. Orthod. **76**:593, 1979.

McNamara, J.A., Jr., Connelly, T.G., and McBride, M.C.: Histological studies of temporomandibular joint adaptations. In McNamara, J.A., Jr., editor: Control mechanisms in craniofacial growth, Monograph 3, Craniofacial growth series, Ann Arbor, 1975, Center for Human Growth and Development, University of Michigan.

McNamara, J.A., Jr., and Huge, S.A.: The Fränkel appliance, Am. J. Orthod. **80**:478, 1981.

McNamara, J.A., Jr., Riolo, M.L., and Enlow, D.H.: Growth of the maxillary complex in the rhesus monkey *(Macaca mulatta)*, Am. J. Phys. Anthropol. **44**:15, 1976.

Meach, C.L.: A cephalometric comparison of bony profile changes in Class II, Division I patients treated with extraoral force and functional jaw orthopaedics, Am. J. Orthod. **52**:353, 1966.

Melsen, B., Melsen, F., and Moss, M.L.: Postural development of the nasal septum studied on human autopsy material. In Carlson, D.S., editor: Craniofacial biology, Monograph 10, Craniofacial growth series, Ann Arbor, 1981, Center for Human Growth and Development, University of Michigan.

Merrifield, L., and Cross, J.: The Kloehn headgear effect, Chicago, 1961, American Association of Orthodontists. (Audiovisual series.)

Milhorn, H.T.: The application of control theory to physiological systems, Philadelphia, 1966, W.B. Saunders Co.

Mills, C.M., Holman, R.G., and Graber, T.M.: Heavy intermittent cervical traction in Class II treatment. A longitudinal cephalometric assessment, Am. J. Orthod. **74**:361, 1978.

Mills, J.R.E.: The long-term results of the proclination of lower incisors, Br. Dent. J. **120**:355, 1966.

Mills, J.R.E.: The effect of orthodontic treatment on the skeletal pattern, Br. J. Orthod. **5**:133, 1978.

Mills, J.R.E., and Vig. K.W.L.: An approach to appliance therapy. II, Br. J. Orthod. **2**:29, 1975.

Milne, J.M., and Cleall, J.F.: Cinefluorographic study of functional adaptation of the oropharyngeal structures, Angle Orthod. **40**:267, 1970.

Moffett, B.C.: A research perspective on craniofacial morphogenesis, Acta Morphol. Neerl. Scand. **10**:91, 1972.

Moiroud, A.: Essai d'utilisation d'une transformation géométrique dans la prévision de la croissance faciale, Orthod. Fr. **52**:725, 1981.

Moss, J.P.: Cephalometric changes during functional appliance therapy, Eur. Orthod. Soc. Trans. **38**:327, 1962.

Moss, M.L.: In First cephalometric workshop, Bolton Brush Foundation, Cleveland, July 1957.

Moss, M.L.: The pathogenesis of artificial cranial deformation, Am. J. Phys. Anthropol. **16**:269, 1958.

Moss, M.L.: Functional analysis of human mandibular growth, J. Prosthet. Dent. **10**:1149, 1960.

Moss, M.L.: The functional matrix. In Kraus, B.S., and Riedel, R.A., editors: Vistas in orthodontics, Philadelphia, 1962, Lea & Febiger.

Moss, M.L.: The role of nasal septal cartilage in mid-face. In McNamara, J.A., Jr., editor: Factors affecting the growth of the mid-face Monograph 6, Craniofacial growth series, Ann Arbor, 1976, Center for Human Growth and Development, University of Michigan.

Moss, M.L.: The dialectics of craniofacial growth research: Is it time for a new synthesis? In McNamara, J.A., Jr., Carlson, D.S., and Ribbens, K.A., editors: The effect of surgical intervention on craniofacial growth, Monograph 12, Craniofacial growth series, Ann Arbor, 1982, Center for Human Growth and Development, University of Michigan.

Moss, M.L., Bromberg, B.E., Song, I.C., and Eisenmann, J.L.: The passive role of nasal septal cartilage in mid-facial growth, Plast. Reconstr. Surg. **41**:536, 1968.

Moss, M.L., and Salentijn, L.: The capsular matrix, Am. J. Orthod. **56**:474, 1969.

Moss, M.L., and Salentijn, L.: The primary role of functional matrices in facial growth, Am. J. Orthod. **55**:566, 1969.

Moss, M.L., and Salentijn, L.: The logarithmic growth of the human mandible, Acta Anat. **77**:341, 1970.

Moss, M.L., Vilmann, H., Dasgupta, G., and Skalak, R.: Craniofacial growth in space and time. In McNamara, J.A., Jr., et al., editors: Craniofacial biology, Monograph 10, Craniofacial growth series, Ann Arbor, 1981, Center for Human Growth and Development, University of Michigan.

Moyers, R.E.: The infantile swallow, Eur. Orthod. Soc. Trans. **40**:180, 1964.

Moyers, R.E.: Handbook of orthodontics, ed. 3, Chicago, 1973, Yearbook Medical Publishers, Inc.

Moyers, R.E.: Skeletal contributions to occlusal development. In McNamara, J.A., Jr., editor: The biology of occlusal development, Monograph 7, Craniofacial growth series, Ann Arbor, 1977, Center for Human Growth and Development, University of Michigan.

Moyers, R.E., Elgoyhen, J., Riolo, M., et al.: Experimental production of Class III in rhesus monkeys, Eur. Orthod. Soc. Rep. Congr. **46**:61, 1970.

Neumann, B.: Funktionskieferorthopädie. Rückblick and Ausblick, Fortschr. Kieferorthop. **36**:73, 1975.

Oppenheim, A.: Die Krise in der Orthodontie, Berlin, 1933, Urban & Schwarzenberg.

O'Ryan, F., Gallagher, D., LaBanc, J., and Epker, B.: The relation between nasorespiratory function and dentofacial morphology: a review, Am. J. Orthod. **82**:403, 1982.

Oudet, C.: Régulations de la longueur anatomique du muscle ptérygoïdien latéral de jeune rat au cours de la croissance. Variations du nombre de sarcomères en série consécutives à des perturbations de la posture de la mandibule. Mémoire de DERBH, Strasbourg, 1979a, Université Louis Pasteur.

Oudet, C.: Rythmes nycthéméral et saisonnier de la vitesse de croissance du squelette et de la susceptibilité du cartilage condylien de la mandibule à l'égard des dispositifs orthopédiques. Doctoral thesis in Human Biology, Université Louis Pasteur, Strasbourg, 1979b.

Oudet, C., and Petrovic, A.: Effets de l'hyperpropulseur postural sur la croissance du cartilage condylien de la mandibule de jeune rat au cours dy cycle circadien, J. Physiol. (Paris) **71**:34, 1975.

Oudet, C., and Petrovic, A.: Effets d'un rétropulseur actif sur la vitesse de croissance du cartilage condylien de jeune rat au cours du nycthémère et de l'année, Orthod. Fr. **47**:15, 1976.

Oudet, C., and Petrovic, A.: Circannual growth variations of the mandibular condylar cartilage in the young rat, J. Interdiscipl. Cycle Res. **8**:338, 1977a.

Oudet, C., and Petrovic, A.: Effects of a postural hyperpropulsor in the growth of the mandibular condylar cartilage of the young rat during circadian cycle (pp. 133-139). In Lassmann, G., and Seitelberger, F., editors: Rhythmische Funktionen in Biologischen Systemen. Ihre Bedeutung f:auur Theorie und Klinik, Vienna 1977b, Facultas-Verlag. vol. 2.

Oudet, C., and Petrovic, A.: Growth rhythms of the cartilage of the mandibular condyle. Effects of orthopedic appliances, Int. J. Chronobiol. **5**:545, 1978a.

Oudet, C., and Petrovic, A.: Variations in the number of sarcomeres in series in the lateral pterygoid muscle as a function of the longitudinal deviation of the mandibular position produced by the postural hyperpropulsor. In Carlson, D., and MacNamara, J.A., Jr., editors: Muscle adaptation in the craniofacial region. Monograph 8, Craniofacial growth series, Ann Arbor, 1978b, Center for Human Growth and Development, University of Michigan.

Oudet, C., and Petrovic, A.: Regulation of the anatomical length of the lateral pterygoid muscle in the growing rat. In Guba, F., Marechal, G., and Takacs, O., editors: Mechanisms of muscle adaptation to functional requirements, Adv. Physiol. Sci. **24**:403, 1981a.

Oudet, C., and Petrovic, A.: Seasonal variations of the growth rate of the condylar cartilage of the mandible in the young rat. In Halberg, F., Scheving, L.E., Powell, E.W., and Hayes, D.K., editors: Proceedings, Twelfth international conference, International Society for Chronobiology, Milan, 1981b, Il Ponte.

Oudet, C., and Petrovic, A.: Tages- und Jahresperiodische Schwankungen der Reakton des Kondylenknorpels bei der kieferorthopädischen Behandlung, Fortschr. Kieferorthop. **42**:1, 1981c.

Oudet, C., and Petrovic, A.: Daytime and seasons are sources of variations for cartilage and bone growth rate. In Dixon, A.D. and Sarnat, B.G., editors: Factors and mechanisms influencing bone growth, Prog. Clin. Biol. Res. **101**:659, 1982.

Oudet, C., Petrovic, A., and Stutzmann, J.J.: Time-dependent effects of a "functional"-type orthopedic appliance on rat mandible growth, Chronobiol. Int., 1985. (In press.)

Pancherz, H.: Long-term effects of activator treatment, Odontol. Rev., vol. 27 (suppl. 35), 1976.

Persson, M.: Structure and growth of facial sutures: histologic microangiographic and arthrographic studies in rats and histologic study in man, Odontol. Rev. **24**(suppl. 26):1, 1973.

Petrovic, A.: Recherches sur les mécanismes histophysiologiques de la croissance osseuse cranio-faciale, Ann. Biol. **9**:303, 1970.

Petrovic, A.: Mechanisms and regulation of mandibular condylar growth, Acta Morphol. Neerl. Scand., **10**:25, 1972.

Petrovic, A.: Control of postnatal growth of secondary cartilages of the mandible by mechanisms regulating occlusion. Cybernetic model, Trans. Eur. Orthod. Soc. **50**:69, 1974.

Petrovic, A.: L'ajustement occlusal: son rôle dans les processus physiologiques de contrôle de la croissance du cartilage condylien, Orthod. Fr. **48**:23, 1977.

Petrovic, A.: Postnatal growth of bone: a perspective of current trends, new approaches, and innovations. In Dixon, A.D., and Sarnat, B.G., editors: Factors and mechanisms influencing bone growth, Prog. Clin. Biol. Res. **101**:297, 1982.

Petrovic, A.: Types d'explication dans les sciences biomédicales et en médecine. In Barreau, H., editor: Séminaire sur les fondements des sciences. L'explication dans les sciences de la vie, Paris, 1983, Editions du CNRS.

Petrovic, A.: An experimental and cybernetic approach to the mechanism of action of functional appliances on the mandibular growth. In McNamara, J.A., Jr., editor: Malocclusion and the periodontium, Monograph 15, Craniofacial growth series, Ann Arbor, 1984a, Center for Human Growth and Development, University of Michigan.

Petrovic, A.: Zweckmässigkeit, Bedeutung und Gültigkeit der experimentellen Forschung auf dem Gebiet der Kieferorthopädie und Orthodontie, Fortschr. Kieferorthop. **45**:165, 1984b.

Petrovic, A., and Charlier, J.P.: La synchondrose sphéno-occipitale de jeune rat en culture de'organes: mise en évidence d'un potentiel de croissance indépendant, C. R. Acad. Sci. (series D) **265**:1511, 1967.

Petrovic, A., Charlier, J.P., and Herrmann, J.: Les mécanismes de croissance du crâne. Recherches sur le cartilage de la cloison nasale et sur les sutures craniennes et faciales de jeunes rats en culture d'organes, Bull. Assoc. Anat. **143**:1376, 1969.

Petrovic, A., and Gasson, N.: Aspects biologiques de la rotation de croissance postérieure ou antérieure de la mandibule, Bull. Orthod. Soc. Yugoslav. **8**:33, 1975.

Petrovic, A., Gasson, N., and Oudet C.: Wirkung der übertriebenen posturalen Vorschubstellung des Unterkiefers auf das Kondylenwachstum der normalen und der mit Wachstumshormon behandelten Ratte, Fortschr. Kieferorthop. **36**:86, 1975a.

Petrovic, A., Gasson, M., and Schlienger, A.: Dissymétrie mandibulaire consécutive à la perturbation occlusale unilatérale provoquée expérimentalement chez le rat. Conception cybernétique des systèmes de contrôle de la croissance des cartilages condylien et angulaire, Orthod. Fr. **45**:409, 1974a.

Petrovic, A., and Heusner, A.: Oxygénation d'un fragment d'organe *in vitro*: principe de la culture organotypique en suspension en phase liquide, C.R. Acad. Sci. (series D) **253**:3066, 1961.

Petrovic, A., Oudet, C., and Gasson, N.: Effets des appareils de propulsion et de rétropulsion mandibulaires sur le nombre de sarcomères en série du muscle ptérygoïdien externe et sur la croissance du cartilage condylien de jeune rat, Orthod. Fr. **44**:191, 1973.

Petrovic, A., Oudet, C., and Gasson, N.: Unterkieferpropulsion durch eine im Oberkiefer fixierte Vorbissführung mit seitlicher Biss-sperre von unterschiedlicher Höhe. Auswirkungen bei Ratten während der Wachstumsperiode und bei erwachsenen Tieren, Fortschr. Kieferorthop. **43:**329, 1982a.

Petrovic, A., Oudet, C., and Shaye, R.: Unterkieferpropulsion durch eine im Oberkiefer fixierte Vorbissführung mit seitlicher Biss-sperre von unterschiedlicher Höhe hinsichtlich der täglichen Dauer der Behandlung, Fortschr. Kieferorthop. **43:**243, 1982b.

Petrovic, A., Oudet, C., and Stutzmann, J.J.: Behandlungsergebnisse in Bezug zur Dauer der über triebenen posturalen Vorschubstellung des Unterkiefers, Fortschr. Kieferorthop. **37:**40, 1976.

Petrovic A.G., Oudet, C.L., and Stutzmann, J.J.: Temporal organization of rat and human skeletal cells: circadian frequency and quantizement of cell generation time. In Edmunds, L., editor: Cell cycle clocks, New York, 1984, Marcel Dekker, Inc.

Petrovic, A., and Shambaugh, G.E., Jr.: Promotion of bone calcification by sodium fluoride, Arch Otolaryngol. **83:**162, 1966.

Petrovic, A., and Shambaugh, G.E., Jr.: Studies on sodium fluoride effects (a) on human sclerotic bone; (b) on prevention of experimental osteoporosis in rats; (c) synergistic action with phosphates, Acta Otolaryngol. **65:**120, 1968.

Petrovic, A., and Stutzmann, J.J.: Le muscle ptérygoïdien externe et la croissance du condyle mandibulaire. Recherches expérimentales chez le jeune rat, Orthod. Fr. **43:**271, 1972.

Petrovic, A., and Stutzmann, J.J.: Further investigations into the functioning of the "comparator" of the servosystem (respective positions of the upper and lower dental arches) in the control of the condylar cartilage growth rate and of the lengthening of the jaw. In McNamara, J.A., Jr., editor: The biology of occlusal development, Monograph 6, Craniofacial growth series, Ann Arbor, 1977, Center for Human Growth and Development, University of Michigan.

Petrovic, A., and Stutzmann, J.J.: Contrôle de la croissance post-natale du squelette facial. Données expérimentales et modèle cybernétique, Actual. Odontostomatol. **128:**811, 1979a.

Petrovic, A., and Stutzmann, J.J.: Die Progenie, experimentelle Untersuchungen über Pathogenese und Therapie, Fortschr. Kieferorthop. **40:**372, 1979b.

Petrovic, A., and Stutzmann, J.J.: Tierexperimentelle Untersuchungen über das Gesichts-Schädelwachstum und seine Beeinflussung. Eine biologische Erklärung der sogenannten Wachstumsrotation des Unterkiefers, Fortschr. Kieferorthop. **40:**1, 1979c.

Petrovic, A., and Stutzmann, J.J.: Experimentelle Untersuchung der kieferorthopädischen Beeinflussbarkeit des Gesichtswachstums, Fortschr. Kieferorthop. **41:**212, 1980a.

Petrovic, A., and Stutzmann, J.J.: Hormone somatotrope: modalités d'action des diverses variétés de cartilage, Pathol. Biol. **28:**43, 1980b.

Petrovic, A., and Stutzmann, J.J.: Hormone somatotrope: modalités d'action sur la croissance des diverses variétés de cartilage, Sem. Hop. **56:**1307, 1980c.

Petrovic, A., and Stutzmann, J.J.: A cybernetic view of facial growth mechanisms. In Kehrer, B., et al., editors: Long-term treatment in cleft lip and palate, Bern, 1981, Hans Huber, Publishers.

Petrovic, A., and Stutzmann, J.J.: Teoría cibernética del cercimiento craneo-facial, post-natal y mecanismos de acción de los aparatos ortopédicos y ortodónticos, Rev. Asoc. Argent. Ortoped. Func. Maxil. **15:**7, 1982.

Petrovic, A., and Stutzmann-Herrmann, J.: Action of rat growth hormone on young rat mandibular condylar cartilage in tissue and organ culture. Presented at the ninth annual meeting of the American Society of Cellular Biologists, Detroit, 1969.

Petrovic, A., Stutzmann, J.J., and Gasson, N.: The final length of the mandible: is it genetically predetermined? In Carlson, D.S., editors: Craniofacial biology, Monograph 10, Craniofacial growth series, Ann Arbor, 1981a, Center for Human Growth and Development, University of Michigan.

Petrovic, A., Stutzmann, J.J., and Oudet, C.: Effets de l'hormone somatotrope sur la croissance du cartilage condylien mandibulaire et de la synchondrose sphéno-occipitale de jeunes rats, en culture organotypique, C. R. Acad. Sci. (series D) **276:**3053, 1973.

Petrovic, A., Stutzmann, J.J., and Oudet, C.: Control processes in post-natal growth of condylar cartilage of the mandible. In McNamara, J.A., Jr., editor: Determinants of mandibular form and growth, Monograph 4, Craniofacial growth series, Ann Arbor, 1975b, Center for Human Growth and Development, University of Michigan.

Petrovic, A., Stutzmann, J.J., and Oudet, C.: Condylectomy and mandibular growth in young rats. A quantitative study, Proc. Finn. Dent. Soc. **77:**139, 1981b.

Petrovic, A., Stutzmann, J.J., and Oudet, C.: Experimentelle Untersuchungen zur Wirkung intraoraler Gummizüge auf den Unter- und Oberkiefer bei wachsenden und ausgewachsenen Ratten, Fortschr. Kieferorthop. **42:**209, 1981c.

Petrovic, A., Stutzmann, J.J., and Oudet, C.: Seasonal variations in the direction of growth of the mandibular condyle (pp. 195-201). In Vidrio, A., editor: Biological rhythms in structure and function, Prog. Clin. Biol. Res. **59C:**195, 1981d.

Petrovic, A., Stutzmann, J.J., and Oudet, C.: Turnover of human alveolar bone removed either in the day or in the night, J. Interdiscipl. Cycle Res. **12:**161, 1981e.

Petrovic, A., Stutzmann, J.J., and Oudet, C.: Defects in mandibular growth resulting from condylectomy and resection of the pterygoid and masseter muscles. In McNamara, J.A., Jr., Carlson, D.S., and Ribbens, K.A., editors: The effect of surgical intervention on craniofacial growth, Monograph 12, Craniofacial growth series, Ann Arbor, 1982c, Center for Human Growth and Development, University of Michigan.

Petrovic, A., Stutzmann, J.J., and Oudet, C.: Orthopedic appliances modulate the bone formation in the mandible as a whole, Swed. Dent. J. **15**(suppl.):197, 1982d.

Petrovic, A., Stutzmann, J.J, and Oudet, C.: La culture organotypique en milieu liquide avec renouvellement continu de l'apport gazeux. Un nouveau moyen d'étude des variations de la formation et de la résorption de l'os humain normal ou pathologique, I.T.B.M. **3:**594, 1982e.

Petrovic, A., Stutzmann, J.J., Oudet, C., and Gasson, N.: Kontrollfaktoren des Kondylenwachstums: Wachstumshormon, musculi pterygoidei laterales, und Vor- und Rückschubgeřte des Unterkiefers, Fortschr. Kieferorthop. **35:**347, 1974b.

Petrovic, A., Stutzmann, J.J., Ozerovic, B., and Vidovic, Z.: Does the Fraenkel appliance produce forward movements of mandibular premolars? Eur. J. Orthod. **4:**173, 1982f.

Pfeiffer, J.P., and Grobety, D.: Simultaneous use of cervical appliance and activator: an orthodontic approach to fixed appliance therapy, Am. J. Orthod. **61:**353, 1972.

Pfeiffer, J.P., and Grobety, D.: The Class II malocclusion: differential diagnosis and clinical application of activators, extraoral traction, and fixed appliances, Am. J. Orthod. **68:**499, 1975.

Pfeiffer, J.P., and Grobety, D.: Removable appliances and extraoral force. In Graber, T.M., and Neumann, B.: Removable orthodontic appliances, ed. 2, Philadelphia, 1984, W.B. Saunders Co.

Plaice, C.H.: A note on the determination of serum beta-glucuronidase activity, J. Clin. Pathol. **14:**661, 1961.

Popper, K.R.: Conjectures and refutations. The growth of scientific knowledge, London, 1963, Routledge & Kegan Paul, Ltd.

Prahl, B.: Sutural growth. Investigations on the growth mechanism of the coronal suture and its relation to cranial growth in the rat. Doctoral Thesis, University of Nijmegan, 1968.

Proffit, W.R.: Equilibrium theory revisited: factors influencing position of the teeth, Angle Orthod. **48:**175, 1978.

Rakosi, T.: Die Ruhelage am Fernröntgenseiten (FRS)-Bild und ihre Bedeutung für die Kieferorthopädie, Fortschr. Kieferorthop. **22:**409, 1961.

Rakosi, T.: Die Bewertung des Zeitfaktors bei der Progeniebehandlung, Fortschr, Kieferorthop. **27**:66, 1966a.

Rakosi, T.: Metrische Untersuchung der Lippen-Lagen bei verschiedenen Gebissanomalien, Fortschr. Kieferorthop. **27**:470, 1966b.

Rakosi, T.: Möglichkeiten und Grenzen der kieferorthopädischen Prävention im Milchgebiss, Dtsch. Zahnaerztl. Z. **21**:848, 1966c.

Rakosi, T.: Röntgenzephalometrische Untersuchungen über die Änderung der Zungenlage bei kieferorthopädischer Therapie, Fortschr. Kieferorthop. **27**:234, 1966d.

Rakosi, T.: Extraktion im Milchgebiss, Fortschr. Kieferorthop. **29**:16, 1968a.

Rakosi, T.: Über die Lippenmorphologie und Lippenfunktion, Zahnaerztl. Welt **77**:671, 1968b.

Rakosi, T.: Heredität, Weichteilmorphologie, und Bewegungsablauf, Fortschr. Kieferorthop. **30**:46, 1969.

Rakosi, T.: Indikation der Extraktion in der kieferorthopädie, Zahnaerztl. Prax. **21**:145, 1970a.

Rakosi, T.: Über die Möglichkeiten der Progenie-Behandlung, Schweiz. Monatsschr. Zahnheilkd. **80**:1021, 1970b.

Rakosi, T.: The significance of roentgenographic cephalometrics in the diagnosis and treatment of Class III malocclusions, Eur. Orthod. Soc. Rep. Congr. p. 155, 1970c.

Rakosi, T.: Variationen des Schluckaktes, Fortschr. Kieferorthop. **31**:81, 1970d.

Rakosi, T.: Die Wirkungsweise und Konstruktionselemente des Funktionsreglers, Zahnaerztl. Prax. **23**:285, 1970e.

Rakosi, T.: Funktionelle Kiefergelenksstörungen bei Kindern, Fortschr. Kieferorthop. **32**:37, 1971a.

Rakosi, T.: Kieferorthopädische Apparate mit apparativer Basis im Mundvorhof, Zahntechnik **29**:125, 1971b.

Rakosi, T.: The scope of orthodontic treatment in adults maintained by oral surgery. Indications, Eur. Orthod. Soc. Rep. Congr., p. 333, 1971c.

Rakosi, T.: Bedeutung des Säuglings- und Kleinkindalters für die Entstehung von Bissanomalien, Zahnaerztl. Prax. **23**:12, 1972a.

Rakosi, T.: Bedeutung der Wachstumsachse des Unterkiefers für die Therapieplanung, Fortschr. Kieferorthop. **33**:31, 1972b.

Rakosi, T.: Über die Schädelbasis-bezüglichen Rotationen des Unterkiefers, Fortschr. Kieferorthop. **33**:177, 1972c.

Rakosi, T.: Über die Problematik der Diagnostik und Behandlung des tiefen Bisses, Fortschr. Kieferorthop. **34**:94, 1973.

Rakosi, T.: Das Problem der Zunge in der Kieferorthopädie, Fortschr. Kieferorthop. **36**:220, 1975a.

Rakosi, T.: The scope of mechanotherapy and functional treatment in the mixed dentition, Trans. Eur. Orthod. Soc., p. 209, 1975b.

Rakosi, T.: Einführung in die Problematik der Befunderhebung in der Kieferorthopädie, Fortschr. Kieferorthop. **38**:115, 1977.

Rakosi, T.: Progenie im Fernröntgenbild, Fortschr. Kieferorthop. **39**:486, 1978.

Rakosi, T.: Therapie der Klasse-II-Dysgnathien: Möglichkeiten und Grenzen, Oesterr. Z. Stomatol. **75**:171, 1978.

Rakosi, T.: Atlas und Anleitung zur praktischen Fernröntgenanalyse, Munich, 1979, C. Hanser Verlag.

Rakosi, T.: Grenzen und Möglichkeiten der kieferorthopädischen Spätbehandlung, Fortschr. Kieferorthop. **41**:590, 1980.

Rakosi, T.: Ätiologie und diagnostische Beurteilung des offenen Bisses, Fortschr. Kieferorthop. **43**:68, 1982a.

Rakosi, T.: An atlas and manual of cephalometric radiography, Philadelphia, 1982b, Lea & Febiger.

Rakosi, T.: Cephalometric radiography, London, 1982c, Wolfe Medical Publications, Ltd.

Rakosi, T.: Therapie des offenen Bisses, Fortschr. Kieferorthop. **43**:171, 1982d.

Rakosi, T.: The principles of functional appliances. In McNamara, J.A., Jr., Ribbens, K.A., Howe, R.P., editors: Clinical alteration of the growing face, Monograph 14, Craniofacial growth series, Ann Arbor, 1983, Center for Human Growth and Development, University of Michigan.

Rakosi, T., and Bäuerle, H.: Retrospektive Beurteilung der Wachstumsprognose nach Holdaway, Fortschr. Kieferorthop. **39**:133, 1978.

Rakosi, T., Jonas, I., and Burgert, R.: Simplified positioner construction, J. Clin. Orthod. **15**:206, 1981.

Rakosi, T., Jonas, I., and Burgert, R.: Vereinfachte Anfertigung von Gaumennaht-Sprengungsplatten, Fortschr. Kieferorthop. **44**:71, 1983.

Rakosi, T., Jonas, I., Keller, H., and Burgert, R.: Vereinfachte Anfertigung eines Positioners, Fortschr. Kieferorthop. **44**:71, 1981.

Rakosi, T., and Rahn, B.A.: Metallimplantate und Knochenwachstum, Fortschr. Kieferorthop. **39**:196, 1978.

Rakosi, T., and Schilli, W.: Class III anomalies: a coordinated approach to skeletal, dental, and soft tissue problems, Oral Surg. **39**:860, 1981.

Rakosi, T., Schmidt, H., and Debrunner, M.: Kriterien für die Beurteilung des Behandlungszieles, Fortschr. Kieferorthop. **37**:405, 1976.

Rakosi, T., and Witt, E.: Grundelemente der festsitzenden Apparaturen, Zahnaerztl. Prax. **22**:19, 1971.

Ramel, U.: Symptome sogenannter Kiefergelenksbeschwerden bei einer Gruppe Schweizer Rekruten. Thesis, 1976, University of Bern.

Randow, K., Carlsson, K., Edlund, J., and Ödberg, T.: The effect of an occlusal interference on the masticatory system, Odontol. Rev. **27**:245, 1975.

Rebholz, K., and Rakosi, T.: Extraorale Kräfte und die Wirbelsäule, Fortschr. Kieferorthop. **38**:324, 1977.

Reitan, K.: Continuous bodily tooth movement and its histological significance, Acta Odontol. Scand. 7:115, 1947.

Reitan, K.: The initial tissue reaction of orthodontic tooth movement, Acta Odontol. Scand. (suppl. 6), p. 240, 1951.

Reitan, K.: Tissue behavior during orthodontic tooth movement, Am. J. Orthod. 46:881, 1960.

Reitan, K.: Effects of force magnitude and direction of tooth movement on different alveolar bone types, Angle Orthod. 34:244, 1964.

Reitan, K.: Initial tissue behavior during apical root resorption, Angle Orthod. 44:68, 1974.

Reitan, K.: Biomechanical principles and reactions. In Graber, T.M., and Swain, B.F., editors: Orthodontics: current principles and techniques, St. Louis, 1985, The C.V. Mosby Co.

Richardson, M.P.: Spontaneous changes in incisor relationship following extraction of lower first permanent molars, Br. J. Orthod. **6**:85, 1979.

Richardson, M.P.: A classification of open bite, Eur. J. Orthod. **3**:289, 1981.

Richardson, M.P.: Measurement of dental base relationship, Eur. J. Orthod. **4**:151, 1982.

Ricketts, R.M.: A study of changes in temporomandibular relations associated with the treatment of Class II malocclusion (Angle), Am. J. Orthod. **38**:918, 1952.

Ricketts, R.M.: Respiratory obstructions and their relation to the tongue posture, Cleft Palate Bull. 8:4, 1958.

Ricketts, R.M.: The influence of orthodontic treatment on facial growth and development, Angle Orthod. **30**:103, 1960.

Ricketts, R.M.: Respiratory obstruction syndrome, Am. J. Orthod. **54**:495, 1968.

Riedel, R.A.: Diagnosis and treatment planning in orthodontics. Dent. Clin. North Am. **12**:175, 1969.

Riolo, M.L., Moyers, R.E., McNamara, J.A., Jr., and Hunter, W.S.: An atlas of craniofacial growth, Monograph 2, Craniofacial growth series, Ann Arbor, 1974, Center for Human Growth and Development, University of Michigan.

Robin, P.: Observation sur un nouvel appareil de redressement, Rev. Stomatol. 9:423, 1902.

Ronning, O.: Alterations in craniofacial morphogenesis induced by parenterally administered papain. An experimental study on the rat, Doctoral dissertation, University of Turku, 1971.

Roux, W.: Gesammelte Abhandlungen über Entwicklungsmechanik der Organismen, Leipzig, 1895, W. Engelmann.

Rygh, P.: Elimination of hyalinized periodontal tissues associated with orthodontic tooth movement, Acta Odontol. Scand. **31:**109, 1973.

Rygh, P.: Orthodontic root resorption occuring during orthodontic treatment, Angle Orthod. **47:**1, 1977.

Sander, F.G.: Zur Frage der Biomechanik des Aktivators: Entwicklung und Erprobung neuer Untersuchungsmethoden, Wiesbaden, 1980, Westdeutscher Verlag, GmbH.

Sander, F.G.: The effects of functional appliances and Class II elastics on masticatory patterns. In McNamara, J.A., Jr., et al., editors: Clinical alteration of the growing face. Monograph 14, Craniofacial growth series, Ann Arbor, 1983, Center for Human Growth and Development, University of Michigan.

Sander, F.G., and Schmuth, G.P.F.: Der Einfluss verschiedener Bisssperren auf die Muskelaktivität bei Aktivatorträgern, Fortschr. Kieferorthop. **40:**107, 1979.

Sassouni, V.: A classification of skeletal facial types, Am. J. Orthod. **55:**109, 1969.

Schlienger, A.: Effets des perturbations unilatérales du niveau du plan d'occlusion sur la vitesse et la direction de croissance du condyle et sur l'allongement de la mandibule. Etude expérimentale chez le jeune rat. Doctoral thesis in Odontological Science, Faculté de Chirurgie Dentaire, Strasbourg, 1978, Université Louis-Pasteur.

Schmuth, G.P.F.: Das Verhalten der Zunge bei verschiedenen Funktionsabläufen, Fortschr. Kieferorthop. **28:**271, 1967.

Schmuth, G.P.F.: Kieferorthopädie, ed. 2, Stuttgart, 1982, Georg Thieme Verlag.

Schmuth, G.P.F.: Milestones in the development and practical application of functional appliances, Am. J. Orthod. **84:**48, 1983.

Schneider, E., Schmidt, H., and Rakosi, T.: Die Korrelation zwischen dem Zungenpressen und dem Aufbau des Gesichtsschädels, Fortschr. Kieferorthop. **36:**379, 1975.

Schwarz, A.M.: Wirkungsweise des Aktivators, Fortschr.·Kieferorthop. **13:**117, 1952.

Schwarz, A.M.: Die Röntgendiagnostik, Vienna, 1958, Urban & Schwarzenberg.

Schwarz, A.M.: Lehrgang der Gebissregelung, Vienna, 1961, Verlag Urban & Schwarzenberg.

Schwarz, A.M., and Gratzinger, M.: Removable orthodontic appliances, Philadelphia, 1966, W.B. Saunders Co.

Scott, J.: Cartilage of the nasal system, Br. Dent. J. **95:**37, 1953.

Scott, J.: The growth of the human face, Proc. R. Soc. Med. **47:**91, 1954.

Scott, J.: Growth at facial sutures, Am. J. Orthod. **42:**381, 1956.

Scott, J.: The growth of the nasal cavities, Acta Otolaryngol. **50:**215, 1959.

Scott, J.: Dento-facial development and growth, Oxford, 1967, Pergamon Press.

Shaye, R.: J.C.O. interviews: Dr. Robert Shaye on functional appliances, J. Clin. Orthod. **17:**330, 1983.

Shaye, R., Schwaninger, B., and Hoffman, D.: Activator construction simplified, J. Clin. Orthod. **13:**773, 1979.

Simon, P.W.: System einer biologisch-mechanischen Therapie der Gesichtsanomalien, Berlin, 1933, Herman Meusser.

Spengeman, W.M.: Personal communications, 1967

Stein, G., and Weinmann, J.: Die physiologische Wanderung der Zahne, Z. Stomatol. **23:**733, 1925.

Stockfisch, H.: The Kinetor. In Graber, T.M., and Neumann, B.: Removable orthodontic appliances, Philadelphia, 1977, W.B. Saunders Co.

Stöckli, P.W., and Dietrich, U.C.: Experimental and clinical findings following functional forward displacement of the mandible, Trans. Eur. Ortho. Soc. p. 435, 1973.

Stöckli, P., and Teuscher, U.M.: The activator-headgear combination in skeletal Class II treatment. Mershon memorial lecture. Presented at the annual meeting of the American Association of Orthodontists, Atlanta, 1982.

Stöckli, P., and Teuscher, U.M.: Combined activator-headgear orthopedics. In Graber, T.M., and Swain, B.F., editors: Orthodontics: current principles and techniques, St. Louis, 1985, The C.V. Mosby Co.

Stöckli, P.W., and Willert, H.G.: Tissue reactions in the temporomandibular joint resulting from anterior displacement of the mandible in the monkey, Am. J. Orthod. **60:**142, 1971.

Storey, E.: Bone changes associated with tooth movement. A histological study of the effect of force for varying duration in the rabbit, guinea pig and rat, Aust. J. Dent. **59:**209, 1955.

Straub, W.: Malfunction of the tongue, Am. J. Orthod. **48:**486, 1962.

Stutzmann, J.J.: Particularités de la croissance postnatale des cartilages secondaires du squelette facial. Recherches in vivo et en culture organotypique chez le jeune rat, sur les processus de commande et de régulation. Doctoral thesis, Université Louis Pasteur, Strasbourg, 1976.

Stutzmann, J.J., and Petrovic, A.: Particularités de croissance de la suture palatine sagittale de jeune rat, Bull. Assoc. Anat. **148:**552, 1970.

Stutzmann, J.J., and Petrovic, A.: Effets de la résection du muscle ptérygoïdien externe sur la croissance du cartilage condylien du jeune rat, Bull. Assoc. Anat. **58:**1107, 1974a.

Stutzmann, J.J., and Petrovic, A.: Le muscle ptérygoïdien externe, un relais de l'action de la langue sur la croissance du condyle mandibulaire. Données expérimentales, Orthod. Fr. **45:**385, 1974b.

Stutzmann, J.J., and Petrovic, A.: Nature et aptitudes évolutives des cellules du compartiment mitotique des cartilages secondaires de la mandibule et du maxillaire de jeune rat. Expériences en culture cytotypique et d'homotransplantation, Bull. Assoc. Anat. **59:**467, 1975a.

Stutzmann, J.J. and Petrovic, A.: Régulation intrinsèque de la croissance du cartilage condylien de la mandibule: inhibition de la prolifération préchondroblastique par les chondroblastes, C.R. Acad. Sci. (series D) **281:**175, 1975b.

Stutzmann, J.J., and Petrovic A.: Tierexperimentelle Untersuchungen über Zusammenhänge zwischen Zunge, Musculus pterygoideus lateralis, mandibulärem Kondylenknorpel, und Gaumennaht, Fortschr. Kieferorthop. **59:**523, 1975c.

Stutzmann, J.J., and Petrovic, A.: Experimental analysis of general and local extrinsic mechanisms controlling upper jaw growth. In McNamara J.A., Jr., editor: Factors affecting the growth of the midface, Monograph 6, Craniofacial growth series, Ann Arbor, 1976, Center for Human Growth and Development, University of Michigan.

Stutzmann, J.J., and Petrovic, A.: Le pic de croissance pubertaire du cartilage condylien chez le mâle: mise en évidence d'une interaction positive entre les effets d'un hyperpropulseur postural et de la testostérone, Orthod. Fr. **48:**12, 1977.

Stutzmann, J.J., and Petrovic, A.: Einfluss von Testosteron auf die Wachstumsgeschwindigkeit des Kondylenknorpels der jungen Ratte. Rolle des "Vergleicher" des Servosystems welches die Verlängerung des Unterkiefers kontrolliert, Fortschr. Kieferorthop. **39:**345, 1978a.

Stutzmann, J.J., and Petrovic, A.: Persistance in organ culture of a growth rate circadian rhythm, Chronobiologia **5:**183, 1978b.

Stutzmann J.J., and Petrovic, A.: Intrinsic regulation of the condylar cartilage growth rate, Eur. J. Orthod. **1:**41, 1979a.

Stutzmann, J.J., and Petrovic, A.: Tierexperimentelle Untersuchungen über das Gesichts-Schädelwachstum und seine Beeinflussung. Eine biologische Erklarung der sogenannte Wachstumsrotation des Unkerkiefers, Fortschr. Kieferorthop. **40:**1, 1979b.

Stutzmann, J.J., and Petrovic, A.: Young rat spheno-occipital synchondrosis: a circadian rhythm of the growth rate and susceptibility to STH and its mediators, Chronobiologia **5:**183, 1979c.

Stutzmann, J.J., and Petrovic, A.: Die Umbaugeschwindigkeit des Alveolarknochens beim Erwachsenen vor und nach orthodontischer Behandlung, Fortschr. Kieferorthop. **42:**386, 1981.

Stutzmann, J.J., and Petrovic, A.: Bone cell histogenesis: the skeletoblast as a stem-cell for preosteoblasts and for secondary-type prechondroblasts. In Dixon, A.D., and Sarnat, B.G., editors: Mechanisms influencing bone growth: progress in clinical and biological research, vol. 101, 1982, A. Liss.

Stutzmann, J.J., and Petrovic, A.: Human alveolar bone turn-over rate. A quantitative study of spontaneous and therapeutically induced variations. In McNamara, J.A., Jr., editor: Malocclusion and the periodontium, Monograph 15, Craniofacial growth series, Ann Arbor, 1984, Center for Human Growth and Development, University of Michigan.

Stutzmann, J.J., Petrovic, A., and George, D.: Effets du rétropulseur actif sur la croissance de la mandibule du jeune rat. Rôle du muscle ptérygoïdien externe et du frein élastique méniscotemporal sur la vitesse et la direction de la croissance condylienne, Orthod. Fr. **47**:1, 1976.

Stutzmann, J.J., Petrovic, A., and George, D.: Life cycle length, number of cell generations, mitotic index, and modal chromsome number as estimated in tissue culture of normal and sarcomatous bone cells. In Donath, A., and Courvoisier, B., editors: Third symposium CEMO, Bone and tumors, Geneva, 1980a, Editions Médecine & Hygiene.

Stutzmann, J.J., Petrovic, A., and Graber, T.M.: Effects of the Fraenkel lateral vestibular shields on the widening of the upper jaw: an experimental investigation in the rat, Stomatol. D.D.R. **33**:753, 1983.

Stutzmann, J.J., Petrovic, A., and Malan, A.: Seasonal variations of the human alveolar bone turnover. A quantitative evaluation in organ culture, J. Interdiscipl. Cycle Res. **12**:177, 1981.

Stutzmann, J.J., Petrovic, A., and Oudet, C.: Effets de la thyroxine sur la croissance du cartilage condylien de jeune rat, J. Physiol. (Paris) **71**:347A, 1975.

Stutzmann, J.J., Petrovic, A., and Shaye, R.: Analyse en culture organotypique de la vitesse de formation-résorption de l'os alvéolaire humain prélevé avant et pendant un traitement comprenant le déplacement des dents: nouvelle voie d'approche en recherche orthodontique, Orthod. Fr. **50**:399, 1979.

Stutzmann, J.J., Petrovic, A., and Shaye, R.: Analyse der Resorptionsbildungsgeschwindigkeit des menschlichen Alveolarknochens in organotypischer Kultur, entnommen vor und während der Durchführung einer Zahnbewegung. Ein neuer Anblick in der orthodontischen Forschung, Fortschr. Kieferorthop. **41**:236, 1980b.

Stutzmann, J.J., Petrovic, A., and Shaye, R.: Extrinsic origin of bone resorbing cells in orthodontic tooth movement, J. Dent. Res. **59**:440, 1980c.

Stutzmann, J.J., Petrovic, A., and Shaye, R.: Relationship between mandibular growth rotation and alveolar bone turnover rate, J. Dent. Res. **59**:448, 1980d.

Symons, N.B.: Studies on the growth and form of the mandible, Dent. Rec., **71**:41, 1951.

Subtelny, J.D.: The significance of adenoid tissue in orthodontia, Angle Orthod. **24**:59, 1954.

Subtelny, J.D., and Daniel, S.: Examination of current philosophies associated with swallowing behavior, Am. J. Orthod. **51**:161, 1965.

Subtelny, J.D., and Sakuda, M.: Open-bite: diagnosis and treatment, Am. J. Orthod. **50**:337, 1964.

Tanner, J.M.: Fetus into man, Cambridge, Mass., 1978, Harvard University Press.

Tennebaum, M., and Gabriel, R.: Orthodontic treatment with removable plates and extraoral forces, Trans. Eur. Orthod. Soc., p. 199, 1973.

Teuscher, U.: Edgewise therapy with cervical and intermaxillary traction—influence on the bony chin, Angle Orthod. **53**:212, 1983.

Thilander, B., and Filipsson, R.: Muscle activity related to activator and intermaxillary traction in Angle Class II, Division 1, malocclusions. An electromyographic study of the temporal, masseter, and suprahyoid muscle, Acta Odontol. Scand. **24**:142, 1966.

Thom, R.: Stabilité structurelle et morphogénèse, Reading, Mass., 1972, W.A. Benjamins, Inc., Advanced Book Program.

Thompson, J.R.: The rest position of the mandible and its significance to dental science, J. Am. Dent. Assoc. **33**:151, 1946.

Todd, J., and Mark, L.: Issues related to the prediction of craniofacial growth, Am. J. Orthod. **79**:63, 1981a.

Todd, J., and Mark, L.: A reply to Dr. Bookstein, Am. J. Orthod. **79**:449, 1981b.

Todd, J., Mark, L., Shaw, R., and Pitenger, J.: The perception of human growth, Sci. Am. **242**:106, 1980.

Tulley, W.J.: Adverse muscle forces—their diagnostic significance, Am. J. Orthod. **42**:801, 1956.

Tulley, W.J.: A critical appraisal of tongue-thrusting, Am. J. Orthod. **55**:640, 1969.

Tulley, W.J.: The scope and limitation of treatment with the activator, Am. J. Orthod. **61**:562, 1972.

Vaes, G., and Jacques, P.: Studies on bone enzymes. The assay of acid hydrolases and other enzymes in bone tissues, Biochem. J. **97**:380, 1965.

Wachsman, C.: Treatment of irregularities of the teeth and jaws by means of activators, Am. J. Orthod. **35**:61, 1949.

Watt, D.D., and Williams, C.H.: The effects of the physical consistency of food on the growth and development of the mandible and the maxilla of the rat, Am. J. Orthod. **37**:895, 1951.

Weinmann, J.P., and Sicher, H.: Bone and bones: fundamentals of bone biology, St. Louis, 1955, The C.V. Mosby Co.

Wexler, M.R., and Sarnat, B.G.: Rabbit snout growth: effect of injury to the septovomeral region, Arch. Otolaryngol. **74**:305, 1961.

Wieslander, L.: The effect of force on cranio-facial development, Am. J. Orthod. **65**:531, 1974.

Wilson, G.H.: The anatomy and physiology of the temporomandibular joint, J. Nat. Dent. Assoc. **7**:414, 1920.

Winders, R.V.: Forces exerted on the dentition by perioral and lingual musculature during swallowing, Angle Orthod. **28**:226, 1958.

Witt, E.: Investigations into orthodontic forces of different appliances, Eur. Orthod. Soc. Rep. Congr. p. 391, 1966.

Witt, E.: Grundprinzipien der Aktivator- und Bionatortherapie, Zahnaerztl. Prax. **22**:1, 1971.

Witt, E., and Gehrle, M.E.: Lietfaden der kieferorthopädischen Technik, Berlin, 1981, Quintessenz Verlag.

Witt, E., and Meyer, U.: Indications for a working action of bimaxillary appliances, Eur. Orthod. Soc. Rep. Congr. p. 321, 1972.

Wolff, J.: Das Gesetz der Transformation der Knochen, Berlin, 1892, Hirschwold.

Woodside, D.G.: Some effects of activator treatment on the mandible and the midface, Trans. Eur. Orthod. Soc. p. 443, 1973.

Woodside, D.G.: The activator: In Salzmann, J.A.: Orthodontics in daily practice, Philadelphia, 1974, J.B. Lippincott Co.

Woodside, D.G.: The Harvold-Woodside activator. In Graber, T.M., and Neumann B.: Removable orthodontic appliances, ed. 2, Philadelphia, 1984, W.B. Saunders Co.

Woodside, D.G., Altuna, G., Harvold, E., et al.: Primate experiments in malocclusion and bone induction, Am. J. Orthod. **83**:460, 1983.

Zeemann, E.C.: Catastrophe theory, Sci. Am. **234**:65, 1976.

INDEX

Abbreviations following page number: *f,* figure; *t,* table.